GLUTATHIONE AND SULFUR AMINO ACIDS IN HUMAN HEALTH AND DISEASE

GLUTATHIONE AND SULFUR AMINO ACIDS IN HUMAN HEALTH AND DISEASE

Edited by

ROBERTA MASELLA
GIUSEPPE MAZZA

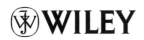

A JOHN WILEY & SONS, INC., PUBLICATION

Published by John Wiley & Sons, Inc., Hoboken, New Jersey
Published simultaneously in Canada

For general information on our other products and services or for technical support, please contact our
Customer Care Department within the United States at (800) 762-2974, outside the United States at
(317) 572-3993 or fax (317) 572-4002.

Wiley also publishes its books in variety of electronic formats. Some content that appears in print may
not be available in electronic format. For more information about Wiley products, visit our web site at
www.wiley.com.

Library of Congress Cataloging-in-Publication Data

Masella, Roberta.
  Glutathione and sulfur amino acids in human health and disease / Roberta Masella, Giuseppe Mazza.
     p. cm.
  Includes index.
  ISBN 978-0-470-17085-4 (cloth)
  1. Glutathione.   2. Sulfur amino acids.   I. Mazza, Giuseppe.   II. Title.
  QP552.G58M37 2009
  612.3'98—dc22
                                    2009011739

Printed in the United States of America

10   9   8   7   6   5   4   3   2   1

CONTENTS

PREFACE

Oxidative stress and antioxidant deficiency have been implicated in the pathogenesis of many diseases and conditions, including atherosclerosis, cancer, aging, and respiratory disease. Glutathione (L-γ-glutamyl-L-cysteinyl-glycine, GSH) is a major antioxidant acting as a free radical scavenger that protects the cell from reactive oxygen species (ROS). In addition, GSH is involved in nutrient metabolism and regulation of cellular metabolic functions ranging from DNA and protein synthesis to signal transduction, cell proliferation, and apoptosis.

By affecting the cellular reduction/oxidation status, GSH may also modulate gene expression and other cellular mechanisms. Glutathione depletion is linked to a number of disease states, including liver cirrhosis, various pulmonary diseases, myocardial ischemia and reperfusion injury, aging, Parkinson's disease, Alzheimer's disease, and sepsis, also called a systemic inflammatory response syndrome. Low intracellular levels of GSH may contribute to the immunodeficiency observed in later stages of HIV infection, as adequate concentrations of GSH are needed for proper lymphocyte function.

Virtually all mammalian cells have capacity to synthesize GSH de novo from glutamate, cysteine, and glycine by two sequential ATP-dependent reactions catalyzed by γ-glutamylcysteine synthetase (γ-GCS), recently renamed glutamate-cysteine ligase, and GSH synthetase. Furthermore, compelling evidence shows that the synthesis depends on γ-GCS activity, cysteine availability, and GSH feedback regulation. The chemical structure of glutathione provides special characteristics ranging from insusceptibility to proteolysis to redox thiols catalysis. These features, together with its high intracellular concentration, make GSH the most important redox-active thiol.

Methionine, cysteine, taurine, and homocysteine are the four common sulfur-containing amino acids. Methionine is nutritionally essential due to the inability of mammals to synthesize its carbon skeleton. It is required for protein synthesis, while its activated form, S-adenosylmethionine, serves as a methyl donor in numerous biological reactions. Methionine is one of the most sensitive amino acids to ROS damage, being converted to methionine sulfoxide [Met(o)]. Since the sulfur atom of Met(o) is a chiral center, oxidation of methionine by ROS results in an equal mixture of both the R and S epimers of Met(o). Further oxidation yields methionine sulfone, which has been detected in tissues, although the mechanism by which it is formed or its relevance remains unknown. One of the recently discovered systems that cells use to protect against oxidative damage is the methionine sulfoxide reductase system (Msr), which can reduce Met(o) in proteins back to methionine.

Cysteine is considered to be semiessential because it is synthesized from methionine, provided that the dietary supply of the latter is sufficient. Methionine catabolism to generate cysteine begins with its activation to *S*-adenosylmethionine, followed by transmethylation and the eventual formation of homocysteine. Thus, homocysteine is synthesized in vivo as an intermediate in methionine metabolism. Elevated plasma homocysteine has been associated with such chronic diseases as atherosclerosis, Alzheimer's disease, and osteoporosis. Homocysteine has been proposed as an additional risk factor related to cardiovascular illness. The theory of a relationship between the sulfur moiety and cardiovascular disease has been present since the late 1960s. However, the evidence presented in this volume indicates that the role of homocysteine as either a mediator or marker of cardiovascular risk remains unclear.

Taurine is synthesized from cysteine by most mammals, but the ability to do so varies markedly. Its synthetic activity is very low in humans and there is evidence that taurine is a conditionally essential nutrient, particularly in premature infants, in patients who are on very long term parenteral nutrition, and possibly in those who are vegans, since fruits, vegetables, grains, legumes, and nuts do not contain measurable amounts of taurine. Taurine is the most abundant free nitrogenous compound in cells, and it has a variety of functions, including its role as a membrane stabilizer, calcium flux regulator, and immune function modulator.

Finally, the nutritional aspects of sulfur compounds must be considered. Amino acid deficiency remains a significant nutritional problem, so new knowledge regarding the utilization and metabolism of dietary amino acids is essential for the development of nutritional strategies. In this regard, the deleterious effects exerted by sulfur amino acids at high intakes must be addressed.

This complex network of roles, functions, and effects makes GSH and sulfur amino acids a fascinating subject for protein chemists, biochemists, nutritionists, and pathologists. However, few publications are targeted at giving a multifaceted view highlighting their biological significance by different focal points.

This book, written by an international panel of experts, is a primary reference book that provides a comprehensive, state-of-the-science, in-depth review of the biochemistry, absorption, metabolism, biological activities, disease prevention, and health promotion of glutathione and sulfur amino acids. The complexity of the relationship between GSH and sulfur amino acids, their physiological role, as well as the possible role exerted by their principal metabolites, in the pathogenesis of chronic-degenerative diseases have been addressed and extensively discussed. In 22 outstanding chapters, this book provides up-to-date information on the following topics:

1. Chemistry, absorption, transport, and metabolism of GSH and sulfur amino acids

2. Antioxidant and detoxification properties of GSH and sulfur amino acids, highlighting the enzymatic systems involved in antioxidant defenses

3. Biological activities of GSH and sulfur amino acids and their role in modulating cell processes

4. Role of GSH and sulfur amino acid deficiency and alteration in the onset of diseases and in aging
5. Protective effects exerted by GSH and sulfur amino acids when used as drugs, functional foods and nutraceuticals in humans and animals

Special attention has been paid to the molecular mechanisms by which sulfur amino acids and GSH can regulate cell processes through the modulation of transcription factors and enzyme activities; and the nutritional and therapeutic significance of dietary sulfur amino acids has been carefully addressed through studies in humans and animal models.

With over 2000 scientific references, this book provides our readers (food scientists, nutritionists, biochemists, food technologists, chemists, molecular biologists, and public health professionals) with a most comprehensive and up-to-date publication on glutathione and sulfur amino acids in human health and disease.

We express our sincere thanks and appreciation to all the contributors who by freely and willingly giving their knowledge and expertise have made this book possible. Our gratitude is also extended to colleagues who have reviewed various chapters, and the editorial staff and publishers at Wiley for their contribution in bringing this work to publication.

We hope that this book will serve to further stimulate the understanding of the role of glutathione and sulfur amino acids in human health and disease, stimulate the development of functional foods and nutraceuticals rich in these important biochemicals and provide consumers worldwide with products that prevent diseases and maintain a healthier life.

G. MAZZA
R. MASELLA

CONTRIBUTORS

KATIA AQUILANO, Department of Biology, University of Rome "Tor Vergata," Rome, Italy

DAVID H. BAKER, Department of Animal Sciences and Division of Nutritional Sciences, University of Illinois, Urbana, IL

NANCY BENIGHT, USDA/ARS Children's Nutrition Research Center, Department of Pediatrics, Baylor College of Medicine, Houston, TX

CÉCILE BOS, INRA, AgroParisTech, Nutrition Physiology and Ingestive Behavior, Paris, France

JOHN T. BROSNAN, Department of Biochemistry, Memorial University of Newfoundland, St. John's, Newfoundland, Canada

MARGARET E. BROSNAN, Department of Biochemistry, Memorial University of Newfoundland, St. John's, Newfoundland, Canada

NATHAN BROT, Center for Molecular Biology and Biotechnology, Florida Atlantic University, Boca Raton, FL and Department of Microbiology and Immunology, Weill Medical College of Cornell University, New York, NY

DOUGLAS G. BURRIN, USDA/ARS Children's Nutrition Research Center, Department of Pediatrics, Baylor College of Medicine, Houston, TX

JULIAN CARRETERO, Department of Physiology, Faculty of Medicine and Odontology, University of Valencia, Spain

MARIA ROSA CIRIOLO, Department of Biology, University of Rome "Tor Vergata," Rome, Italy

MASSIMO D'ARCHIVIO, Department of Veterinary Public Health and Food Safety, Istituto Superiore di Sanità, Rome, Italy

JAYANTA R. DAS, Division of Cardiology, Cedars-Sinai Medical Center, and David Geffen School of Medicine, University of California, Los Angeles, CA

RICHARD DEKHUIJZEN, Department of Pulmonary Diseases, Radboud University, Nijmegen, The Netherlands

RYAN N. DILGER, Department of Animal Sciences and Division of Nutritional Sciences, University of Illinois, Urbana, IL

PAOLO DI SIMPLICIO, Department of Neuroscience, Pharmacology Unit, University of Siena 53100 Siena, Italy

JOSÉ M. ESTRELA, Department of Physiology, Faculty of Medicine and Odontology, University of Valencia, Spain

GIUSEPPE FILOMENI, Department of Biology, University of Rome "Tor Vergata," Rome, Italy

ENRICO GARACI, Department of Experimental Medicine and Biochemical Sciences, University of Rome "Tor Vergata," Rome, Italy

CLAIRE GAUDICHON, INRA, AgroParisTech, Nutrition Physiology and Ingestive Behavior, Paris, France

PIETRO GHEZZI, Chair in Experimental Medicine, Trafford Centre, Brighton & Sussex Medical School, Brighton, UK

ROBERT GRIMBLE, B.Sc., PH.D., R.NUTR., Professor of Nutrition, Institute of Human Nutrition, Institute of Developmental Sciences Building, School of Medicine, University of Southampton, Southampton, UK

RAMESH C. GUPTA, Department of Chemistry, SASRD, Nagaland University, Nagaland, India

JEAN-FRANÇOIS HUNEAU, INRA, AgroParisTech, Nutrition Physiology and Ingestive Behavior, Paris, France

NILS-ERIK HUSEBY, Institute of Medical Biology and Department of Pharmacy, University of Tromsø, Norway

HIERONIM JAKUBOWSKI, Department of Microbiology and Molecular Genetics UMDNJ-New Jersey Medical School, International Center for Public Health, Newark, NJ, and Institute of Bioorganic Chemistry, Polish Academy of Sciences, Poznań, Poland

SANJAY KAUL, Division of Cardiology, Cedars-Sinai Medical Center, and David Geffen School of Medicine, University of California, Los Angeles, CA

JELENA MARKOVIC, Department of Physiology, Faculty of Medicine, University of Valencia, Valencia, Spain

ROBERTA MASELLA, Department of Veterinary Public Health and Food Safety, Istituto Superiore di Sanità, Rome, Italy.

JOHN J. MIEYAL, Department of Pharmacology, Case Western Reserve University, School of Medicine, Cleveland, OH

JACKOB MOSKOVITZ, University of Kansas, School of Pharmacy, Department of Pharmacology and Toxicology, Lawrence, KS

LUCIA NENCIONI, Department of Public Health Sciences, University of Rome "La Sapienza," Rome, Italy

DEREK B. OIEN, University of Kansas, School of Pharmacy, Department of Pharmacology and Toxicology, Lawrence, KS

ANGEL ORTEGA, Department of Physiology, University of Valencia, Valencia, Spain

ANNA TERESA PALAMARA, Department of Public Health Sciences, University of Rome "La Sapienza," Rome, Italy

FEDERICO V. PALLARDÒ, Department of Physiology, Faculty of Medicine, University of Valencia, Valencia, Spain

RODICA E. PETREA, Alzheimer Disease Center, Boston University, Boston, MA

ELLINOR RISTOFF, Department of Pediatrics, Children's Hospital, Karolinska University Hospital Huddinge, Stockholm, Sweden

ELIZABETH A. SABENS, Department of Pharmacology, Case Western Reserve University School of Medicine, Cleveland, OH

KEVIN L. SCHALINSKE, Department of Food Science and Human Nutrition, Iowa State University, Ames, IA

SUDHA SESHADRI, Alzheimer Disease Center, Boston University, Boston, MA

ROSSELLA SGARBANTI, Department of Public Health Sciences, Pharmaceutical Microbiology Section, University of Rome "La Sapienza," Rome, Italy

BARBARA STOLL, USDA/ARS Children's Nutrition Research Center, Department of Pediatrics, Baylor College of Medicine, Houston, TX

ELISABETH SUNDKVIST, Institute of Medical Biology and Department of Pharmacy, University of Tromsø, Norway

GUNBJØRG SVINENG, Institute of Medical Biology and Department of Pharmacy, University of Tromsø, Norway

HAIM TAPIERO, Universite de Paris—Faculté de Pharmacie CNRS UMR 8612, Chatenay Malabry, France

KENNETH D. TEW, Department of Cell and Molecular Pharmacology, Medical University of South Carolina, Charleston, SC

DANYELLE M. TOWNSEND, Department of Pharmaceutical Sciences Medical University of South Carolina, Charleston, SC

JOSÉ VIÑA, Department of Physiology, Faculty of Medicine, University of Valencia, Valencia, Spain

HERBERT WEISSBACH, Center for Molecular Biology and Biotechnology, Florida Atlantic University, Boca Raton, FL

PART I

INTRODUCTION

CHAPTER 1

GLUTATHIONE AND THE SULFUR-CONTAINING AMINO ACIDS: AN OVERVIEW

JOHN T. BROSNAN and MARGARET E. BROSNAN

1.1 INTRODUCTION

Methionine and cysteine are two of the canonical amino acids that are incorporated into proteins, where they can be quite abundant. According to the Massachusetts Nutrient Data Bank, the sulfur amino acid content (methionine plus cysteine) for animal proteins, cereals, and nuts is between 37 and 41 mg/g protein. Legumes and fruits/vegetables average 25 and 23 mg/g protein, respectively [1]. Taurine, a non-protein β-amino sulfonic acid, is present in many animal tissues but is absent from most plants [2]. In addition, homocysteine is synthesized in vivo as an intermediate in methionine metabolism. Elevated plasma homocysteine has been associated with such chronic diseases as atherosclerosis, Alzheimer's disease, and osteoporosis [3–5]. Homocysteine thiolactone is synthesized by methionyl-tRNA synthetase when an elevated concentration of homocysteine leads to its selection for charging of tRNA^{met} in place of methionine [6]. Structures of these amino acids are shown in Fig. 1.1.

The names of these amino acids recall their structure or discovery. Methionine reflects the fact that this amino acid contains a methyl group attached to a sulfur atom. The history of cysteine and cystine is particularly interesting. We first meet it on July 5, 1810 when William Hyde Wollaston, MD, secretary to the Royal Society, read a paper entitled "On Cystic Oxide, a New Species of Urinary Calculus," to that august body [7]. The bladder stone, which had been removed from a five-year-old boy, was named cystic oxide from the Greek word for bladder, *kystis*. We now know that such stones are largely comprised of cystine, which is quite insoluble, particularly at low pH. Subsequent work revealed that the substance was not an oxide and the terms cysteine (for the reduced form) and cystine (for the disulfide)

Glutathione and Sulfur Amino Acids in Human Health and Disease. Edited by R. Masella and G. Mazza
Copyright © 2009 John Wiley & Sons, Inc.

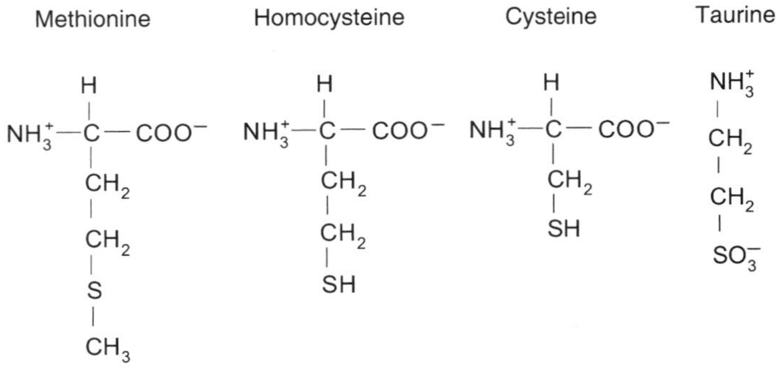

Methionine   Homocysteine   Cysteine   Taurine

$$
\begin{array}{cccc}
& H & & H & & H & & NH_3^+ \\
& | & & | & & | & & | \\
NH_3^+\!-\!C\!-\!COO^- & & NH_3^+\!-\!C\!-\!COO^- & & NH_3^+\!-\!C\!-\!COO^- & & CH_2 \\
& | & & | & & | & & | \\
& CH_2 & & CH_2 & & CH_2 & & CH_2 \\
& | & & | & & | & & | \\
& CH_2 & & CH_2 & & SH & & SO_3^- \\
& | & & | & & & & \\
& S & & SH & & & & \\
& | & & & & & & \\
& CH_3 & & & & & &
\end{array}
$$

Figure 1.1   Structures of the common, sulfur-containing amino acids.

came into use. Cysteine (or more accurately, cystine) has the distinction of being our oldest known amino acid.

Homocysteine is a homolog of cysteine. Its discovery dates from 1932, when du Vigneaud was examining the nature of the sulfur in insulin. He found that treatment of methionine with strong acid yielded homocysteine [8]. Subsequent work showed that homocysteine fed to animals could produce cysteine and that homocysteine could be produced after ingestion of methionine [9]. Taurine was discovered in 1824, just a few years after cystine, by Tiedemann and Gmelin [10]. Since it was originally isolated from ox bile, the name taurine reflects its bovine origin (*Bos taurus*).

Methionine cannot be produced, de novo, by animals and is therefore a dietary essential amino acid. Cysteine is not an essential amino acid, as it may be readily produced from methionine [11]. Taurine is an essential nutrient, during development, in some species [12].

1.2   WHY SULFUR-CONTAINING AMINO ACIDS?

Perhaps the most fundamental question that can be asked about these compounds is why they contain sulfur. The question may be better stated as: what properties of sulfur are fundamental to the functions of these amino acids? Methionine and cysteine are incorporated into proteins and also play important metabolic roles. However, we consider their roles in proteins to be primary and key to their selection; the metabolic roles are likely to have evolved subsequently. Sulfur belongs to group VIA of the periodic table. This group also includes oxygen and selenium. An appreciation of the importance of sulfur chemistry to the function of these amino acids is revealed by considering the roles of these amino acids in proteins and how these roles would be affected if the sulfur atom were replaced by an oxygen atom.

Cysteine's most distinctive role in proteins lies in its ability to form a disulfide linkage with another cysteine residue, thus providing a readily reversible covalent bond in vivo. Extracellular proteins are particularly rich in these disulfide linkages, which may be either intrachain or interchain and which play a fundamental role in determining the stability of proteins [13]. In fact, one of the earliest examples of bioengineering involved cysteine. It occurred in 1906 when Karl Nessler designed a machine to curl a woman's hair by reducing the disulfide bonds in keratin. If the hair was then twisted around a series of rods and the disulfide bonds allowed to reform, the hair would be "curled." The original design was less than satisfactory (his wife lost considerable hair) but eventually the design was so improved that every woman could afford a "Toni" permanent at home if she wished.

The amino acid serine is a structural analogue of cysteine in which the sulfur atom is replaced by oxygen but serine shows no comparable tendency to form dioxides. This important difference may be explained by the acid dissociation of H_2O and H_2S since serine and cysteine may be regarded as derivatives of these compounds (Fig. 1.2). H_2S is a much stronger acid than is H_2O (pKa 7.04 and 15.74, respectively) (Fig. 1.2a), which means that, of the two conjugate bases, SH^- will be formed much more readily than OH^-. The reason for the difference in these dissociation constants is straightforward. Although both oxygen and sulfur share the same number of electrons in their outer orbitals ($2p^4$ and $3p^4$, respectively), because of oxygen's much smaller size these electrons are held much more closely and, therefore, more tightly to the positive nucleus in an oxygen atom than in a sulfur atom. Indeed, oxygen is much more electronegative than sulfur (3.44 and 2.58, respectively, on the Pauling scale). Applying these considerations to cysteine and serine, it is evident that cysteine will dissociate to H^+ and the corresponding thiolate anion much more readily than serine will dissociate to H^+ and the corresponding oxide (pK$_{SH}$ of cysteine 8.3 and pK$_{OH}$ of serine ~ 13) (Fig. 1.2b). The pK values for these amino acids in proteins may vary somewhat but the principle remains. Since the formation of disulfide linkages first requires the dissociation of two cysteines, followed by the reaction of the two thiolate anions, we can appreciate that the formation of interchain linkages between two cysteine residues is feasible, whereas the formation of comparable interchain linkages between serine residues is highly unfavored. The same argument applies to other functions of cysteine, which require thiol dissociation. For example,

(a) Hydrogen sulfide is a stronger acid than water

$$pK_a \qquad H_2O = 15.74 \qquad H_2S = 7.04$$

(b) Cysteine is a stronger acid than serine

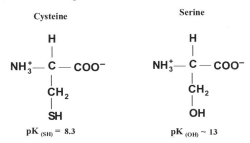

Figure 1.2 The importance of the sulfur atom to the chemistry of cysteine.

substitution of serine for cysteine in glutathione would provide a molecule that would essentially be incapable of becoming oxidized and unable to play a physiological role in oxidation-reduction reactions.

There are many other roles played by cysteine in proteins and they all rely on the unique chemistry of sulfur. Giles et al. [14] draw our attention to the multiple roles played by cysteine in biocatalysis, which include disulfide formation, metal binding, electron donation, and redox catalysis. Beinert and coworkers [15, 16] emphasize the role of iron-sulfur clusters in proteins, including their involvement in nitrogen fixation, electron transfer, the catalysis of homolytic reactions, and acting as sensors of iron and oxygen.

We may also enquire about the effects of substitution of methionine's sulfur with oxygen and how this would affect methionine's role in proteins. Methionine is among the most hydrophobic of amino acids; substitution of its sulfur with the much more electronegative oxygen would result in a δ^- charge at the oxygen atom, making the side chain much less hydrophobic. This would affect methionine's function in a number of ways. For example, methionine is the initiating amino acid in the synthesis of eukaryotic proteins. *N*-formylmethionine serves the same function in prokaryotes. As most of these methionine residues are subsequently removed, it is evident that their function lies in the initiation of translation rather than in the structure of the mature protein. In eukaryotic cells, the initiation of translation requires the association of the charged initiator tRNA (met-tRNA^{met}) with the initiation factor, eIF-2, and the 40S ribosomal subunit, together with a molecule of the mRNA that is to be translated. Drabkin and RajBhandary [17] have studied this reaction in detail and suggest that the hydrophobic nature of methionine is key to the binding of the initiator tRNA to eIF-2. Using appropriate double mutations (in codon and anticodon), they were able to show that the hydrophobic valine could be effective for initiation in mammalian cells but that the polar glutamine was very poor. The hydrophobicity of methionine also has an important effect on the role played by this amino acid in protein structure. Most of the methionine residues in globular proteins are found in the interior hydrophobic core; in membrane-spanning protein domains, methionine is often found to interact with the lipid bilayer [18]. The sulfur atom of methionine is key to its hydrophobicity and, therefore, to its functions in protein structure.

Not all methionine residues are buried in the interiors of proteins. In *Escherichia coli* glutamine synthetase, as much as one third of them are found on the protein surface, many clustered around the active site. These residues are susceptible to oxidation by certain reactive oxygen species (ROS), producing methionine sulfoxide. Figures 1.3a and 1.3b show the reaction of such a methionine residue with hydrogen peroxide. Levine et al. [19] view these methionine residues as playing the role of molecular lightning rods, in that they protect access of ROS to the active site. In line with this view is the fact that they report that oxidation of these residues has little effect on the catalytic activity of the enzyme. These oxidized methionine residues may be reduced to methionine by the enzyme methionine sulfoxide reductase. This is dealt with, in detail, in the chapters by Weissbach and by Moskovitz, including the roles played by this system in age-related diseases. What concerns us here, however, is the suitability of sulfur for this role. The production of the sulfoxide employs a

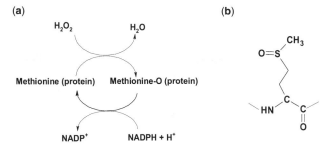

Figure 1.3 Methionine sulfoxide in proteins. (a) Oxidation of a methionine residue to methionine sulfoxide and its reduction back to methionine. (b) Structure of a methionine sulfoxide residue in a protein.

hybrid δ orbital that is available to sulfur. However, electrons in oxygen cannot access such orbitals, so that a methionine analog in which oxygen replaced the sulfur would be unable to employ this mechanism to protect against ROS.

1.3 *S*-ADENOSYLMETHIONINE, NATURE'S WONDER COFACTOR

S-adenosylmethionine (SAM) (Fig. 1.4) is an extraordinarily versatile cofactor; it has been said that it is second only to ATP in the number of reactions in which it is involved. Genomic and metabolic studies indicate that SAM is required by all organisms that have been studied. It may, therefore, be regarded as one of life's essential molecules. Nevertheless, not all organisms contain methionine adenosyltransferase

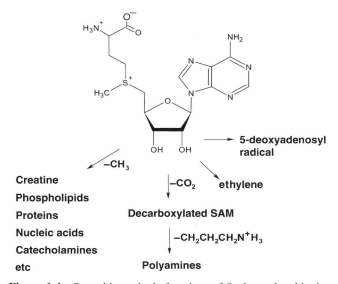

Figure 1.4 Some biosynthetic functions of *S*-adenosylmethionine.

and, therefore, not all organisms can synthesize SAM [20]. It appears that organisms without this enzyme can acquire SAM via transport from their surroundings. For example *Pneumocystis carinii*, an opportunistic fungal pathogen associated with AIDS, is a SAM auxotroph that actively transports this molecule [21].

SAM was discovered in the early 1950s by Cantoni [22] as the activated methyl donor required for a number of methylation reactions. It is known primarily for its role as a donor of methyl groups. No fewer than 60 different methyltransferases have been identified but the number is likely to be much higher. Analysis of seven completely sequenced genomes, including the human genome, suggests that class-1 SAM-dependent methyltransferases account for between 0.6% and 1.6% of open reading frames [23]. In mammals, this would indicate about 300 class-1 methyltransferases, to which must be added an unknown number of class-2 and class-3 enzymes. It is clear that we must expect the discovery of many new methyltransferases in the coming years.

The key to the function of SAM as a methyl donor lies in the sulfonium ion (Fig. 1.4). In particular, the electrophilic nature of the carbon atoms adjacent to the sulfur atom causes them to withdraw electrons and facilitate their transfer to suitable nucleophilic acceptors. In the case of methyltransferases, the methyl group is transferred, to produce the methylated product and *S*-adenosylhomocysteine (Fig. 1.5). In this context, it is of interest to enquire about the importance of sulfur. Why is sulfur so appropriate for these reactions? An answer becomes evident by considering the situation with two possible analogs of methionine, one in which an oxygen replaces the sulfur and one in which a methylene group replaces the sulfur. In the latter case, the molecule would be essentially inert in methyl transfer reactions as the methyl carbon would not be electrophilic. Considering the situation with oxygen, due to the very high electronegativity of this atom, the analogous oxonium compound would be so reactive that it would react promiscuously, without the need for an enzyme. The ideal biological methylating agent should be potentially reactive but not so highly reactive per se, that it would display an appreciable rate of uncatalyzed methylation reactions. With *S*-adenosylmethionine there is a very low level of background "noise" in the form of random, undesired methyl transfer reactions. A catalytic acceleration of 12 or so orders of magnitude by appropriate enzymes

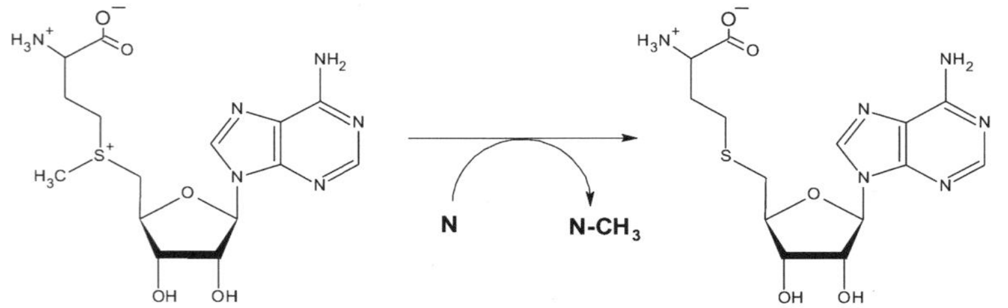

S-Adenosylmethionine   *S*-Adenosylhomocysteine

Figure 1.5   A typical methyltransferase reaction. N represents a suitable nucleophile.

enables the transfer of a methyl group to a specific nucleophile to occur at a rate that is physiologically relevant, and with a high signal-to-noise ratio (Richard Schowen, personal communication). We can compare *S*-adenosylmethionine to Goldilocks' sampling of the bowls of porridge. The oxonium compound is too hot, the compound in which sulfur is replaced by a methylene group is too cold but the sulfur-containing compound, *S*-adenosylmethionine, is just right.

S-adenosylmethionine is regarded as a high-energy molecule. More properly, it may be stated that SAM has a high methyl group-transfer potential. In fact, the ΔG^0 for SAM-dependent methylation reactions is greater than that for ATP hydrolysis [24]. Not surprisingly, therefore, the synthesis of SAM requires a considerable input of chemical energy, as is apparent from the reaction catalyzed by methionine adenosyltransferase,

$$\text{L-Methionine} + \text{ATP} + \text{H}_2\text{O} \longrightarrow \text{SAM} + \text{PPi} + \text{Pi}$$

The pyrophosphate produced is hydrolyzed to two molecules of inorganic phosphate, which tends to pull the reaction to the right. The synthesis of one molecule of SAM, therefore, requires the removal of all three phosphoryl groups from ATP.

Recent work has clarified quantitative aspects of methyl transfer in humans [25]. Application of stable isotope methodology which involves the constant infusion of [methyl-^{2}H$_3$] and [1-^{13}C] methionine permits the estimation of total methyl fluxes. Consensus values are 16.7 to 23.4 mmol/day per 70 kg body weight for young adults. These estimates are reduced by almost 10% in elderly subjects. Progress has also been made in delineating the quantitatively major methyltransferases. These are creatine synthesis, involving guanidinoacetate methyltransferase, and phosphatidylcholine synthesis, via phosphatidylethanolamine methyltransferase. Together, these may account for some 80% of total methyl transfer reactions in individuals who ingest customary North American diets, which may provide some 4 to 8 mmol creatine per day [26]. The other quantitatively major methyltransferase reaction is glycine *N*-methyl transferase, particularly in situations of high methionine intake. All three of these enzymes are either predominantly, or exclusively, found in the liver, which points to this organ as the major site of SAM utilization in mammals. In addition to these quantitatively major reactions, SAM can transfer its methyl group to a variety of nucleophilic acceptors, including amino acid residues in proteins, bases in DNA and RNA, small molecules, and even a metal oxide, arsenite [27, 28]. Methylation, therefore, plays a role in such diverse events as fetal development, hormone and phospholipid synthesis, protein repair, detoxification, and the regulation of gene expression.

SAM is, however, involved in a wide variety of reactions other than methylation. The arguments made for the importance of the sulfonium ion for facilitating methyl transfer are equally valid for the transfer of the other substituents to the sulfur. Polyamine synthesis involves the transfer of aminopropyl groups from decarboxylated SAM. For example, the addition of an aminopropyl group to putrescine results in the synthesis of spermidine and 5′-methylthioadenosine [29]. The 5′-deoxyadenosyl group of SAM may be transferred to the fluoride ion to produce the organofluorine,

5'-fluorodeoxyadenosine [30]. S-adenosylmethionine is also employed in such other alkylation reactions as the synthesis of the fruit-ripening hormone ethylene and the production of new methylene groups in cyclopropane fatty acids [29]. SAM can also be used as a source of ribosyl groups in the biosynthetic pathway for the synthesis of queuosine, a modified tRNA nucleoside [29].

Perhaps the most exciting recent finding related to SAM has been the identification of the superfamily of radical SAM enzymes. It has been predicted that this superfamily may contain more than 600 different enzymes, particularly in plants [31]. Radical SAM enzymes carry out the cleavage of relatively unreactive carbon-hydrogen bonds within alkyl groups [32]. Such reactions had hitherto been regarded as the province of hemoproteins or vitamin B12-containing enzymes. It seems that electron transfer from these clusters to SAM is critical to the formation of the SAM radical and is followed by its reductive cleavage to methionine and the 5'-deoxyadenosyl radical. The strongly oxidizing 5'-deoxyadenosyl radical can abstract a hydrogen atom from the carbon atom of various substrate molecules to produce 5'-deoxyadenosine and a radical substrate. The radical substrate may be converted to the final product of the enzyme-catalyzed reaction [31]. In some situations, SAM is not consumed in the overall reaction but is regenerated when the radical product abstracts a hydrogen from 5'-deoxyadenosine which facilitates its reaction with methionine, to yield SAM [31]. In most cases, however, 5'-deoxyadenosine is the final product so that these radical SAM enzymatic reactions reflect a net utilization of SAM.

SAM radical enzymes are involved in biotin synthesis, in which a sulfur atom is inserted across two carbon-hydrogen bonds to produce biotin's sulfur-containing ring. Lipoic acid synthesis also requires a SAM radical enzyme; in this case, two sulfur atoms are added to two poorly reactive C-H bonds, to produce the dihydrolipoyl group. Radical SAM enzymes are also involved in heme biosynthesis, thiamin biosynthesis, and bacterial lysine metabolism [32, 33]. The review by Wang and Frey should be consulted for a partial list of radical SAM enzymes [32].

S-adenosylmethionine is not the only sulfonium compound involved in methyl group metabolism. S-methylmethionine is a sulfonium compound in which an additional methyl group is linked to the sulfur atom of methionine; in effect, it is an analog of S-adenosylmethionine in which the adenosyl group is replaced by a methyl group. Plants contain significant quantities of this unusual amino acid, where it plays a role in their one-carbon metabolism [34]. S-methylmethionine can be metabolized in animal tissues. It has choline-sparing activity in chickens [35]. It has been suggested that this finding may result from the use of S-methylmethionine as a methyl-group donor in animals, either for betaine-homocysteine methyltransferase or phosphatidylethanolamine methyltransferase, or both [35]. Certainly, it is important to determine, at the enzymatic level, the role of this intriguing plant product in animals, particularly its potential role as a direct methyl donor.

1.4 GLUTATHIONE

Glutathione was discovered in 1922 by Sir Frederick Gowland Hopkins, the first professor of biochemistry at the University of Cambridge and future Nobelist.

To his considerable embarrassment, Hopkins proposed that glutathione was a dipeptide of glutamate and cysteine [36]. Nevertheless, from the very outset, Hopkins appreciated the key role of glutathione in oxidation-reduction reactions. His 1922 paper states: "When a tissue is washed until it has lost its power of reducing methylene blue the subsequent addition of glutathione to a buffer solution in which the tissue residue is suspended restores reducing power. This is the case when the dipeptide [sic] is added in its oxidized (disulfide) form. The tissue residue first reduces the sulfur group and a system is thus established which under anaerobic conditions continuously reduces methylene blue until an equilibrium" [37]. It is clear that Hopkins understood the role of glutathione as a biological reducing agent, and that there must be a means of reducing oxidized glutathione so as to regenerate the reduced form.

We have come a long way from Hopkins' era and now appreciate the very many functional roles played by glutathione. In addition to its role in oxidation-reduction reactions, glutathione plays a role in leukotriene synthesis, in the covalent modification of proteins, in the conjugation and excretion of lipophilic xenobiotics, and in the detoxification of methylglyoxal. These issues are dealt with, in depth, in this volume. Glutathione's most important function, however, lies in oxidation-reduction reactions and we will, therefore, highlight a few key features of its role in these reactions.

Schafer and Buettner have done considerable work to put our understanding of glutathione on a quantitative footing [38]. They emphasize the fact that glutathione is the major intracellular thiol-disulfide redox buffer. They point out that this depends both on the redox potential of the GSSG/2GSH redox pair:

$$GSSG + 2H^+ + 2e^- \longrightarrow 2GSH,$$

and on the total cellular concentrations of these compounds. Cytosolic GSH concentrations are in the region of 1 to 11 mM, which is much higher than most other redox-active compounds. In addition, they emphasize the fact that the redox potential of the glutathione system is quite dependent on the absolute concentrations of the redox species. This is so because in the calculation of the redox potential of the glutathione system, [GSH] enters as a squared term. Thus, the Nernst equation for glutathione half-cell is given by:

$$Ehc = -240 - (59.1/2) \log\left(\frac{[GSH]^2}{[GSSG]}\right) mV$$

These considerations both emphasize the importance of the total concentration of glutathione as well as the errors that can be introduced by employing the GSH/GSSG ratio, rather than $[GSH]^2/[GSSG]$ as the indicator of redox potential.

Schafer and Buettner [38] also emphasize the cellular compartmentation of glutathione. There are a number of compartments that are quite distinct from each other. The cytosol is the site of glutathione synthesis and usually contains the highest concentration of glutathione. Mitochondria have a separate pool, which, together with superoxide dismutase, plays an important role in protecting against oxidative damage brought about by the superoxide produced during oxidative phosphorylation.

A separate nuclear pool of glutathione is important for maintaining the redox state of crucial sulfhydryls in proteins required for DNA repair and gene expression. The glutathione pool within the lumen of the endoplasmic reticulum is relatively oxidized ($E_{hc} = -180\,mV$, compared with $-232\,mV$ in the cytosol). This appears to be important for the formation of disulfide linkages in proteins that are destined for export into the extracellular space.

Finally, it is important to consider the constancy, or lack thereof, of the glutathione redox buffer. We are conditioned, of course, to regard a "buffer" as something to be functionally defended by cells. This is certainly true if we restrict ourselves to a particular functional or developmental window, but it is not necessarily the case when we have a broader perspective. Indeed, alterations in the functional properties of the "buffer" may have, or reflect, important and pleiotropic consequences. Schafer and Buettner [38] suggest that the glutathione system may be a useful indicator of the redox environment of cells. "Redox environment" is used as a general term for a linked set of cellular redox couples. It encompasses both the redox potentials and the concentrations of the different redox couples. It is apparent that, as reflected by the glutathione system, the cellular redox environment changes, in significant ways, during the life of a cell. Evidence for this idea comes from a variety of systems (slime mold, sea urchin eggs, NIH/3T3 cells), so that it appears to be a fundamental property. It appears that the cellular redox potential is relatively reduced during proliferative phases and becomes more oxidized with differentiation. Apoptosis occurs in a more oxidized cellular redox environment, which becomes even more oxidized during cell necrosis. These changes in the glutathione system are thought to reflect parallel changes in the redox state of critical protein sulfhydryl groups. Sulfhydryl groups, per se, are reduced but may become oxidized by virtue of forming

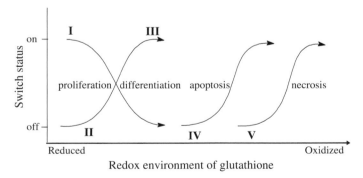

Figure 1.6   Protein nano-switches, in which protein sulfhydryl groups may be oxidized or reduced as a function of the redox potential of the cellular glutathione system. These switches may control regulatory programs that determine cells' fates. During the proliferative phase (**I**), the glutathione redox system is most reduced and the nano-switches that control this process are fully on. At **II**, the glutathione system becomes somewhat more oxidized, the proliferation switches are turned off and the differentiation switches are turned on, until most cells are differentiating (**III**). If the glutathione redox system becomes even more oxidized then death programs, such as apoptosis (**IV**) or necrosis (**V**) become activated. After Schafer and Buettner [38].

disulfide linkages with other cysteine residues or a mixed disulfide with other thiols, of which GSH is quantitatively the most important. The reduction potential of the various cellular redox potentials may be regarded as a means of activating or inhibiting broad programs of cellular activity. Modulation of the S-thiolation/dethiolation status of critical protein sulfhydryl groups can alter their activity with regard to signal transduction, nucleic acid synthesis, gene expression and cell cycle regulation. Schafer and Buettner [38] regard the redox states of certain critical sulfhydryl groups as acting as nano switches that can facilitate broad programs of cellular activity (Fig. 1.6). In this view, the cellular redox environment may determine whether a cell enters a proliferation or differentiation program or whether it enters a cell death program.

1.5 TAURINE—THE SECOND ESSENTIAL SULFUR-CONTAINING AMINO ACID?

Taurine is synthesized from cysteine by most mammals, but the ability to do so varies markedly. Although rodents have a large capacity for taurine synthesis, cats do not [39]; thus taurine is an essential nutrient for cats. The inability to synthesize the required amount of taurine was probably not a problem for feral cats since they are carnivores and their food supply would be expected to contain ample taurine but the same is not always true for the family pet, which may be fed a home-cooked diet [40]. Although most dogs do synthesize sufficient taurine, in some situations, especially with certain larger breeds, like Newfoundlands, taurine can become deficient, resulting in dilated cardiomyopathy [41]. Taurine synthetic activity is also very low in human liver [42] and there is evidence that taurine is a conditionally essential nutrient, particularly in premature infants [43], in patients who are on very long term parenteral nutrition [44], and possibly in those who are vegans [45], since fruits, vegetables, grains, legumes, and nuts do not contain measurable amounts of taurine [40]. In fact, taurine has been referred to as a "carninutrient," a nutrient that is provided in the diet primarily by animal products [46].

The amino acids we think of as essential are all incorporated into protein during its synthesis, but this is not the case for taurine. It does, however, play many roles and more are being recognized all the time. It is the most abundant free amino acid in animal tissues. For example, it represents more than 50% of free amino acids in muscle [18]; it has been reported to act as an antioxidant and a membrane stabilizer [42]. It has long been known to be essential for conjugation of bile acids to give taurocholic acid and taurochenodeoxycholic acid for excretion of cholesterol degradation products into the bile. Most of the bile salts are reabsorbed so this pathway does not normally represent much loss of taurine, but cystic fibrosis patients do have a marked decrease in recycling of bile salts [47] and thus may need a taurine supplement [48]. The cholesterol-lowering anion-exchange resin cholestyramine lowers reabsorption of bile salts and thus patients on this drug may also need supplementary taurine [2]. Taurine is also well known for its roles in immunomodulation [49] and in lowering of elevated blood pressure, possibly by an antisympathetic effect [50]. Recently, several new functions of taurine have been proposed.

One of the major classes of function recently ascribed to taurine is that of signaling molecule. In some cases, free taurine itself serves the role, for example as modulator of the glycine receptor in retinal progenitor cells to direct some of these cells to become rod photoreceptors [51]. Activation of glycine receptors in hypothalamus may also play a role in osmoregulation [52]. In other cases, taurine is conjugated to another small molecule, such as an amino acid or fatty acid. In 1985, Marnela et al. [53] reported on the isolation of γ-glutamyltaurine as a major taurine-containing peptide from calf's brain. This role of taurine will be discussed later in this volume (see Chapter 22). While looking for an endogenous ligand for the cannabinoid receptor, Devane et al. [54] isolated N-acylethanolamine, the first of a newly recognized family of lipid transmitters. In 2006, Saghatelian et al. [55] identified a new member of the family in mouse tissues, N-acyltaurine (NAT). In brain the acyl group is usually a long-chain saturated fatty acid (especially 24 : 0), whereas in liver and kidney it is a polyunsaturated fatty acid, such as 20 : 4 and 22 : 6. NATs were able to activate three different members of the transient receptor potential family of calcium channels [55], which may in part explain the known effects of taurine on calcium movement across cell membranes (as reviewed in [2]).

Although taurine has not been found as a constituent of proteins, it is found as a posttranscriptional modification of two mitochondrial tRNA molecules in humans [56]. Suzuki et al. found that the uridine at the anticodon first or wobble position of tRNA^{lys} and tRNA$^{leu(UUR)}$ is modified by covalent addition of taurine through its amino group to a methyl at C5 of the uracil base, leaving a free sulfonic acid group. In tRNA$^{leu(UUR)}$, the modified uridine is 5-taurinomethyluridine and in tRNA^{lys} it is 5-taurinomethyl 2-thiouridine [56] (Fig. 1.7). Suzuki and coworkers have shown that lack of modification with taurine causes defective translation in general for tRNA^{lys} and specifically of UUG-rich genes for tRNA$^{leu(UUR)}$ [57]. In certain mito-chondrial myopathies, the uridine modification is missing and this deficit has been suggested as the key factor responsible for the phenotypic features of these disorders [58]. Although there are no data at present, one could speculate that the cardio-myopathy observed in taurine-deficient dogs [59] is also due in part to incomplete modification of these mitochondrial tRNAs [56], due to lack of substrate, taurine.

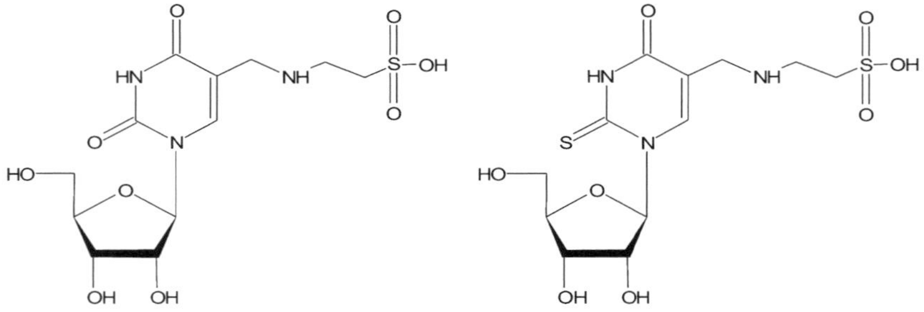

5-Taurinomethyl uridine   5-Taurinomethyl 2-thiouridine

Figure 1.7   Chemical structures of the taurine-modified bases 5-taurinomethyl uridine and 5-taurinomethyl 2-thiouridine, in mitochondrial tRNA [56].

1.6 CONCLUSIONS

The fields of glutathione and the sulfur-containing amino acids continue to offer great opportunities for innovative research. The importance of reactive oxygen species, as both physiological and pathological agents, and the importance of defence against their deleterious effects are now apparent. Our understanding of the relative roles of the various intracellular glutathione pools, and how these different redox potentials are maintained, is in its infancy. The pleiotropic effects of changes in cellular redox environment are likely to become even more important to the fates of cells, including neoplastic cells. We know a great deal about the different taurine pools and their potential functions but our mechanistic understanding of these functions is very incomplete. However, we do appreciate that the roles of glutathione and the sulfur-containing amino acids are dependent on the singular chemical properties of sulfur. Much remains to be learned and we should recall the words of Hamlet,

> There are more things in heaven and earth, Horatio,
> Than are dreamt of in your philosophy.

ACKNOWLEDGMENTS

Work cited from the authors' laboratories was supported by grants from the Canadian Institutes for Health Research. We thank Dr. G.D. Markham for providing us with Fig. 1.4.

REFERENCES

1. Pellett, P.L. (1996). World essential amino acid supply with special attention to South-East Asia. *Food and Nutrition Bulletin, 17*, 204–234.
2. Huxtable, R.J. (1992). Physiological actions of taurine. *Physiological Reviews, 72*, 101–163.
3. Seshadri, N., Robinson, K. (1999). Homocysteine and coronary risk. *Current Cardiology Reports, 1*, 91–98.
4. Seshadri, S. (2006). Elevated plasma homocysteine levels: Risk factor or risk marker for the development of dementia and Alzheimer's disease. *Journal of Alzheimer's Disease, 9*, 393–398.
5. Herrmann, M., Widmann, T., Herrmann, W. (2005). Homocysteine: A newly recognized risk factor for osteoporosis. *Clinical Chemistry and Laboratory Medicine, 43*, 1111–1117.
6. Jakubowski, H. (2006). Pathophysiological consequences of homocysteine excess, *Journal of Nutrition, 136*, 1741S–1749S.
7. Wollaston, W.H. (1810). On cystic oxide, a new species of urinary calculus. *Philosophical Transactions of the Royal Society of London, 100*, 223–230.
8. Butz, L.W., du Vigneaud, V. (1932). The formation of a homologue of cystine by the decomposition of methionine with sulfuric acid. *Journal of Biological Chemistry, 99*, 135–142.

9. Finkelstein, J.D. (2000). Homocysteine: A history in progress. *Nutrition Reviews*, *58*, 193–204.

10. Tiedemann, F., Gmelin, L. (1827). Einige neue Bestandteile der Galle des Ochsen. *Annalen der Physik und Chemie*, *9*, 326–337.

11. Stipanuk, M.H. (2004). Sulfur amino acid metabolism: Pathways for production and removal of homocysteine and cysteine. *Annual Review of Nutrition*, *24*, 539–577.

12. Sturman, J.A. (1988). Taurine in development. *Journal of Nutrition*, *118*, 1169–1176.

13. Wetzel, R., Perry, L.J., Baase, W.A., Becktel, W.J. (1988). Disulfide bonds and thermal stability in T4 lysozyme. *Proceedings of the National Academy of Sciences of the United States of America*, *85*, 401–405.

14. Giles, N.M., Giles, G.I., Jacob, C. (2003). Multiple roles of cysteine in biocatalysis. *Biochemical and Biophysical Research Communications*, *300*, 1–4.

15. Beinert, H. (2000). A tribute to sulfur. *European Journal of Biochemistry*, *267*, 5657–5664.

16. Beinert, H., Holm, R.H., Munck, E. (1997). Iron-sulfur clusters: Nature's modular, multi-purpose structures. *Science*, *277*, 653–659.

17. Drabkin, H.J., RajBhandary, U.L. (1998). Initiation of protein synthesis in mammalian cells with codons other than AUG and amino acids other than methionine. *Molecular and Cellular Biology*, *18*, 5140–5147.

18. Brosnan, J.T., Brosnan, M.E. (2006). The sulfur-containing amino acids: An overview. *Journal of Nutrition*, *136*, 1636S–1640S.

19. Levine, R.L., Mosoni, L., Berlett, B.S., Stadtman, E.R. (1996). Methionine residues as endogenous antioxidants in proteins. *Proceedings of the National Academy of Sciences of the United States of America*, *93*, 15036–15040.

20. Tamas, I., Klasson, L.M., Sandstrom, J.P., Andersson, S.G. (2001). Mutualists and parasites: How to paint yourself into a (metabolic) corner. *FEBS Letters*, *498*, 135–139.

21. Merali, S., Vargas, D., Franklin, M., Clarkson, A.B., Jr. (2000). S-adenosylmethionine and *Pneumocystis carinii*. *Journal of Biological Chemistry*, *275*, 14958–14963.

22. Cantoni, G.L. (1953). S-adenosylmethionine; a new intermediate formed enzymatically from L-methionine and adenosinetriphosphate. *Journal of Biological Chemistry*, *204*, 403–416.

23. Katz, J.E., Dlakic, M., Clarke, S. (2003). Automated identification of putative methyltransferases from genomic open reading frames. *Molecular and Cellular Proteomics*, *2*, 525–540.

24. Schubert, H.L., Blumenthal, R.M., Cheng, X. (2003). Many paths to methyl transfer: A chronicle of convergence. *Trends in Biochemical Sciences*, *28*, 329–335.

25. Mudd, S.H., Brosnan, J.T., Brosnan, M.E., Jacobs, R.L., Stabler, S.P., Allen, R.H., Vance, D.E., Wagner, C. (2007). Methyl balance and transmethylation fluxes in humans. *American Journal of Clinical Nutrition*, *85*, 19–25.

26. Stead, L.M., Brosnan, J.T., Brosnan, M.E., Vance, D.E., Jacobs, R.L. (2006). Is it time to reevaluate methyl balance in humans? *American Journal of Clinical Nutrition*, *83*, 5–10.

27. Clarke, S., Banfield, K. S-adenosylmethionine-dependent methyltransferases. In Carmel, R., Jacobsen, D.W., eds., *Homocysteine in health and disease*. Cambridge University Press, Cambridge, 2001, pp. 63–76.

28. Aposhian, H.V. (1997). Enzymatic methylation of arsenic species and other new approaches to arsenic toxicity. *Annual Review of Pharmacology and Toxicology, 37,* 397–419.

29. Fontecave, M., Atta, M., Mulliez, E. (2004). S-adenosylmethionine: Nothing goes to waste. *Trends in Biochemical Sciences, 29,* 243–249.

30. O'Hagan, D., Schaffrath, C., Cobb, S.L., Hamilton, J.T.G., Murphy, C.D. (2002). Biosynthesis of an organofluorine molecule. *Nature, 416,* 279.

31. Roje, S. (2006). S-adenosyl-L-methionine: Beyond the universal methyl group donor. *Phytochemistry, 67,* 1686–1698.

32. Wang, S.C., Frey, P.A. (2007). S-adenosylmethionine as an antioxidant: The radical SAM superfamily. *Trends in Biochemical Sciences, 32,* 101–110.

33. Frey, P.A. (1993). Lysine 2,3-aminomutase: Is adenosylmethionine a poor man's adenosyl-cobalamin? *FASEB Journal, 7,* 662–670.

34. Hanson, A.D., Roje, S. (2001). One-carbon metabolism in higher plants. *Annual Review of Plant Physiology and Plant Molecular Biology, 52,* 119–137.

35. Augspurger, N.R., Scherer, C.S., Garrow, T.A., Baker, D.H. (2005). Dietary S-methylmethionine, a component of foods, has choline-sparing activity in chickens. *Journal of Nutrition, 135,* 1712–1717.

36. Simoni, R.D., Hill, R.L., Vaughan, M. (2002). The discovery of glutathione by F. Gowland Hopkins and the beginning of biochemistry at Cambridge University. *Journal of Biological Chemistry, 277,* e13.

37. Hopkins, F.G., Dixon, M. (1922). On glutathione. II. A thermostable oxidation-reduction system. *Journal of Biological Chemistry, 54,* 527–563.

38. Schafer, F.Q., Buettner, G.R. (2001). Redox environment of the cell as viewed through the redox state of the glutathione disulfide/glutathione couple. *Free Radicals in Biology and Medicine, 30,* 1191–1212.

39. Sturman, J.A. (1991). Dietary taurine and feline reproduction and development. *Journal of Nutrition, 121,* S166–S170.

40. Spitze, A.R., Wong, D.L., Rogers, Q.R., Fascetti, A.J. (2003). Taurine concentrations in animal feed ingredients: Cooking influences taurine content. *Journal of Animal Physiology and Animal Nutrition, 87,* 251–262.

41. Backus, R.C., Ko, K.S., Fascetti, A.J., Kittleson, M.D., MacDonald, K.A., Maggs, D.J., Berg, J.R., Rogers, Q.R. (2006). Low plasma taurine concentration in Newfoundland dogs is associated with low plasma methionine and cyst(e)ine concentrations and low taurine synthesis. *Journal of Nutrition, 136,* 2525–2533.

42. Wright, C.E., Tallan, H.H., Lin, Y.Y., Gaull, G.E. (1986). Taurine: Biological update. *Annual Review of Biochemistry, 55,* 427–453.

43. Heird, W.C. (2004). Taurine in neonatal nutrition-revisited. *Archives of Disease in Childhood-Fetal and Neonatal Edition, 89,* 473–474.

44. Geggel, H.S., Ament, M.E., Heckenlively, J.R., Martin, D.A., Kopple, J.D. (1985). Nutritional requirement for taurine in patients receiving long-term parenteral nutrition. *New England Journal of Medicine, 17,* 142–146.

45. Laidlaw, S.A., Schultz, T.D., Cecchino, J.T., Kopple, J.D. (1988). Plasma and urine taurine levels in vegans. *American Journal of Clinical Nutrition, 47,* 660–663.

46. McCarty, M.F. (2004). Sub-optimal taurine status may promote platelet hyperaggregability in vegetarians. *Medical Hypotheses, 63*, 426–433.

47. Weber, A.M., Roy, C.C. (1985). Bile acid metabolism in children with cystic fibrosis. *Acta Paediatrica Scandinavica Supplement, 317*, 9–15.

48. Thompson, G.N. (1988). Excessive fecal taurine loss predisposes to taurine deficiency in cystic fibrosis. *Journal of Pediatric Gastroenterology and Nutrition, 7*, 214–219.

49. Bouckenooghe, T., Remacle, C., Reusens, B. (2006). Is taurine a functional nutrient? *Current Opinion in Clinical Nutrition and Metabolic Care, 9*, 728–733.

50. Militante, J.D., Lombardini, J.B. (2002). Treatment of hypertension with oral taurine: Experimental and clinical studies. *Amino Acids, 23*, 381–393.

51. Young, T.L., Cepko, C.L. (2004). A role for ligand-gated ion channels in rod photoreceptor development. *Neuron, 41*, 867–879.

52. Hussy, N., Deleuze, C., Pantaloni, A., Desarménien, M.G., Moos, F. (1997). Agonist action of taurine on glycine receptors in rat supraoptic magnocellular neurons: Possible role in osmoregulation. *Journal of Physiology, 502*, 609–621.

53. Marnela, K.M., Morris, H.R., Panico, M., Timonen, M., Lähdesmäki, P. (1985). Glutamyl-taurine is the predominant synaptic taurine peptide. *Journal of Neurochemistry, 44*, 752–754.

54. Devane, W.A., Hanus, L., Breuer, A., Pertwee, R.G., Stevenson, L.A., Griffin, G., Gibson, D., Mandelbaum, A., Etinger, A., Mechoulam, R. (1992). Isolation and structure of a brain constituent that binds to the cannabinoid receptor. *Science, 258*, 1946–1949.

55. Saghatelian, A., McKinney, M.K., Bandell, M., Patapoutian, A., Cravatt, B.F. (2006). A FAAH-regulated class of N-acyl taurines that activates TRP ion channels. *Biochemistry, 45*, 9007–9015.

56. Suzuki, T., Suzuki, T., Wada, T., Saigo, K., Watanabe, K. (2002). Taurine as a constituent of mitochondrial tRNAs: New insights into the functions of taurine and human mitochondrial diseases. *EMBO Journal, 21*, 6581–6589.

57. Kirino, Y., Yasukawa, T., Ohta, S., Akira, S., Ishihara, K., Watanabe, K., Suzuki, T. (2004). Codon-specific translational defect caused by a wobble modification deficiency in mutant tRNA from a human mitochondrial disease. *Proceedings of the National Academy of Sciences of the United States of America, 101*, 15070–15075.

58. Kirino, Y., Goto, Y., Campos, Y., Arenas, J., Suzuki, T. (2005). Specific correlation between the wobble modification deficiency in mutant tRNAs and the clinical features of a human mitochondrial disease. *Proceedings of the National Academy of Sciences of the United States of America, 102*, 7127–7132.

59. Kittleson, M.D., Keene, B., Pion, P.D., Loyer, C.G. (1997). Results of the multicenter spaniel trial (MUST): Taurine- and carnitine-responsive dilated cardiomyopathy in American cocker spaniels with decreased plasma taurine concentration. *Journal of Veterinary Internal Medicine, 11*, 204–211.

PART II

CHEMISTRY AND METABOLISM OF GSH AND SULFUR AMINO ACIDS

CHAPTER 2

SULFUR AMINO ACIDS CONTENTS OF DIETARY PROTEINS: DAILY INTAKE AND REQUIREMENTS

CÉCILE BOS, JEAN-FRANÇOIS HUNEAU, and CLAIRE GAUDICHON

2.1 INTRODUCTION

Methionine and cysteine are generally present at low levels in dietary proteins and are limiting amino acids of legume protein. However, diets based on different protein sources are seldom considered to provide insufficient amounts of sulfur amino acids, when compared to their nutritional requirement. Although only methionine is nutritionally indispensable, the requirement is usually assessed for both amino acids due to their tight metabolic link.

For the past two decades the importance of sulfur amino acids, and especially cysteine, in dietary protein has been addressed because of increasing knowledge of the impact of sulfur amino acids on human health. However, it is important to keep in mind the technical difficulties that can be encountered when attempting to quantify these amino acids in proteins.

2.2 SULFUR AMINO ACIDS (SAA) CONTENT OF DIETARY PROTEIN

2.2.1 Measurement of SAA in Proteins

Although sequencing has been used to determine amino acid profiles in proteins, the methods that are usually referenced for amino acid quantification are based on analytical procedures. The first step of this measurement is the release of amino acids after protein hydrolysis using chemical agents (usually HCl) and heating. The method of Moore and Stein [1] is the most frequently used, consisting of a 24 h reaction with 6 N HCl at 110°C. Sulfur amino acids (SAA) cannot be analyzed simultaneously with other amino acids because the HCl hydrolysis results in dramatic losses in SAA. A previous oxidation step with performic acid is thus required and leads to the production of cysteic acid from both cysteine and cystine, and methionine sulfone from methionine [1]. The duration of hydrolysis is a critical point since the different amino acids are released at different rates [2]. The optimal duration ranges from 12 to 48 h. For cysteine, the hydrolysis step cannot exceed 24 h. Due to the different efficiency ratios for each amino acid depending on hydrolysis conditions, several chromatographic profiles must be realized from different hydrolysates. The use of DTDPA (dithiodipropionic acid) has been reported as a hydrolysis method allowing for the release of every amino acid in a single hydrolysate [3]. Tuan and Phillips [4] described a rapid method for protein hydrolysis and analysis and, under their experimental conditions, found an optimal cysteine content after 75 and 50 min of DTDPA hydrolysis of a sorghum and a casein diet, respectively. However, for methionine, the optimal yield was obtained after 540 min of reaction for the casein diet, showing that each amino acid must be analyzed separately depending on its interaction with the hydrolytic agents.

Once the amino acids are released from the protein, several methods can be used to quantify amino acids in protein hydrolysates. The reference methods involve cation-exchange chromatography coupled with post-column ninhydrine or o-phtalaldehyde (OPA) derivatization [5]. However, reverse phase HPLC can also be used to determine the amino acid content in protein hydrolysates.

These methodological points are important because variations in analytical procedures can partly explain why protein composition tables are sometimes free from sulfur amino acids values as well as the differences observed among different references for a same protein.

2.2.2 Dietary Sources of SAA

Sulfur amino acids are present at relatively low levels in dietary proteins (Table 2.1). They do not exceed 5% of total amino acids. Among plant proteins, cereal proteins contain 3% to 5% of sulfur amino acids, whereas sulfur amino acids in legume proteins range from 2% to 3.5%. Legume proteins are generally considered as having limiting values of these amino acids. Although not yet used for human nutrition, rapeseed protein exhibits interesting profiles in sulfur amino acids. This is also true for leaf proteins such as Rubisco. Animal proteins generally bring higher amounts of sulfur amino acids when compared to vegetable sources. Total milk proteins contain 3.6% of sulfur amino acids, but with notable variations among the different fractions: caseins are the poorest in these amino acids (3.3%) and soluble proteins contain 4.1%. Among milk soluble proteins, α-lactalbumin, which represents only 25% of soluble proteins, exhibits a remarkably high content of sulfur amino acids that reaches more than 7% when calculated on the basis of amino acid sequence. Eggs are also rich in sulfur amino acids, which exceed 5% of the total amino acid content.

The ratio between cysteine and methionine also varies between 0.5 and 1 for the main protein sources. The higher cysteine to methionine ratio is observed in rapeseed proteins (in particular the napin fraction) and α-lactalbumin (ratio >3), whereas the egg proteins, caseins, and meat exhibit lower ratios. However, because the latter proteins are widely consumed by humans, they provide more cysteine than the former.

TABLE 2.1   Amino Acid Composition of Various Proteins

Protein Source	Methionine (g/100 g Protein)	Cysteine (eq. Cysteine, g/100 g Protein)
Meat (beef)	2.5	1.4
Poultry (chicken)[1]	1.5	1.4
Fish (salmon)[1]	2.9	1.1
Egg[1]	3.2	2.3
White[2]	3.9	2.5
Yolk[2]	2.5	1.8
Milk[3]	2.9	0.7
Casein[3]	3	0.3
Soluble protein[3]	2.1	2
Wheat[4]	1.5	2.6
Rice[4]	2.7	1.6
Maize[4]	2.2	2.5
Soy[4]	1.5	1.6
Pea[4]	0.9	1.7
Bean[4]	1.1	1.1
Lupin[4]	0.7	1.7
Rapeseed[4]	2	2.7

Sources: [1]USDA database (http://www.naI.usda.gov/foic/foodcomp/searchy).
[2]Reference 49.
[3]Reference 50.
[4]Reference 51.

The question as to whether sulfur amino acids are partially destroyed during heat treatments is poorly documented. During heating or alkaline treatments, dehydroalanine can be produced from amino acids such as phosphoserin or cysteine [6]. Cysteine can then react with dehydroalanine to form lanthionine. Thus, it can be assumed that cooking processes or industrial heat treatments decrease the cysteine content of protein and that the values given in food composition tables are overestimated. Amino acid composition of milk proteins was described depending on different heat treatments such as pasteurization, ultra high temperature (UHT) and spray and no dramatic losses in cysteine or methionine were reported [7]. After cooking of eggs, meat or fish, the assessment of cysteine losses is not easy to perform due to the absence of dedicated literature on this topic. The U.S. Department of Agriculture (USDA) provides a huge list of amino acid composition in foods (http://www.ars.usda.gov). In this case, amino acids profiles are given in grams per 100 g of food, instead of grams per 100 g of proteins, which adds a difficulty due to the variation of water content before and after cooking. However, amino acid values are extrapolated from a unique determination for each source of protein and from the specific protein content in the product.

For plant proteins, significant losses of sulfur amino acids may occur depending on the heat treatment. For instance, boiling beans in water for 1 or 2 hours leads to cysteine loss of 16% and 20%, respectively, and to methionine losses of 19% and 29% [8]. Among all amino acids, sulfur amino acids exhibited the highest rate of loss. Similarly, autoclaving seems to moderately alter cysteine content of proteins. Kim and Barbeau [9] reported a decrease of cysteine content in soy protein after

30 min of autoclaving (from 1.09 g/100 g of protein to 0.87 g/100 g), the loss being more pronounced after 140 min of treatment (0.67 g/100 g). Methionine content was unaffected by the treatment. Ouédraogo et al. [10] found no difference of sulfur amino acid content of soy proteins after either 15 or 25 min of roasting at 100°C.

Finally, the sulfur amino acid content of proteins is generally assessed for purified sources of proteins and then extrapolated to food products. Neither the impact of the matrix containing the protein nor the influence of the processes applied to food products are really documented.

2.3 SULFUR AMINO ACID INTAKE

Data concerning sulfur amino acids in humans are scarce, and mainly relate to developed countries, while little is known concerning methionine and cysteine intake in developing and emerging countries.

Sulfur amino acids are consumed as part of dietary proteins. In Western countries, mean dietary protein intake is close to $1.5 \text{ g} \cdot \text{kg}^{-1} \cdot \text{d}^{-1}$ in adults, with a sulfur amino acid content of proteins in the 2% to 5% range, resulting in an average sulfur amino acid intake exceeding $30 \text{ mg} \cdot \text{kg}^{-1} \cdot \text{d}^{-1}$. This value is above the average requirement for methionine + cysteine in adults ($15 \text{ mg} \cdot \text{kg}^{-1} \cdot \text{d}^{-1}$) [11, 12]. Because most dietary protein sources have a Cys to Met ratio between 0.5 and 1, methionine is expected to account for 50% to 70% of sulfur amino acid intake in developed countries.

In the U.S. population, the sulfur amino acid intake of adults has been estimated from the food intake data of the third national examination survey (NHANES III). The average intakes of Met and Cys are 2.3 and $1.3 \text{ g} \cdot \text{d}^{-1}$ for men and 1.6 and 0.9 $\text{g} \cdot \text{d}^{-1}$ in women, respectively [13]. For the French population, the average methionine intake in adults is $2.1 \text{ g} \cdot \text{d}^{-1}$, close to the U.S. value [14]. According to this last study, the proportion of individuals with methionine intake below the mean dietary requirement for sulfur amino acids is close to 0 in the French population, while the 90th percentile of methionine intake is approximately $3 \text{ g} \cdot \text{d}^{-1}$ ($45 \text{ mg} \cdot \text{kg}^{-1} \cdot \text{d}^{-1}$). In school-aged children, due to the very high protein intake observed in Western countries, sulfur amino acid intake is even higher than in adults, with for instance a median intake of $60 \text{ mg} \cdot \text{kg}^{-1} \cdot \text{d}^{-1}$ and a 90th percentile close to $100 \text{ mg} \cdot \text{kg}^{-1} \cdot \text{d}^{-1}$ in France [14].

In developing countries, the average protein intake in adults is $68 \text{ g} \cdot \text{d}^{-1}$ according to FAO STAT, and may even fall below $50 \text{ g} \cdot \text{d}^{-1}$ for central and southern Africa [15]. In this context of a low protein diet, sulfur amino acid availability may become limiting for glutathione synthesis and compromise the antioxidant defence of the body [16].

2.4 NUTRITIONAL REQUIREMENT FOR TOTAL SULFUR AMINO ACIDS

2.4.1 The Biological Basis for SAA Requirement

The essential nature of methionine in humans was first evidenced in 1949 by Rose and colleagues in their series of experiments in rats and humans to identify and quantify the nutritional requirements for amino acids [17]. They showed that a diet devoid in methionine but adequate in other amino acids and total N led to a negative N balance as soon as the second day after the methionine is removed from the diet. Hence, this work provided evidence that methionine cannot be synthesized by mammalian organisms and requires the consumption of sufficient amounts to compensate for daily losses of methionine.

Methionine and cysteine belong to the 20 amino acid precursors for protein synthesis and must be available at the sites of synthesis in sufficient amounts to permit whole-body protein homeostasis. Methionine disappearance from the free amino acid pool occurs through two principal pathways: transmethylation and transsulfuration [18]. Transmethylation reactions result in the transfer of the methionine methyl group to methyl acceptors, such as creatine, DNA, RNA, and carnitine. This pathway is reversible since homocysteine can be remethylated to produce methionine. The transsulfuration pathway results in the transfer of a homocysteine sulfur group to a serine residue to form cystathionine and then cysteine by an irreversible reaction. Hence, cysteine can be synthesized from methionine (donor of the S group) and serine (C skeleton) and is not an indispensable amino acid. However, cysteine is often termed conditionally indispensable because the production rate from methionine and serine can be limiting in some instances where the cysteine requirement is increased [19, 20]. Moreover, cysteine is a precursor of glutathione, a major cellular antioxidant, for which homeostasis is better achieved when cysteine rather than its precursor methionine is provided [21]. Cysteine is also the precursor of taurine and sulfate. Catabolism of cysteine occurs through a transamination reaction followed by the loss of the S group to form pyruvate or by a dehydrogenation to form 3-mercaptolactate. The complexity of methionine and cysteine metabolism, as well as their implication in several other metabolic pathways, explains part of the difficulties encountered in the determination of the nutritional regulation of SAA homeostasis.

2.4.2 Definitions

Sulfur amino acid requirements are usually treated as a whole because of the link between methionine and cysteine metabolism. To clarify the different available estimates of SAA requirements, the principal definitions are presented below, as recently proposed by Ball et al. [22].

- *Total Sulfur Amino Acid Requirement (TSAA)*: TSAA refers to the level of methionine, in the absence of cysteine, that must be supplied to satisfy the requirement, as assessed by different criteria, depending on the method used (e.g., N balance, tracer oxidation or balance). TSAA can only be measured by testing the effects of graded methionine intakes in the absence of cysteine. To further estimate the portion of the requirement that can be provided as cysteine instead of methionine, it is then necessary to measure the minimum obligatory requirement for methionine and the sparing of methionine by cysteine, as detailed below.

- *Minimum Obligatory Requirement for Methionine (MORM)*: This value represents that part of the methionine requirement that cannot be supplied in a form other than methionine, the remainder being provided as cysteine. Hence, this minimum obligatory requirement for methionine must be measured in conditions of excess of both dietary cysteine and factors affecting the requirement of SAA (vitamins, cofactor, methyl donors) by testing the effects of graded methionine intakes on the criterion that it is monitored to judge of the fulfilment of the requirement.
- *Cysteine Sparing*: The sparing of a portion of the methionine requirement by cysteine is measured by testing graded intakes of cysteine and a sufficient intake of methionine, corresponding to the MORM. The sparing effect is usually expressed as a percentage of the TSAA. The possibility to substitute part of the methionine intake by cysteine has to be reasoned on a molar basis, because of the difference in molecular weight between the two amino acids (one mole of methionine is 23% heavier than one mole of cysteine).

2.4.3 Quantification of the Total SAA Nutritional Requirement

As for the other indispensable amino acids, the requirement for total SAA was first determined by testing the influence of different methionine levels, in the absence of cyst(e)ine in the diet, on N balance and by defining the minimal requirement as the level allowing for a zero or positive N balance. The proposed value was 1.1 g per day for young male adults weighing 60 to 80 kg [23]. The requirement in women was later determined as 0.55 g/d, or ~9 mg/kg/d [24] (Table 2.2).

The first estimates of methionine requirement based on N balance data served as a basis for the recommendations published by the FAO/WHO in 1973 [25] and again in the expert consultation held by FAO/WHO/UNU in 1985 for indispensable amino acids [26]. The requirement of methionine was expressed as a global level for SAA and reached 13 mg/kg/d for adults.

Due to the well-known limitations in N balance studies [27], many reassessments of indispensable amino acids requirements in humans have been conducted based on isotopic studies. Several approaches have been developed by the groups of Vernon Young at the Massachusetts Institute of Technology (Boston) and Paul Pencharz in Toronto [28]. The first group first verified whether supplying 13 mg/kg/d of methionine in the absence of cysteine fulfilled the requirements of healthy adults by measuring the balance between intake and oxidation of a ^{2}H, ^{13}C tracer of methionine infused intravenously [29]. They concluded that TSAA requirement was probably superior to the FAO recommendation and confirmed this finding in elderly subjects based on the effects of graded intakes of methionine on the rate of oxidation of tracers of methionine or cysteine infused intravenously, that is, the short-term indicator amino acid balance method (IAAB) [30]. Another approach used by the same group consisted in estimating the TSAA requirement from the obligatory amino acid losses, as measured in conditions of protein-free feeding in healthy adults [31]. The requirement for TSAA was found to reach 12 mg/kg/d using this approach (Table 2.2).

TABLE 2.2   Total SAA Requirement in Humans Measured Using Different Approaches and Published Values

References	Method	Subjects	TSAA Requirement (mg/kg/d)[1]
Experimental Studies			
Rose et al. [23]	N balance	Healthy young men	13
Young et al. [29]	Short-term IAAB	Healthy young men	12
Fukagawa et al. [30]	Short-term IAAB	Healthy elderly men	13
Raguso et al. [31]	OAAL	Healthy young men	13
Raguso et al. [12]	Short-term IAAB	Healthy young men	13
Di Buono et al. [33]	IAAO	Healthy young man	13
Kurpad et al. [11]	24 h IAAB	Healthy young men	15
Kurpad et al. [36]	24 h IAAB	Undernourished young men	16
Turner et al. [34]	IAAO	Healthy school children	13
Recommendations for TSAA Requirement			
FAO/WHO [25]			13
FAO/WHO/UNU [26]			13
FAO/WHO/UNU [37]			15
FNB/IOM [13]			13

[1]TSAA requirement is measured with no cyst(e)ine intake.
IAAB: indicator amino acid balance; OAAL: oxidative amino acid losses; IAAO: indicator amino acid oxidation; FAO: food and agriculture organization; WHO: world health organization; UNU: united nations university; FNB: food and nutrition board; IOM: institute of medicine.

The indicator amino acid technique (IAAO) developed by the Toronto group to measure indispensable amino acid requirements in humans uses the oxidation of an indicator amino acid (usually ^{13}C-phenylalanine, infused intravenously), measured in subjects submitted to graded intakes of the amino acid under study, to assess the requirement of this amino acid [32]. The oxidation of the tracer is high for intakes of the amino acid tested below the requirement and it decreases then stabilizes for intakes above the requirement. The requirement is thus characterized by the breakpoint occurring in the tracer oxidation curve. The TSAA requirement has been quantified to 13 mg/kg/d by this technique in both young men and healthy children [33, 34].

Finally, a series of studies conducted by V. Young and A. Kurpad have used an improved experimental design based on both short-term IAAB and IAAO approaches to quantify indispensable amino acid requirement, including that of SAA [11, 35, 36]. Human subjects are submitted for one week periods to graded intakes of the amino acid of interest, while receiving otherwise equal amounts of the other amino acids and energy macronutrients. At the end of each period, they are infused an indicator amino acid tracer (^{13}C-leucine) and the 24 h oxidation and balance are assessed. The requirement of the test amino acid is determined by the minimal intake value allowing for a null or positive tracer balance. This very robust design has demonstrated a TSAA requirement of 15 mg/kg/d in healthy Indian male subjects [11]. Against the observations for lysine requirement, the same design applied to chronically undernourished Indian subjects did not result in a significantly increased estimate of TSAA requirement (16 mg/kg/d) [36] (Table 2.2).

In conclusion, the results of these studies demonstrate that the requirement for TSAA ranges between 13 and 15 mg/kg/d. At the last meeting of FAO/WHO/ UNU, held in Geneva in 2002, the requirement for TSAA was reassessed at 15 mg/ kg/d, a value that can also be expressed as 22 mg/g of protein when taking into account the protein requirement [37]. In contrast to most of the other indispensable amino acids, the SAA requirement, when reassessed by isotopic methods, was not found very different from the first data obtained by basic N balance studies.

The TSAA requirement of 13 to 15 mg/kg/d is an assessment of the mean requirement of the population, implying that 50% of the population has a lower requirement whereas 50% has a higher requirement. To estimate the safe intake and calculate the recommended intake that warrants the fulfilment of the TSAA requirement for 97.5% of the population, it is necessary to know the variability of the requirement in the general population. The IAAO method allows this estimation to be done because it measures the requirement in each subject and calculates an interindividual variability of the response. Hence, TSAA safe intake was reported to reach 21 mg/kg/d [33]. On a more theoretical basis, the American Food and Nutrition Board RDA (Recommended Dietary Allowances) for indispensable amino acids, including for TSAA, is 19 mg/kg/d [13].

2.4.4 The Sparing Effect of Dietary Cyst(e)ine on Methionine Requirement

The possibility of meeting part of the requirement for TSAA by dietary cysteine, referred to as the "sparing" effect of cysteine, as previously explained, is much more controversial than the determination of TSAA per se. Supplying excess dietary cysteine is thought to decrease the utilization of methionine through the transulfuration pathway and therefore sparing a portion of the methionine intake. This effect is clearly established in a number of animal species [22, 38, 39]. It was also demonstrated in humans in the first N balance study by Rose and colleagues, who observed the ability of L-cystine to replace 80% to 89% of the TSAA [40] and confirmed the finding in women using the same methodology [24]. However, the existence of this sparing effect is not apparent from all the studies that have examined this question and when demonstrated, the extent of this effect differs greatly from one study to another (Table 2.3). For instance, most of the studies based on the IAAB approach did not evidence any significant sparing effect [30, 41, 42], or when an effect was observed, the authors were unable to quantify its magnitude [35]. On the other hand, IAAO studies were able to detect such an effect in both adults and children [43, 44], amounting to 64% and 55% of the TSAA, respectively. This group also reported a methionine-sparing effect by dietary cysteine in neonatal piglets [45].

In the human studies, the intake of cysteine allowing this methionine-sparing effect was 21 mg/kg/d [43, 44]. As outlined by Young, the nutritional significance of this

TABLE 2.3   Minimal Obligatory Methionine Requirement and Sparing Effect of Cysteine on Methionine Requirement

References	Method	Minimal Obligatory Methionine Requirement[1]	Evidence for a Cysteine Sparing Effect	Extent of the Sparing Effect
Rose et al. [23]	N balance	0.1 g/d	Yes	80%–89%
Reynolds et al. [24]	N balance	4.8	Yes	47%
Hiramatsu et al. [41]	Short-term IAAB	ND	No	–
Fukagawa et al. [30]	Short-term IAAB	ND	Yes	Modest
Raguso et al. [12]	Short-term IAAB	13.0 mg/kg/d	No	–
Di Buono et al. [33]	IAAO	4.5 mg/kg/d	Yes	64%
Kurpad et al. [36]	24 h IAAB	10.0 mg/kg/d	Yes	No quantification
Humayun et al. [44]	IAAO	5.8 mg/kg/d	Yes	55%

[1]Measured with excess cysteine.
IAAB: indicator amino acid balance; IAAO: indicator amino acid oxidation; ND: not determined.

sparing of methionine by cysteine is thus difficult to appreciate because the ratio of cys:met ($\sim$3 to 4) necessary to observe this effect is far from that naturally observed in dietary protein and in current diets [46], as presented in the first part of this chapter. Moreover, based on the absence of modification of cysteine flux under a large range of cysteine intakes [12, 41], Young hypothesized that increasing cysteine intake was buffered by the important first-pass uptake of this amino acid, as evidenced in other studies [47, 48]. Hence, this question is still under debate [22, 39].

2.5 CONCLUSIONS

Studies dedicated to quantify the requirement for total SAA agree on a mean requirement in humans ranging between 13 and 15 mg/kg/d. The corresponding safe intake that warrants the fulfilment of the TSAA requirement for 97.5% of the population is estimated between 19 and 21 mg/kg/d. Given the level of SAA intake in Western populations ($>$2 g/kg/d), it seems that these amino acids are not limiting among dietary sources, although a more precise study to record the intake distribution is necessary. In contrast, the situation in developing countries may constitute a problem due to the low protein intake and the lower animal protein consumption. Hence, this situation deserves further investigations. An unresolved question remains with respect to the methionine-sparing effect, which is only demonstrated using excess cysteine intakes and of which the significance is under debate.

REFERENCES

1. Moore, S., Stein, W. (1963). Chromatographic determination of amino acids by the use of automatic recording equipment. *Methods in Enzymology*, *6*, 819–831.

2. Rowan, A., Moughan, P., Wilson, M. (1992). Effect of hydrolysis time on the determination of the amino acid composition of diet, ileal digesta and feces samples and on the determination of dietary amino acid digestibility coefficients. *Journal of Agricultural and Food Chemistry*, *40*, 981–985.

3. Barkholt, V., Jensen, A.L. (1989). Amino acid analysis: Determination of cysteine plus half-cystine in proteins after hydrochloric acid hydrolysis with a disulfide compound as additive. *Analytical Biochemistry*, *177*, 318–322.

4. Tuan, Y., Phillips, R. (1997). Optimized determination of cystine/cysteine and acid-stable amino acids from a single hydrolysate of casein and sorghum-based diet and digesta samples. *Journal of Agricultural and Food Chemistry*, *45*, 3535–3540.

5. FAO (Food and Agriculture Organization). (1970). Amino acid content of foods and biological data of proteins, bulletin no. 24. Rome: FAO.

6. Mauron, J. (1990). Influence of processing on protein quality. *Journal of Nutritional Science and Vitaminology (Tokyo)*, *36*, S57–S69.

7. Lacroix, M., Leonil, J., Bos, C., Henry, G., Airinei, G., Fauquant, J., Tome, D., Gaudichon, C. (2006). Heat markers and quality indexes of industrially heat-treated [(15)N] milk protein measured in rats. *Journal of Agricultural and Food Chemistry*, *54*, 1508–1517.

8. Hardy, J., Parmentier, M., Fanni, J. (1999). Functionality of nutrients and thermal treatments of food. *Proceedings of the Nutrition Society*, *58*, 579–585.

9. Kim, Y.A., Barbeau, W.E. (1991). Changes in the nutritive value of soy protein concentrate during autoclaving. *Plant Foods for Human Nutrition*, *41*, 179–192.

10. Ouédraogo, C.L., Combe, E., Lalles, J.P., Toullec, R., Treche, S., Grongnet, J.F. (1999). Nutritional value of the proteins of soybeans roasted at a small-scale unit level in Africa as assessed using growing rats. *Reproduction, Nutrition, Development*, *39*, 201–212.

11. Kurpad, A.V., Regan, M.M., Varalakshmi, S., Vasudevan, J., Gnanou, J., Raj, T., Young, V.R. (2003). Daily methionine requirements of healthy Indian men, measured by a 24-h indicator amino acid oxidation and balance technique. *American Journal of Clinical Nutrition*, *77*, 1198–1205.

12. Raguso, C.A., Regan, M.M., Young, V.R. (2000). Cysteine kinetics and oxidation at different intakes of methionine and cystine in young adults. *American Journal of Clinical Nutrition*, *71*, 491–499.

13. FNB/IOM (Food and Nutrition Board of the Institute of Medicine). (2005). *Dietary Reference Intakes for Energy, Carbohydrate, Fiber, Fat, Fatty Acids, Cholesterol, Protein, and Amino Acids (Macronutrients)*. Washington, D.C.: National Academy Press, pp. 1–143.

14. Martin, A., Touvier, M., Volatier, J.-L. (2004). The basis for setting the upper range of adequate intake for regulation of macronutrient intakes, especially amino acids. *Journal of Nutrition*, *134*, 1625S–1629S.

15. FAO (Food and Agriculture Organization). (2007). *FAO Statistical Year Book 2005–2006*. Rome: FAO.

16. Jackson, A.A., Gibson, N.R., Lu, Y., Jahoor, F. (2004). Synthesis of erythrocyte glutathione in healthy adults consuming the safe amount of dietary protein. *American Journal of Clinical Nutrition*, *80*, 101–107.

17. Rose, W.C., Johnson, J.E., Haines, W.J. (1950). The amino acid requirements of man. I. The role of valine and methionine. *Journal of Biological Chemistry*, *182*, 541–556.

18. Stipanuk, M.H. (1986). Metabolism of sulfur-containing amino acids. *Annual Review of Nutrition*, *6*, 179–209.

19. Laidlaw, S.A., Kopple, J.D. (1987). Newer concepts of the indispensable amino acids. *American Journal of Clinical Nutrition*, *46*, 593–605.

20. Reeds, P.J. (2000). Dispensable and indispensable amino acids for humans. *Journal of Nutrition*, *130*, 1835S–1840S.

21. Stipanuk, M.H., Coloso, R.M., Garcia, R.A., Banks, M.F. (1992). Cysteine concentration regulates cysteine metabolism to glutathione, sulfate and taurine in rat hepatocytes. *Journal of Nutrition*, *122*, 420–427.

22. Ball, R.O., Courtney-Martin, G., Pencharz, P.B. (2006). The in vivo sparing of methionine by cysteine in sulfur amino acid requirements in animal models and adult humans. *Journal of Nutrition*, *136*, 1682S–1693S.

23. Rose, W.C., Coon, M.J., Lockhart, H.B., Lambert, G.F. (1955). The amino acid requirements of man. XI. The threonine and methionine requirements. *Journal of Biological Chemistry*, *215*, 101–110.

24. Reynolds, M.S., Steel, D.L., Jones, E.M., Baumann, C.A. (1958). Nitrogen balances of women maintained on various levels of methionine and cystine. *Journal of Nutrition*, *64*, 99–111.

25. FAO/WHO (Food and Agriculture Organization/World Health Organization). (1973). Energy and protein requirements: Report of a joint FAO/WHO *Ad Hoc* Expert Committee, FAO Nutrition Meetings Report Series, No. 52. Rome: FAO.

26. FAO/WHO/UNU (Food and Agriculture Organization/World Health Organization/United Nations University). (1986). Energy and protein requirements. Report of a joint FAO/WHO/UNU Expert Consultation, World Health Organization Technical Report Series, No. 724. Geneva: WHO.

27. Young, V.R., Bier, D.M., Pellett, P.L. (1989). A theoretical basis for increasing current estimates of the amino acid requirements in adult man, with experimental support. *American Journal of Clinical Nutrition*, *50*, 80–92.

28. Young, V.R., Borgonha, S. (2000). Nitrogen and amino acid requirements: The Massachusetts Institute of Technology amino acid requirement pattern. *Journal of Nutrition*, *130*, 1841S–1849S.

29. Young, V.R., Wagner, D.A., Burini, R., Storch, K.J. (1991). Methionine kinetics and balance at the 1985 FAO/WHO/UNU intake requirement in adult men studied with L-[2H3-methyl-1-13C]methionine as a tracer. *American Journal of Clinical Nutrition*, *54*, 377–385.

30. Fukagawa, N.K., Yu, Y.M., Young, V.R. (1998). Methionine and cysteine kinetics at different intakes of methionine and cysteine in elderly men and women. *American Journal of Clinical Nutrition*, *68*, 380–388.

31. Raguso, C.A., Pereira, P., Young, V.R. (1999). A tracer investigation of obligatory oxidative amino acid losses in healthy, young adults. *American Journal of Clinical Nutrition*, *70*, 474–483.

32. Pencharz, P.B., Ball, R.O. (2003). Different approaches to define individual amino acid requirements. *Annual Review of Nutrition, 23,* 101–116.

33. Di Buono, M., Wykes, L.J., Ball, R.O., Pencharz, P.B. (2001). Total sulfur amino acid requirement in young men as determined by indicator amino acid oxidation with L-[1-13C]phenylalanine. *American Journal of Clinical Nutrition, 74,* 756–760.

34. Turner, J.M., Humayun, M.A., Elango, R., Rafii, M., Langos, V., Ball, R.O., Pencharz, P.B. (2006). Total sulfur amino acid requirement of healthy school-age children as determined by indicator amino acid oxidation technique. *American Journal of Clinical Nutrition, 83,* 619–623.

35. Kurpad, A.V., Regan, M.M., Varalakshmi, S., Gnanou, J., Lingappa, A., Young, V.R. (2004). Effect of cystine on the methionine requirement of healthy Indian men determined by using the 24-h indicator amino acid balance approach. *American Journal of Clinical Nutrition, 80,* 1526–1535.

36. Kurpad, A.V., Regan, M.M., Varalakshmi, S., Gnanou, J., Young, V.R. (2004). Daily requirement for total sulfur amino acids of chronically undernourished Indian men. *American Journal of Clinical Nutrition, 80,* 95–100.

37. FAO/WHO/UNU (Food and Agriculture Organization/World Health Organization/United Nations University). (2007). Protein and amino acid requirements in human nutrition. Report of a joint FAO/WHO/UNU Expert Consultation, World Health Organization Technical Report, No. 935. Geneva: WHO.

38. Finkelstein, J.D., Martin, J.J., Harris, B.J. (1986). Effect of dietary cystine on methionine metabolism in rat liver. *Journal of Nutrition, 116,* 985–990.

39. Fukagawa, N.K. (2006). Sparing of methionine requirements: Evaluation of human data takes sulfur amino acids beyond protein. *Journal of Nutrition, 136,* 1676S–1681S.

40. Rose, W.C., Wixom, R.L. (1955). The amino acid requirements of man. XIII. The sparing effect of cystine on the methionine requirement. *Journal of Biological Chemistry, 216,* 753–773.

41. Hiramatsu, T., Fukagawa, N.K., Marchini, J.S., Cortiella, J., Yu, Y.M., Chapman, T.E., Young, V.R. (1994). Methionine and cysteine kinetics at different intakes of cystine in healthy adult men. *American Journal of Clinical Nutrition, 60,* 525–533.

42. Raguso, C.A., Ajami, A.M., Gleason, R., Young, V.R. (1997). Effect of cystine intake on methionine kinetics and oxidation determined with oral tracers of methionine and cysteine in healthy adults. *American Journal of Clinical Nutrition, 66,* 283–292.

43. Di Buono, M., Wykes, L.J., Ball, R.O., Pencharz, P.B. (2001). Dietary cysteine reduces the methionine requirement in men. *American Journal of Clinical Nutrition, 74,* 761–766.

44. Humayun, M.A., Turner, J.M., Elango, R., Rafii, M., Langos, V., Ball, R.O., Pencharz, P.B. (2006). Minimum methionine requirement and cysteine sparing of methionine in healthy school-age children. *American Journal of Clinical Nutrition, 84,* 1080–1085.

45. Shoveller, A.K., Brunton, J.A., House, J.D., Pencharz, P.B., Ball, R.O. (2003). Dietary cysteine reduces the methionine requirement by an equal proportion in both parenterally and enterally fed piglets. *Journal of Nutrition, 133,* 4215–4224.

46. Young, V.R. (2001). Got some amino acids to spare? *American Journal of Clinical Nutrition, 74,* 709–711.

47. Bos, C., Stoll, B., Fouillet, H., Gaudichon, C., Guan, X., Grusak, M.A., Reeds, P.J., Tome, D., Burrin, D.G. (2003). Intestinal lysine metabolism is driven by the enteral availability of

dietary lysine in piglets fed a bolus meal. *American Journal of Physiology. Endocrinology and Metabolism, 285,* E1246–E1257.

48. Stoll, B., Henry, J., Reeds, P.J., Yu, H., Jahoor, F., Burrin, D.G. (1998). Catabolism dominates the first-pass intestinal metabolism of dietary essential amino acids in milk protein-fed piglets. *Journal of Nutrition, 128,* 606–614.

49. Thapon, J., Bourgeois, C. (1994). *L'oeuf et les ovoproduits,* TEC & DOC, Lavoisier, Paris, 260–274.

50. Rutherfurd, S.M., Moughan, P.J. (1998). The digestible amino acid composition of several milk proteins: Application of a new bioassay. *Journal of Dairy Sciences, 81,* 909–917.

51. Bodwell, C., Petit, L. (1983). *Plant Proteins for Human Foods.* The Hague: Martinus Nijhoff/Dr W. Junk, pp. 225–245.

CHAPTER 3

CELLULAR COMPARTMENTALIZATION OF GLUTATHIONE

FEDERICO V. PALLARDÓ, JELENA MARKOVIC, and JOSÉ VIÑA

3.1 INTRODUCTION

Tripeptide glutathione (L-γ-glutamyl-L-cysteinyl-glycine, GSH) performs many physiological functions [1] in part due to its widespread localization within cells and also due to its high concentration in cells and tissues. Due to its redox properties it plays a major role in protecting the cell against oxidants and electrophiles.

In addition, GSH takes part in other important functions, such as the regulation of DNA and protein synthesis. The control of basic cellular functions, such as apoptosis or cell cycle regulation, has also been reported.

Pioneer work from Alton Meister [2] linked GSH synthesis and its degradation throughout the so-called γ-glutamyl cycle, a cytosolic process. The importance of cellular compartmentalization of GSH is twofold, first because it plays an important role in fighting against reactive oxygen species (ROS). It is well known that these molecules have a very short half life and exert their action close to the place they are produced. Thus, the presence or absence of GSH could determine the development of localized oxidative damage for the cell structure or metabolic function located in the vicinity. The second reason GSH compartmentalization is of paramount importance is because of its role as a cellular detoxifying agent. It is known that tumors that have high glutathione levels are more resistant to chemotherapy.

To review the compartmentalization of glutathione in mammal cells is an intricate matter. This is due to the presence in the literature of a number of contradictory reports. The reason for the controversy is mainly methodological. Until very recently most reports were based mainly on cell fractionation techniques. These techniques appear to be reliable for mitochondrial studies; however, their usefulness in nuclear or even endoplasmic reticulum measurements is at least controversial.

Glutathione and Sulfur Amino Acids in Human Health and Disease. Edited by R. Masella and G. Mazza
Copyright © 2009 John Wiley & Sons, Inc.

Although knowledge on cellular GSH distribution is not completely established, a considerable number of experiments depict a consistent scenario, which is described in this chapter.

3.2 GLUTATHIONE CONTENT IN CELLS

3.2.1 Whole Cells

Glutathione concentration in cells may be as high as 10 mM. Cellular glutathione status may be modified under both physiological and pathological conditions. Lowering the concentration of the reduced form of glutathione (GSH) may or may not be accompanied by an increase in the levels of the oxidized form (GSSG), depending on whether it is caused by oxidative stress. Thus, accurate determination of glutathione in biological samples is of critical importance and is largely dependent on proper treatment of the sample. The GSSG concentration is usually very low compared to the GSH concentration [3, 4]. Pioneer work by Tateishi and coworkers [5] and Akerboom and Sies [4] showed that rat liver GSH ranges from 2.0 to 7.0 μmol/g of tissue and GSSG from 0.007 to 0.084 μmol/g of tissue. In isolated rat hepatocytes GSH concentration is 4 μmol/g of wet weight [3].

Most of the glutathione is maintained in its reduced form by glutathione reductase. As mentioned above, glutathione synthesis and its degradation are linked by the γ-glutamyl cycle, which involves cytosolic steps and one membrane-bound enzyme, γ-glutamyl transferase (Fig. 3.1).

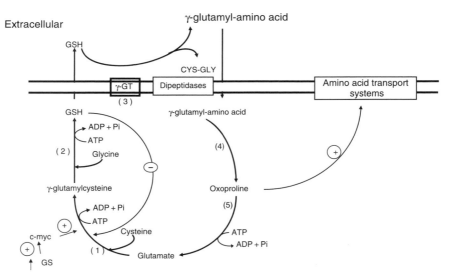

Figure 3.1 The γ-glutamyl cycle. (1) γ-glutamylcysteine synthetase; (2) GSH synthetase; (3) γ-glutamyltranspeptidase; (4) γ-glutamylcyclotransferase; (5) oxoprolinase. CYS-GLY, cysteinyl glycine; γ-GT, γ-glutamyl transferase.

The main cellular localizations that have been described for glutathione are the cytosol, the mitochondria, the endoplasmic reticulum (ER), and the cell nucleus.

3.2.2 Cytosol

As pointed out above, GSH synthesis occurs by two sequential, ATP-dependent reactions in the cytoplasm, catalyzed by glutamate cysteine ligase (formerly known as γ-glutamylcysteine synthase) and GSH synthetase. Almost all cellular GSH is synthesized in the cytosol with little if any production in other organelles, including the mitochondria [6, 7]. The capacity for GSH synthesis is present in almost all mammalians cells. Degradation of GSH is mediated by a different pathway. However not all mammalian cell types can degrade GSH [8]. Cleavage of the γ-glutamyl-peptide bond by γ-glutamyl transferase (γ-GT) takes place mainly in epithelial cells but its expression is very low in parenchymal cells. The cytosolic concentration of GSH depends not only on the rate of synthesis and degradation but also its efflux through the plasma membrane. Recently a number of plasma membrane proteins capable of exporting GSH out of the cell have been described in tumor cells. These are ATP-binding cassette C1 (ABCC1) and cystic fibrosis transmembrane conductance regulator (CFTR) [9, 10]. ABCC1 is a member of the ABC transmembrane proteins that function as efflux pumps, with diverse substrate specificity. It is involved in the extrusion of several endogenous cell metabolites, including leukotriene C4 (LTC4) and GSH. CFTR forms an ion channel that is permeable both to Cl^- and to larger organic anions, among them GSH. In airway epithelial cells CFTR exports GSH to the airway surface fluid. Thus, a new avenue of research on the regulation of cytosolic GSH has been opened by different families of membrane transporters.

3.2.3 Mitochondria

Mitochondria are major sources of ROS, thus it is a cellular priority to maintain high glutathione levels within mitochondria. In fact, their function is closely linked to maintenance of the redox balance since mitochondria are the main consumers of oxygen within the cell. The generation of ROS as a by-product of mitochondrial physiological metabolism is due to the partial reduction reactions that take place during the four-electron reduction of molecular oxygen (O_2) to water.

Increased ROS production by mitochondria could induce a positive feedback that would establish chronic oxidative stress, impaired mitochondrial function, and further production of ROS. This inevitably leads to mitochondrial damage and even to lesions in other cellular structures [11–13]. Not only oxygen-derived free radicals, but also reactive nitrogen species (RNS) like nitric oxide (NO) and peroxynitrite (ONOO) are produced inside mitochondria. Thus, formation of *S*-nitrosoglutathione (GSNO) takes place during normal mitochondrial metabolism. The formation of GSNO has been reported to play a regulatory role in mitochondrial homeostasis.

Mitochondrial GSH concentration is usually similar to that of the cytoplasm [14]. In hepatocytes, 15% of all cellular glutathione is in the mitochondria [15].

Initial studies on mitochondrial GSH transport were performed by Kurosava et al. [16] in the early 1990s. These authors found higher GSH levels in mitochondria than in the cytosol and described the presence of mitochondrial transport activity that was dependent on the respiratory state of the mitochondria. The highest transport activity was found under state 4 conditions.

Martensson and coworkers [17] found a two-kinetic component when studying isolated mitochondria from rat liver. Similar results, using different approaches, where reported by Garcia-Ruiz and coworkers in 1995 [18] and Schenellmann [19].

Nowadays a clear picture has emerged, where at least two anion carrier proteins, the dicarboxylate carrier (DIC) and the 2-oxoglutarate carrier (OGC), play a major role in the transport of GSH to mitochondria (for a review see Reference 13). According to Lash [20] approximately 60% of the total amount of GSH transport in renal cortical mitochondria is mediated by DIC and around 40% is mediated by OGC, and the presence of other unidentified carriers was not excluded. It is known that DIC is responsible for the transport of dicarboxylates from the cytoplasm to mitochondria, thereby supplying substrates for the Krebs cycle [21, 22]. Thus, GSH would compete for the carrier and could explain the reported correlation between GSH transport and the mitochondrial state.

3.2.4 Endoplasmic Reticulum

The endoplasmic reticulum (ER) plays a major role in the folding of native proteins. By contrast to the cytosol the ER contains a relatively higher concentration of oxidized glutathione (GSSG) [23]. This allows the formation of native disulfide-bonds in the ER. This process is catalyzed by protein disulfide isomerases and GSSG is believed to be involved in the oxidation of protein disulfide isomerases [24]. It has also been shown, however, that the ER flavoprotein Erol catalyzes the oxidation of protein disulfide isomerases in vivo and in vitro [25–28].

The folding of many proteins depends on the formation of disulfide bonds. Recent advances in genetics and cell biology have outlined a core pathway for disulfide bond formation in the ER of eukaryotic cells. In this pathway, oxidizing equivalents flow from the recently identified ER membrane protein Ero1p to secretory proteins. The reaction is catalyzed by the protein disulfide isomerase (PDI) [29].

Despite the vital importance of redox regulation in the ER, we have little knowledge about the mechanisms responsible for the ER redox balance. Furthermore, very little information is available on the effects of different pathological conditions on the thiol metabolism and redox folding in the ER. For instance, when Nardai et al. [30] were examining the role of molecular chaperones in the cellular pathology of diabetes mellitus, they found that the ER redox environment moved to a more reducing state. This has importance in the pathophysiology of the late-onset complications of the disease.

3.2.5 Nucleus

Mercury orange, monochlorobimane, and 5-chloromethylfluorescein diacetate (CMFDA) are the most commonly used probes for GSH determination, but the results obtained by these methods are conflicting. Pioneer work by Bellomo et al. [31] using monochlorobimane-GSH conjugation showed a $3:1$ nucleus:cytoplasm ratio. However, a more recent report by Briviba et al. [32] showed that the high nuclear fluorescence was due to an influx of the fluorescent bimane-GSH adduct into the nucleus. Thomas et al. [33] used fractionation techniques and flow cytometry with mercury orange as this probe readily forms fluorescent adducts with GSH and other nonprotein sulfydryls (NPSH), but reacts much more slowly with protein sulfydryls. Contrary to previous reports they found lower GSH levels in the nucleus than in the cytoplasm. The mean nucleus:cytoplasmic ratio they found was 0.57 ± 0.05. They suggested that there is a distinct pool of GSH in the nucleus since it was partially resistant to buthionine sulfoximine (BSO) depletion compared with the cytoplasm. More recently, Söderdahl et al. [34] showed the highest GSH staining in a perinuclear mitochondrial-rich compartment and low nuclear GSH staining using mercury orange and a specific GSH antibody. Finally, Voehringer et al., using CMFDA which binds in 95% to GSH, showed that GSH was mainly distributed in the cytoplasm although Bcl-2 overexpression was able to increase nuclear GSH levels [35].

In recent years new methods have become available for measuring the nuclear redox state. These have been reviewed by Hansen et al. [15]. Two forms of the redox blot have been developed to separate nuclear proteins on the basis of different charge or mass oxidized. Other techniques include antibodies that only bind to the oxidized form of the protein [36], and mass spectrometry [37]. Another recent approach to determine the nuclear redox state is the use of redox-sensitive green fluorescent proteins (roGFP). Although it is a promising step, so far no physiological oxidative treatment has been able to cause detectable changes in the excitation ratios of roGFP [38].

Although the nuclear redox state (mainly thioredoxin) can be determined, measurement of nuclear GSH concentrations is limited, and no methods are available to measure nuclear GSSG [38].

In order to study glutathione compartmentalization in 3T3 fibroblasts during cell growth, we used a triple staining (CMFDA-Hoechst-propidium iodide) or (CMFDA-Hoechst-mitotracker) by confocal microscopy [39]. Figure 3.2 shows how GSH colocalizes with nuclear DNA when cells are proliferating. However, when cells were confluent at 3 and 5 days after plating no differences between nucleus and cytoplasm could be seen. The images obtained at 3 or 5 days in culture are similar to those reported previously by Söderdahl et al. 2002 [34] using GSH antibody and mercury orange. Thus, our results may explain the apparent discrepancies in the GSH distribution. It is very important to take into account the exact point of the cell cycle, since cells that are preparing to divide have high nuclear GSH levels and quiescent cells have similar (or even lower) GSH levels in the nucleus and the cytoplasm. Figure 3.3 shows higher GSH levels in the nucleus of the cells soon after plating.

How GSH enters the nucleus and how it is regulated during the different phases of the cell cycle are still matters of debate. The regulation of such interactions is also unclear. According to Smith and colleagues [36], the possible biochemical mechanisms responsible for the turnover of nuclear GSH are the following: (1) GSH may be taken up from the cytoplasm into the nuclei either passively or through energy-dependent processes. (2) GSH may be synthesized de novo in the nucleus by the enzymes glutamate cysteine ligase and GSH synthetase. (3) GSH may function to

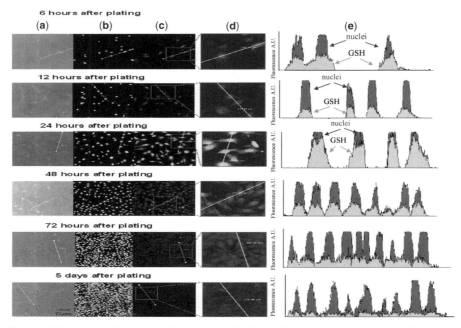

Figure 3.2   Confocal microscopic images of 3T3 fibroblasts during cell growth. Cells were plated in chamber slides 5 days, 72 h, 48 h, 24 h, 12 h, and 6 h before the experiment and were stained and analyzed the same day. Triple staining was performed on living cells: Hoechst 33342 to localize nuclei, CMFDA to mark GSH, and propidium iodide to exclude dead cells. During microscopic confocal analysis cells were maintained in the chamber provided with 5% CO_2 and at 37°C. Images were taken by light microscopy (panel A) and by confocal microscopy, to capture blue fluorescence of nuclei (panel B), green fluorescence that marks GSH (panel C), and red fluorescence of dead cells (results not shown). Maximum projection images were analyzed by profile of fluorescence, where a cross section white line of $200 \pm 20 \mu m$ was drawn through a cell field (best shown on amplified detail on panel D) to compare distribution of green CMFDA fluorescence (levels of GSH) along the line (green area under the curves on E panels) with blue Hoechst fluorescence (nuclei localization) (blue area under the curve in E panels). (See color insert.)

transport γ-glu-cys-cys. Ho and Guenthner [37], using nuclear fractions, concluded that GSH is taken up by the nucleus by passive diffusion and no evidence for an ATP-dependent mechanism for GSH concentration was observed. Glutamate cysteine ligase and GSH synthetase activities were found in nuclei [37]. Four to eight percent of cell GSH synthetic activity is found in the nucleus and is able to maintain nuclear GSH levels [37].

The role of ATP-dependent mechanisms in maintaining the nuclear/cytoplasmic GSH concentration was studied by Bellomo and coworkers [40]. We have not found an ATP-dependent mechanism in 3T3 fibroblasts or glutamate cysteine ligase in the cell nucleus [39]. We suggest that during the changes in the nuclear membrane

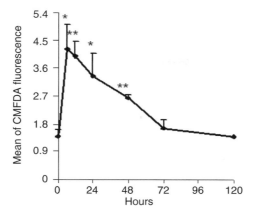

Figure 3.3 Nucleus : cytoplasm GSH ratio obtained by confocal microscopy. Analysis of the cellular distribution of GSH. Cells were plated, stained, and images obtained as described in Fig. 3.2. To quantify the changes in GSH distribution in cells along the cell cycle, cells were analyzed by area (as described in materials and methods). Nucleus : cytoplasm ratio for GSH in every cell analyzed was established by dividing the mean of green CMFDA fluorescence of nucleus area by the mean of CMFDA fluorescence in cytoplasm area. Results are mean $\pm$ SD from three independent experiments, where 100 cells in at least five different fields were analyzed.

that precede cell division nuclear pores could allow the specific translocation of selected substances, among them glutathione.

It is generally believed that the nuclear pore complex is the biochemical machinery that controls the molecular traffic across the nuclear envelope [41, 42]. Although free diffusion of ions and small hydrophilic molecules across the nuclear pore has been described [43], ion gradients and transnuclear ATP-dependent membrane potential have been reported [42].

A number of pathophysiological situations show the importance of nuclear GSH. Atzori et al. [44] showed variations in the amount and redox state of cellular thiols, particularly reduced glutathione, supporting a role for thiols in the regulation of growth and squamous differentiation of human bronchial epithelial cells. In another example, depletion of nuclear GSH to 50%–60% of initial values prior to irradiation (400 cGy) resulted in nuclear DNA fragmentation and apoptosis, suggesting that GSH plays a critical protective role in maintaining nuclear functional integrity, determining the intrinsic radiosensitivity of cells [45].

Thalidomide produces human birth defects, mainly limb reduction malformations (phocomielia) [46]. A rat thalidomide-resistant and a rabbit thalidomide-sensitive species were used to compare potential differences among limb bud cells [47]. Confocal microscopy revealed that glutathione distribution determined by CMFDA staining was different in both cell types. Thalidomide induced cytosolic GSH depletion in both cell lines; however, nuclear GSH levels remained high in the rat thalidomide-resistant cells but not in the rabbit thalidomide-sensitive cells. Thus, a redox shift in the nucleus may result in the misregulation of interactions between transcription factors and DNA, causing defective growth and development. Nowadays, thalidomide is still used in clinical practice as an inhibitor of angiogenesis and tumor growth.

Although the role of nuclear GSH in the synthesis of DNA [48] and in the protection against oxidative damage or ionizing radiation [49] is well established, little is known about GSH concentration in the nucleus and its possible regulation. This may be due to two main factors, the first of which is methodological: it is impossible to determine the nuclear concentration of GSH using standard cell fractionation and analytical approaches [30]. The second factor is that most, if not all, reports share the common view of nuclear GSH distribution in a static situation. Cells are usually studied under steady-state conditions, that is, when they are confluent (G_0/G_1 phase of the cell cycle), but the nucleus changes dramatically during the different phases of the cell cycle. Thus, studies to determine nuclear GSH distribution must take into account cell cycle physiology.

We recently reported [39] that GSH concentrates in the nucleus in early phases of cell growth, when most of the cells are in an active division phase, and it redistributes uniformly between nucleus and cytoplasm when they reach confluence.

In conclusion, cells need a reduced nuclear environment (provided by glutathione) to proliferate. Indeed, the nucleus : cytoplasm ratio is high several hours after plating. Thus, before exponential cell growth glutathione translocates to the nucleus. When cells reach confluence at 72 h and 5 days after plating, GSH distribution is similar in both the nucleus and the cytoplasm.

It appears that the study of cellular compartmentalization of GSH may be advantageous to understand cell physiology and the metabolic changes that take place during the different phases of the cell cycle.

REFERENCES

1. Viña, J. (1990). *Glutathione: Metabolism and Physiological Functions.* Boca Raton, FL: CRC Press.

2. Meister, A., Anderson, M.E. (1983). Glutathione. *Annual Review of Biochemistry, 52,* 711–760.

3. Viña, J., Hems, R., Krebs, H.A. (1978). Maintenance of glutathione content in isolated hepatocyctes. *Biochemical Journal, 170,* 627–630.

4. Akerboom, T.P.M., Sies, H. (1981). Assay of glutathione, glutathione disulfide, and glutathione mixed disulfides in biological samples. *Methods in Enzymology, 77,* 373–382.

5. Tateishi, N., Higashi, T., Shinya Naruse, A., Sakamoto, Y. (1974). Studies on the regulation of glutathione level in rat liver. *Journal of Biochemistry (Tokyo), 75,* 93–103.

6. Griffith, O.W., Meister, A. (1985). Origin and turnover of mitochondrial glutathione. *Proceedings of the National Academy of Sciences USA, 82,* 4668–4672.

7. McKernan, T.M., Woods, E.B., Lash, L.H. (1991). Uptake of glutathione by renal cortical mitochondria. *Archives of Biochemistry and Biophysics, 288,* 653–663.

8. Hinchman, C.A., Ballatori, N. (1990). Glutathione-degrading capacities of liver and kidney in different species. *Biochemical Pharmacology, 40,* 1131–1135.

9. Laberge, R., Karwatsky, J., Lincoln, M.C., Leimanis, M.L., Georges, E. (2007). Modulation of GSH levels in ABCC1 expressing tumor cells triggers apoptosis through oxidative stress. *Biochemical Pharmacology*, *73*, 1727–1737.

10. Linsdell, P., Hanrahan, J.W. (1998). Glutathione permeability of CFTR. *American Journal of Physiology*, *275*, C323–C326.

11. Sastre, J., Serviddio, G., Pereda, J., Minana, J.B., Arduini, A., Vendemiale, G., Poli, G., Pallardo, F.V., Vina, J. (2007). Mitochondrial function in liver disease. *Frontiers in Bioscience*, *12*, 1200–1209.

12. Monsalve, M., Borniquel, S., Valle, I., Lamas, S. (2007) Mitochondrial dysfunction in human pathologies. *Frontiers in Bioscience*, *12*, 1131–1153.

13. Passos, J.F., Von Zglinicki, T. (2006). Oxygen free radicals in cell senescence: Are they signal transducers? *Free Radical Research*, *40*, 1277–1283.

14. Garcia-Ruiz, C., Morales, A., Ballesta, A., Rodes, J., Kaplowitz, N., Fernandez-Checa, J.C. (1994). Effect of chronic ethanol feeding on glutathione and functional integrity of mitochondria in periportal and perivenous rat hepatocytes. *Journal of Clinical Investigation*, *94*, 193–201.

15. Hansen, J.M., Go, Y.M., Jones, D.P. (2006). Nuclear and mitochondrial compartmentalization of oxidative stress and redox signaling. *Annual Review of Pharmacology and Toxicology*, *46*, 215–234.

16. Kurosawa, K., Hayashi, N., Sato, N., Kamada, T., Tagawa, K. (1990). Transport of glutathione across the mitochondrial membranes. *Biochemical and Biophysical Research Communication*, *167*, 367–372.

17. Martensson, J., Lai, J.C.K., Meister, A. (1990). High-affinity transport of glutathione is part of a multicomponent system essential for mitochondrial function. *Proceedings of the National Academy of Sciences USA*, *87*, 7185–7189.

18. Garcia-Ruiz, C., Morales, A., Cole, A., Rodes, J., Kaplowitz, N., Fernandez-Checa, J.C. (1995). Evidence that the rat hepatic mitochondrial carrier is distinct from the sinusoidal and canalicular transporters for reduced glutathione. *Journal of Biological Chemistry*, *270*, 15946–15949.

19. Schnellmann, R.G. (1991). Renal mitochondrial glutathione transport. *Life Science*, *49*, 393–398.

20. Lash, L.H. (2006). Mitochondrial glutathione transport: Physiological, pathological and toxicological implications. *Chemico-Biological Interactions*, *163*, 54–67.

21. Klingenberg, M. (1979). Overview on mitochondrial metabolite transport systems. *Methods in Enzymology*, *56*, 245–252.

22. Palmieri, F. (2004). The mitochondrial transporter family (SLC25): Physiological and pathological implications. *Pflügers Archives*, *447*, 689–709.

23. Hwang, C., Sinskey, A.J., Lodish, H.F. (1992). Oxidized redox state of glutathione in the endoplasmic reticulum. *Science*, *257*, 1496–1502.

24. Chakravarthi, S., Jessop, C.E., Bulleid, N.J. (2006). The role of glutathione in disulphide bond formation and endoplasmic-reticulum-generated oxidative stress. *EMBO Reports*, *7*, 271–275.

25. Frand, A.R., Kaiser, C.A. (1998). The ERO1 gene of yeast is required for oxidation of protein dithiols in the endoplasmic reticulum. *Molecular Cell*, *1*, 161–170.

26. Pollard, M.G., Travers, K.J., Weissman, J.S. (1998). Ero1p: A novel and ubiquitous protein with an essential role in oxidative protein folding in the endoplasmic reticulum. *Molecular Cell, 1,* 171–182.

27. Tu, B.P., Weissman, J.S. (2002). The FAD- and O_2-dependent reaction cycle of Ero1-mediated oxidative protein folding in the endoplasmic reticulum. *Molecular Cell, 10,* 983–994.

28. Weissman, J.S., Kim, P.S. (1993). Efficient catalysis of disulphide bond rearrangements by protein disulphide isomerase. *Nature, 365,* 185–188.

29. Frand, A.R., Kaiser, C.A. (1999). Ero1p oxidizes protein disulfide isomerase in a pathway for disulfide bond formation in the endoplasmic reticulum. *Molecular Cell, 4,* 469–477.

30. Nardai, G., Korcsmaros, T., Papp, E., Csermely, P. (2003). Reduction of the endoplasmic reticulum accompanies the oxidative damage of diabetes mellitus. *Biofactors, 17,* 259–267.

31. Bellomo, G., Vairetti, M., Stivala, L., Mirabelli, F., Richelmi, P., Orrenius, S. (1992). Demonstration of nuclear compartmentalization of glutathione in hepatocytes. *Proceedings of the National Academy of Sciences USA, 89,* 4412–4416.

32. Briviba, K., Fraser, G., Sies, H., Ketterer, B. (1993). Distribution of the monochlorobimane-glutathione conjugate between nucleus and cytosol in isolated hepatocytes. *Biochemical Journal, 294,* 631–633.

33. Thomas, M., Nicklee, T., Hedley, D.W. (1995). Differential effects of depleting agents on cytoplasmic and nuclear non-protein sulphydryls: A fluorescence image cytometry study. *British Journal of Cancer, 72,* 45–50.

34. Söderdahl, T., Enoksson, M., Lundberg, M., Holmgren, A., Ottersen, O.P., Orrenius, S., Bolcsfoldi, G., Cotgreave, I.A. (2003). Visualization of the compartmentalization of gluta-thione and protein-glutathione mixed disulfides in cultured cells. *FASEB Journal, 17,* 124–126.

35. Voehringer, D.W., McConkey, D.J., McDonnell, T.J., Birsbay, S., Meyn, R.E. (1998). Bcl-2 expression causes redistribution of glutathione to the nucleus. *Proceedings of the National Academy of Sciences USA, 95,* 2956–2960.

36. Smith, C.V., Jones, D.P., Guenthner, T.M., Lash, L.H., Lauterburg, B.H. (1996). Compartmentation of glutathione: Implications for the study of toxicity and disease. *Toxicology and Applied Pharmacology, 140,* 1–12.

37. Ho, Y.F., Guenthner, T.M. (1994). Uptake and biosynthesis of glutathione by isolated hepatic nuclei. *Toxicologist, 14,* 178.

38. Kim, J.R., Lee, S.M., Cho, S.H., Kim, J.H., Kim, B.H., Kwon, J., Choi, C.Y., Kim, Y.D., Lee, S.R. (2004). Oxidation of thioredoxin reductase in HeLa cells stimulated with tumor necrosis factor-alpha. *FEBS Letters, 567,* 189–196.

39. Markovic, J., Borras, C., Ortega, A., Sastre, J., Vina, J., Pallardo, F.V. (2007). Glutathione is recruited into the nucleus in early phases of cell proliferation. *Journal of Biological Chemistry, 282,* 20416–20424.

40. Bellomo, G., Palladini, G., Vairetti, M. (1997). Intranuclear distribution, function and fate of glutathione and glutathione-S-conjugate in living rat hepatocytes studied by fluorescence microscopy. *Microscopy Research and Technique, 36,* 243–252.

41. Hinshaw, J.E. (1992). Architecture and design of the nuclear pore complex. *Cell, 69,* 1133–1141.

42. Mazzanti, M., Innocenti, B., Rigatelli, M. (1994). ATP-dependent ionic permeability on nuclear envelope in in situ nuclei of Xenopus oocytes. *FASEB Journal, 8,* 231–236.

43. Mazzanti, M., Bustamante, J.O., Oberleithner, H. (2001). Electrical dimension of the nuclear envelope. *Physiology Reviews*, *81*, 1–19.

44. Atzori, L., Dypbukt, J.M., Hybbinette, S.S., Moldeus, P., Grafstrom, R.C. (1994). Modifications of cellular thiols during growth and squamous differentiation of cultured human bronchial epithelial cells. *Experimental Cell Research*, *211*, 115–120.

45. Morales, A., Miranda, M., Sanchez-Reyes, A., Biete, A., Fernandez-Checa, J.C. (1998). Oxidative damage of mitochondrial and nuclear DNA induced by ionizing radiation in human hepatoblastoma cells. *International Journal of Radiation Oncology Biology and Physics*, *42*, 191–203.

46. McBride, W.G. (1961). Thalidomide and congenital abnormalities. *Lancet*, *2*, 1358.

47. Hansen, J.M., Harris, K.K., Philbert, M.A., Harris, C. (2002). Thalidomide modulates nuclear redox status and preferentially depletes glutathione in rabbit limb versus rat limb. *Journal of Pharmacology and Experimental Therapeutics*, *300*, 768–776.

48. Thelander, L., Reichard, P. (1979). Reduction of ribonucleotides. *Annual Review in Biochemistry*, *48*, 133–158.

49. Biaglow, J.E., Varnes, M.E., Clark, E.P., Epp, E.R. (1983). The role of thiols in cellular response to radiation and drugs. *Radiation Research*, *95*, 437–455.

CHAPTER 4

INTESTINAL METABOLISM OF SULFUR AMINO ACIDS

NANCY BENIGHT, DOUGLAS G. BURRIN, and BARBARA STOLL

4.1 INTRODUCTION

The gastrointestinal tract (GIT) serves a key function in the digestion of dietary protein and absorption of amino acids. However, the GIT is also an important site of amino acid metabolism in the body. Methionine is an indispensable amino acid and must be supplied in the diet (Fig. 4.1). In addition, considerable attention in recent years has been focused homocysteine, a product of methionine transmethylation. Numerous clinical studies have shown that elevated plasma homocysteine levels are strongly associated with increased risk for several diseases, including atherosclerosis, Alzheimer's disease [1, 2], ischemic and hemorrhagic stroke [3, 4], and most recently inflammatory bowel disease (IBD) [5]. However, another intermediate formed during the initial step in transmethylation of methionine is S-adenosylmethionine (SAM), which has been shown to play a pivotal role in hepatic injury, regeneration, and alcohol-induced liver cancer [6]. As the major methyl donor in the body [7], SAM also plays an integral role in the regulation of DNA methylation, which is an important epigenetic determinant of gene expression and has been implicated in the inverse relationship between folate status and various cancers, particularly colorectal cancer [8]. Cysteine is considered semidispensable, as it can be synthesized by all tissues in the body via transmethylation of methionine, yet requires an adequate source of methionine and serine precursors. Cysteine is the essential constituent amino acid in the functional (CXXC) motif of the major cellular antioxidant families, including glutathione, glutaredoxins, thioredoxins, and peroxiredoxins [9]. As such, the bioavailability of cysteine, derived from methionine transsulfuration, proteolysis, or the diet, has a critical influence on cellular redox function and the susceptibility to oxidant stress.

Glutathione and Sulfur Amino Acids in Human Health and Disease. Edited by R. Masella and G. Mazza
Copyright © 2009 John Wiley & Sons, Inc.

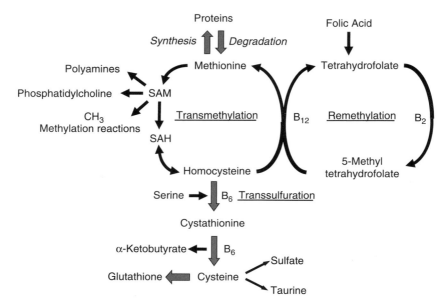

Figure 4.1 Overview of methionine and cysteine metabolism. SAM, *S*-adenosylmethionine; SAH, *S*-adenosylhomocysteine.

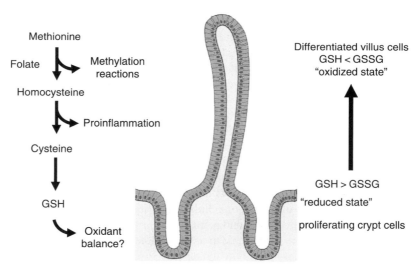

Figure 4.2 Functional importance of sulfur amino acids in the gastrointestinal tract (GIT). Sulfur amino acid metabolism and its required cofactors influence many aspects of GIT physiology, including production of methyl donor groups, oxidant balance, and inflammatory response.

In this chapter, we will discuss the evidence for sulfur amino acid metabolism in the gastrointestinal tract (GIT) and its functional importance in health and disease. There are several reports indicating that the methionine metabolic cycle is active in intestinal epithelial cells and these have an effect on maintaining homeostasis in the GIT (Fig. 4.2). The intermediate S-adenosylmethionine (SAM) is not only critical in methionine metabolism, but also serves as the one carbon donor in the majority of cellular methylation reactions. Deregulated or reduced SAM concentrations are implicated in many diseases, including colorectal cancer. Other metabolic products whose production requires a functional methionine metabolism, such as polyamines, are critical for the continual replacement of enterocytes as well as colonocytes, both of which are part of the mucosal surface of the GIT and are subject to high cellular turnover rates. Methylthioadenosine, a secondary product of polyamine conversion, has been shown to have numerous critical functions within cells. Therefore, the GIT serves a more diverse function than simply providing an entry and processing point for sulfur amino acids from dietary and microbial sources. The GIT is a significant consumer of sulfur amino acids and relies on this metabolic cycle to support normal growth and maintenance; this becomes evident when examining diseases that affect the GIT, such as IBD and colorectal cancer.

4.2 ISOTOPIC APPROACHES TO STUDY METABOLISM

Isotopic amino acids have been used extensively to elucidate the fundamental biochemical pathways, key enzymes, and major tissues involved in sulfur amino acid metabolism in mammals. Early studies in rodents and isolated tissue extracts mainly used radioisotopes [10–14]. However, in the past 20 years, stable isotopes have been used to quantify sulfur amino acid metabolism in vivo in humans and animals [15–19]. A particularly important series of studies was reported by Storch and coworkers using multiple isotopomers of methionine (Fig. 4.3) in adult humans [20–22]. In these studies, infusion and measurements of steady-state plasma enrichment of 1-$[^{13}C]$methionine and methyl-$[^2H_3]$methionine were used to establish an in vivo kinetic model of sulfur amino acid metabolism that provided estimates of transmethylation, remethylation, and transsulfuration. These studies demonstrated the role of feeding, fasting, and the sparing action of dietary cysteine on kinetics of methionine catabolism in humans. More recently the Storch–Young model has been modified using homocysteine enrichment as the precursor for intracellular methionine kinetics [23, 24]. These reports and subsequent studies have revealed that the rates of methionine metabolism are substantially higher than previous estimates and markedly stimulated by insulin [25–27]. Others have used alternative isotopomers of methionine, namely U-$[^{13}C]$methionine, to quantify methionine cycle kinetics in humans, animals, and intestinal epithelial cells [27–29] and also found relatively higher rates of homocysteine remethylation and evidence for homocysteine synthesis in the gut.

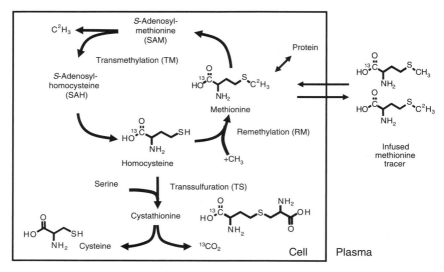

Figure 4.3   Storch–Young kinetic model of methionine metabolism. This illustrates the fates of the two labeled isotopomers used in the studies by Storch and coworkers, 1-[^{13}C]methionine and methyl-[^{2}H$_3$]methionine. The [^{2}H$_3$]-methyl group is lost during transmethylation from SAM to SAH, whereas the [^{13}C]-carbon group is transferred to 1-[^{13}C]homocysteine, 1-[^{13}C]cystathionine and finally oxidized to ^{13}CO$_2$ via α-ketobutyrate in the TCA cycle [20].

4.3   EVIDENCE OF GUT SULFUR AMINO ACID METABOLISM

Early studies by Mudd et al. [10] using rat models were the first to identify the mucosa of the small intestine as a site for transsulfuration, as indicated by the presence of all three required enzymes for transsulfuration; however, the small intestine possessed reduced activity of one or more of these enzymes when compared to the liver. Stegink and den Besten [30] were first to show that the splanchnic organs are an important site of transmethylation and transsulfuration of dietary methionine for the synthesis of cysteine. They found that the circulating cystine concentration was higher in adults given a cystine-free nutrient solution via the nasogastric compared to intravenous route (Fig. 4.4). Since then, others have demonstrated that intravenous feeding without or with minimum cysteine supplementation results in low circulating levels of cystine in human infants [31] and piglets [32]. Circulating plasma total cysteine concentrations were significantly greater in enterally than in parenterally fed piglets receiving methionine as the sole dietary sulfur amino acid and were positively associated with sulfur amino acid intake in enterally but not parenterally fed piglets [33]. These data agree with the data from Stegink and den Besten [30] and suggest that first-pass splanchnic metabolism is important for the synthesis of cysteine in neonates as well as adults. Other studies with isotopic tracers have shown indirectly that, in the fed state, a substantial fraction of the dietary methionine transsulfuration occurs via first-pass splanchnic metabolism in adult humans [15, 34]. These studies

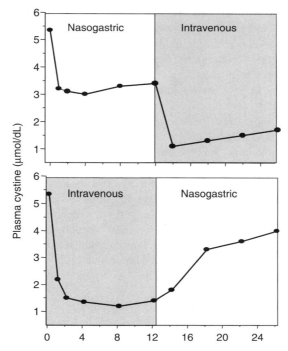

Figure 4.4   Steginck and den Besten results. Studies by Steginck and den Besten found that circulating plasma cystine was higher in humans receiving a cysteine-free nutrient solution via the nasogastric route than by the intravenous route [30].

suggest that first-pass splanchnic metabolism, and predominantly the intestinal tissue, is a potentially important site of transmethylation and transsulfuration of dietary methionine. However, the extent to which this occurs in the liver versus the GIT has not been characterized extensively.

Pig models have been utilized extensively to study in vivo amino acid metabolism in the gut as they have similar physiology to humans, especially neonates. Our studies in infant pigs showed that the net portal absorption of several indispensable amino acids, including methionine, was significantly less than 100% of the dietary intake, ranging from 40% to 70% [35]. The importance of the gut also was demonstrated in studies where the whole body methionine requirement was 30% greater in enterally fed than parenterally fed piglets [33, 36]. Most recently, our pig studies combined the Storch–Young isotopic tracer model and demonstrated that ∼20% of the dietary methionine intake is metabolized by the GIT and released as either homocysteine or completely oxidized to CO_2 [37]. This study made several important findings; first, the net release of homocysteine into the portal circulation indicated that the GIT contributes to the circulating homocysteine load and that a majority (∼70%) of the methionine used by the GIT was metabolized via transmethylation and transsulfuration. Further, GIT metabolism accounted for ∼25% of the transmethylation and transsulfuration in the whole body. We also found evidence for mRNA expression and enzymatic activity of cystathionine β-synthase in isolated intestinal epithelial cells. These results provided compelling evidence that methionine metabolism in the GIT is substantial and may be important for normal gut function.

Other animal models provide support for the notion that the gut is a site of methionine metabolism. In vivo studies showed kinetic evidence that transmethylation, remethylation, and transsulfuration occur in the ruminant GIT [18, 29]. A recent series of stable isotopic tracer studies in sheep demonstrated that the GIT is capable of methionine synthesis via transamination from the dietary 2-hydroxy-4-methylbutanoic acid (HMB), a hydroxy form of methionine keto-acid 2-ketomethylbutanoic acid [38, 39]. These studies showed that while nearly all (87%) of the $[^{13}C]$-HMB infused into the abomasum was absorbed into the blood, substantial enrichment of $[^{13}C]$-methionine occurred in the small and large intestinal tissue. These studies indicate that, at least in sheep, the enzymes necessary for conversion of HMB stereoisomers (L-α-hydroxy acid oxidase and D-hydroxy acid dehydrogenase) to 2-ketomethylbutanoic acid and transamination to methionine exist in the gut. This work is consistent with early studies in rat tissues [40] that demonstrated methionine oxidation occurs via an alternate pathway of transamination that is independent of transmethylation and formation of SAM. Further, studies in young chicks have shown that use of DL-HMB in the context of a methionine deficient diet is an effective source for the production of L-methionine to maintain growth [41]. This study also indicated that addition of DL-HMB in a methionine-sufficient diet results in similar growth depression and toxicity as excessive L-methionine only, indicating that the transamination reaction in young chicks is highly efficient. The extent to which this alternate methionine oxidative pathway is metabolically significant in humans has been questioned, however, since accumulation of 2-ketomethylbutanoic acid occurred in the urine of CBS-deficient patients only during hypermethioninemia [42]. These studies provide good evidence that explains the high bioavailability and widespread use of DL-HMB as a feed additive to meet the methionine requirements in domestic livestock species.

With respect to cysteine in the GIT, in vivo studies showed that less than 100% of the dietary cysteine load appears in the portal blood, suggesting extensive intestinal utilization of cysteine [35, 43]. However, these estimates of plasma cysteine may be flawed by the analytical methods used for amino acid analysis, since cysteine readily dimerizes to cystine and can be bound to proteins via disulfide linkage, indicating that these values may underestimate actual plasma cysteine levels. The first step in cysteine catabolism is conversion to cysteine sulfinate via the enzyme cysteine dioxygenase. Approximately 70% to 90% of cysteine sulfinate is subsequently decarboxylated via cysteine sulfinate decarboxylase to produce hypotaurine, which is then oxidized to taurine via a poorly characterized enzymatic reaction [1]. Rodent studies with ^{14}C-labeled cysteine demonstrated significantly higher oxidation when given via the intragastric (70%) than intraperitoneal (41%) route, suggesting that nearly half of the whole body cysteine oxidation occurs in splanchnic tissues [1]. More importantly, subsequent work demonstrated that intestinal enterocytes extensively metabolize cysteine to cysteine sulfinate via cysteine dioxygenase. In vivo rodent studies with intravenous infusion of isotopically labeled [^{15}N]-cysteine indicate that an important metabolic fate of cysteine in the gut is incorporation into glutathione (GSH) [44]. Thus, it appears that the intestine has the enzymatic capacity for transmethylation, remethylation, and transsulfuration of methionine, and for conversion of cysteine into GSH and taurine. Additional kinetic evidence for methionine transmethylation, remethylation, and transsulfuration within the gut epithelium comes from cell culture studies. Specifically, studies in human colon carcinoma cells (Caco-2) demonstrate significant release of homocysteine and cystathionine, further suggesting that the intestine exports homocysteine and contributes to the plasma homocysteine load [27]. These studies also found that the production of homocysteine by epithelial cells was suppressed by increased folate availability in the media, suggesting active remethylation via methionine synthase activity.

Additional clinical evidence of methionine and cysteine metabolism in the gut is available in the context of disease states. For example, normal mucosal biopsies from patients with endoscopically determined colonic disease (i.e., IBD, colon cancer, diverticulosis) as well as patients with no colonic disease all show measurable production of homocysteine, cysteine, and glutathione [45]. These results correlate to the animal findings mentioned above which indicate that the key enzymes for transmethylation and transsulfuration are present in the human colon. Nutritional epigenetic studies further implicate GIT methionine metabolism with the risk of colon cancer. Epigenetic modifications of DNA and DNA binding proteins via methylation of CpG islands within DNA is largely mediated by the product of methionine metabolism, namely *S*-adenosylmethionine (SAM), which serves as the major methyl donor in the body. Further, a current topic of debate is the role of folate in colon cancer prevention.

4.4 OTHER KEY PLAYERS IN INTESTINAL SULFUR AMINO ACID METABOLISM

4.4.1 Folate

As a critical component of homocysteine remethylation via methionine synthase, folate is intricately linked to methionine metabolism (Fig. 4.5). The main role of folate is to provide one carbon units needed to perform various cellular functions, including DNA methylation and DNA synthesis as well as protein synthesis. Folate is derived from the diet in the form of polyglutamate and absorption in the proximal jejunum occurs after brush border enzymes hydrolyze into a monoglutamate form [46]. 5-Methyltetrahydrofolate (MTHF) is the methyl donor for the reaction catalyzed by the enzyme methionine synthase. Evidence indicates that the enzymes necessary for folate utilization via remethylation are active in the GIT. Animal and cell culture studies have characterized the activity of methionine synthase in the small [47] and large intestine [48]. Further, genetic studies in colorectal cancer have examined the polymorphisms found in both methionine synthase and methyltetrahydrofolate reductase (MTHFR) [49, 50]. Dietary folate deficiency or mutations in genes in the

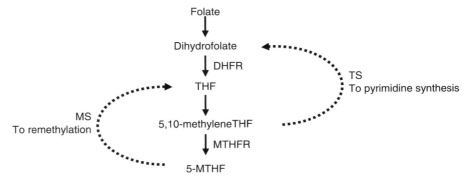

Figure 4.5   Folate pathway. Folate can be acquired either from the diet or from production via gastrointestinal tract lumen bacteria. Once inside the cell, it exists in multiple isoforms, each of which serves as an important constituent of other metabolic pathways. DHFR, dihydrofolate reductase; MS, methionine synthase; MTHF, 5,10-methylene-THF; MTHFR, 5,10-methylene-THF, reductase; THF, tetrahydrofolate; TS, thymidylate synthase.

folate pathway can lead to alterations in multiple pathways, including the methionine cycle. Intracellular SAM controls the rate of remethylation. Thus, in cases of reduced SAM concentration, remethylation is upregulated to replenish the supply of methionine via homocysteine, which is then transmethylated to form additional SAM. However, in states of folate deficiency, there is a lack of MTHF to provide methyl groups for remethylation of homocysteine to methionine.

Folate also plays a critical role in pyrimidine synthesis, as the 5,10-methylenetetrahydrofolate form is a one carbon donor for the formation of dTMP from dUMP. This reaction is the rate limiting step in de novo DNA synthesis and requires the enzyme thymidylate synthase (TS) [51]. As an essential enzyme in DNA synthesis, TS is found in all cells. Deficiencies in folate lead to an imbalance in the dTMP precursor pool for incorporation into newly synthesized DNA. In the face of such deficiency, dUMP will be incorporated in place of dTMP, which is the equivalent of a mutational event [51]. This leads to continuous DNA repair cycles, as multiple dUMPs can be incorporated, and ultimately to DNA strand breakage. This process has been confirmed in the GIT; studies in isolated colonocytes from rats receiving dietary restriction of folate or methionine and choline showed an increase in DNA strand breakage when compared to colonocytes from rats on a control diet [52].

4.4.2 *S*-Adenosylmethionine

Although it is an intermediate of methionine metabolism, SAM is metabolized via other pathways that are important to a variety of cellular functions. Figure 4.6 outlines the possible fates of SAM. Generation of SAM occurs via action of methionine adenosyltransferase (MAT) enzymes, which in humans are encoded by the genes MAT1A and MAT2A [53]. In humans, the MAT2A (MAT II) is ubiquitously expressed, whereas the products of MAT1A (MAT I and MAT III) are liver specific.

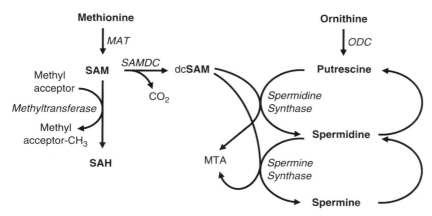

Figure 4.6 *S*-adenosylmethionine (SAM) metabolism. SAM serves as a substrate for several pathways critical to cellular function, including as a methyl donor for many more than 100 methylation reactions, as well as for polyamine synthesis. A product of SAM from polyamine synthesis is MTA, which has been indicated as a regulator of transmethylation. MAT, methionine adenosyltransferase; MTA, methylthioadenosine; ODC, ornithine decarboxylase; SAH, *S*-adenosylhomocysteine; SAMDC, *S*-adenosylmethionine decarboxylase.

Indirect evidence of the presence of remethylation enzymes in the GIT comes from piglet methionine kinetic studies, which found significant production of ^{13}C-homocysteine after intraduodenal administration of 1-^{13}C-methionine [37]. Further, expression of MAT2A has been confirmed in human as well as mouse colonic tissue biopsies and has been shown to be regulated by leptin and growth factors such as IGF-1 and EGF in colonic cell lines [53].

Once SAM is produced, it can be processed via two pathways. The first involves a variety of methyltransferases that can transfer a one carbon unit to a methyl acceptor group, whereas the second pathway involves metabolism of SAM for polyamine synthesis. There is a large number of methyltransferases that have been identified in human tissues. However, bioinformatic analysis suggests that we have only identified 25% of human methyltransferases [54]. More than 100 identified methylation reactions use SAM as the methyl donor [55]. Examples include methylation of CpG islands in DNA as well as methylation of RNA or proteins. SAM is also involved in xenobiotic detoxification, as well as inhibition of neurotransmitters and formation of small molecules. With regard to the GIT, areas of hypermethylation or hypomethylation within DNA may lead to altered gene expression of the affected or neighboring genes as well as changes in recombination patterns, leading to DNA strand breaks and altered physiology. SAM depletion may also alter methylation patterns of RNA or proteins, which can lead to further changes in normal cell function.

SAM has recently been shown to play an important role in the formation of phosphatidylcholine (PC) in the liver. Figure 4.7 shows the formation of PC, which occurs through the addition of methyl groups from three molecules of SAM to phosphatidylethanolamine via the enzyme phosphatidylethanolamine *N*-methyltransferase

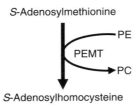

Figure 4.7   Phosphatidylcholine synthesis. Three molecules of *S*-adenosylmethionine (SAM) are required to form phosphatidylcholine (PC) from phosphatidylethanolamine (PE) using the enzyme phosphatidylethanolamine *N*-methyltransferase (PEMT). PC has been shown as a substantial consumer of methyl groups from SAM; therefore, its production and utilization is dependent on adequate methionine absorption and distribution in the gastrointestinal tract.

(PEMT). This usage of SAM leads to increased *S*-adenosylhomocysteine and subsequently homocysteine. Studies in PEMT − / − mice fed a high fat diet showed a 50% decrease in plasma homocysteine concentrations when compared to wild type mice on the same diet [56], indicating that PC production is utilizing a substantial amount of SAM in the liver. As methionine is an essential amino acid, the ability of the GIT to acquire it from dietary sources and the efficiency of the pathway will have an effect on PC production and its downstream actions, such as choline and acetylcholine production, incorporation into cellular membranes and cholesterol removal.

SAM is a key intermediate in polyamine formation. Figure 4.6 depicts the polyamine synthesis pathway and the essential role of SAM in this process. First, ornithine is used to form putrescine; next SAM is required to convert putrescine to spermine and spermidine. In conversion of putrescine, the first step in synthesis is to form decarboxylated SAM (dcSAM) via *S*-adenosylmethionine decarboxylase (SAMDC). The intracellular concentration of dcSAM is low in mammalian cells, so this step is essential in activating polyamine synthesis via this pathway. Spermidine synthase or spermine synthase catalyzes the release of the remainder of the methionine backbone from SAM and this is used to form either spermidine or spermine, respectively, from putrescine. A secondary metabolic product of these reactions is methylthioadenosine (MTA), which is an inhibitor of cellular processes, including cell proliferation and apoptosis [57].

Polyamines carry multiple basic charges and therefore are able to strongly bind and stabilize DNA. This trait also affords polyamines a role in the stabilization of RNA secondary structure as well as a modulator of specific enzyme activities. Beyond its role in nucleic acid stabilization, polyamines are important in all cells and function in various processes involved in cell growth and differentiation [58]. Large quantities of polyamines are consumed in the typical diet, yet studies have shown that the quantity of polyamines in serum remains constant and in the micromolar range [59]. This indicates that the GIT is utilizing or degrading a substantial amount of the ingested polyamines and only releases what is needed to maintain low circulating serum levels. Indeed, the GIT is known for its large requirement of polyamines, as it is one of the most rapidly proliferating tissues in the body [59], due to the short life span of epithelial cells. Polyamine uptake from the intestinal lumen has been shown to be highest in epithelial cells as well as colon cancer cells and this occurs due to mitogenic activation of SAMDC [59].

As polyamines are critical for intestinal epithelial cell growth and are implicated in colon cancer, several studies have examined the effects of polyamine depletion on specific oncogenes. Studies examining c-Myc expression in an intestinal epithelial cell line (IEC-6) found that polyamines do regulate the expression of c-myc, which is known to be a key regulator of cell cycle progression [60]. Other studies from this group have found that a reduction of polyamines in IEC-6 cells led to inhibition of mucosal cell growth by stabilization of p53 [61]. Further, this same group recently published information regarding the involvement of polyamines in innate immunity. They showed that polyamine depletion in IEC-6 cells reduced the expression of toll-like receptor 2 (TLR-2); this reduction was associated with reduced epithelial barrier integrity [62]. Clearly, polyamines play a pivotal role in intestinal epithelial cell function through modulation of specific gene products in multiple pathways. This indicates that the status of the methionine cycle and therefore polyamines is critical in GIT health and disturbances may play a role in intestinal disease.

The secondary production of MTA via polyamine synthesis increases the importance of SAM and therefore methionine metabolism in normal cell function. MTA can be formed by two pathways; however, both rely on SAM as precursor. MTA is degraded via methylthioadenosine phosphorylase (MTAP) to produce adenosine and a precursor that can be used by the methionine salvage pathway to provide additional methionine. MTAP is important, as MTA is known to block polyamine synthesis via inhibition of spermidine and spermine synthases [63].

It is well established that intracellular concentrations of SAM control the rate of transmethylation under normal conditions. Studies in colorectal cancer cell line (HT-29) showed that MTA is more potent at preventing mitogen activation of MAT2A than SAM [53], indicating that MTA may in fact exert control over SAM and therefore activation of the transmethylation. To this end, a recent study found that MTAP mRNA expression is reduced in liver biopsies of patients with hepatocellular carcinoma (HCC) or cirrhosis when compared to healthy liver biopsies [64]. This reduction in MTAP mRNA was attributed to changes in epigenetic regulation, specifically hypermethylation, as shown in HCC cell lines; further, work in rat models of liver damage showed that SAM concentrations were reduced in the cirrhotic livers of these rats. Taken together, these ideas indicate that a hypermethylation event induced by damage to hepatocytes leads to reduction of MTAP mRNA expression and this inhibits the removal of MTA. The high concentration of MTA may lead to reduction in methionine cycling by blocking MAT2A activity, thereby leading to hypomethylation of DNA and reduced polyamine synthesis. These changes could lead to epigenetic modification of DNA and altered gene expression and may play a role in the initial stages of carcinoma formation. There is limited information on the function of MTA in the GIT and this warrants further exploration.

4.5 CYSTEINE IN REDOX FUNCTION AND OXIDANT STRESS IN THE GUT

Sulfur amino acids, principally cysteine, play a key role in cellular redox function and susceptibility to oxidant stress [65, 66]. The biology of cellular redox function has expanded dramatically in recent years and now encompasses multiples families, such as glutaredoxins, thioredoxins, peroxiredoxins, and most recently sulfiredoxin [9, 67]. Cysteine is a constituent amino acid of the tripeptide glutathione that is well known as a major cellular antioxidant in mammals; however, it is also the essential constituent amino acid in the functional (CXXC) motif of the other major cellular antioxidant families. Cysteine is also a component of numerous regulatory and catalytic domains of transcription factors, kinases and phosphatases [68, 69]. A key signaling kinase involved in intracellular redox sensing is apoptosis signal-regulating kinase (ASK1), which exists in cells bound with reduced forms of thioredoxin and glutaredoxin [68]. Upon oxidation by reactive oxygen species, thioredoxin dissociates from ASK1, thereby activating it and major downstream kinase pathways involved in cell stress and functions, namely p38 and c-Jun N-terminal kinases (JNK). In addition to intracellular redox function, new findings have shown that the concentrations of free cysteine and its oxidized disulfide form, cystine, together with GSH/GSSG have a dominant role in regulating the extracellular redox state, including the plasma pool [66, 70]. Thus, the cellular bioavailability of cysteine derived from the diet, methionine transsulfuration, or proteolysis is important for maintaining cellular redox function. Mediating oxidant stress and maintaining normal redox status is especially important in intestinal epithelial cells, which are exposed to high levels of oxidant stress due to the high rate of oxidative metabolism as well as exposure to luminal toxins and oxidants derived from the diet.

Studies with human colonic epithelial cells (Caco-2) indicated that as differentiation proceeds, cell GSH and cysteine concentrations and proliferation rate decrease, whereas the rate of apoptosis increases [71]. Additional intestinal cell culture studies showed that increased oxidant stress and redox imbalance suppress cell proliferation and induce apoptosis and are associated with a more oxidized glutathione and cysteine state [72–74]. In vitro studies with colonic epithelial cells showed that cells grown in cysteine-deficient media have suppressed GSH concentrations and cell proliferation rates, both of which are increased with cysteine supplementation [75–77]. This phenomenon also occurred in vivo where rats fed sulfur amino acid-deficient diets had reduced concentrations of GSH and cysteine and a more oxidized redox state in both the plasma and intestinal mucosa [78]. Collectively, these studies suggest that cysteine availability and local GSH concentration have a direct influence on epithelial cell proliferation and survival and are inversely proportional to cellular differentiation state. However, the role of extracellular cysteine in cell redox function appears to be regulated independently of GSH and thioredoxins.

In addition to dietary cysteine, there also may be a functional role for intracellular cysteine synthesis via methionine transsulfuration in intestinal epithelial cells. It is evident that cysteine availability is important for maintenance of epithelial cell GSH level and cell survival; however, it is unknown whether methionine transsulfuration can affect cysteine availability and epithelial cell function.

4.6 PATHOPHYSIOLOGY OF SULFUR AMINO ACID METABOLISM IN THE GIT

4.6.1 Mechanisms of Deficiency

The most obvious method for developing a deficiency of a required substance is through poor diet; this has greater implications in Westernized societies. With the coming of the industrial revolution and modern agricultural processes, the diets of individuals living in these societies have changed significantly. Increases in the amount of processed refined grains, refined sugars and vegetable oils, salts and fatty meat [79] affect the nutritional values of the foods we eat. This is further exacerbated by high prevalence of fast food in the Western diet and also a reduction in exercise. Poor daily food choices may be enough to influence levels of critical vitamins and minerals, such as those needed for sulfur amino acid metabolism.

Another expected path to deficiency is via genetic variation in enzymes required for a pathway to function. In sulfur amino acid metabolism, it is well established that allelic variation in genes involved in folate metabolism as well as transsulfuration can lead to reduced activity of these enzymes and therefore reduced efficiency of methionine metabolism. For example, cystathionine-β-synthase (CBS) deficiency results in reduced transsulfuration in individuals who have one defective copy of the enzyme, leading to elevated homocysteine. However, homozygosity for the defective enzyme is the most common cause of homocysteinemia in inherited cases, as transsulfuration is effectively blocked with no functioning CBS.

Other GIT-specific deficiencies can occur due to alterations in the anatomy of the absorptive surfaces within the GIT. As the small intestine is the major location for nutrient absorption, changes in physiological function can cause deficiency even when an adequate supply of nutrients is consumed in the diet. For example, intestinal inflammation is common in celiac disease and inflammatory bowel disease (IBD), as well as during bacterial and viral infections. Inflammation can lead to changes in epithelial cell physiology, which can cause reduced functioning of specific nutrient receptors, or diarrhea, which leads to rapid loss of intestinal contents. Loss of portions of the small intestine can also leave individuals susceptible to nutrient deficiencies. For example, surgical resection of the intestine is a standard treatment option to remove damaged portions of the intestine due to chronic diseases such as IBD. Further, medications used to treat conditions of intestinal inflammation in a chronic setting can interfere with nutrient absorption receptors within the lumen of the intestine. Other medications can interfere directly with methionine metabolism. Methotrexate (MTX), which is used as an immunosuppressor for treatment of IBD, is an inhibitor of folate metabolism. MTX blocks the action of dihydrofolate reductase, which converts dihydrofolate to tetrahydrofolate, as well as MTHF reductase. MTX is generally used for maintenance of remission of IBD; however, the exact mechanism of action by which it suppresses the immune system is unknown [80]. Use of methotrexate for treatment of other inflammatory diseases, such as rheumatoid arthritis, has been linked to an increase in plasma homocysteine [81], although this association has not been studied in IBD patients.

4.6.2 Inflammatory Bowel Disease

The strong direct association between homocysteine and incidence of several human diseases, including cardiovascular disease and stroke, has led to a burgeoning literature on the biological effects of homocysteine in numerous tissues and cells, especially the vascular endothelium [82]. However, recent publications have begun to elucidate links to two common classes of intestinal disease.

Inflammatory bowel disease refers to chronic intestinal inflammatory diseases, specifically Crohn's disease and ulcerative colitis. These diseases are distinctly different with respect to disease location within the intestine, etiology and treatment options, but patients tend to present with similar symptoms, such as diarrhea, abdominal pain, and rectal bleeding. Recently, a possible novel link between inflammatory effects of homocysteinemia and IBD was demonstrated in studies showing increased homocysteine concentrations in plasma and mucosa biopsies from patients with Crohn's disease and ulcerative colitis [5, 45, 83]. Interestingly, the study by Danese et al. [5] also showed increased homocysteine production by cultured lamina propria mononuclear cells isolated from mucosal biopsies from IBD versus normal patients. Other studies in IBD patients have shown that increased plasma homocysteine is associated with decreased B-vitamin levels, particularly those involved in methionine metabolism (folate, B6, and B12) [83–85]. Multiple factors can lead to malnutrition of these vitamins in IBD patients, including drug interactions, reduced nutrient intake, and reduced ability of the small intestine to absorb nutrients [86]. Further indirect clinical evidence in support of this theory is a recent study in which IBD patients had a higher risk of early atherosclerosis than healthy controls as shown by greater carotid intima-media thickness and this was independently associated with plasma homocysteine level [87]. Other reports indicate that patients with IBD also have a substantially increased risk of thromboembolism due to a hypercoagulable state and prothrombotic condition [88]; this risk is a specific feature in patients with IBD, as other chronic inflammatory diseases (rheumatoid arthritis and celiac disease) do not show this increased risk for thromboembolism [89]. The increased risk may be associated with the increase in plasma homocysteine levels, as ex vivo examination of platelets from non-IBD patients with homocysteinemia showed functional alteration of platelets when compared to patients with normal plasma homocysteine levels [90].

Animal models of IBD have been successful in identifying factors that are disrupted during IBD, including immune system components, signaling molecules, and adhesion molecules. Many rodent models of IBD have been developed [91], yet one model is of particular interest when examining IBD in the context of homocysteinemia. The dextran sulfate sodium (DSS) model is a well-established approach to induce intestinal inflammation and mucosal injury similar to what is seen in human ulcerative colitis. Recent studies have used this model to investigate the effect on microvascular function using intravital video microscopy, which allows for the study of microvessels in live animals to identify changes in vessel morphology and function [92, 93]. Studies using DSS-treated mice to examine changes in colonic venule function have shown that experimental colitis induces a prothrombogenic condition in the colonic microcirculation, as indicated by increased platelet and leukocyte adhesion; the molecular mechanism of this response involves upregulation of adhesion molecules in intestinal venules [93]. This correlates to studies in cultured human intestinal microvascular endothelial cells which found increased leukocyte adhesion and upregulation of VCAM-1 [5]. DSS-treated mice also show constriction of arterioles in the submucosa of the terminal ileum and proximal colon when the arterioles were located close to venules that showed increased platelet adhesion [94]. Together, these studies demonstrate that experimental colitis causes vascular dysfunction in the mouse intestine. These results are similar to findings in human studies that indicate that vascular perfusion of mucosal surfaces is diminished in patients with IBD, with the extent of vascular damage correlated to severity of injury [95]. Loss of endothelium integrity may lead to increased vascular permeability and facilitate greater extravasation of blood leukocytes into the submucosal tissue of the gut, thereby increasing the number of immune cells involved in activation and maintenance of inflammation in IBD.

We postulate that the increase in homocysteine found in patients with IBD may be the causal link to occurrences such as increased vascular permeability, increased risk of atherosclerosis as well as thromboembolism, and changes in platelet and endothelial cell function. Studies of homocysteine involvement in other organs and diseases have indicated similar physiological changes. For example, Yi et al. [96] found that high plasma homocysteine is associated with glomerular injury in the kidney due to podocyte damage and changes in expression of podocyte-specific proteins involved in filtration barrier function. Further, human macrophage cell lines exposed to moderate concentrations of homocysteine had increased expression of monocyte chemoattractant protein 1 (MCP-1) as well as increased chemotaxis; these events were mediated by activation of NF-κB via increased phosphorylation of IκB-α [97]. Interestingly, similar results have been shown in other cell types. Studies in primary and immortalized human osteoblast cells exposed to physiologically high concentrations of homocysteine had enhanced apoptosis through the mitochondrial pathway that was shown to be mediated via IκB-α phosphorylation and subsequent NF-κB activation [98]. The authors speculated that the homocysteine led to an increase in reactive oxygen species (ROS), which in turn led to NF-κB activation. Studies in endothelial cells have confirmed that homocysteine exposure increased cellular ROS and activated NF-κB [99]. Further, they showed homocysteine led to increased mitochondrial biogenesis by modification of nuclear encoded proteins required for mitochondrial DNA replication, altering mitochondrial gene expression and causing damage. Finally, examination of TNF-α-resistant carcinoma cell lines showed that addition of homocysteine and adenosine altered the SAH : SAM ratio, which in turn led to reduced methylation. In combination with low amounts of TNF-α, the trio (adenosine, homocysteine, and TNF-α) was sufficient to induce TNF-α-mediated cytotoxicity through destruction of the mitochondrial membrane potential. Taken together, these papers

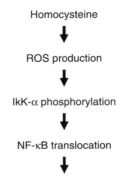

Homocysteine

⬇

ROS production

⬇

IκK-α phosphorylation

⬇

NF-κB translocation

⬇

Changes in mitochondrial biogenesis

Figure 4.8 Hypothesized influence of homocysteine on apoptosis. Studies in other cell types have demonstrated that excess homocysteine leads to increased reactive oxygen species (ROS) which phosphorylate IκK-α, activating NF-κB and causing changes in mitochondrial biogenesis. These changes lead to destruction of the mitochondrial membrane potential and activate apoptosis.

strongly suggest a role for homocysteine in mediating apoptosis in a variety of cell types through activation of NF-κB (Fig. 4.8). Although this idea has not been investigated in intestinal epithelial cells, it is plausible to hypothesize that homocysteine is capable of activating the same pathways in these cells. This has implications for IBD patients, where homocysteine production has been shown to be upregulated in isolated intestinal lymphoid cells [5]. The increase in homocysteine in these cells may lead to mitochondrial dysfunction and apoptosis, resulting in increased permeability of the epithelium. This would allow for invasion of microbes from the intestinal lumen, further activating the immune system. It has been shown that lamina propria mononuclear cells derived from IBD patient samples produce more homocysteine when stimulated by anti-CD3 [5]. Therefore, increased immune activity due to microbial invasion may lead to more homocysteine production, leading to more mitochondrial dysfunction and apoptosis, further damaging the epithelium and increasing permeability, creating a futile cycle of epithelial cell damage (Fig. 4.9).

4.6.3 Colorectal Cancer

Another GI disease that has been linked with sulfur amino acid metabolism is colorectal cancer, based on the relationship between low folate status and increased risk of tumorigenesis [8]. Studies in humans, animals, and cell culture indicate that the cellular mechanisms that mediate the effects of low folate availability with tumorigenesis include alterations in DNA methylation, as well as cell proliferation and repair [100]. Recent studies in two genetic lines of mice with targeted disruption of folate transport genes demonstrated that low folate status was associated with increased incidence of colonic cell proliferation, aberrant crypt foci, adenocarcinomas, and local

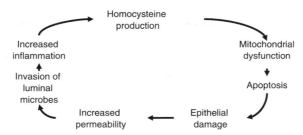

Figure 4.9   Effects of increased apoptosis influenced by homocysteine production. Activation of apoptosis as a consequence of high concentrations of homocysteine causes cell death and increased permeability of the intestinal epithelium. This allows for invasion of luminal microbes, which trigger increased inflammation and more homocysteine production, leading to an unregulated cycle of epithelial damage.

inflammatory lesions [101]. Studies with cultured colon carcinoma cells (Caco-2 and HT-29) are conflicting, however, with some showing that folate deficiency suppresses cell growth [102], whereas others found that added folate suppressed cell growth and proliferation based on measures of bromodeoxyuridine incorporation [103]; interestingly, the latter study found that physiological homocysteine concentrations stimulated cell proliferation and this was inhibited by addition of folate.

It is remarkable that the debate on folate and colorectal cancer has received considerably less attention as to how the key metabolites of methionine transmethylation, namely homocysteine and SAM, directly affect cell function since folate regulates these indirectly via remethylation pathways. There is an extant literature describing a strong direct link between intracellular SAM concentrations and alcohol-induced hepatocellular carcinoma [6, 104]; however, there have been very few investigations of the role of SAM in colorectal cancer. One recent investigation by Chen et al. examined the role of MAT2A and SAM in colonic cell lines as well as human and animal colon biopsies [53]. Their studies in HT-29 and RKO cell lines indicated that addition of exogenous SAM or MTA reduced the expression of MAT2A and prevented its induction by growth factors. Data in human biopsies showed that MAT2A was upregulated in cancerous regions when compared to regions of healthy colonocytes from the same patient. Further, the cancerous colonocytes also had upregulated SAM. These results were also duplicated in Min mice, an established mouse model of colorectal cancer. These data are slightly confusing when considered in the global context of SAM regulation. Although Chen et al. showed that SAM is increased in colorectal cancer, it is also well known that a reduction of SAM due to folate deficiency can lead to DNA hypomethylation, which may increase the risk of cancer as well. This is similar to the folate controversy described above. As recent commentary on folate and its use as a chemopreventative agent in colorectal cancer suggested, timing of folate administration may be a critical determinant of cancer susceptibility [105]; this may be also true for SAM supplementation. It is now established that SAM plays a role in proliferation during colorectal cancer. However, the role of cellular homocysteine should also be considered in colorectal cancer. Patients with IBD have not only increased plasma homocysteine levels [83, 106–109], but also an increased risk of developing colorectal cancer [110]. Whether cellular homocysteine levels play a direct role in the regulation of proliferation and apoptosis in colonocytes warrants further study.

4.7   CONCLUSIONS

It has become increasingly evident that the GIT is a metabolically significant site of sulfur amino acid metabolism in the body. The evidence for a functional methionine cycle and production of SAM and homocysteine raises the issue of how these molecules function in the GIT in health and disease states (Fig. 4.10). In regard to inflammatory bowel disease patients, the circulating homocysteine concentrations are increased and may be derived from increased synthesis within intestinal mucosal epithelial cells and mononuclear cells and may exacerbate the disease. Further study is warranted to establish whether the association between homocysteine and inflammatory bowel injury are causally linked or precipitated by poor nutritional status, mainly B vitamins. These intriguing findings along with literature linking folate status and colorectal carcinogenesis imply that metabolic regulation of the methionine cycle occurs in intestinal epithelial cells. Yet we still have a limited understanding of major factors that determine the production of homocysteine and SAM, and how these influence the proliferation, survival, and gene expression in epithelial cells. Epigenetic regulation of gene expression via modulation DNA methylation may be the critical role of SAM in intestinal cells. It is becoming well established that cysteine availability is a key metabolic determinant in the regulation of intestinal cell redox status. It remains to be seen whether augmentation of cysteine availability by nutritional means can be an effective strategy for treatment of diseases linked to oxidant injury in the GIT. Clearly, we are just beginning to fully understand sulfur amino acid metabolism within the GIT and its implications in health and disease states.

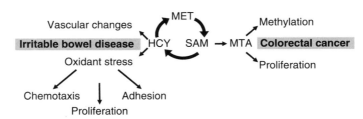

Figure 4.10   Effects of methionine metabolism on intestinal disease states. Methionine (MET) metabolism is intricately related with two of the major disease states in the gastrointestinal tract, inflammatory bowel disease and colorectal cancer. Intermediates such as S-adenosylmethionine (SAM) and homocysteine (HCY) exert substantial influence on the course of these diseases through downstream and related pathways. MTA, methylthioadenosine.

REFERENCES

1. Stipanuk, M.H. (2004). Sulfur amino acid metabolism: Pathways for production and removal of homocysteine and cysteine. *Annual Review of Nutrition, 24*, 539–577.

2. Selhub, J. (1999). Homocysteine metabolism. *Annual Review of Nutrition, 19*, 217–246.

3. Hogeveen, M., Blom, H.J., Van Amerongen, M., Boogmans, B., Van Beynum, I.M., Van De, B.M. (2002). Hyperhomocysteinemia as risk factor for ischemic and hemorrhagic stroke in newborn infants. *Journal of Pediatrics, 141*, 429–431.

4. Van Beynum, I.M., Smeitink, J.A., den Heijer, M., te Poele Pothoff, M.T., Blom, H.J. (1999). Hyperhomocysteinemia: A risk factor for ischemic stroke in children. *Circulation, 99*, 2070–2072.

5. Danese, S., Sgambato, A., Papa, A., Scaldaferri, F., Pola, R., Sans, M., Lovecchio, M., Gasbarrini, G., Cittadini, A., Gasbarrini, A. (2005). Homocysteine triggers mucosal microvascular activation in inflammatory bowel disease. *American Journal of Gastroenterology, 100*, 886–895.

6. Martinez-Chantar, M.L., Garcia-Trevijano, E.R., Latasa, M.U., Pérez-Mato, I., Sánchez del Pino, M.M., Corrales, F.J., Avila, M.A., Mato, J.M. (2002). Importance of a deficiency in S-adenosyl-L-methionine synthesis in the pathogenesis of liver injury. *American Journal of Clinical Nutrition, 76*, 1177S–1182S.

7. Stead, L.M., Brosnan, J.T., Brosnan, M.E., Vance, D.E., Jacobs, R.L. (2006). Is it time to reevaluate methyl balance in humans? *American Journal of Clinical Nutrition, 83*, 5–10.

8. Kim, Y.I. (2005). Nutritional epigenetics: Impact of folate deficiency on DNA methylation and colon cancer susceptibility. *Journal of Nutrition, 135*, 2703–2709.

9. Holmgren, A., Johansson, C., Berndt, C., Lonn, M.E., Hudemann, C., Lillig, C.H. (2005). Thiol redox control via thioredoxin and glutaredoxin systems. *Biochemical Society Transactions, 33*, 1375–1377.

10. Mudd, S.H., Finkelstein, J.D., Irreverre, F., Laster, L. (1965). Transsulfuration in mammals. Microassays and tissue distributions of three enzymes of the pathway. *Journal of Biological Chemistry, 240*, 4382–4392.

11. Aguilar, T.S., Benevenga, N.J., Harper, A.E. (1974). Effect of dietary methionine level on its metabolism in rats. *Journal of Nutrition, 104*, 761–771.

12. Stipanuk, M.H., Benevenga, N.J. (1977). Effect of cystine on the metabolism of methionine in rats. *Journal of Nutrition, 107*, 1455–1467.

13. Stipanuk, M.H. (1979). Effect of excess dietary methionine on the catabolism of cysteine in rats. *Journal of Nutrition, 109*, 2126–2139.

14. Stipanuk, M.H., Rotter, M.A. (1984). Metabolism of cysteine, cysteinesulfinate and cysteinesulfonate in rats fed adequate and excess levels of sulfur-containing amino acids. *Journal of Nutrition, 114*, 1426–1437.

15. Hiramatsu, T., Fukagawa, N.K., Marchini, J.S., Cortiella, J., Yu, Y.M., Chapman, T.E., Young, V.R. (1994). Methionine and cysteine kinetics at different intakes of cystine in healthy adult men. *American Journal of Clinical Nutrition, 60*, 525–533.

16. Fukagawa, N.K., Yu, Y.M., Young, V.R. (1998). Methionine and cysteine kinetics at different intakes of methionine and cysteine in elderly men and women. *American Journal of Clinical Nutrition, 68*, 380–388.

17. Raguso, C.A., Regan, M.M., Young, V.R. (2000). Cysteine kinetics and oxidation at different intakes of methionine and cystine in young adults. *American Journal of Clinical Nutrition, 71,* 491–499.

18. Lobley, G.E., Shen, X., Le, G., Bremner, D.M., Milne, E., Calder, A.G., Anderson, S.E., Dennison, N. (2003). Oxidation of essential amino acids by the ovine gastrointestinal tract. *British Journal of Nutrition, 89,* 617–630.

19. Mercier, S., Breuille, D., Mosoni, L., Obled, C., Patureau, M.P. (2002). Chronic inflammation alters protein metabolism in several organs of adult rats. *Journal of Nutrition, 132,* 1921–1928.

20. Storch, K.J., Wagner, D.A., Burke, J.F., Young, V.R. (1988). Quantitative study in vivo of methionine cycle in humans using [methyl-2H3]- and [1-13C]methionine. *American Journal of Physiology, 255,* E322–E331.

21. Storch, K.J., Wagner, D.A., Burke, J.F., Young, V.R. (1990). [1-13C; methyl-2H3]methionine kinetics in humans: Methionine conservation and cystine sparing. *American Journal of Physiology, 258,* E790–E798.

22. Storch, K.J., Wagner, D.A., Young, V.R. (1991). Methionine kinetics in adult men: Effects of dietary betaine on L-[2H3-methyl-1-13C]methionine. *American Journal of Clinical Nutrition, 54,* 386–394.

23. MacCoss, M.J., Fukagawa, N.K., Matthews, D.E. (2001). Measurement of intracellular sulfur amino acid metabolism in humans. *American Journal of Physiology. Endocrinology and Metabolism, 280,* E947–E955.

24. MacCoss, M.J., Fukagawa, N.K., Matthews, D.E. (1999). Measurement of homocysteine concentrations and stable isotope tracer enrichments in human plasma. *Analytical Chemistry, 71,* 4527–4533.

25. Tessari, P., Kiwanuka, E., Coracina, A., Zaramella, M., Vettore, M., Valerio, A., Garibotto, G. (2005). Insulin in methionine and homocysteine kinetics in healthy humans: Plasma vs. intracellular models. *American Journal of Physiology. Endocrinology and Metabolism, 288,* E1270–E1276.

26. Tessari, P., Coracina, A., Kiwanuka, E., Vedovato, M., Vettore, M., Valerio, A., Zaramella, M., Garibotto, G. (2005). Effects of insulin on methionine and homocysteine kinetics in type 2 diabetes with nephropathy. *Diabetes, 54,* 2968–2976.

27. Townsend, J.H., Davis, S.R., Mackey, A.D., Gregory, J.F., III. (2004). Folate deprivation reduces homocysteine remethylation in a human intestinal epithelial cell culture model: Role of serine in one-carbon donation. *American Journal of Physiology. Gastrointestinal and Liver Physiology, 286,* G588–G595.

28. Davis, S.R., Stacpoole, P.W., Williamson, J., Kick, L.S., Quinlivan, E.P., Coats, B.S., Shane, B., Bailey, L.B., Gregory, J.F., III. (2004). Tracer-derived total and folate-dependent homocysteine remethylation and synthesis rates in humans indicate that serine is the main one-carbon donor. *American Journal of Physiology. Endocrinology and Metabolism, 286,* E272–E279.

29. Lobley, G.E., Connell, A., Revell, D. (1996). The importance of transmethylation reactions to methionine metabolism in sheep: Effects of supplementation with creatine and choline. *British Journal of Nutrition, 75,* 47–56.

30. Stegink, L.D., Den Besten, L. (1972). Synthesis of cysteine from methionine in normal adult subjects: Effect of route of alimentation. *Science, 178,* 514–516.

31. Zlotkin, S.H., Bryan, M.H., Anderson, G.H. (1981). Cysteine supplementation to cysteine-free intravenous feeding regimens in newborn infants. *American Journal of Clinical Nutrition*, *34*, 914–923.

32. Shoveller, A.K., House, J.D., Brunton, J.A., Pencharz, P.B., Ball, R.O. (2004). The balance of dietary sulfur amino acids and the route of feeding affect plasma homocysteine concentrations in neonatal piglets. *Journal of Nutrition*, *134*, 609–612.

33. Shoveller, A.K., Brunton, J.A., Pencharz, P.B., Ball, R.O. (2003). The methionine requirement is lower in neonatal piglets fed parenterally than in those fed enterally. *Journal of Nutrition*, *133*, 1390–1397.

34. Raguso, C.A., Ajami, A.M., Gleason, R., Young, V.R. (1997). Effect of cystine intake on methionine kinetics and oxidation determined with oral tracers of methionine and cysteine in healthy adults. *American Journal of Clinical Nutrition*, *66*, 283–292.

35. Stoll, B., Henry, J., Reeds, P.J., Yu, H., Jahoor, F., Burrin, D.G. (1998). Catabolism dominates the first-pass intestinal metabolism of dietary essential amino acids in milk protein-fed piglets. *Journal of Nutrition*, *128*, 606–614.

36. Shoveller, A.K., Brunton, J.A., House, J.D., Pencharz, P.B., Ball, R.O. (2003). Dietary cysteine reduces the methionine requirement by an equal proportion in both parenterally and enterally fed piglets. *Journal of Nutrition*, *133*, 4215–4224.

37. Riedijk, M.A., Stoll, B., Chacko, S., Schierbeek, H., Sunehag, A.L., van Goudoever, J.B., Burrin, D.G. (2007). Methionine transmethylation and transsulfuration in the piglet gastrointestinal tract. *Proceedings of the National Academy of Sciences USA*, *104*, 3408–3413.

38. Lobley, G.E., Wester, T.J., Calder, A.G., Parker, D.S., Dibner, J.J., Vazquez-Anon, M. (2006). Absorption of 2-hydroxy-4-methylthiobutyrate and conversion to methionine in lambs. *Journal of Dairy Science*, *89*, 1072–1080.

39. Lobley, G.E., Wester, T.J., Holtrop, G., Dibner, J.J., Parker, D.S., Vazquez-Anon, M. (2006). Absorption and digestive tract metabolism of 2-hydroxy-4-methylthiobutanoic acid in lambs. *Journal of Dairy Science*, *89*, 3508–3521.

40. Mitchell, A.D., Benevenga, N.J. (1978). The role of transamination in methionine oxidation in the rat. *Journal of Nutrition*, *108*, 67–78.

41. Dilger, R.N., Kobler, C., Weckbecker, C., Hoehler, D., Baker, D.H. (2007). 2-keto-4-(methylthio)butyric acid (keto analog of methionine) is a safe and efficacious precursor of L-methionine in chicks. *Journal of Nutrition*, *137*, 1868–1873.

42. Tangerman, A., Wilcken, B., Levy, H.L., Boers, G.H., Mudd, S.H. (2000). Methionine transamination in patients with homocystinuria due to cystathionine beta-synthase deficiency. *Metabolism*, *49*, 1071–1077.

43. Bos, C., Stoll, B., Fouillet, H., Guan, X., Grusak, M.A., Reeds, P.J., Tome, D., Burrin, D.G. (2003). Intestinal lysine metabolism is driven by the enteral availability of dietary lysine in piglets fed a bolus meal. *American Journal of Physiology. Endocrinology and Metabolism*, *285*, E1246–E1257.

44. Malmezat, T., Breuille, D., Capitan, P., Mirand, P.P., Obled, C. (2000). Glutathione turnover is increased during the acute phase of sepsis in rats. *Journal of Nutrition*, *130*, 1239–1246.

45. Morgenstern, I., Raijmakers, M.T., Peters, W.H., Hoensch, H., Kirch, W. (2003). Homocysteine, cysteine, and glutathione in human colonic mucosa: Elevated levels of

homocysteine in patients with inflammatory bowel disease. *Digestive Diseases and Sciences*, *48*, 2083–2090.

46. Gregory, J.F. III, Quinlivan, E.P. (2002). In vivo kinetics of folate metabolism. *Annual Review of Nutrition*, *22*, 199–220.

47. Keating, J.N., Weir, D.G., Scott, J.M. (1985). Demonstration of methionine synthetase in intestinal mucosal cells of the rat. *Clinical Sciences (London)*, *69*, 287–292.

48. Ortiou, S., Alberto, J.M., Gueant, J.L., Merten, M. (2004). Homocysteine increases methionine synthase mRNA level in Caco-2 cells. *Cellular Physiology and Biochemistry*, *14*, 407–414.

49. Chen, J., Giovannucci, E., Kelsey, K., Rimm, E.B., Stampfer, M.J., Colditz, G.A., Spiegelman, D., Willett, W.C., Hunter, D.J. (1996). A methylenetetrahydrofolate reductase polymorphism and the risk of colorectal cancer. *Cancer Research*, *56*, 4862–4864.

50. Ma, J., Stampfer, M.J., Christensen, B., Giovannucci, E., Hunter, D.J., Chen, J., Willett, W.C., Selhub, J., Hennekens, C.H., Gravel, R., Rozen, R. (1999). A polymorphism of the methionine synthase gene: Association with plasma folate, vitamin B12, homocyst(e)ine, and colorectal cancer risk. *Cancer Epidemiology, Biomarkers & Prevention*, *8*, 825–829.

51. Lamprecht, S.A., Lipkin, M. (2003). Chemoprevention of colon cancer by calcium, vitamin D and folate: Molecular mechanisms. *Nature Reviews. Cancer*, *3*, 601–614.

52. Duthie, S.J., Narayanan, S., Brand, G.M., Grant, G. (2000). DNA stability and genomic methylation status in colonocytes isolated from methyl-donor-deficient rats. *European Journal of Nutrition*, *39*, 106–111.

53. Chen, H., Xia, M., Lin, M., Yang, H., Kuhlenkamp, J., Li, T., Sodir, N.M., Chen, Y.H., Josef-Lenz, H., Laird, P.W., Clarke, S., Mato, J.M., Lu, S.C. (2007). Role of methionine adenosyltransferase 2A and S-adenosylmethionine in mitogen-induced growth of human colon cancer cells. *Gastroenterology*, *133*, 207–218.

54. Brosnan, J.T., da Silva, R., Brosnan, M.E. (2007). Amino acids and the regulation of methyl balance in humans. *Current Opinion in Clinical Nutrition and Metabolic Care*, *10*, 52–57.

55. Mato, J.M., Alvarez, L., Ortiz, P., Pajares, M.A. (1997). S-adenosylmethionine synthesis: Molecular mechanisms and clinical implications. *Pharmacology & Therapeutics*, *73*, 265–280.

56. Noga, A.A., Stead, L.M., Zhao, Y., Brosnan, M.E., Brosnan, J.T., Vance, D.E. (2003). Plasma homocysteine is regulated by phospholipid methylation. *Journal of Biological Chemistry*, *278*, 5952–5955.

57. Avila, M.A., Garcia-Trevijano, E.R., Lu, S.C., Corrales, F.J., Mato, J.M. (2004). Methylthioadenosine. *International Journal of Biochemistry and Cell Biology*, *36*, 2125–2130.

58. Yerlikaya, A. (2004). Polyamines and S-adenosylmethionine decarboxylase. *Turkish Journal of Biochemistry*, *29*, 208–214.

59. Milovic, V. (2001). Polyamines in the gut lumen: Bioavailability and biodistribution. *European Journal of Gastroenterology and Hepatology*, *13*, 1021–1025.

60. Liu, L., Li, L., Rao, J.N., Zou, T., Zhang, H.M., Boneva, D., Bernard, M.S., Wang, J.Y. (2005). Polyamine-modulated expression of c-myc plays a critical role in stimulation of normal intestinal epithelial cell proliferation. *American Journal of Physiology. Cell Physiology*, *288*, C89–C99.

61. Li, L., Rao, J.N., Guo, X., Liu, L., Santora, R., Bass, B.L., Wang, J.Y. (2001). Polyamine depletion stabilizes p53 resulting in inhibition of normal intestinal epithelial cell proliferation. *American Journal of Physiology. Cell Physiology, 281*, C941–C953.

62. Chen, J., Rao, J.N., Zou, T., Liu, L., Marasa, B.S., Xiao, L., Zeng, X., Turner, D.J., Wang, J.Y. (2007). Polyamines are required for expression of Toll-like receptor 2 modulating intestinal epithelial barrier integrity. *American Journal of Physiology. Gastrointestinal and Liver Physiology, 293*, G568–G576.

63. Grillo, M.A., Colombatto, S. (2008). S-adenosylmethionine and its products. *Amino Acids, 34*(2), 187–193.

64. Berasain, C., Hevia, H., Fernandez-Irigoyen, J., Larrea, E., Caballeria, J., Mato, J.M., Prieto, J., Corrales, F.J., Garcia-Trevijano, E.R., Avila, M.A. (2004). Methylthioadenosine phosphorylase gene expression is impaired in human liver cirrhosis and hepatocarcinoma. *Biochimica and Biophysica Acta, 3*, 276–284.

65. Deplancke, B., Gaskins, H.R. (2002). Redox control of the transsulfuration and glutathione biosynthesis pathways. *Current Opinion in Clinical Nutrition and Metabolic Care, 5*, 85–92.

66. Jones, D.P. (2006). Extracellular redox state: Refining the definition of oxidative stress in aging. *Rejuvenation Research, 9*, 169–181.

67. Winyard, P.G., Moody, C.J., Jacob, C. (2005). Oxidative activation of antioxidant defence. *Trends in Biochemical Sciences, 30*, 453–461.

68. Matsukawa, J., Matsuzawa, A., Takeda, K., Ichijo, H. (2004). The ASK1-MAP kinase cascades in mammalian stress response. *Journal of Biochemistry (Tokyo), 136*, 261–265.

69. Conour, J.E., Graham, W.V., Gaskins, H.R. (2004). A combined in vitro/bioinformatic investigation of redox regulatory mechanisms governing cell cycle progression. *Physiological Genomics, 18*, 196–205.

70. Moriarty-Craige, S.E., Jones, D.P. (2004). Extracellular thiols and thiol/disulfide redox in metabolism. *Annual Review of Nutrition, 24*, 481–509.

71. Nkabyo, Y.S., Gu, L.H., Jones, D.P., Ziegler, T.R. (2002). Glutathione and thioredoxin redox during differentiation in human colon epithelial (Caco-2) cells. *American Journal of Physiology. Gastrointestinal and Liver Physiology, 6*, G1352–G1359.

72. Pias, E.K., Aw, T.Y. (2002). Apoptosis in mitotic competent undifferentiated cells is induced by cellular redox imbalance independent of reactive oxygen species production. *FASEB Journal, 16*, 781–790.

73. Noda, T., Iwakiri, R., Fujimoto, K., Aw, T.Y. (2001). Induction of mild intracellular redox imbalance inhibits proliferation of CaCo-2 cells. *FASEB Journal, 15*, 2131–2139.

74. Jonas, C.R., Ziegler, T.R., Gu, L.H., Jones, D.P. (2002). Extracellular thiol/disulfide redox state affects proliferation rate in a human colon carcinoma (Caco2) cell line. *Free Radical Biology and Medicine, 33*, 1499–1506.

75. Miller, L.T., Watson, W.H., Kirlin, W.G., Ziegler, T.R., Jones, D.P. (2002). Oxidation of the glutathione/glutathione disulfide redox state is induced by cysteine deficiency in human colon carcinoma HT29 cells. *Journal of Nutrition, 132*, 2303–2306.

76. Noda, T., Iwakiri, R., Fujimoto, K., Rhoads, C.A., Aw, T.Y. (2002). Exogenous cysteine and cystine promote cell proliferation in CaCo-2 cells. *Cell Proliferation, 35*, 117–129.

77. Nkabyo, Y.S., Go, Y.M., Ziegler, T.R., Jones, D.P. (2005). Extracellular cysteine/cystine redox regulates the p44/p42 MAPK pathway by metalloproteinase-dependent epidermal

growth factor receptor signaling. *American Journal of Physiology. Gastrointestinal and Liver Physiology, 289,* G70–G78.

78. Nkabyo, Y.S., Gu, L.H., Jones, D.P., Ziegler, T.R. (2006). Thiol/disulfide redox status is oxidized in plasma and small intestinal and colonic mucosa of rats with inadequate sulfur amino acid intake. *Journal of Nutrition, 5,* 1242–1248.

79. Cordain, L., Eaton, S.B., Sebastian, A. Mann, N., Lindeberg, S., Watkins, B.A., O'Keefe, J.H., Brand-Miller, J. (2005). Origins and evolution of the Western diet: Health implications for the 21st century. *American Journal of Clinical Nutrition, 81,* 341–354.

80. Pierik, M., Rutgeerts, P., Vlietinck, R., Vermeire, S. (2006). Pharmacogenetics in inflammatory bowel disease. *World Journal of Gastroenterology, 12,* 3657–3667.

81. van Ede, A.E., Laan, R.F., Blom, H.J., Boers, G.H., Haagsma, C.J., Thomas, C.M., De Boo, T.M., van de Putte, L.B. (2002). Homocysteine and folate status in methotrexate-treated patients with rheumatoid arthritis. *Rheumatology (Oxford), 41,* 658–665.

82. Zou, C.G., Banerjee, R. (2005). Homocysteine and redox signaling. *Antioxidants and Redox Signaling, 7,* 547–559.

83. Romagnuolo, J., Fedorak, R.N., Dias, V.C., Bamforth, F., Teltscher, M. (2001). Hyperhomocysteinemia and inflammatory bowel disease: Prevalence and predictors in a cross-sectional study. *American Journal of Gastroenterology, 96,* 2143–2149.

84. Saibeni, S., Cattaneo, M., Vecchi, M., Zighetti, M.L., Lecchi, A., Lombardi, R., Meucci, G., Spina, L., de Franchis, R. (2003). Low vitamin B(6) plasma levels, a risk factor for thrombosis, in inflammatory bowel disease: Role of inflammation and correlation with acute phase reactants. *American Journal of Gastroenterology, 98,* 112–117.

85. Mahmood, A., Needham, J., Prosser, J., Mainwaring, J., Trebble, T., Mahy, G., Ramage, J. (2005). Prevalence of hyperhomocysteinaemia, activated protein C resistance and prothrombin gene mutation in inflammatory bowel disease. *European Journal of Gastroenterology and Hepatology, 17,* 739–744.

86. Goh, J., O'Morain, C.A. (2003). Review article: nutrition and adult inflammatory bowel disease. *Alimentary Pharmacology & Therapeutics, 17,* 307–320.

87. Papa, A., Danese, S., Urgesi, R., Grillo, A., Guglielmo, S., Roberto, I., Bonizzi, M., Guidi, L.I., Santoliquido, A., Fedeli, G., Gasbarrini, G., Gasbarrini, A. (2006). Early atherosclerosis in patients with inflammatory bowel disease. *European Reviews for Medical and Pharmacological Sciences, 10,* 7–11.

88. Danese, S., Papa, A., Saibeni, S., Repici, A., Malesci, A., Vecchi, M. (2007). Inflammation and coagulation in inflammatory bowel disease: The clot thickens. *American Journal of Gastroenterology, 102,* 174–186.

89. Miehsler, W., Reinisch, W., Valic, E., Osterode, W., Tillinger, W., Feichtenschlager, T., Grisar, J., Machold, K., Scholz, S., Vogelsang, H., Novacek, G. (2004). Is inflammatory bowel disease an independent and disease specific risk factor for thromboembolism? *Gut, 53,* 542–548.

90. Riba, R., Nicolaou, A., Troxler, M., Homer-Vaniasinkam, S., Naseem, K.M. (2004). Altered platelet reactivity in peripheral vascular disease complicated with elevated plasma homocysteine levels. *Atherosclerosis, 175,* 69–75.

91. Jurjus, A.R., Khoury, N.N., Reimund, J.M. (2004). Animal models of inflammatory bowel disease. *Journal of Pharmacological and Toxicological Methods, 50,* 81–92.

92. Mori, M., Stokes, K.Y., Vowinkel, T., Watanabe, N., Elrod, J.W., Harris, N.R., Lefer, D.J., Hibi, T., Granger, D.N. (2005). Colonic blood flow responses in experimental colitis:

Time course and underlying mechanisms. *American Journal of Physiology. Gastro-intestinal and Liver Physiology, 289*, G1024–G1029.

93. Mori, M., Salter, J.W., Vowinkel, T., Krieglstein, C.F., Stokes, K.Y., Granger, D.N. (2005). Molecular determinants of the prothrombogenic phenotype assumed by inflamed colonic venules. *American Journal of Physiology. Gastrointestinal and Liver Physiology, 288*, G920–G926.

94. Harris, N.R., Whatley, J.R., Carter, P.R., Specian, R.D. (2005). Venular constriction of submucosal arterioles induced by dextran sodium sulfate. *Inflammatory Bowel Diseases, 11*, 806–813.

95. Hatoum, O.A., Binion, D.G., Gutterman, D.D. (2005). Paradox of simultaneous intestinal ischaemia and hyperaemia in inflammatory bowel disease. *European Journal of Clinical Investigation, 35*, 599–609.

96. Yi, F., dos Santos, E.A., Xia, M., Chen, Q.Z., Li, P.L., Li, N. (2007). Podocyte injury and glomerulosclerosis in hyperhomocysteinemic rats. *American Journal of Nephrology, 27*, 262–268.

97. Wang, G., Siow, Y.L., O, K. (2001). Homocysteine induces monocyte chemoattractant protein-1 expression by activating NF-κB in THP-1 macrophages. *American Journal of Physiology. Heart and Circulatory Physiology, 280*, H2840–H2847.

98. Kim, D.J., Koh, J.M., Lee, O., Kim, N.J., Lee, Y.S., Kim, Y.S., Park, J.Y., Lee, K.U., Kim, G.S. (2006). Homocysteine enhances apoptosis in human bone marrow stromal cells. *Bone, 39*, 582–590.

99. Perez-de-Arce, K., Foncea, R., Leighton, F. (2005). Reactive oxygen species mediates homocysteine-induced mitochondrial biogenesis in human endothelial cells: Modulation by antioxidants. *Biochemical and Biophysical Research Communications, 338*, 1103–1109.

100. Jang, H., Mason, J.B., Choi, S.W. (2005). Genetic and epigenetic interactions between folate and aging in carcinogenesis. *Journal of Nutrition, 135*, 2967S–2971S.

101. Ma, D.W., Finnell, R.H., Davidson, L.A., Callaway, E.S., Spiegelstein, O., Piedrahita, J.A., Salbaum, J.M., Kappen, C., Weeks, B.R., James, J., Bozinov, D., Lupton, J.R., Chapkin, R.S. (2005). Folate transport gene inactivation in mice increases sensitivity to colon carcinogenesis. *Cancer Research, 65*, 887–897.

102. Novakovic, P., Stempak, J.M., Sohn, K.J., Kim, Y.I. (2006). Effects of folate deficiency on gene expression in the apoptosis and cancer pathways in colon cancer cells. *Carcinogenesis, 27*, 916–924.

103. Akoglu, B., Milovic, V., Caspary, W.F., Faust, D. (2004). Hyperproliferation of homocysteine-treated colon cancer cells is reversed by folate and 5-methyltetrahydrofolate. *European Journal of Nutrition, 43*, 93–99.

104. Lu, S.C., Martinez-Chantar, M.L., Mato, J.M. (2006). Methionine adenosyltransferase and S-adenosylmethionine in alcoholic liver disease. *Journal of Gastroenterology and Hepatology, 21*(Suppl 3), S61–S64.

105. Ulrich, C.M., Potter, J.D. (2007). Folate and cancer: Timing is everything. *Journal of the American Medical Association, 297*, 2408–2409.

106. Koutroubakis, I.E., Dilaveraki, E., Vlachonikolis, I.G., Vardas, E., Vrentzos, G., Ganotakis, E., Mouzas, I.A., Gravanis, A., Emmanouel, D., Kouroumalis, E.A. (2000). Hyperhomocysteinemia in Greek patients with inflammatory bowel disease. *Digestive Diseases and Sciences, 45*, 2347–2351.

107. Cattaneo, M., Vecchi, M., Zighetti, M.L., Saibeni, S., Martinelli, I., Omodei, P., Mannucci, P.M., de Franchis, R. (1998). High prevalence of hyperhomocysteinemia in patients with inflammatory bowel disease: A pathogenic link with thromboembolic complications? *Thrombosis and Haemostasis, 80*, 542–545.

108. Nakano, E., Taylor, C.J., Chada, L., McGaw, J., Powers, H.J. (2003). Hyperhomocystinemia in children with inflammatory bowel disease. *Journal of Pediatric Gastroenterology and Nutrition, 37*, 586–590.

109. Chowers, Y., Sela, B.A., Holland, R., Fidder, H., Simoni, F.B., Bar-Meir, S. (2000). Increased levels of homocysteine in patients with Crohn's disease are related to folate levels. *American Journal of Gastroenterology, 95*, 3498–3502.

110. Munkholm, P., Loftus, E.V., Jr., Reinacher-Schick, A., Kornbluth, A., Mittmann, U., Esendal, B. (2006). Prevention of colorectal cancer in inflammatory bowel disease: Value of screening and 5-aminosalicylates. *Digestion, 73*, 11–19.

CHAPTER 5

HEPATIC SULFUR AMINO ACID METABOLISM

KEVIN L. SCHALINSKE

5.1 INTRODUCTION

The liver plays a key role in the metabolism of the sulfur amino acids methionine and cysteine. Hepatic methionine and cysteine are important essential amino acids for protein synthesis. However, cysteine is a conditionally essential amino acid, as it can be synthesized from methionine via hepatic pathways that are also important in other metabolic processes and biosynthetic reactions. The role of the liver with respect to sulfur amino acid metabolism is unique in that the complete scope of reactions relevant to their metabolism is liver-specific. A number of recent studies have shown that other nutritional and physiologic factors may have an impact on hepatic sulfur amino acid metabolism. A basic understanding of sulfur amino acid metabolism and identifying modulating factors is critically important, as perturbation of sulfur amino acid metabolism along with related metabolic pathways has been shown to be linked to numerous pathological conditions.

5.2 DIETARY RELATION BETWEEN METHIONINE AND CYSTEINE

Both dietary methionine and cysteine are essential amino acids critical for protein synthesis, as well as other biological processes such as the synthesis of glutathione (Fig. 5.1). One of the most important uses for methionine, particularly in the liver, is that it provides the methyl groups necessary for a large number of transmethylation reactions. Cysteine is considered a conditionally essential amino acid as methionine can be metabolized by the liver to generate cysteine when dietary sources are inadequate, provided there is sufficient methionine. Methionine catabolism to generate cysteine begins with its activation to S-adenosylmethionine (SAM), followed by

Glutathione and Sulfur Amino Acids in Human Health and Disease. Edited by R. Masella and G. Mazza
Copyright © 2009 John Wiley & Sons, Inc.

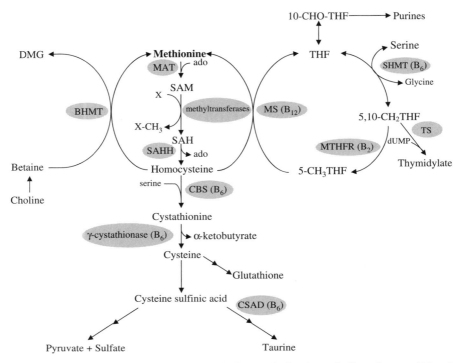

Figure 5.1   Hepatic sulfur amino acid metabolism and related metabolic pathways. Abbreviations: ado, adenosine; BHMT, betaine-homocysteine S-methyltransferase; CBS, cystathionine β-synthase; CSAD, cysteine sulfinic acid decarboxylase; DMG, dimethylglycine; MAT, methionine adenosyltransferase; MS, methionine synthase; MTHFR, 5,10-methylene-THF reductase; SAH, S-adenosylhomocysteine; SAHH, S-adenosylhomocysteine hydrolase; SAM, S-adenosylmethionine; SHMT, serine hydroxymethyltransferase; THF, tetrahydrofolate; TS, thymidylate synthase.

transmethylation and the eventual formation of homocysteine. Homocysteine exists at a metabolic branch point in that it can be remethylated back to methionine, or be irreversibly catabolized via the transsulfuration pathway to generate cystathionine and subsequently cysteine. Mudd and Poole [1] demonstrated that approximately half of the homocysteine is metabolized by transsulfuration to cystathionine and the other half is remethylated back to methionine.

The methionine-sparing effect of dietary cyste(i)ne has been known for nearly 70 years [2] and has been examined further in a number of studies by Finkelstein and coworkers [3, 4]. These studies helped define the metabolic relation between methionine and cysteine, in that dietary cysteine serves not to replace methionine, but rather conserve methionine by promoting the homocysteine-methionine cycle (i.e., remethylation) and spare it from being used for cysteine synthesis via the irreversible transsulfuration of homocysteine. A more detailed discussion of the pathways related to methionine and cysteine metabolism, and their regulation, is presented later in this chapter.

5.3 METABOLIC RELATION BETWEEN HEPATIC SULFUR AMINO ACIDS, B VITAMINS, AND METHYL GROUP METABOLISM

Sulfur amino acid metabolism is critically important in the liver as it is intimately related to a number of important biosynthetic and regulatory processes, including biological methylation and epigenetic control of gene expression. Moreover, these processes are dependent on a variety of other essential nutrients, including folate, choline, B12, B6, and riboflavin (Fig. 5.1). The relation between all of these nutrients is critical as perturbation of these metabolic processes is associated with a number of pathological conditions, including cardiovascular disease, cancer development, birth defects, and neurological disorders [5–8].

5.3.1 Folate-Dependent One-Carbon Metabolism

Methionine is the primary donor of methyl groups, in the form of SAM, for biological methylation reactions. Approximately half of the body folate pool is hepatic and the folate-dependent one-carbon pool is a significant source of methionine methyl groups, as well as being intimately linked to homocysteine metabolism and methyl group regulation [9]. Serine is the major source of one-carbon groups through the action of the B6-dependent enzyme serine hydroxymethyltransferase (SHMT), which generates the folate coenzyme 5,10-methylene-tetrahydrofolate (5,10-CH_2-THF) and the amino acid glycine. The methylene group of 5,10-CH_2-THF has a number of metabolic fates. The methylene carbon can be oxidized to other folate coenzymes, or it can be directly used for the synthesis of thymidylate, a reaction catalyzed by thymidylate synthase, the rate limiting step in the synthesis of DNA. Alternatively and more relevant to sulfur amino acid metabolism, 5,10-CH_2-THF can be reduced to 5-CH_3-THF by the enzyme 5,10-methylene-THF reductase (MTHFR), a FAD-dependent reaction that is irreversible under physiological conditions. The methyl group from 5-CH_3-THF ultimately can be used for the remethylation of homocysteine, derived from all SAM-dependent transmethylation reactions, to regenerate methionine. Folate-dependent remethylation of homocysteine is catalyzed by the B12-dependent enzyme methionine synthase. Thus, hepatic folate-dependent remethylation serves as a means to conserve and recycle the homocysteine moiety of methionine and concomitantly provide methyl groups for critical SAM-dependent transmethylation reactions.

5.3.2 SAM-Dependent Transmethylation

Methionine, from the diet or by folate-dependent homocysteine remethylation, is essential for other biosynthetic reactions and regulatory processes via SAM-dependent transmethylation, a large variety of reactions that are heavily dependent on the liver. The initial step in methionine utilization is activation to SAM in an ATP-dependent reaction catalyzed by methionine adenosyltransferase (MAT) [10–13]. The enzyme MAT exists in a number of hepatic and extrahepatic isoforms that display unique enzyme kinetics. For liver, the tetramer MAT I and dimer MAT

III, derived from the *MAT1A* gene, exhibit a higher K_m than MAT II, the isoform present in extrahepatic tissues that is derived from the *MAT2A* gene. Thus, the liver possesses a tremendous capacity to convert methionine to SAM even under conditions of high methionine concentrations. SAM is the universal methyl donor in a number of transmethylation reactions, including the methylation of small molecules, proteins, lipids, and nucleic acids. The role and regulation of SAM-dependent transmethylation reactions will be discussed in more detail later in this chapter, particularly with respect to reactions that are predominantly liver-specific.

5.3.3   Homocysteine Remethylation and Transsulfuration

Following all SAM-dependent transmethylation reactions, S-adenosylhomocysteine (SAH) is generated, which is a potent inhibitor of most methyltransferases [14]. Because SAM is a positive modulator of methyltransferase activity, the intracellular ratio of SAM to SAH is considered an index of transmethylation potential [15, 16]. SAH is hydrolyzed to adenosine and homocysteine by the action of SAH hydrolase (SAHH). Homocysteine has a number of metabolic fates in the liver. As mentioned, homocysteine can be remethylated back to methionine using a methyl group from 5-CH_3-THF. Conversely, hepatic homocysteine remethylation can also occur by the folate-independent use of betaine, derived from the oxidation of choline, as a methyl donor. This reaction is catalyzed by betaine-homocysteine S-methyltransferase (BHMT), an enzyme that exists predominantly in the liver, and for some species, in the kidney [17, 18]. It has been estimated that folate-dependent and folate-independent mechanisms contribute equally to remethylation of homocysteine in the liver [19]. For both remethylation reactions, hepatic conversion of homocysteine to methionine provides a means to supply methyl groups for SAM-dependent transmethylation reactions, as well as prevent homocysteine pools from accumulating. This latter aspect of homocysteine metabolism is critical, because the accumulation of hepatic homocysteine and its subsequent link to elevated circulating concentrations of homocysteine (i.e., hyperhomocysteinemia) has been shown to be an independent risk factor for cardiovascular disease [5, 20], as well as being associated with other pathologies [6–8]. In contrast to remethylation, homocysteine can be irreversibly catabolized by the transsulfuration pathway present in the liver. This involves a number of B6-dependent steps, including the initial condensation of homocysteine with serine to form cystathionine, followed by the subsequent generation of cysteine. These two reactions are catalyzed by the enzymes cystathionine β-synthase (CBS) and γ-cystathionase, respectively. The transsulfuration pathway largely exists in the liver, but can also be found in the kidney, pancreas, and intestine [21].

5.3.4   Cysteine Metabolism

Besides protein synthesis, a major use of cysteine is for the generation of the tripeptide glutathione, an important compound for oxidative defense. This hepatic biosynthetic reaction involves the initial synthesis of glutamylcysteine, catalyzed by the enzyme γ-glutamylcysteine synthetase and utilization of ATP, followed by a second

ATP-dependent reaction that catalyzes the addition of glycine via the action of glutathione synthetase to form glutathione. Although most cells can synthesize glutathione, the liver represents a major site for its production. Besides glutathione synthesis, cysteine can be catabolized to cysteine sulfinic acid and subsequently used in the generation of taurine. Cysteine sulfinic acid decarboxylase (CSAD) is a key initial enzyme in this process that requires vitamin B6 as a cofactor. Taurine is a β-amino sulfonic acid that functions in the liver as an essential conjugate for the synthesis of bile salts, and can be circulated to other tissues, where it has a number of proposed functions, including osmoregulation, as an antioxidant, and as a neurotransmitter [22]. Conversely, cysteine can be converted to pyruvate and inorganic sulfate as a means to meet energy needs by gluconeogenesis and remove sulfur from the body via the urine, respectively. Alternative to transsulfuration, the actions of CBS and γ-cystathionase can be used to generate reduced sulfur, in the form of hydrogen sulfide (H_2S), from cysteine [23, 24]. The production of H_2S from cysteine has received considerable attention recently as new physiologic roles for H_2S have emerged, including the regulation of muscle function and pancreatic beta-cell maintenance [25].

5.3.5 Sulfur Amino Acids as an Energy Source

Related to the methionine to cysteine conversion, both sulfur amino acids can be catabolized to specific keto acids as a means to meet energy needs, as mentioned above. Following the generation of cystathionine from the condensation of homocysteine and serine, the next reaction by γ-cystathionase results in the formation of cysteine and -ketobutyrate, wherein three carbons originating from the five-carbon methionine skeleton are contained within the latter four-carbon compound. α-Ketobutyrate can then be decarboxylated to form propionyl-CoA, which subsequently enters the TCA cycle as succinyl-CoA following its conversion to methylmalonyl-CoA. The other product of the γ-cystathionase reaction, cysteine, can be directly catabolized to pyruvate and thus serve as a substrate for gluconeogenesis in the liver.

5.4 REGULATION OF SULFUR AMINO ACID METABOLISM AND RELATED METABOLIC PATHWAYS IN THE LIVER

The proper metabolic partitioning of methionine and cysteine is critical to meet protein synthesis requirements, provide methyl groups for important transmethylation reactions, and to maintain homocysteine homeostasis. Besides resulting in an inability to synthesize essential biological compounds, disruption of either methyl group and/or homocysteine is associated with numerous pathological conditions, including cardiovascular disease, cancer development, birth defects, and neurological disorders [5–8]. Thus, regulation of sulfur amino acid metabolism and the related balance of methyl groups and homocysteine are critical for optimizing health and preventing disease. The following discussion will focus on proteins that function as liver-specific users of SAM, as well as regulators of methyl group and homocysteine balance.

5.4.1 Liver-Specific Proteins Involved in the Regulation of Sulfur Amino Acid Metabolism and Related Biosynthetic Processes

Methionine serves as a major source of methyl groups for SAM-dependent transmethylation reactions, a process that is highly predominant in the liver. In addition to catalyzing important biosynthetic reactions, a number of key proteins, all methyltransferases, are also instrumental in controlling methyl group and homocysteine metabolism. Moreover, these proteins and their respective functions are tissue specific, with the liver being the primary site for their expression.

5.4.1.1 Guanidinoacetate N-Methyltransferase (GAMT) GAMT is a liver-specific enzyme that catalyzes the final step in the synthesis of creatine, an important molecule in meeting energy needs as a component of creatine phosphate in muscle. Creatine phosphate is utilized during initial anaerobic energy bursts by serving as a source of phosphate for the generation of ATP from ADP. The initial step in creatine synthesis occurs in the kidney, where arginine-glycine amidinotransferase converts arginine and glycine to ornithine and guanidinoacetate. In turn, guanidinoacetate circulates to the liver to generate creatine by SAM-dependent transmethylation, requiring ATP and the action of GAMT. Until recently, the utilization of SAM-derived methyl groups by GAMT has been considered the largest biosynthetic requirement for methyl groups from SAM, representing nearly 75% of SAM-methyl group usage [1, 26]. Because GAMT represents such a significant source of SAM-methyl group utilization, it concomitantly presents itself as a major contributor to hepatic homocysteine pools. Thus, the demand for creatine synthesis is intimately linked to methionine and cysteine metabolism. This relation is readily apparent by the observation that dietary provision of guanidinoacetate, the substrate for SAM-dependent creatine synthesis, increased homocysteine production, whereas dietary creatine diminished homocysteine concentrations [27].

5.4.1.2 Glycine N-Methyltransferase (GNMT) Although GNMT has an enzymatic function, that being conversion of glycine to sarcosine (i.e., N-methylglycine) using a methyl group from SAM, its primary role has been proposed to be a regulator of methyl group metabolism [9]. The basis for this is supported by several lines of evidence: (1) sarcosine synthesis appears to be a nonsignificant reaction as it has no known physiological function; (2) GNMT is extremely abundant in the cell, representing nearly 1% to 3% of the total cytosolic protein; (3) GNMT is not product-inhibited by SAH to nearly the same extent as other SAM-dependent methyltransferases; and (4) the binding of GNMT by 5-CH_3-THF inhibits its activity. Thus, GNMT is considered a key regulatory protein that controls both the supply of methyl groups from the folate-dependent one-carbon pool and utilization of methyl groups for transmethylation reactions by optimizing the intracellular ratio of SAM to SAH [28, 29]. Phosphorylation of GNMT appears to be another component to posttranslationally regulate its activity and the binding affinity of 5-CH_3-THF [28, 29]. This regulatory role for GNMT can be illustrated by examining how it functions to maintain methyl group balance, as intracellular methionine concentrations fluctuate.

Under conditions of methionine excess, the concomitant increase in SAM serves to inhibit the activity of MTHFR allosterically [30, 31], thereby decreasing 5-CH$_3$-THF concentrations, which results in diminishing the inhibitory impact of 5-CH$_3$-THF on GNMT. The increase in GNMT activity allows for disposal of excess methyl groups as sarcosine. Conversely, low methionine and/or methyl group supply results in decreased SAM concentrations, increased MTHFR activity, and subsequent elevations in 5-CH$_3$-THF pools, resulting in the inhibition of GNMT activity and serving to conserve methyl groups for SAM-dependent transmethylation reactions. It should be further noted that expression of GNMT is tissue specific, with the majority of its abundance being hepatic. Depending on the species, GNMT has also been shown to be present in significant quantities in the kidney, pancreas, and small intestine [32].

5.4.1.3 *Phosphatidylethanolamine N-Methyltransferase (PEMT)*
Adequate synthesis of phosphatidylcholine (PC) is dependent on two pathways: the CDP-choline (i.e., Kennedy) pathway, present in all nucleated cells, and the PEMT pathway, which is primarily hepatic and has been estimated to be responsible for approximately 20% to 40% of the total PC synthesis that is required [33]. For the latter, the hepatic synthesis of PC involves the PEMT-dependent transfer of three methyl groups from SAM to phosphatidylethanolamine (PE). The synthesis of PC by SAM-dependent methylation of PE is considered to be primarily a hepatic process, although recent reports have found detectable levels of PEMT mRNA in other tissues [34]. Nonetheless, hepatic PC synthesis is well recognized to be an essential process in the ultimate generation of very low density lipoprotein (VLDL) particles required for transport of triglycerides from the liver to extrahepatic tissues, a lack of which is known to result in the development of hepatic steatosis [35]. Because the hepatic synthesis of PC from PEMT involves the use of three SAM methyl groups and concomitantly generates three molecules of homocysteine, it has recently been suggested that PEMT may represent a more significant source of methyl group use than previously thought [36, 37], and, thus, may be a key regulator in homocysteine balance [38, 39]. Using knockout mice representing both the PEMT and CDP-choline pathways for PC synthesis, it has been shown that a lack of these metabolic processes has a significant influence on the regulation of plasma homocysteine concentrations [38, 39].

5.4.1.4 *Serine Hydroxymethyltransferase (SHMT)*
SHMT is not a SAM-dependent methyltransferase, but rather a B6-dependent enzyme that transfers the three-carbon from serine to THF to form 5,10-CH$_2$-THF and glycine, a reaction that is considered to be the primary source of carbon moieties for the folate-dependent one-carbon pool and subsequent methyl group metabolism. Although not liver specific, because half of the total body folate pool is hepatic the action of SHMT to regulate one-carbon usage by the folate-dependent one-carbon pool is important. Besides enzymatically providing one-carbon units for biosynthetic reactions, the expression of SHMT has been shown to be a regulatory signal for differentiating the use of the methylene carbon group (i.e., 5,10-CH$_2$-THF) for DNA synthesis

as opposed to committing it to its utilization as a source of methyl groups for SAM-dependent transmethylation reactions [40]. A number of nutrients or nutritional conditions, such as iron deficiency and retinoic acid treatment, have been shown to influence SHMT expression, thus potentially linking them to sulfur amino acid metabolism as well [41, 42].

5.4.2 Allosteric Regulation of Sulfur Amino Acid Metabolism

Hepatic methionine catabolism is also regulated allosterically by a number of relevant metabolites (Fig. 5.2). As mentioned, SAM inhibits the activity of MTHFR

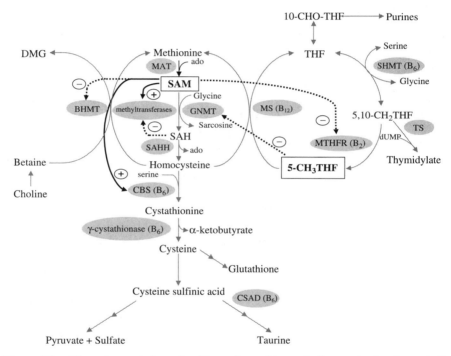

Figure 5.2 Allosteric regulation of sulfur amino acid metabolism and related metabolic pathways. S-adenosylmethionine (SAM), S-adenosylhomocysteine (SAH), and 5-methyl-tetrahydrofolate (5-CH$_3$-THF) exert allosteric control over a number of key enzymes involved in sulfur amino acid metabolism and the folate-dependent one-carbon pool, particularly under fluctuating methionine concentrations. Solid arrows denoted with a $\oplus$ symbol indicate positive modulation of the enzyme, whereas dashed arrows denoted with a $\ominus$ symbol indicate allosteric inhibition. Abbreviations: ado, adenosine; BHMT, betaine-homocysteine S-methyltransferase; CBS, cystathionine β-synthase; CSAD, cysteine sulfinic acid decarboxylase; DMG, dimethyl-glycine; GNMT, glycine N-methyltransferase; MAT, methionine adenosyltransferase; MS, methionine synthase; MTHFR, 5,10-methylene-THF reductase; SAHH, S-adenosylhomocysteine hydrolase; SHMT, serine hydroxymethyltransferase; THF, tetrahydrofolate; TS, thymidylate synthase.

allosterically, thereby reducing 5-CH$_3$THF production and alleviating its inhibition of GNMT activity [28–31]. This allows for the control of GNMT based on methyl group supply and optimizing the ratio of SAM to SAH. SAM also controls folate-independent remethylation of homocysteine by allosteric inhibition of BHMT [43]. In contrast to inhibition, SAM is a positive modulator of CBS activity [44], effectively promoting methionine catabolism to cysteine production under conditions of high methionine and concomitant elevated SAM concentrations in the cell. Taken together, this ensures that excessive methionine concentrations are adequately handled such that the sulfur amino acid metabolic pathway remains relatively constant, depending on the needs of the cell. Conversely, this regulatory network also functions to ensure methyl group supply is met by recycling homocysteine and optimizing the SAM : SAH ratio.

5.4.3 Other Uses of Methionine as SAM

In addition to the liver-specific methyltransferase reactions mentioned above, there are a number of other important SAM-dependent transmethylation reactions that occur in hepatic and or extrahepatic tissues, as well as non-transmethylation uses for SAM, and thus are dependent on an adequate supply of methionine. SAM-dependent methyltransferase reactions include the synthesis of carnitine from lysine, the activation and inactivation of neurotransmitters, and the methylation of DNA for epigenetic control of gene expression. This latter use of SAM-derived methyl groups has emerged as an extremely important aspect of sulfur amino acid metabolism that has significant implications in disease development, including cancer development, diabetes, and vascular disease [45, 46]. Besides transmethylation, SAM also serves as a precursor for the synthesis of the polyamines spermine, spermidine, and putrescine [47] following the initial catalytic action of SAM decarboxylase [48].

5.5 IMPACT OF PHYSIOLOGIC AND NUTRITIONAL FACTORS ON SULFUR AMINO ACID METABOLISM

Numerous nutrients, nutritional conditions, hormones, and other physiologic factors can impact sulfur amino acid metabolism. Perturbation of sulfur amino acid metabolism can be associated with a number of adverse health consequences, including vascular disease, birth defects, cancer development, and other pathologies. Similarly, this association may be a metabolic link between specific chronic problems and their relation to secondary complications and disease.

5.5.1 Adaptation to Excess Dietary Sulfur Amino Acids

The liver has a tremendous capacity to handle excess dietary methionine [49], although high concentrations of methionine can be quite toxic [50]. This ability to adapt to high methionine concentrations resides in the control and function of MAT, GNMT, MTHFR, CBS, and SAM, as has been discussed throughout this chapter. In brief, the excess methionine is activated to SAM, which exerts its allosteric control on methyltransferases, MTHFR, and CBS (Fig. 5.2). Collectively, this results in the increased catabolism of methionine through the transmethylation and transsulfuration pathway, diminishes methionine generation by homocysteine remethylation, and disposes of excess methyl groups by activation of GNMT. Recently, it has been shown that GNMT activation is not only the result of diminished inhibitory binding of 5-CH$_3$-THF, but also the result of increased abundance of the GNMT protein that is dose (i.e., dietary methionine intake) dependent and liver specific [51]. As discussed, increased dietary intake of cyst(e)ine spares methionine catabolism by transsulfuration and promotes the methionine cycle. The relative dietary intake of methionine and cysteine is an important issue, as dietary proteins can vary tremendously in their absolute sulfur amino acid content, and the ratio of methionine to cysteine. When the capacity of the adaptive network described above to handle increasing methionine intake levels is exceeded, methionine can have toxic effects, including diminished food intake, lack of growth, and tissue damage [50]. This may be due to the fact that excess methionine can be metabolized by transamination, an alternative catabolic route [52] where the production of metha-nethiol from methionine transamination is the basis for the toxic effects of excess methionine [53].

The aforementioned discussion has focused on the metabolism of excessive dietary methionine; however, it should be noted that elevations in circulating methionine concentrations (i.e., hypermethioninemia) can also be the result of genetic disorders. For example, it has been documented in humans [54] and recently been shown in a knockout mouse model [55] that a lack of GNMT expression results in extremely high circulating levels of both methionine and SAM. A genetic defect in the hepatic form of MAT I/III has also been identified in humans and shown to be characterized by hypermethioninemia [56, 57]. Thus, the toxic effects of methionine owing to inherited disorders, albeit rare, are an important and recognized aspect of hepatic sulfur amino acid metabolism.

5.5.2 Nutritional Deficiencies and Ethanol Intake

As is clearly evident from Fig. 5.1, a nutritional deficiency of B vitamins (folate, B6, B12, riboflavin) and/or methyl donors (choline, methionine) has a profound effect on sulfur amino acid metabolism and subsequently is a significant factor in disease risk. For the liver, a methyl group-deficient condition has been well documented to result in the development of hepatocarcinogenesis, likely related in part to the improper control of gene expression through epigenetic mechanisms such as SAM-dependent methylation of DNA, as well as inadequate PC synthesis [45, 58–62]. Conversely, established neoplastic tissues have a high requirement for methionine, and thus methionine deprivation has been shown to reduce cancerous growth [63]. Ethanol consumption is also well known to perturb methyl group metabolism in a fashion similar to methyl/B vitamin deficiency [64–68]. More recent comprehensive reviews have been reported on hepatic sulfur amino acid metabolism as a function of methyl group deficiency, ethanol administration, and liver disease [46, 66, 69–73].

5.5.3 Nutrient Regulation

Retinoids are a seemingly unrelated group of nutrients that appear to exert control over the metabolism of sulfur amino acids, and thus impact transmethylation, remethylation, transsulfuration, and the folate-dependent one-carbon pool. Early observations in this regard were a series of studies that demonstrated retinol pretreatment prior to excessive methionine intake was protective against the ensuing toxic effects, owing in part to enhanced catabolism of methionine in the liver [74, 75]. More recently, it has been shown that mechanistically all-*trans*-retinoic acid, as well as other retinoid compounds, induces the expression and subsequent activity of GNMT, as well as an increase in the activity of MS [76–78]. This resultant condition of methyl group loss was evident by a decrease in circulating methionine concentrations and hypomethylation of DNA [77, 78]. Moreover, the impact of retinoic acid on altering sulfur amino acid metabolism was most predominant in the liver, and female rats were more sensitive to the effects of retinoic acid as compared to males [79]. Therefore, retinoid compounds appear to have the ability to regulate hepatic sulfur amino acid and methyl group metabolism by controlling the expression and activity of key enzymes, thus providing potential links between retinoid administration and disease states associated with sulfur amino acid metabolism.

5.5.4 Hormonal Factors

Clearly, an emerging area of research is directed at understanding the link between diabetes and sulfur amino acid metabolism, particularly in the liver. Animal models for both type 1 and type 2 diabetes, as well as glucocorticoid-treated hepatic cell lines, have shown that methionine catabolism was enhanced during the diabetic and gluconeogenic states [80–87]. Using a streptozotocin (STZ)-induced rat model, it has been shown that an acute type 1 diabetic state leads to hepatic induction of GNMT, PEMT, BHMT, and CBS, whereas the activity of MS was significantly diminished. Hypohomocysteinemia was consistently noted in these studies as a result of a diabetic state. Likewise, treatment of rats or hepatic cell lines with glucocorticoids (e.g., dexamethasone) also induced expression of GNMT and CBS. Insulin administration has been shown to prevent these alterations in both rats and cell lines, indicating that these metabolic alterations were likely due to a lack of insulin or elevated counterregulatory hormones. Consistent observations have been reported for type 2 diabetes using the Zucker diabetic fatty (ZDF) rat, indicating insulin resistance produces a similar effect. Most importantly, these findings using rodent models closely reflect what has been reported in type 1 and type 2 human studies [88–90]. Hypohomocysteinemia in type 1 diabetic patients is thought to be explained, at least in part, by enhanced transsulfuration [91]. However, plasma homocysteine levels in both type 1 and 2 diabetics increased with the severity of renal dysfunction [92]. This hyperhomocysteinemia has recently been attributed to suppressed homocysteine clearance, as indicated by kinetic studies in type 2 diabetics with nephropathy [93]. This novel relation between diabetes and disruption of important metabolic processes serves as a potential link between diabetes and its complications, such as cardiovascular disease.

5.5.5 Other Factors

It is beyond the scope of this review to address the entire body of literature regarding the metabolism of sulfur amino acids; however, there are a number of other factors or conditions that clearly impact sulfur amino acid metabolism that deserve mention. Thyroid status, both hyper- and hypothyroidism, has been shown to perturb both the hepatic folate-dependent one-carbon pool and regulatory proteins involved in sulfur amino acid metabolism, such as GNMT [94–98]. Using Ames dwarf mice, it has been shown that age is characterized by enhanced catabolism of methionine in the liver [99, 100]. Lastly, genetic polymorphisms, particularly those that have a well-established metabolic link to sulfur amino acid metabolism such as the MTHFR C677T mutation [101], are continuously being examined to determine their impact on health and disease related to methionine, methyl groups, homocysteine, cysteine, and the B vitamins.

5.6 CONCLUSIONS

The hepatic metabolism of the sulfur amino acids methionine and cysteine is critical for the maintenance of a number of essential biosynthetic processes and genetic regulation. Besides protein synthesis, the methyl group of methionine is critical for the numerous SAM-dependent transmethylation reactions, many if which are unique to the liver. Methylation is also an epigenetic mechanism to control gene expression, and an inability to adequately support DNA methylation results in the aberrant gene expression which can be a major factor in diseases such as cancer. Adequate cysteine pools, whether directly from the diet or via methionine catabolism, is also important in a number of biosynthetic reactions, most notably the synthesis of the antioxidant glutathione. The metabolism of homocysteine, an intermediate in the methionine-cysteine pathway and a by-product of all SAM-dependent transmethylation reactions, must be tightly controlled as its accumulation is associated with a number of adverse conditions, including cardiovascular disease, cancer development, birth defects, and neurological disorders. Identifying physiologic and nutrition factors that impact methionine metabolism, such as diabetes and specific nutrient deficiencies, will continue to be an important avenue of investigation to better understand the relation between sulfur amino acid metabolism and disease, and subsequently develop intervention strategies.

REFERENCES

1. Mudd, S.H., Poole, J.R. (1975). Labile methyl balances for normal humans on various dietary regimens. *Metabolism, 24*, 721–735.
2. Womack, M., Rose, W.C. (1941). Partial replacement of dietary methionine by cysteine for purposes of growth, *Journal of Biological Chemistry, 141*, 375–379.
3. Finkelstein, J.D., Martin, J.J., Harris, B.J. (1988). Methionine metabolism in mammals. The methionine sparing effect of cysteine. *Journal of Biological Chemistry, 263*, 11750–11754.

4. Finkelstein, J.D., Mudd, S.H. (1967). Transsulfuratioin in mammals. The methionine sparing effect of cysteine. *Journal of Biological Chemistry, 242*, 873–880.

5. Kang, S.-S., Wong, P.W., Malinow, M.R. (1992). Hyperhomocyst(e)inemia as a risk factor for occlusive vascular disease. *Annual Review of Nutrition, 12*, 279–298.

6. Mattson, M.P., Shea, T.B. (2003). Folate and homocysteine metabolism in neural plasticity and neurodegenerative disorders. *Trends in Neuroscience, 26*, 137–146.

7. Newberne, P.M., Rogers, A.E. (1986). Labile methyl groups and the promotion of cancer. *Annual Review of Nutrition, 6*, 407–432.

8. Scott, J.M., Kirke, P.N., Weir, D.G. (1990). The role of nutrition in neural tube defects. *Annual Review of Nutrition, 10*, 277–295.

9. Wagner, C. (1995). Biochemical role of folate in cellular metabolism. In Bailey, L.B., ed., *Folate in Health and Disease*, pp. 23–42. New York: Marcel Dekker.

10. Chou, J.Y. (2000). Molecular genetics of hepatic methionine adenosyltransferase deficiency. *Pharmacological Therapy, 85*, 1–9.

11. Mato, J.M., Alvarez, L., Ortiz, P., Pajares, M.A. (1997). S-adenosylmethionine synthesis: Molecular mechanisms and clinical implications. *Pharmacological Therapy, 3*, 265–280.

12. Okada, G., Teraoka, H., Isukada, K. (1981). Multiple species of mammalian S-adenosyl-methionine synthetase. Partial purification and characterization. *Biochemistry, 20*, 934–940.

13. Sullivan, D.M., Hoffman, J.L. (1983). Fractionation and kinetic properties of rat liver and kidney methionine adenosyltransferase isozymes. *Biochemistry, 22*, 1636–1641.

14. Kerr, S.J. (1972). Competing methyltransferase systems. *Journal of Biological Chemistry, 247*, 4248–4252.

15. Cantoni, G.L. (1982). S-adenosylamino acids thirty years later: 1951–1981. In Usdin, E., Borchardt, R.T., and Creveling, C.R., eds., *The Biochemistry of S-Adenosylmethionine and Related Compounds*, pp. 3–10. London: MacMillan.

16. Cantoni, G.L., Chiang, P.K. (1980). The role of S-adenosylhomocysteine and S-adenosyl-homocysteine hydrolase in the control of biological methylations. In Cavallini, D., Gaull, G.E., and Zappia, V., eds., *Natural Sulfur Compounds*, pp. 67–80. New York: Plenum Press.

17. Delgado-Reyes, C.V., Wallig, M.A., Garrow, T.A. (2001). Immunohistochemical detection of betaine-homocysteine S-methyltransferase in human, pig, and rat liver and kidney. *Archives of Biochemistry and Biophysics, 74*, 761–766.

18. Mudd, S.H., Finkelstein, J.D., Irreverr, F., Laster, L. (1965). Transsulfuration in mammals: Microassays and tissue distributions of three enzymes of the pathway. *Journal of Biological Chemistry, 240*, 4382–4392.

19. McKeever, M.P., Weir, D.G., Molloy, A., Scott, J.M. (1991). Betaine-homocysteine methyltransferase: Organ distribution in man, pig and rat and subcellular distribution in the rat. *Clinical Sciences, 81*, 551–556.

20. Clarke, R., Daly, L., Robinson, K., Naughten, E., Cahalane, S., Fowler, B., Graham, I. (1991). Hyperhomocysteinemia: An independent risk factor for vascular disease. *New England Journal of Medicine, 324*, 1149–1155.

21. Finkelstein, J.D. (1990). Methionine metabolism in mammals. *Journal of Nutritional Biochemistry, 1*, 228–234.

22. Hayes, K.C., Sturman, J.A. (1981). Taurine in metabolism. *Annual Review of Nutrition, 1*, 401–425.

23. Dominy, J.E., Stipanuk, M.H. (2004). New roles for cysteine and transsulfuration enzymes: Production of H_2S, a neuromodulator and smooth muscle relaxant. *Nutrition Reviews, 62*, 348–353.

24. Stipanuk, M.H. (2004). Sulfur amino acid metabolism: Pathways for production and removal of homocysteine and cysteine. *Annual Review of Nutrition, 24*, 539–577.

25. Yang, G., Yang, W., Wu, L., Wang, R. (2007). H_2S, endoplasmic reticulum stress, and apoptosis of insulin-secretin beta cells. *Journal of Biological Chemistry, 282*, 16567–16576.

26. Mudd, S.H., Ebert, M.H., Scriver, C.R. (1980). Labile methyl group balances in the human: The role of sarcosine. *Metabolism, 29*, 707–720.

27. Stead, L.M., Au, K.P., Jacobs, R.L., Brosnan, M.E., Brosnan, J.T. (2001). Methylation demand and homocysteine metabolism: Effects of dietary provision of creatine and gua-nidinoacetate. *American Journal of Physiology: Endocrinology and Metabolism, 281*, E1095–E1100.

28. Wagner, C., Briggs, W.T., Cook, R.J. (1985). Inhibition of glycine N-methyltransferase by folate derivatives: Implications for regulation of methyl group metabolism. *Biochemical and Biophysical Research Communications, 127*, 746–752.

29. Wagner, C., Decha-Umphai, W., Corbin, J. (1989). Phosphorylation modulates the activity of glycine N-methyltransferase, a folate binding protein. *In vitro* phosphorylation is inhibited by the natural folate ligand. *Journal of Biological Chemistry, 264*, 9638–9642.

30. Kutzbach, C., Stokstad, E.L.R. (1967). Feedback inhibition of methylenetetrahydrofolate reductase. Partial purification, properties, and inhibition by S-adenosylmethionine. *Biochimica Biophysica Acta, 250*, 459–477.

31. Matthews, R.G. (1986). Methylenetetrahydrofolate reductase from pig liver. *Methods in Enzymology, 122*, 372–381.

32. Yeo, E.-J., Wagner, C. (1994). Tissue distribution of glycine N-methyltransferase, a major folate-binding protein in liver. *Proceedings of the National Academy of Sciences, U.S.A. 91*, 210–214.

33. Sundler, R., Akesson, B. (1975). Regulation of phospholipid biosynthesis in isolated rat hepatocytes. Effect of different substrates. *Journal of Biological Chemistry, 250*, 3359–3367.

34. Zhu, X., Ziesel, S.H. (2005). Gene expression profiling in phosphatidylethanolamine N-methyltransferase knockout mice. *Brain Research and Molecular Brain Research, 134*, 239–255.

35. Yao, Z.M., Vance, D.E. (1988). The active synthesis of phosphatidylcholine is required for very low density lipoprotein secretion from rat hepatocytes. *Journal of Biological Chemistry, 263*, 2998–3004.

36. Stead, L.M., Brosnan, J.T., Brosnan, M.E., Vance, D.E, Jacobs, R.L. (2006). Is it time to reevaluate methyl balance in humans? *American Journal of Clinical Nutrition, 83*, 5–10.

37. Mudd, S.H., Brosnan, J.T., Brosnan, M.E., Jacobs, R.L., Stabler, S.P., Allen, R.H., Vance, D.E., Wagner, C. (2007). Methyl balance and transmethylation fluxes in humans. *American Journal of Clinical Nutrition, 85*, 19–25.

38. Jacobs, R.L., Stead, L.M., Devlin, C., Tabas, I., Brosnan, M.E., Brosnan, J.T., Vance, D.E. (2005). Physiological regulation of phospholipid methylation alters plasma homocysteine in mice. *Journal of Biological Chemistry, 280*, 28299–28305.

39. Noga, A.A., Zhao, Y., Vance, D.E. (2002). An unexpected requirement for phosphatidylethanolamine N-methyltransferase in the secretion of very low density lipoproteins. *Journal of Biological Chemistry, 277*, 42358–42365.

40. Herbig, K., Chiang, E.-P., Lee, L.-R., Hills, J., Shane, B., Stover, P.J. (2002). Cytoplasmic serine hydroxymethyltransferase mediates competition between folate-dependent deoxyribonucleotide and S-adenosylmethionine biosyntheses. *Journal of Biological Chemistry, 277*, 38381–38389.

41. Nakshatri, H., Bouillet, P., Bhat-Nakshatri, P., Chambon, P. (1996). Isolation of retinoic acid-repressed genes from P19 embryonal carcinoma cell. *Gene, 174*, 79–84.

42. Oppenheim, E.W., Adelman, C., Liu, X., Stover, P.J. (2001). Heavy chain ferritin enhances serine hydroxymethyltransferase expression and de novo thymidine biosynthesis. *Journal of Biological Chemistry, 276*, 19855–19861.

43. Finkelstein, J.D., Martin, J.J. (1984). Inactivation of betaine-homocysteine methyltransferase by adenosylmethionine and adenosylhomocysteine. *Biochemical and Biophysical Research Communications, 118*, 14–19.

44. Finkelstein, J.D., Kyle, W.E., Martin, J.J., Pick, A. (1975). Activation of cystathionine synthase by adenosylmethionine and adenosylmethionine. *Biochemical and Biophysical Research Communications, 66*, 81–87.

45. Ross, S.A. (2003). Diet and DNA methylation interactions in cancer prevention. *Annals of the New York Academy of Sciences, 983*, 197–207.

46. Williams, K.T., Schalinske, K.L. (2007). New insights into the regulation of methyl group and homocysteine metabolism. *Journal of Nutrition, 137*, 311–314.

47. Tabor, C.W., Tabor, H. (1984). Polyamines. *Annual Review of Biochemistry, 53*, 749–790.

48. Pegg, A.E. (1984). S-adenosylmethionine decarboxylase: A brief review. *Cell Biochemistry and Function, 2*, 11–15.

49. Finkelstein, J.D., Martin, J.J. (1986). Methionine metabolism in mammals. Adaptation to methionine excess. *Journal of Biological Chemistry, 261*, 1582–1587.

50. Benevenga, N.J., Steele, R.D. (1984). Adverse effects of excessive consumption of amino acids. *Annual Review of Nutrition, 4*, 157–181.

51. Rowling, M.J., McMullen, M.H., Chipman, D.C., Schalinske, K.L. (2002). Hepatic glycine N-methyltransferase is up-regulated by methionine in rats. *Journal of Nutrition, 132*, 2545–2549.

52. Benevenga, N.J. (1984). Evidence for alternative pathways of methionine catabolism. *Advances in Nutrition Research, 6*, 1–18.

53. Steele, R.D., Benevenga, N.J. (1979). The metabolism of 3-methylthiopropionate in rat liver homogenates. *Journal of Biological Chemistry, 254*, 8885–8890.

54. Mudd, S.H., Cerone, R., Schiaffino, M.C., Fantasia, A.R., Minniti, G., Caruso, U., Lorini, R., Watkins, D., Matiaszuk, N., Rosenblatt, D.S., Schwahn, B., Rozen, R., LeGros, L., Koth, M., Capdevilia, A., Lika, Z., Finkelstein, J.D., Tangerman, A., Stabler, S.P., Allen, R.H., Wagner, C. (2001). Glycine N-methyltransferase deficiency: A novel inborn error causing persistent isolated hypermethioninemia. *Journal of Inheritable Metabolic Diseases, 24*, 448–464.

55. Luka, Z., Capdevila, A., Mato, J.M., Wagner, C. A. (2006). Glycine N-methyltransferase knockout mouse model for humans with deficiency of this enzyme. *Transgenic Research*, *15*, 393–397.

56. Chamberlin, M.E., Ubagai, T., Mudd, S.H., Thomas, J., Pao, V.Y., Nguyen, T.K., Levy, H.L., Greene, C., Freehauf, C., Chou, J.Y. (2000). Methionine adenosyltransferase I/III deficiency: Novel mutations and clinical variations. *American Journal of Human Genetics*, *66*, 347–355.

57. Ubagai, T., Lei, K.J., Huang, S., Mudd, S.H., Levy, H.L., Chou, J.Y. (1995). Molecular mechanisms of an inborn error of methionine pathway: Methionine adenosyltransferase deficiency. *Journal of Clinical Investigation*, *96*, 1943–1947.

58. Christman, J.K., Sheikhnejad, G., Dizik, M., Abileah, S., Wainfan, E. (1993). Reversibility of changes in nucleic acid methylation and gene expression induced in rat liver by severe dietary methyl deficiency. *Carcinogenesis*, *14*, 551–557.

59. Ghoshal, A.K., Farber, E. (1984). The induction of liver cancer by dietary deficiency of choline and methionine without added carcinogens. *Carcinogenesis*, *5*, 1367–1370.

60. Pogribny, I.P., Basnakian, A.G., Miller, B.J., Lopatina, N.G., Poirier, L.A., James, S.J. (1995). Breaks in genomic DNA and within the *p53* gene are associated with hypomethylation in livers of folate/methyl-deficient rats. *Cancer Research*, *55*, 1894–1901.

61. Wainfan, E., Dizik, M., Stender, M., Christman, J.K. (1989). Rapid appearance of hypomethylated DNA in livers of rats fed cancer-promoting, methyl-deficient diets. *Cancer Research*, *49*, 4094–4097.

62. Wainfan, E., Poirier, L.A. (1992). Methyl groups in carcinogenesis: Effects on DNA methylation and gene expression. *Cancer Research*, *52*, 2071S–2077S.

63. Mecham, J.O., Rowitch, D., Wallace, C.D., Stern, P.H., Hoffman, R.M. (1983). The metabolic defect of methionine dependence occurs frequently in human tumor cell lines. *Biochemical and Biophysical Research Communications*, *117*, 429–434.

64. Barak, A.J., Beckenhauer, H.C., Tuma, D.J., Badakhsh, S. (1987). Effects of prolonged ethanol feeding on methionine metabolism in rat liver. *Biochemistry and Cell Biology*, *65*, 230–233.

65. Finkelstein, J.D., Cello, J.P., Kyle, W.E. (1974). Ethanol-induced changes in methionine metabolism in rat liver. *Biochemical and Biophysical Research Communications*, *61*, 525–531.

66. Schalinske, K.L., Nieman, K.M. (2005). Disruption of methyl group metabolism by ethanol. *Nutrition Reviews*, *63*, 387–391.

67. Trimble, K.C., Molloy, A.M., Scott, J.M., Weir, D.G. (1991). The effect of ethanol on one-carbon metabolism: Increased methionine catabolism and lipotrope methyl-group wastage. *Hepatology*, *18*, 984–989.

68. Villanueva, J.A., Halsted, C.H. (2004). Hepatic transmethylation reactions in micropigs with alcoholic liver disease. *Hepatology*, *439*, 1303–1310.

69. Davis, C.D., Uthus, E.O. (2004). DNA methylation, cancer susceptibility, and nutrient interactions. *Experimental Biology and Medicine*, *229*, 988–995.

70. Lieber, C.S. (2000). Alcohol: Its metabolism and interaction with nutrients. *Annual Review of Nutrition*, *20*, 395–430.

71. Mato, J.M., Martinez-Chantar, M.L., Lu, S.C. (2008). Methionine metabolism and liver disease. *Annual Review of Nutrition*, *28*, 273–293.

72. Nagy, L.E. (2004). Molecular aspects of alcohol metabolism: Transcription factors involved in early ethanol-induced liver injury. *Annual Review of Nutrition*, *24*, 55–78.

73. Van den Veyver, I.B. (2002). Genetic effects of methylation diets. *Annual Review of Nutrition*, *22*, 255–282.

74. Peng, Y.-S., Evenson, J.K. (1979). Alleviation of methionine toxicity in young male rats fed high levels of retinol. *Journal of Nutrition*, *109*, 281–290.

75. Peng, Y.-S., Russell, D.H., Evenson, J.K. (1981). Alleviation of methionine toxicity by glycine and serine in rats pretreated with excess retinol. *Nutrition Reports International*, *23*, 303–311.

76. Ozias, M.K., Schalinske, K.L. (2003). All-*trans*-retinoic acid rapidly induces glycine N-methyltransferase in a dose-dependent manner and reduces circulating methionine and homocysteine levels in rats. *Journal of Nutrition*, *133*, 4090–4094.

77. Rowling, M.J., McMullen, M.H., Schalinske, K.L. (2002). Vitamin A and its derivatives induce hepatic glycine N-methyltransferase and hypomethylation of DNA in rats. *Journal of Nutrition*, *132*, 365–369.

78. Rowling, M.J., Schalinske, K.L. (2001). Retinoid compounds activate and induce hepatic glycine N-methyltransferase in rats. *Journal of Nutrition*, *131*, 1914–1917.

79. McMullen, M.H., Rowling, M.J., Ozias, M.K., Schalinske, K.L. (2002). Activation and induction of glycine N-methyltransferase by retinoids are tissue- and gender-specific. *Archives of Biochemistry and Biophysics*, *401*, 73–80.

80. Hartz, C.S., Nieman, K.M., Jacobs, R.L., Vance, D.E., Schalinske, K.L. (2006). Hepatic phosphatidylethanolamine *N*-methyltransferase expression is increased in diabetic rats. *Journal of Nutrition*, *136*, 3005–3009.

81. Nieman, K.M., Hartz, C.S., Szegedi, S.S., Garrow, T.A., Sparks, J.D., Schalinske, K.L. (2006). Folate status modulates the induction of hepatic glycine N-methyltransferase and homocysteine metabolism in diabetic rats. *American Journal of Physiology: Endocrinology and Metabolism*, *291*, E1235–E1242.

82. Nieman, K.M., Rowling, M.J., Garrow, T.A., Schalinske, K.L. (2004). Modulation of methyl group metabolism by streptozotocin-induced diabetes and all-*trans*-retinoic acid. *Journal of Biological Chemistry*, *279*, 45708–45712.

83. Ratnam, S., Maclean, K.N., Jacobs, R.L., Brosnan, M.E., Kraus, J.P., Brosnan, J.T. (2002). Hormonal regulation of cystathionine β-synthase expression in liver. *Journal of Biological Chemistry*, *277*, 42912–42918.

84. Ratnam, S., Wijekoon, E.P., Hall, B., Garrow, T.A., Brosnan, M.E., Brosnan, J.T. (2006). Effects of diabetes and insulin on betaine-homocysteine S-methyltransferase expression in rat liver. *American Journal of Physiology: Endocrinology and Metabolism*, *290*, E933–E939.

85. Rowling, M.J., Schalinske, K.L. (2003). Retinoic acid and glucocorticoid treatment induces hepatic glycine *N*-methyltransferase and lowers plasma homocysteine concentrations in the rat and rat hepatoma cells. *Journal of Nutrition*, *133*, 3392–3398.

86. Wijekoon, E.P., Hall, B.N., Ratnam, S., Brosnan, M.E., Zeisel, S.H., Brosnan, J.T. (2005). Homocysteine metabolism in ZDF (type 2) diabetic rats. *Diabetes*, *54*, 3245–3251.

87. Schalinske, K.L. (2003). Interrelationship between diabetes and homocysteine metabolism: Hormonal regulation of cystathionine β-synthase. *Nutrition Reviews*, *61*, 136–138.

88. Hofmann, M.A., Kohl, K., Zumbach, M.S., Borcea, V., Bierhaus, A., Henkels, A., Amiral, J., Fiehn, W., Ziegler, R., Wahl, P., Nawroth, P.P. (1997). Hyperhomocyst(e)inemia and endothelial dysfunction in IDDM. *Diabetes Care*, *20*, 1880–1886.

89. Hoogeveen, E.K., Kostense, P.J., Jakobs, C., Dekker, J.M., Nijpels, G., Heine, R.J., Bouter, L.M., Stehouwer, C.D. (2000). Hyperhomocysteinemia increases risk of death, especially in type 2 diabetes: 5-year follow-up of the Hoorn Study. *Circulation*, *101*, 1506–1511.

90. Robillon, J.F., Canivet, B., Candito, M., Sadoul, J.L., Jullien, D., Morand, P., Chambon, P., Freychet, P. (1994). Type 1 diabetes mellitus and homocyst(e)ine. *Diabete Metabolism*, *20*, 494–496.

91. Abu-Lebdeh, S.H., Barazzoni, R., Meek, S.E., Bigelow, M.L., Persson, X.-M.T., Nair, K.S. (2006). Effects of insulin deprivation and treatment on homocysteine metabolism in people with type 1 diabetes. *Journal of Clinical Endocrinology and Metabolism*, *91*, 3344–3348.

92. Poirier, L.A., Brown, A.T., Fink, L.M., Wise, C.K., Randolph, C.J., Delongchamp, R.R., Fonseca, V.A. (2001). Blood S-adenosylmethionine concentrations and lymphocyte methylenetetrahydrofolate reductase activity in diabetes mellitus and diabetic nephropathy. *Metabolism*, *50*, 1014–1018.

93. Tessari, P., Coracina, A., Kiwanuka, E., Vedovato, M., Vettore, M., Valerio, A., Zaramella, M., Garibotto, G. (2005). Effects of insulin on methionine and homocysteine kinetics in type 2 diabetes with nephropathy. *Diabetes*, *54*, 2968–2976.

94. Finkelstein, J.D., Martin, J.J., Kyle, W.E., Harris, B.J. (1978). Methionine metabolism in mammals: Regulation of methylenetetrahydrofolate reductase content of rat tissues. *Archives of Biochemistry and Biophysics*, *191*, 153–160.

95. Jacobs, R.L., Stead, L.M., Brosnan, M.E., Brosnan, J.T. (2000). Plasma homocysteine is decreased in the hypothyroid rat. *Canadian Journal of Physiology and Pharmacology*, *78*, 565–570.

96. Keating, J.N., Kusano, G., Stokstad, E.L.R. (1988). Effect of thiouracil in modifying folate function in severe vitamin B_{12} deficiency. *Archives of Biochemistry and Biophysics*, *267*, 119–124.

97. Stokstad, E.L.R., Nair, C.P.P. (1988). Effect of hypothyroidism on methylmalonate excretion and hepatic vitamin B-12 levels in rats. *Journal of Nutrition*, *118*, 1495–1501.

98. Tanghe, K.A., Garrow, T.A., Schalinske, K.L. (2004). Triiodothyronine treatment attenuates the induction of hepatic glycine *N*-methyltransferase by retinoic acid and elevates plasma homocysteine concentrations in rats. *Journal of Nutrition*, *134*, 2913–2918.

99. Uthus, E.O., Brown-Borg, H.M. (2003). Altered methionine metabolism in long living Ames dwarf mice. *Experimental Gerontology*, *38*, 491–498.

100. Uthus, E.O., Brown-Borg, H.M. (2006). Methionine flux to transsulfuration is enhanced in the long living Ames dwarf mouse. *Mechanisms in Ageing and Development*, *127*, 444–450.

101. Chen, Z., Karplis, A.C., Ackerman, S.L., Progribny, I.P., Melnyk, S. et al. (2001). Mice deficient in methylenetetrahydrofolatereductase exhibit hyperhomocysteinemia and decreased methylation capacity, with neuropathology and aortic lipid deposition. *Human Molecular Genetics*, *10*, 433–443.

PART III

ANTIOXIDANT AND DETOXIFICATION ACTIVITIES

CHAPTER 6

GLUTATHIONE AND SULFUR CONTAINING AMINO ACIDS: ANTIOXIDANT AND CONJUGATION ACTIVITIES

NILS-ERIK HUSEBY, ELISABETH SUNDKVIST, and GUNBJØRG SVINENG

6.1 INTRODUCTION

Cells in the human body are constantly exposed to highly reactive oxygen-derived free radicals and peroxides. These oxidants are either produced as by-products of mitochondrial metabolism or intracellular enzyme systems, or they can originate from external sources such as inhaled oxygen and pollutants. Such reactive oxidant species (ROS) may oxidize and damage cellular lipids, proteins, and DNA, which will result in impaired macromolecular function and can also initiate programmed cell death.

For living cells to function properly, an equilibrium must exist between oxidizing and reducing agents. The level of oxidants is kept in a regulated, narrow range by the action of several antioxidant systems that have evolved in aerobic organisms [1, 2]. A central element in what can be regarded as the first line of defense acting at a gross level is glutathione (GSH; L-γ-glutamyl-L-cysteinyl-glycine) [3, 4]. This thiol acts as a reducing cofactor, for example, in the glutathione peroxidase reaction to reduce hydroperoxides, and also as a direct scavenger of radicals. In the second line of defense specialized proteins, including thioredoxins, glutaredoxins, heme oxygenases, and reductases, are involved at a more subtle level in cellular adaptation and protection. These latter ones will only be mentioned briefly in this review.

GSH is the most abundant intracellular nonprotein thiol. Its central role in maintaining the redox environment and homeostasis will be the major topic of this chapter. GSH acts together with other defense mechanisms, including chemical and enzymatic antioxidants, precise pO_2 regulation, and alterations in gene expression, to lessen the

Glutathione and Sulfur Amino Acids in Human Health and Disease. Edited by R. Masella and G. Mazza
Copyright © 2009 John Wiley & Sons, Inc.

oxidant toxicity in cells. The level of intracellular GSH is regulated by several mechanisms, including cysteine availability and transport, rates of synthesis and regeneration, GSH utilization, efflux to extracellular fluids, and scavenging [2, 4–6].

Another important neutralization function of GSH is the detoxification of xenobiotics. The body is also exposed to a variety of endogenous and exogenous electrophilic compounds that are conjugated to GSH for necessary elimination. In this chapter the glutathione transferase reactions catalyzing the conjugation of GSH to xenobiotics and the elimination of these conjugates through receptors are described.

There are two other important redox couples that act together with GSH in regulating the redox environment, the cysteine (Cys/CySS) and thioredoxin-1 (Trx1) systems. The three systems are maintained at different redox potentials in cells, and are independently regulated. In this review, we focus on the role of GSH in redox balance, but will also refer to recent data on the role of cysteine/cystine.

ROS are also produced by various enzyme systems such as NADPH oxidase and lipoxygenase as part of cellular signaling pathways that regulate energy production, cell proliferation, and apoptosis. In this way local and subtle changes in the redox balance have significant effects on the function of several signaling factors. This system senses oxidative and chemical stress and will initiate repair mechanisms. It will be discussed briefly.

High ROS levels will therefore have profound effects on cell function and signaling pathways. The term oxidative stress describes an oxidizing environment that may be harmful and deleterious to macromolecules and will also strongly disrupt redox-regulated signaling pathways [7–9].

Oxidative stress situations have been associated with several human diseases, such as development of neoplastic cells and cancer, chronic inflammations, lung diseases, aging, neurodegenerative diseases, and cardiovascular disorders. The last part of this chapter will briefly describe just a few such disease processes.

6.2 REACTIVE OXYGEN SPECIES AND ANTIOXIDANTS

6.2.1 Reactive Oxygen Species (ROS)

The term ROS embraces a wide range of molecules, which are partially reduced metabolites of oxygen, and with higher reactivity than oxygen. They include superoxide ($\cdot O_2^-$), hydrogen peroxide (H_2O_2), hydroxyl radical ($\cdot OH$), and lipid peroxides (LOO$\cdot$). ROS are formed constantly in the cell, mainly in the mitochondria and peroxisomes. In aerobic metabolism, oxygen is the final acceptor for electrons being produced from the electron transport chain in the mitochondria during ATP production. It has been estimated that 1% to 3% of the total oxygen taken up by the mitochondria is reduced to superoxide by side reactions of complex I and III. ROS are also generated in the metabolism of foreign compounds, toxins or drugs by the cytochrome p450 system, and from enzyme systems such as lipoxygenase, cyclooxygenase, xanthine oxidase, and the NADPH oxidase (NOX) complexes [3, 9]. The NADPH oxidases are activated in response to growth factors, cytokines, and other signaling molecules, such as insulin, and produce superoxide in regulated and controlled processes. In phagocytes, ROS are produced by NADPH oxidase as part of the host defense mechanisms against invasion of foreign organisms such as bacteria and fungi, and also in inflammatory processes [10].

Superoxide has been considered to be the primary ROS and can be converted to other and secondary oxygen species through various reactions as indicated in Fig. 6.1. Superoxide has a short lifetime, and is converted to H_2O_2 either spontaneously or by superoxide dismutase (SOD) catalysis (Fig. 6.1; reaction 1).

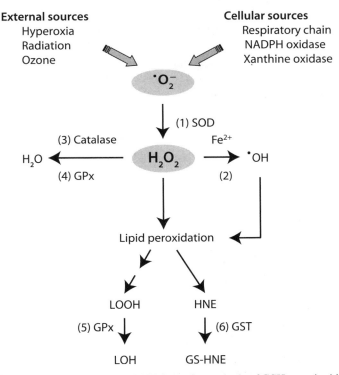

Figure 6.1   Reactive oxygen species (ROS) formation and role of GSH as antioxidant. ROS in the form of superoxide ($\cdot O_2^-$) arise either through activation of oxygen by external processes, or from cellular and metabolic processes. Superoxide is converted to H_2O_2 by superoxide dismutase (SOD) (reaction 1). H_2O_2 can be converted to the hydroxyl radical ($\cdot OH$) in the Fenton reaction (reaction 2), which is catalyzed by transition metals such as Fe^{2+}. H_2O_2 can be decomposed or reduced enzymatically by catalase (reaction 3) into water and oxygen, or by glutathione peroxidase (GPx) to water (reaction 4). GPx uses GSH as reducing agent, which is then oxidized to glutathione disulfide (GSSG). H_2O_2 and $\cdot OH$ can also initiate lipid peroxidation, which generates products such as lipid hydroperoxides (LOOH) and 4-hydroxynonenal (HNE). LOOH are reduced to alcohols and oxygen by glutathione peroxidase (catalyzed by the GPx isoform GPx4) (reaction 5), wheras 4-hydroxynonenal (HNE) is conjugated to GSH by glutathione transferase (GST) to a glutathiyl adduct (reaction 6).

$$\text{Superoxide dismutase}$$
$$(1) \quad 2\,^{\bullet}O_2^- + 2H^+ \longrightarrow H_2O_2 + O_2$$

H_2O_2 is a less potent oxidant than superoxide but can diffuse across membranes and throughout the cell. In higher concentrations (during oxidative stress situations) it will damage proteins, lipids, and DNA and may induce programmed cell death. In lower, regulated and physiological concentrations, H_2O_2 may act as a signaling agent (see below).

The hydroxyl radical ($^{\bullet}OH$) can be generated from H_2O_2 in the presence of metals such as iron in the Fenton reaction (Fig. 6.1; reaction 2).

$$(2) \quad Fe^{2+} + H_2O_2 \longrightarrow Fe^{3+} + \,^{\bullet}OH + OH^-$$

This radical has a high reactivity and will therefore react close to its site of formation. However, as this reaction requires free Fe^{2+}, its significance in vivo is not clear [9].

Radicals are also produced during lipid peroxidation (Fig. 6.1). Polyunsaturated fatty acids are sensitive to oxidation and during various stress situations, including oxidative stress, increased peroxidation of polyunsaturated fatty acids may occur. These processes may generate reactive products, including the highly reactive peroxyl radicals ($LOO^{\bullet}$), lipid hydroperoxides (LOOH), and α,β-unsaturated hydroxyalkenals such as 4-hydroxynonenal (HNE) and malondialdehyde (MDA) [11, 12]. Several of the products formed can act as mutagens, or form adducts with various macromolecules. HNE has received much attention recently as a signaling molecule that activates signaling pathways, including the mitogen-activated protein kinase (MAPK) pathway [13, 14].

Reactive nitrogen species (RNS) are derivates of nitric oxide (NO). NO is a radical generated by nitric oxide synthases which convert arginine to citrulline and form NO via oxidative reactions. NO readily diffuses through the cytoplasm and across cell membranes. It has been shown that NO has several biological signaling effects, including blood pressure regulation, neurotransmission, smooth muscle relaxation, and immune regulation. Overproduction of RNS (nitrosative stress) will result in nitrosylation, which can alter properties of many proteins. In oxidative bursts, NO may react with superoxide to produce peroxynitrite ($ONOO^-$) which is a very active oxidant and may cause DNA fragmentation and lipid oxidation [1, 9, 15].

6.2.2 Antioxidants

GSH has a central role in maintaining the redox environment [8]. GSH acts together with the glutathione peroxidase reactions to detoxify H_2O_2 and various lipid hydroperoxides and can also act as an antioxidant in scavenging hydroxyl radical and singlet oxygen directly.

GSH is produced in large quantities in all cells and is distributed into subcellular pools: the cytosolic (1–11 mM) in which GSH is synthesized, the nucleic (3–15 mM) where GSH maintains a functional redox state for DNA repair and gene expression, and the mitochondrial (5–11 mM) where the oxidative stress is high [7]. The extracellular concentration of GSH is low, and the concentration in plasma is around 0.002 mM.

The cellular antioxidant defense system includes other *molecular* antioxidants in the form of vitamins such as vitamin A, C (ascorbic acid), and E (α-tocopherol), carotenoids and flavonoids. The defense also involves *enzymatic* systems such as superoxide dismutase (SOD), catalase, and glutathione peroxidase (GPx) coupled with glutathione reductase (GR). Other oxidant scavengers are thioredoxin coupled with thioredoxin reductase, and glutaredoxin which uses GSH as cosubstrate.

Two major antioxidant systems will reduce H_2O_2, the catalase and the glutathione peroxidase (GPx) reactions (Fig. 6.1; reactions 3 and 4). Catalase is found in peroxisomes and in the cytoplasm of most cells, particularly in liver and erythrocytes. GPx uses GSH as a reducing cofactor, which is oxidized to glutathione disulfide (GSSG).

Catalase

(3) $2H_2O_2 \longrightarrow 2H_2O + O_2$

Glutathione peroxidase

(4) $H_2O_2 + 2GSH \longrightarrow 2H_2O + GSSG$

GSH is also involved in neutralization of lipid peroxidation products. Both lipid hydroperoxide (LOOH) and 4-hydroxynonenal (HNE), being derived from phospholipid and fatty acids, can be neutralized with GSH by GPx (Fig. 6.1; reaction 5) or glutathione transferase (GST) (Fig. 6.1; reaction 6). It has also been shown that the human alpha class of GST can reduce lipid hydroperoxides using GSH as a reducing agent (reaction 7).

Glutathione peroxidase

(5) $LOOH + 2GSH \longrightarrow LOH + GSSG + O_2$

Glutathione transferase

(6) $HNE + GSH \longrightarrow GS\text{-}HNE$

Glutathione transferase A1

(7) $LOOH + 2GSH \longrightarrow LOH + GSSG + H_2O$

In addition, GSH is an important protective agent against RNS as it reacts with peroxynitrite (reaction 8). Both GCL and GST expression have been reported to be increased after peroxynitrite exposure [16–18], as has the expression of γ-glutamyltransferase [19].

Glutathione peroxidase

(8) $ONOO^- + 2GSH \longrightarrow NO_2^- + GSSG + H_2O$

6.3 GLUTATHIONE REDOX CYCLE

6.3.1 Glutathione Peroxidase

Glutathione peroxidases (GPx) catalyze the reduction of H_2O_2 to H_2O using reduced glutathione (GSH) as the electron donor (Figs. 6.1 and 6.2; reaction 4). The glutathione disulfide (GSSG) generated in this reaction can be reduced back to GSH by glutathione reductase and NADPH (Fig. 6.2; reaction 9).

Glutathione reductase

(9) $GSSG + NADPH + H^+ \longrightarrow 2GSH + NADP^+$

The two reactions (reactions 4 and 9) constitute the glutathione redox cycle (Fig. 6.2) and this recycling prevents the depletion of cellular GSH (for a review see Reference 20). The role of GSH and GPx in the reduction of H_2O_2 has been known for 50 years; the protective role of the enzyme and GSH was characterized in a study in 1957 on oxidative reactions and damage in erythrocytes [21]. Fifteen years later it was reported that selenium is a cofactor in the GPx reaction [22] (for reviews, see References 23 and 24).

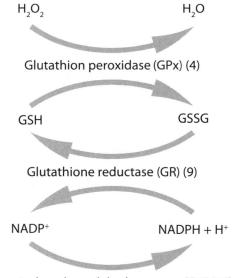

Figure 6.2   The GSH redox cycle. The reduction of H_2O_2 to H_2O is catalyzed by glutathione peroxidases (GPx) using GSH as reducing agent (reaction 4). The oxidized glutathione disulfide (GSSG) can be reduced back to GSH with glutathione reductase (GR) using NADPH as reducing agent (reaction 9). The oxidized $NADP^+$ can be reduced in the pentose phosphate shunt, using the oxidation of glucose 6-phosphate to 6-phosphogluconlactone catalyzed by glucose 6-phosphate dehydrogenase (G6PDH) (reaction 10).

Glutathione peroxidases comprise a family of enzymes present in the cytosol of most cells. They include five genetically distinct, selenium-dependent isoforms and two selenium-independent forms. The seven enzymes are termed GPx1-7 (Table 6.1). The selenium-dependent forms (GPx1-4, and GPx6) have selenium bound to the cysteine at the active site and this modified amino acid appears to be essential for the catalytic function of these enzymes. During translation, the selenium-cysteine amino acid residue is incorporated into the protein through a specific SeCys-tRNA [24]. Two forms, GPx3 and 5 are secreted from various cells and are present in body fluids such as plasma and epithelial lining fluid [24, 25]. The human GPx5 and GPx7 are non-selenium-dependent GPx, presenting a cysteine-residue and not SeCys in the active site [26].

The availability of selenium is an important factor for the expression of the various GPx genes, which may reflect their relative biological importance. Biochemically, this is related to mRNA stability. The GPx1 isoform is vulnerable and its mRNA disappears rapidly in moderate selenium deficiency. When compared to GPx1, the GPx2 and the GPx4 isoforms are significantly more stable in selenium deficiency [27].

The GPx isoforms differ with respect to cellular and tissue distribution, substrate specificity, and genetic regulation. High levels of activity are found in tissues exposed to high oxygen levels, such as lungs and red blood cells, but the activity is also high in liver, kidney, and pancreas. Recent studies indicate that the GPx isoforms have adopted different biological functions. GPx can reduce both H_2O_2 and various organic hydroperoxides. The K_m values for all hydroperoxides depend on the GSH concentration, and are in the micromolar range. This makes the GPxs very effective hydroperoxide scavengers even at low GSH concentrations.

The GPx1, the classical or cytosolic GPx (cGPx), was the first to be described and its major role as an antioxidant enzyme is to reduce hydroperoxides, including H_2O_2, using GSH as electron donor. The GPx1 activity is upregulated after oxidative stress and is also regulated during development, being increased at birth. In some parenchymal organs the enzyme regulation is clearly under hormonal control. The activity may also increase after exposure to xenobiotics and toxins [28, 29]. The enzyme is induced in human umbilical cord cells by increased oxygen tension when cells were grown in selenium-supplemented media. This upregulation resulted from both increased transcription and increased mRNA stabilization [30]. The antioxidant role of the enzyme was clearly demonstrated in GPx1 knockout animals, which were vulnerable to severe oxidative stress, although the enzyme appeared not to be indispensable. On the other hand, GPx1-overexpressing mice were more resistant to oxidative stress [31].

The GPx2 isoform is frequently called gastrointestinal GPx (GI-GPx). This isoform is highly expressed in the gastrointestinal system but is also present in other epithelial cells. GPx2 has been suggested to function as a barrier against the absorption of lipid hydroperoxide derived from the diet in the intestinal epithelium [32]. An important role for the enzyme in fighting inflammatory responses in the GI system was indicated from studies of GPx2 knockout mice [33]. Its activity is also detected in colon and skin cancer and in cultured cancer cells. Studies on the transcriptional regulation of this subtype in such cells indicate that the GPx2 can be classified as part of the

TABLE 6.1 Glutathione Peroxidase Properties of Human Subtypes

Systemic Name	GPx1	GPx2	GPx3	GPx4	GPx5	GPx6	GPx7
Trivial name	cGPx, classical or cytosolic GPx	GI-GPx, gastrointestinal GPx	pGPx, plasmatic GPx	PH-GPx, phospholipid GPx	e-GPx, epididymal GPx	OMP, olfactory GPx	NPGPx, nonseleno phospholipid GPx
Tissue distribution	Most cell types; erythrocytes, liver, lung	Stomach, liver, intestine	Several organs	Testis, liver, spermatozoa	Epididymis, spermatozoa	Olfactory epithelium	Mammary
Localization	Cytosol, nucleus, mitochondria	Cytosol, nucleus	Secreted, cytosol	Cytosol, nucleus, mitochondria, membrane-bound	Secreted		Cytosol
SeCys residue	Yes	Yes	Yes	Yes	No	Yes	No

cell's protection against oxidant-induced apoptosis, especially in the preneoplastic state, making the cells procarcinogenic [34].

GPx3 is also called plasma or extracellular GPx (eGPx). The activity of GPx3 is detected in plasma, amniotic fluid, and breast milk, but its function in these fluids is unknown [23]. This GPx subform is glycosylated, which indicates that the enzyme is indeed exported and not passively released from cells or released after cell damage. It is a monomer, in contrast to the tetramer composition of most other GPxs. GPx3 can reduce H_2O_2, organic and free fatty acid hydroperoxides, and to some extent phospholipid hydroperoxides. The enzyme is produced by bronchial epithelial cells and alveolar macrophages, and may be secreted from these cells into the epithelial lining fluid. The enzyme has been well studied in epithelial lining fluid of the lung and clearly is an important participant in detoxification of ROS in the lungs. GPx3 has apparently a significant role in preventing oxidant-mediated lung diseases [25]. It has been shown that GPx3 can be upregulated in the lungs in response to stress or disease. This is also supported by in vitro studies showing upregulation of GPx3 mRNA after oxidative stress. Interestingly, nitrosylated GSH (GSNO) is an effective cosubstrate for GPx3, and GSNO also induces expression of the GPx3 gene. It has been suggested that upregulation of GPx3 in the lung can be an important mechanism for neutralizing both ROS and RNS [25].

GPx4 is also termed phospholipid hydroperoxide GPx (PH-GPx) as this isoform may protect membranes through its ability to reduce phospholipid hydroperoxides and in this way reduce the damage to membranes. However, as lipid hydroperoxides as well as H_2O_2 have signaling functions, the action of PGx4 will also affect the regulation of signaling pathways. In particular, PGx4 will interfere with the regulation of eicosanoid and leukotriene biosynthesis as lipid peroxides are required for activity of enzymes in these pathways [23, 35]. Genetic overexpression of GPx4 resulted in a specific reduction of cyclooxygenase (COX) and lipoxygenase (LOX) activities and thus eicosanoid synthesis. The nuclear factor-κB (NF-κB) transcription factor system was consistently inhibited as GPx4 interferes with NF-κB activation of interleukin-1 [36]. Through these mechanisms the GPx4 complements the anti-inflammatory function of GPx2. Overexpression of GPx4 in tumor cells reduced eicosanoid synthesis, and this resulted in both reduced solid tumor growth and malignant progression [35]. GPx4 may thus be an interesting target for anticancer agents. Another crucial role for GPx4 has been demonstrated in sperm maturation and embryogenesis [37].

The GPx5 is expressed in the epididymis in the male genital tract and in spermatozoa. This subform contains cysteine instead of selenocysteine in the active site and shows a low peroxidase activity. It has been indicated from studies of their biochemical and physiological functions that they may not be true GSH peroxidases. Spermatozoa are prone to oxidative damage, but ROS are also important in sperm maturation. GPx5 may, in this fine balance of ROS production and recycling, act as ROS sensors in various signaling pathways [24].

GPx6 has been found in the olfactory epithelium, where it may act together with GSH in antioxidant defense of the nasal cavity [23].

GPx7, another nonselenocysteine peroxidase, was identified in breast cancer cells but is expressed in several tissues [38], including developing mammary glands. This enzyme appears to be a novel phospholipid hydroperoxide glutathione peroxidase, playing a role in alleviating oxidative stress generated from polyunsaturated fatty acids.

6.3.2 Glutathione Reductase

GSH is regenerated from the oxidized GSSG in the glutathione reductase (GR) reaction with NADPH as reducing agent (Fig. 6.2; reaction 9). In this way, the GSH/GSSG ratio is maintained in a mainly reduced form. The NADPH is derived mainly from the pentose phosphate pathway shunt (Fig. 6.2; reaction 10).

$$\text{Glutathione reductase}$$
$$(9) \quad GSSG + NADPH + H^+ \longrightarrow 2GSH + NADP^+$$

$$\text{Glucose-6-phophate dehydrogenase}$$
$$(10) \quad \text{Glucose-6-P} + NADP^+ \longrightarrow \text{6-phospho-gluconlactone} + NADPH + H^+$$

The importance of the NADPH production in maintaining a reduced environment has been of special focus in erythrocytes. Patients with a genetic defect in glucose-6-phosphate dehydrogenase are prone to suffer serious medical consequences [39]. Exposing cells to oxidative stress resulted in increased expression of glutathione reductase. Interestingly, small stress proteins such as Hsp27 may modulate the ability of cells to respond to oxidative stress. It has been shown that the expression of this molecular chaperon correlates with a reduced level of ROS, apparently through a reduction in intracellular level of iron, and thus reduction of $\cdot$OH formation. This will result in a significant increase in the activities of glucose-6-dehydrogenase, glutathione reductase, and glutathione transferase [40].

6.4   REGULATION OF GSH AND CYSTEINE LEVELS

6.4.1   GSH Biosynthesis and Glutamate Cysteine Ligase (GCL)

There is a dynamic balance between the rate of synthesis and the rate of consumption of GSH within the cell. GSH biosynthesis must therefore be regulated to cope with loss of GSH which is not only its oxidation to GSSG and eventual export of GSSG, but also to that being used for conjugation reactions and mercapturic acid production and export, as well as for glutathionylation.

GSH synthesis is an intracellular, two-step process catalyzed by the enzymes glutamate cysteine ligase (GCL, Fig. 6.3; reaction 11) and GSH synthase (GS, Fig. 6.3; reaction 12).

$$\text{Glutamate-cysteine ligase}$$
$$(11) \quad \text{glutamate} + \text{cysteine} + ATP \longrightarrow \gamma\text{-glutamylcysteine} + ADP + P_i$$

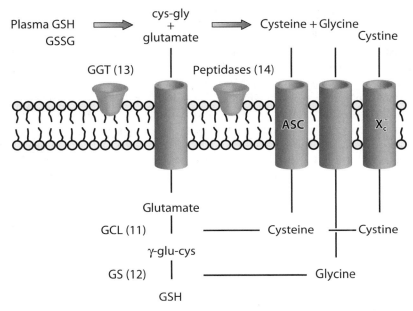

Figure 6.3 GSH biosynthesis and salvage. GSH is synthesized from the constituent amino acids in two reactions, which are catalyzed by glutamate cysteine ligase (GCL, reaction 11) and glutathione synthase (GS, reaction 12). Each reaction needs ATP. For synthesis, cysteine is obtained through uptake of extracellular cysteine or cystine through the ASC and the X_c^- transporters, respectively. Extracellular GSH is also a cysteine reservoir, being degraded by γ-glutamyltransferase, GGT (reaction 13) and various peptidases (reaction 14).

Glutathione synthase

$$(12) \quad \text{γ-glutamylcysteine} + \text{glycine} + \text{ATP} \longrightarrow \text{GSH} + \text{ADP} + P_i$$

The rate of biosynthesis is controlled primarily by cysteine availability, GCL activity which is feedback inhibited by GSH, and by the expression level of GCL. Oxidative stress situations may increase the expression of GCL and thereby the GSH level, and may occur first through a short-term increase in GSH synthesis due to reduced feedback inhibition of the synthesis, followed by transcriptional upregulation of GCL [5, 41, 42]. Additionally, various oxidants can increase the cysteine/ cystine uptake and concomitantly increase the GSH production [43].

The GCL enzyme is a heterodimer, with a catalytic (heavy) subunit (GCLC) that exhibits the active site, and a lighter subunit that is a regulator or modulator subunit (GCLM). The subunits are encoded by separate genes and transcription of both is upregulated after oxidative stress [41, 44]. The activity of GCL may also be regulated by posttranslational modifications including phosphorylation and nitrosylation [45, 46].

6.4.2 GSH Salvage and γ-Glutamyltransferase (GGT)

Only a few cell types have transport systems for direct uptake of GSH, but most cells, particularly those with absorptive or secretory functions, express γ-glutamyltransferase (GGT). This enzyme initiates the hydrolysis of extracellular GSH (Fig. 6.3; reaction 13). GGT is bound to the external side of the plasma membrane [47] and cleaves the gamma linkage between glutamate and cysteine, which is resistant to degradation by other peptidases or proteinases. This enzyme also acts as a transferase, transferring the γ-glutamyl groups to various acceptors including cystine. The remaining cys-gly moiety of GSH is hydrolyzed by various peptidases (Fig. 6.3; reaction 14). The resulting products of these reactions are taken up by the cell and become substrates for renewed GSH synthesis (Fig. 6.3; reactions 11 and 12). For more details, see References 48 to 50.

$$\text{GGT}$$
$$(13) \quad \text{GSH} \longrightarrow \text{glutamate} + \text{cysteinyl-glycine}$$

$$\text{peptidases}$$
$$(14) \quad \text{cysteinyl-glycine} \longrightarrow \text{cysteine} + \text{glycine}$$

The enzyme GGT was first described in 1948 when it was reported that rat kidneys contained an enzyme that could hydrolyse the γ-glutamyl bond in GSH [51]. Expression of GGT is a significant advantage for the cell, particularly when the cellular level of cysteine is low, as the enzyme will degrade circulating GSH and thus increase the availability of cysteine [6, 19, 52, 53]. The importance of GGT in maintaining cellular cysteine levels and GSH homeostasis, and thus for cellular antioxidant capacity, has been confirmed in GGT knockout mice. Such mice showed high levels of GSH both in serum and urine, and decreased levels in tissues and cells. The animals suffered from cysteine deficiency and were susceptible to oxygen-induced injury in the lungs [54, 55].

GGT has a complex gene structure and regulation. Increased expression has been demonstrated in several cell types after oxidative stress and also in cells exposed to xenobiotics, drugs, alcohol, and anticancer drugs [56, 57].

6.4.3 Cysteine Availability

The availability of cysteine is a significant rate-limiting factor in GSH biosynthesis [20]. The plasma cysteine level is kept within a narrow range, below its threshold for toxicity and tendency to react with proteins in disulfide exchange. Cysteine has also low solubility in plasma [58]. However, both plasma cystine and plasma GSH may be used for GSH biosynthesis (Fig. 6.3). Cystine is taken up by the cell through the glutamate-cystine antiporter (X_c^-) and inside, cystine can be reduced to cysteine for GSH biosynthesis. Cysteine is taken up by a sodium-dependent neutral amino acid transporter (ASC).

The synthesis of GSH occurs in almost all cells but liver has a major role in converting cysteine into GSH. This is related to the important function of liver in removing the major part of dietary cysteine from the portal blood. Liver regulates the intracellular free cysteine pool tightly, even when dietary intake of sulfur amino acid or protein is high. This ensures that liver cells maintain enough cysteine for protein and GSH synthesis, and avoiding levels above the threshold of cell toxicity. The liver is releasing significant amounts of GSH to the circulation as a part of the interorgan transportation of GSH. Circulating GSH is therefore a significant reservoir for cysteine [48, 59], being degraded by extracellular γ-glutamyltransferase (GGT, Fig. 6.3; reaction 13) as part of the γ-glu cycle [48]. A major part of circulating GSH is removed by the kidneys [60, 61]. Methionine can be converted to cysteine via the transsulfuration pathway in the liver and, therefore, dietary methionine can replace cysteine to support GSH biosynthesis in liver. Tissue GSH may be strongly reduced if the intake of sulfur amino acid is marginal. Chronically high levels of cysteine have been associated with various diseases, including rheumatoid arthritis and Parkinson's disease. At low or marginal cysteine levels, an increase in GCL has been reported [58].

6.4.4 Redox Environment

The maintenance of a balanced redox state or redox environment is dependent on a linked set of redox couples both within and outside the cell. These redox couples and reactions 1 and 3 to 8 described above will neutralize and regulate ROS, thus avoiding cell damage. The systems are also important in redox signaling mechanisms to sense stress and danger and to repair oxidative damage. The major systems are GSH/GSSG, cysteine/cystine, and thioredoxin. In addition, the glutaredoxin system is gaining increasing attention. The thioredoxin and glutaredoxin systems will be described in another chapter.

The plasma GSH/GSSG ratio has been used to estimate the redox state in biological systems. A reduced state of the GSH/GSSG couple appears to correlate with the proliferating state of the cell, whereas an increasingly more oxidized state is characteristic for cells during differentiation and apoptosis. The ratio is decreased with age, and plasma GSH also becomes more oxidized with age-related diseases such as type 2 diabetes and cardiovascular diseases [7, 62].

The cysteine/cystine (Cys/CySS) ratio is another central parameter in maintaining the redox environment. The plasma Cys/CySS pool is significantly larger and more oxidized than the plasma GSH/GSSG couple, and the two couples are not in equilibrium [63]. In a report on human colon carcinoma cells (HT29) it was demonstrated that the extracellular Cys/CySS redox state was regulated by mechanisms that are independent of intracellular GSH levels [64].

The importance of the Cys/CySS couple as a discrete major regulator of cell survival was emphasized in a recent study on Burkitt's lymphoma cells [65]. This study confirmed that GSH level alone is not a decisive factor for cell survival. In lymphoma cells overexpressing the cystine transporter (glutamate/cystine antiporter; X_c^-) an increased uptake of cystine was noted, and these cells also became highly resistant towards oxidative stress. This did not affect the intracellular GSH content, but was followed by an increased level in the extracellular cysteine concentration. Thus, a reducing environment was obtained. The Cys/CySS couple must therefore be viewed as a discrete regulator of cell survival [63, 65].

A third major redox couple in cells is the thioredoxin system $(TrxSS/Trx(SH)_2)$, which plays an important role in regulating the oxidative state of protein sulfhydryl groups. Apparently, the GSH system is more effective in reducing small disulfide molecules and in reacting directly with ROS, whereas Trx reduces primarily the exposed disulfides on proteins [66]. The three thiol systems act as independent antioxidant systems in equilibrating the redox state, and they also function independently in cellular compartments such as the cytoplasm, nucleus, and mitochondria [67, 68].

6.4.5 Oxidative Stress

An increase in intracellular levels of oxidants will lead to damage to macromolecules and thus impair cell function, and can lead to cell death. The term oxidative stress has been used for many years to describe such a situation and has been defined as an imbalance of peroxidants and antioxidants, in favor of the former [69]. This will therefore describe a situation of high levels of oxidants and/or reduced levels of antioxidants. It has become clear that subtle variations occurring in the intracellular redox environment have profound effects on a large number of signaling molecules in the cell, thereby changing cell function. Such control events occur through discrete and regulated redox reactions and not by global thiol/disulfide balances or imbalances. Based on this understanding, oxidative stress has now been suggested to be defined as a disruption of redox signaling and control [70]. Furthermore, measurement of oxidative stress and red/ox balance cannot be defined by a single entity such as GSH/GSSG, but depends at least also on the Cys/CySS and thioredoxin systems [62, 70].

6.5 BIOTRANSFORMATION

Humans are constantly exposed to drugs and compounds from the environment that may pose health problems. A collective name for these drugs and nonessential compounds are xenobiotics. The physical property that enables many xenobiotics to be absorbed is their lipophilicity, but this also makes their direct elimination more difficult. The elimination of xenobiotics often depends on their conversion to water-soluble substances by a process known as biotransformation, which is catalyzed by enzymes in the liver and other tissues. The result of this biotransformation is that the physical properties of a xenobiotic are generally changed from favoring absorption to favoring excretion in urine and feces. These biochemical processes are usually enzymatic processes, and are divided into phase I and phase II reactions. Phase I reactions expose or introduce a functional group and include hydrolysis, oxidation, and reduction. The phase I enzymes include cytochrome P450 and are located primarily in the endoplasmic reticulum membrane. These will not be discussed further in this chapter. Phase II reactions include glucuronidation, sulfation, acetylation, methylation, conjugation with glutathione, and conjugation with amino acids. The phase II enzymes are located mainly in the cytosol [71].

The enzymes or enzyme systems that catalyze the biotransformation are widely distributed throughout the body, but in humans the liver is their main location. This is not surprising since substances absorbed from the gastrointestinal tract go through the liver before they enter the general circulation. Other locations where these enzymes are expressed are, for example, skin, lungs, nasal and oral cavity, eye, and gastrointestinal tract, which all represent sites that may be exposed to xenobiotics. Phase I and phase II biotransformation enzymes are often referred to as detoxification enzymes. This is only partly true, since in a number of cases the metabolic products are more toxic than the parent compound. This process is often referred to as bioactivation. Extrahepatic tissues have limited abilities with respect to the diversity of substances they can process. Hence, biotransformation of a compound within the extrahepatic tissues may have important toxicological consequence for that particular tissue [72].

Genetic variability (polymorphism) in biotransformation enzymes may have an influence on the conjugation activity. This may cause an individual response to drugs, drug interactions, and drug toxicity. Physiological factors may also influence the response to a given xenobiotic. Age is one factor, and very young and old humans often have dissimilar metabolism. Other factors are hormones, sex differences, pregnancy, changes in the intestinal microflora, diseases, and nutrition [69].

6.5.1 Glutathione Conjugation

The glutathione transferases used to be called glutathione *S*-transferases and this gave rise to the widely used abbreviation GST. Glutathione conjugation is of particular importance for detoxification, because substrates of these reactions often are potent electrophiles that could bind covalently to macromolecules such as proteins or nucleic acids, and cause cellular damage and genetic mutations. The glutathione conjugation reaction may occur spontaneously, but it is much more efficient when catalyzed by the glutathione transferases. The effectiveness of conjugation to glutathione depends on multiple factors. First, the cellular content and production ability for glutathione must be sufficient and, second, the cells need transporters that are able to export glutathione conjugates from the cells.

Glutathione transferases catalyze the first of four steps in the formation of *N*-acetylcysteine derivatives (mercapturic acid) of a diverse group of compounds. The mercapturic conjugates are thereafter excreted into the urine. Three major families of proteins that are widely distributed exhibit glutathione transferase activity; cytosolic-, mitochondrial-, and microsomal glutathione transferases [73], although more recent investigations have shown that several of the proteins included in this family are not transferases at all [74]. Besides catalyzing conjugation, reduction and isomerization reactions, cytosolic glutathione transferases also bind hydrophobic nonsubstrate ligands covalently or noncovalently. This contributes to intracellular transport and deposition of xenobiotics and hormones [73]. Microsomal glutathione transferases are now referred to as membrane-associated proteins in eicosanoid and glutathione (MAPEG) metabolism. Most MAPEGs are involved in the synthesis of eicosanoids, leucotriens, and prostaglandins [74]. As with most biotransformation enzymes, the various glutathione transferases demonstrate different but overlapping substrate selectivity.

6.5.2 Glutathione Transferase Families

Isolation and characterization of these enzymes have shown that they are composed of either identical or nonidentical subunits that associate in dimers to form the catalytic unit. The enzymes are ubiquitously expressed, with the highest activity found in liver, intestine, kidney, testis, and adrenal gland. Based on amino acid sequence similarities seven classes of cytosolic glutathione transferases are found in mammalian species. These are named alpha-, mu-, omega-, pi-, sigma-, theta-, and zeta-glutathione transferase. Other classes of cytosolic glutathione transferases are identified in nonmammalian species [73]. Cytosolic glutathione transferases are subject to significant genetic polymorphisms in the human population [75]. This most likely contributes to interindividual differences in responses to xenobiotics and may have effects on tumorigenesis, neurodegenerative diseases, and inflammatory diseases [20].

The mammalian mitochondrial glutathione transferase isoenzyme comprises one single enzyme named kappa-glutathione transferase. In human this enzyme is widely and uniformly expressed. Six human MAPEGs are characterized and genetic polymorphisms among MAPEG members have been identified. The biological significance of these findings need to be confirmed in further studies [74].

6.5.3 Transport of Glutathione Conjugates

Before glutathione conjugated xenobiotics and metabolites (e.g., cysteinyl leukotriene C_4) can be eliminated from the body or act on cellular targets, they need to be exported out of the cells. Proteins belonging to the ATP-binding cassette (ABC) superfamily of transport proteins often mediate this efflux process. ABC transporters are found in cells of all species from bacteria to man [76]. In humans, the ABC superfamily contains 48 members, which are organized into seven subfamilies (ABCA–ABCG) based on their amino acid sequence homology [77]. Typically, ABC transporters utilize the energy from ATP hydrolysis to pump substrates across the cell membrane against a concentration gradient. The functional unit of the ABC transporters consists of two transmembrane domains (TMD) and two nucleotide-binding domains (NBD) where ATP binds. Some of the new members of the ABC superfamily do not contain transmembrane domains, and therefore may not be involved in transport across membranes. This includes members of the ABCE and ABCF superfamilies where functions are still unknown.

Multidrug resistance protein-1 and -2 (MRP1 and MRP2) are important contributors to cellular extrusion and elimination of phase II conjugates. They both belong to the ABCC subfamily that contains 12 members, including the multidrug resistance protein 1-9 (MRP1-9). In addition to the common four-domain structure (two TMD and two NBD), some of the MRPs contain a third N-terminal membrane spanning region. MRP transporters with this extra domain are referred to as long

MRPs, while the others are referred to as short MRPs. The MRP family has been identified as active membrane transporters for various compounds, including glutathione, glutathione conjugates, and other products of phase II metabolism [77, 78].

MRP1 is overexpressed in many drug-resistant tumor cell lines. Although there has been extensive research on how the binding and hydrolysis of ATP are coupled to substrate binding, translocation, and release, detailed molecular knowledge of the structure and transport mechanism of MRP1 is still lacking [78].

Glutathione is linked to the transport across cell membranes in many complex mechanisms. Indeed, glutathione is required for the transport of drugs and other xenobiotics by MRP1, although conjugation to glutathione is not taking place in all cases. Drugs such as the vinca alkaloids (cytostatic) seem to be co-exported and not conjugated to glutathione. MRP1 also mediates glutathione disulfide (GSSG) efflux during oxidative stress in several cell types, including astrocytes (glial cells), endothelial cells, and probably erythrocytes [77].

6.5.4 Non-ABC Glutathione Transport

The non-ABC drug transporter RLIP76, also called Ral binding protein-1 (RalBP-1), has been shown to play a role in drug resistance. It was initially cloned as a Ral binding protein that was proposed to be a link between Ral and Ras pathways. It has recently been shown in addition that RLIP76 is a multispecific transporter of chemotherapeutic agents and glutathione conjugates. One such conjugate is the adduct of GSH and 4-hydroxynonenal (HNE), which is a major end product of lipid peroxidation and also a cell signaling molecule [14]. However, the transport mechanisms are yet to be defined [79].

6.6 ROS-MEDIATED CELLULAR SIGNALING

The redox environment affects diverse cell responses such as cell growth, differentiation, and apoptosis. The role of H_2O_2 as a signal molecule in these processes is now well accepted. This oxidant takes part not only in host defense reactions (oxidative bursts), oxidative biosynthesis, and oxidative stress, but can also stimulate or regulate central factors in signal transduction pathways (for recent reviews, see References 66 and 80 to 82). The concept that H_2O_2 may function as a signaling agent is also central for understanding molecular mechanisms in a variety of human diseases [3, 82].

4-Hydroxynonenal (HNE) is another ROS-derived molecule, being formed during lipid peroxidation. It has been used as a mediator of oxidative damage. HNE is also involved in signal transduction and affects the cell cycle in a concentration-dependent manner [14], and may at low concentrations upregulate the transcription of several genes involved in GSH homeostasis and metabolism, including glutamate cysteine ligase (GCL) and γ-glutamyltransferase (GGT) and glutathione transferases (GSTs) [57, 83–85].

Several signaling pathways are sensitive to changes in ROS levels due to modifications of redox sensitive cysteinyl residues in various receptor tyrosine kinases

(RTKs), protein tyrosine phosphatases (PTPs), and transcription factors. After stimulation by various external factors, including growth factors and cytokines, cells will produce a controlled oxidative burst and generate a low concentration of ROS [10, 81]. This occurs through activation of enzymes, including lipoxygenase and NADPH oxidases, that produce superoxide ($\cdot O_2^-$). The superoxide is converted into H_2O_2 by superoxide dismutase (SOD), which may then diffuse across the plasma membrane and inactivate susceptible signaling molecules, including PTPs [86]. The thiolate form of cysteine residue in the active site of PTP is oxidized, resulting in reversible inactivation of the phosphatase. The oxidized residue can be reduced back to an active form by glutaredoxin, thioredoxin, or by GSH but the mechanisms have not been established [10, 87]. Inactivation of PTP will prolong and strengthen the external signal and will be a significant part of the activation of tyrosine kinase signaling cascades.

The NADPH oxidase systems (NOX) were studied originally in phagocytic leukocytes as the generator of ROS for host defense against bacterial and fungal pathogens. NADPH oxidase is now recognized as a central system in many redox regulated processes with important biological functions [10, 66, 88, 89]. Overexpression of NADPH oxidase is a frequent finding in cancer cells, which was first indicated from observations of increased H_2O_2 in cancer cells [10]. NADPH oxidase systems are also involved in other diseases such as atherosclerosis, defective immune function, and inflammatory bowel diseases, and may be important when searching for new treatment approaches.

6.7 TRANSCRIPTION REGULATION OF ANTIOXIDANT AND CONJUGATION ENZYMES

Cells will respond to oxidative and chemical stress by increasing the expression of several antioxidant and phase II drug-metabolizing enzymes. In this way, cells may restore their redox balance, increase the xenobiotic detoxification, and thus increase their survival chances. The upregulated transcription of these genes occurs in a coordinated and integrated fashion and has at least one common enhancer; termed the antioxidant response element, ARE (also called the electrophile response element, EpRE). This element is found in the promoter region of most genes that are induced by oxidative and chemical stress, and includes glutathione peroxidase (GPx), both subunits of the enzyme glutamate cysteine ligase (GCL), glutathione synthase (GS), glutathione reductase (GR), γ-glutamyltransferase (GGT), the light subunit of the cystine transporter (cystine/glutamate antiporter, X_c^-), glutathione transferase (GST), as well as peroxiredoxins and thioredoxins [8, 57, 82, 90].

Central transcription factors that are redox regulated include activator protein-1 (AP-1), nuclear factor-κB (NF-κB), and nuclear factor erythroid 2 (NF-E2) related factors 1 and 2 (Nrf1, Nrf2). AP-1 and NF-κB proteins are well known in regulation of the antioxidant enzymes mentioned above. However, the principal and essential ARE-binding proteins are the (NF-E2) related factors Nrf1 and mainly Nrf2. Data from both in vivo and in vitro studies shows that Nfr2 is essential in maintaining redox balance and thus cell survival after oxidative stress [8, 34, 91]. Nrf2 is activated by diverse oxidants and chemicals, and after phosphorylation and dissociation from a cytoplasmic inhibitor (Keap1), it translocates to the nucleus and binds to ARE in the promoter of multiple antioxidant enzymes and defense proteins [91, 92]. Nrf2 appears to involve several signal transcription pathways, including MAPK, PKC, and PI-3K pathways [8, 93–95]. An improved understanding of Nrf2 antioxidant pathways will provide new therapeutic strategies for treatment of human disorders in which oxidative and chemical stress are involved.

6.8 OXIDATIVE STRESS AND DISEASES

The redox environment can frequently be altered during diseases and changes in the redox state may also result in diseases. Changes in GSH levels and metabolism have been associated with various illnesses, including lung diseases, cancer, neurodegenerative diseases, cardiovascular diseases, liver diseases, and diabetes. Antioxidants as part of nutritional therapies to improve GSH status show great promise.

6.8.1 Lungs and Oxidative Injuries

The lungs are constantly exposed to atmospheric oxygen. Exposure to polluted air containing reactive oxygen and nitrogen species, mineral dust, or tobacco smoke can result in airway inflammation followed by increased oxidant burden due to accumulation of macrophages and leukocytes. On the other hand, oxidants are crucial for host defense against infections, also in the lungs. These oxidants may inactivate antiproteases, induce apoptosis, regulate cell proliferation, and modulate the immune system in the lungs [3, 96]. At the molecular level, the oxidants have been implicated in initiating inflammatory responses via activation of transcription factors such as NF-κB and AP-1 and regulating pro-inflammatory processes [97]. Aberrations in the redox balance can lead to various diseases, including asthma, acute respiratory distress syndrome, and chronic obstructive pulmonary diseases [3].

There is a very high concentration of GSH in the alveolar epithelial lining fluid, which also contains large amounts of glutathione peroxidase (both GPx1 and the extracellular GPx3) [98]. Expression of both subtypes can be induced by increased oxygen tension [28]. The fluid also contains glutathione reductase and NADPH for maintaining GSH in its reduced form [98]. In cystic fibrosis patients, a reduced level of GSH in the lower airways has been reported and oxidative stress may play a significant role in the pathophysiology of cystic fibrosis, and a higher intake of antioxidants has been recommended for these patients [99].

Increased lung damage has been reported in *nrf2* gene deficiency after exposure to oxidants such as cigarette smoke, diesel exhaust particles, and to hyperoxia. Apparently, Nrf2 is critical in pulmonary protection and it is suggested that the Nrf2 pathway can provide new therapeutic strategies for acute respiratory distress syndrome, cancer, and emphysema [93].

6.8.2 GSH Metabolism in Neurodegenerative Diseases

Distinct alterations in the redox state have been reported in neurodegenerative diseases such as Alzheimer's disease and Parkinson's disease. Several reports have described that GSH declines with age as well as in neurodegenerative diseases. This has been connected to a downregulation of glutamylcysteine ligase (GCL) and glutathione synthase (GS) expression. There are also reports on mitochondrial dysfunction, oxidative stress, and GSH depletion in brain tissue from patients with neurodegenerative diseases [82].

In brain tissue from Alzheimer's patients, an increase in mRNA level of both glutathione peroxidase (GPx) and glutathione reductase (GR) has been reported, whereas glutathione transferase (GST) and multidrug resistance protein-1 (MRP1) were apparently oxidatively damaged and dysfunctional [100]. Increased levels of the lipid oxidation product 4-hydroxynonenal (HNE) have been reported in brain tissue from such patients and from experimental animals, and a link between HNE and increased damage of mitochondria and subsequent GSH depletion has been suggested [85, 101]. The potential causative agent of Alzheimer's disease, amyloid β-peptide, results in oxidative stress and neurotoxicity both in vitro and in synaptosomes in vivo [101]. Injections of GSH and antioxidants increased the level of GSH and reduced the oxidative damage. Studies also indicate that increasing the antioxidative capacity through dietary or pharmacological intake of antioxidants can be beneficial in treatment of Alzheimer's disease [100, 101].

In Parkinson's disease less is known regarding enzymes involved but there is strong evidence of dysfunction in GSH metabolism in the development of the disease [82]. A number of studies have found that GSH is reduced in the substantia nigra of these patients, and there is a strong correlation between the severity of the disease and loss of GSH [102]. Both clinical findings and experiments on cultured dopaminergic cells have strongly indicated that a depletion of GSH will result in oxidative stress and decreased mitochondrial functions, probably due to an oxidation of complex I. Increased levels of peroxynitrite, usually neutralized by GSH, have been reported in Parkinson's disease [102].

6.8.3 GSH Metabolism in Cancer

The concept that GSH can protect against oxidative stress and against electrophiles has significant importance in cancer. In carcinogenesis, during tumor spread and metastasis as well as during tumor treatment, GSH metabolism in both cancer cells and in host cells is of central importance.

Several reports point to a direct involvement of GSH in inhibiting tumor initiation, promotion, and progression. A role of oxidative stress in cancer formation has been demonstrated in several epidemiological and clinical investigations [103, 104]. Factors such as tobacco, ethanol, and age may result in local oxidative stress and thus increased risk for cancer [105–107]. However, high levels of GSH in the host appear to protect against cancer development [108]. This must be due to the ability of GSH to bind and inactivate carcinogens and DNA damaging free radicals [109].

An inverse association has been observed between dietary intake of GSH from fruit and vegetables and a decreased risk of cancer in the oral cavity [110]. In prostate cancer, increased ROS levels due to androgens have been linked to cancer initiation [111].

On the other hand, high levels of GSH are frequently demonstrated in various cancer types. This includes tumors with multidrug and/or radiation resistance, such as melanoma, and cancer in colon, breast, and lung [112–116]. As tumors progress they tend to increase their resistance towards oxidative stress. In experimental metastasis a high number of circulating tumor cells are trapped in liver microvasculature. Endothelial cells will release harmful ROS in response to cancer cell contact, and kill the major portion of the cells. However, tumor cells surviving this oxidative stress situation show higher level of GSH, or increased ability to resynthesize GSH (for a review see Reference 6). In another study, selection of tumor cells through repeated in vivo passages showed higher levels of GSH and increased ability to resist oxidative stress [117].

Tumors with increased levels of GSH have higher resistance towards radiation and therapy. To sensitize cells to chemotherapy and radiotherapy, a combined strategy for depletion of GSH has been suggested [6]. This is based on reduction of the anti-apoptotic protein Bcl-2, inhibition of γ-glutamyltransferase (GGT), and accelerated efflux of GSH from malignant cells. In addition, improved knowledge regarding the mechanisms involved in ROS signaling and redox environment regulation will clearly offer improved treatment regimes.

REFERENCES

1. Halliwell, B. (1999). Antioxidant defence mechanisms: From the beginning to the end (of the beginning). *Free Radical Research*, *31*, 261–272.
2. Hayes, J.D., McLellan, L.I. (1999). Glutathione and glutathione-dependent enzymes represent a co-ordinately regulated defence against oxidative stress. *Free Radical Research*, *31*, 273–300.
3. Rahman, I., Biswas, S.K., Kode, A. (2006). Oxidant and antioxidant balance in the airways and airway diseases. *European Journal of Pharmacology*, *533*, 222–239.
4. Meister, A., Anderson, M.E. (1983). Glutathione. *Annual Review of Biochemistry*, *52*, 711–760.
5. Dickinson, D.A., Forman, H.J. (2002). Cellular glutathione and thiols metabolism. *Biochemical Pharmacology*, *64*, 1019–1026.
6. Estrela, J.M., Ortega, A., Obrador, E. (2006). Glutathione in cancer biology and therapy. *Critical Reviews in Clinical Laboratory Sciences*, *43*, 143–181.
7. Schafer, F.Q., Buettner, G.R. (2001). Redox environment of the cell as viewed through the redox state of the glutathione disulfide/glutathione couple. *Free Radical Biology and Medicine*, *30*, 1191–1212.
8. Masella, R., Di Benedetto, R., Varì, R., Filesi, C., Giovannini, C. (2005). Novel mechanisms of natural antioxidant compounds in biological systems: Involvement of glutathione and glutathione-related enzymes. *Journal of Nutritional Biochemistry*, *16*, 577–586.

9. Valko, M., Leibfritz, D., Moncol, J., Cronin, M.T., Mazur, M., Telser, J. (2007). Free radicals and antioxidants in normal physiological functions and human disease. *International Journal of Biochemistry & Cell Biology, 39*, 44–84.

10. Lambeth, J.D. (2004). NOX enzymes and the biology of reactive oxygen. *Nature Reviews. Immunology, 4*, 181–189.

11. Spiteller, G. (2006). Peroxyl radicals: Inductors of neurodegenerative and other inflammatory diseases. Their origin and how they transform cholesterol, phospholipids, plasmalogens, polyunsaturated fatty acids, sugars, and proteins into deleterious products. *Free Radical Biology and Medicine, 41*, 362–387.

12. Negre-Salvayre, A., Coatrieux, C., Ingueneau, C., Salvayre, R. (2008). Advanced lipid peroxidation end products in oxidative damage to proteins. Potential role in diseases and therapeutic prospects for the inhibitors. *British Journal of Pharmacology, 153*, 6–20.

13. Dianzani, M.U. (2003). 4-Hydroxynonenal from pathology to physiology. *Molecular Aspects of Medicine, 24*, 263–272.

14. Awasthi, Y.C., Yang, Y., Tiwari, N.K., Patrick, B., Sharma, A., Li, J., Awasthi, S. (2004). Regulation of 4-hydroxynonenal-mediated signaling by glutathione S-transferases. *Free Radical Biology and Medicine, 37*, 607–619.

15. Cohen, R.A., Adachi, T. (2006). Nitric-oxide-induced vasodilatation: Regulation by physiologic S-glutathiolation and pathologic oxidation of the sarcoplasmic endoplasmic reticulum calcium ATPase. *Trends in Cardiovascular Medicine, 16*, 109–114.

16. Kang, K.W., Choi, S.H., Kim, S.G. (2002). Peroxynitrite activates NF-E2-related factor 2/antioxidant response element through the pathway of phosphatidylinositol 3-kinase: The role of nitric oxide synthase in rat glutathione S-transferase A2 induction. *Nitric Oxide, 7*, 244–253.

17. Lim, S.Y., Jang, J.H., Na, H.K., Lu, S.C., Rahman, I., Surh, Y.J. (2004). 15-Deoxy-Delta12,14-prostaglandin J(2) protects against nitrosative PC12 cell death through up-regulation of intracellular glutathione synthesis. *Journal of Biological Chemistry, 279*, 46263–46270.

18. Li, M.H., Jang, J.H., Na, H.K., Cha, Y.N., Surh, Y.J. (2007). Carbon monoxide produced by upregulated heme oxygenase-1 in response to nitrosative stress induces expression of glutamate cysteine ligase in PC12 cells via activation of PI3K-Akt and Nrf2-ARE signaling. *Journal of Biological Chemistry, 282*, 28577–28586.

19. Huseby, N.E., Asare, N., Wetting, S., Mikkelsen, I.M., Mortensen, B., Sveinbjornsson, B., Wellman, M. (2003). Nitric oxide exposure of CC531 rat colon carcinoma cells induces γ-glutamyltransferase which may counteract glutathione depletion and cell death. *Free Radical Research, 37*, 99–107.

20. Townsend, D.M., Tew, K.D., Tapiero, H. (2003). The importance of glutathione in human disease. *Biomedicine & Pharmacotherapy, 57*, 145–155.

21. Mills, G.C. (1957). Hemoglobin catabolism. I. Glutathione peroxidase, an erythrocyte enzyme which protects hemoglobin from oxidative breakdown. *Journal of Biological Chemistry, 229*, 189–197.

22. Flohe, L., Gunzler, W.A., Schock, H.H. (1973). Glutathione peroxidase: A selenoenzyme. *FEBS Letters, 32*, 132–134.

23. Brigelius-Flohe, R. (2006). Glutathione peroxidases and redox-regulated transcription factors. *Biological Chemistry, 387*, 1329–1335.

24. Herbette, S., Roeckel-Drevet, P., Drevet, J.R. (2007). Seleno-independent glutathione peroxidases. More than simple antioxidant scavengers. *FEBS Journal, 274,* 2163–2180.

25. Comhair, S.A., Erzurum, S.C. (2005). The regulation and role of extracellular glutathione peroxidase. *Antioxidants & Redox Signaling, 7,* 72–79.

26. Papp, L.V., Lu, J., Holmgren, A., Khanna, K.K. (2007). From selenium to selenoproteins: Synthesis, identity, and their role in human health. *Antioxidants & Redox Signaling, 9,* 775–806.

27. Wingler, K., Bocher, M., Flohe, L., Kollmus, H., Brigelius-Flohe, R. (1999). mRNA stability and selenocysteine insertion sequence efficiency rank gastrointestinal glutathione peroxidase high in the hierarchy of selenoproteins. *European Journal of Biochemistry, 259,* 149–157.

28. Jornot, L., Junod, A.F. (1997). Hyperoxia, unlike phorbol ester, induces glutathione peroxidase through a protein kinase C-independent mechanism. *Biochemical Journal, 326,* 117–123.

29. Moscow, J.A., Morrow, C.S., He, R., Mullenbach, G.T., Cowan, K.H. (1992). Structure and function of the 5'-flanking sequence of the human cytosolic selenium-dependent glutathione peroxidase gene (hgpx1). *Journal of Biological Chemistry, 267,* 5949–5958.

30. Jornot, L., Junod, A.F. (1995). Differential regulation of glutathione peroxidase by selenomethionine and hyperoxia in endothelial cells. *Biochemical Journal, 306,* 581–587.

31. Cheng, W.H., Ho, Y.S., Valentine, B.A., Ross, D.A., Combs, G.F., Lei, X.G. (1998). Cellular glutathione peroxidase is the mediator of body selenium to protect against paraquat lethality in transgenic mice. *Journal of Nutrition, 128,* 1070–1076.

32. Brigelius-Flohe, R. (1999). Tissue-specific functions of individual glutathione peroxidases. *Free Radical Biology and Medicine, 27,* 951–965.

33. Esworthy, R.S., Yang, L., Frankel, P.H., Chu, F.F. (2005). Epithelium-specific glutathione peroxidase, Gpx2, is involved in the prevention of intestinal inflammation in selenium-deficient mice. *Journal of Nutrition, 135,* 740–745.

34. Banning, A., Deubel, S., Kluth, D., Zhou, Z., Brigelius-Flohe, R. (2005). The GI-GPx gene is a target for Nrf2. *Molecular and Cellular Biology, 25,* 4914–4923.

35. Heirman, I., Ginneberge, D., Brigelius-Flohe, R., Hendrickx, N., Agostinis, P., Brouckaert, P., Rottiers, P., Grooten, J. (2006). Blocking tumor cell eicosanoid synthesis by GPx4 impedes tumor growth and malignancy. *Free Radical Biology and Medicine, 40,* 285–294.

36. Banning, A., Schnurr, K., Bol, G.F., Kupper, D., Muller-Schmehl, K., Viita, H., Yla-Herttuala, S., Brigelius-Flohe, R. (2004). Inhibition of basal and interleukin-1-induced VCAM-1 expression by phospholipid hydroperoxide glutathione peroxidase and 15-lipoxygenase in rabbit aortic smooth muscle cells. *Free Radical Biology and Medicine, 36,* 135–144.

37. Conrad, M., Moreno, S.G., Sinowatz, F., Ursini, F., Kolle, S., Roveri, A., Brielmeier, M., Wurst, W., Maiorino, M., Bornkamm, G.W. (2005). The nuclear form of phospholipid hydroperoxide glutathione peroxidase is a protein thiol peroxidase contributing to sperm chromatin stability. *Molecular and Cellular Biology, 25,* 7637–7644.

38. Utomo, A., Jiang, X., Furuta, S., Yun, J., Levin, D.S., Wang, Y.C., Desai, K.V., Green, J. E., Chen, P.L., Lee, W.H. (2004). Identification of a novel putative non-selenocysteine containing phospholipid hydroperoxide glutathione peroxidase (NPGPx) essential for

alleviating oxidative stress generated from polyunsaturated fatty acids in breast cancer cells. *Journal of Biological Chemistry, 279,* 43522–43529.

39. Beutler, E. (1994). G6PD deficiency. *Blood, 84,* 3613–3636.

40. Arrigo, A.P., Virot, S., Chaufour, S., Firdaus, W., Kretz-Remy, C., Diaz-Latoud, C. (2005). Hsp27 consolidates intracellular redox homeostasis by upholding glutathione in its reduced form and by decreasing iron intracellular levels. *Antioxidants & Redox Signaling, 7,* 414–422.

41. Liu, R.M., Hu, H., Robison, T.W., Forman, H.J. (1996). Increased γ-glutamylcysteine synthetase and γ-glutamyl transpeptidase activities enhance resistance of rat lung epithelial L2 cells to quinone toxicity. *American Journal of Respiratory Cell and Molecular Biology, 14,* 192–197.

42. Shi, M.M., Kugelman, A., Iwamoto, T., Tian, L., Forman, H.J. (1994). Quinone-induced oxidative stress elevates glutathione and induces γ-glutamylcysteine synthetase activity in rat lung epithelial L2 cells. *Journal of Biological Chemistry, 269,* 26512–26517.

43. Bannai, S., Sato, H., Ishii, T., Sugita, Y. (1989). Induction of cystine transport activity in human fibroblasts by oxygen. *Journal of Biological Chemistry, 264,* 18480–18484.

44. Dickinson, D.A., Moellering, D.R., Iles, K.E., Patel, R.P., Levonen, A.L., Wigley, A., Darley-Usmar, V.M., Forman, H.J. (2003). Cytoprotection against oxidative stress and the regulation of glutathione synthesis. *Biological Chemistry, 384,* 527–537.

45. Griffith, O.W. (1999). Biologic and pharmacologic regulation of mammalian glutathione synthesis. *Free Radical Biology and Medicine, 27,* 922–935.

46. Sun, W.M., Huang, Z.Z., Lu, S.C. (1996). Regulation of γ-glutamylcysteine synthetase by protein phosphorylation. *Biochemical Journal, 320,* 321–328.

47. Tate, S.S., Meister, A. (1981). γ-glutamyl transpeptidase: Catalytic, structural and functional aspects. *Molecular and Cellular Biochemistry, 39,* 357–368.

48. Orlowski, M., Meister, A. (1970). The γ-glutamyl cycle: A possible transport system for amino acids. *Proceedings of the National Acadamy of Sciences USA, 67,* 1248–1255.

49. Curthoys, N.P., Hughey, R.P. (1979). Characterization and physiological function of rat renal γ-glutamyltranspeptidase. *Enzyme, 24,* 383–403.

50. Zhang, H., Forman, H.J., Choi, J. (2005). γ-glutamyl transpeptidase in glutathione biosynthesis. *Methods in Enzymology, 401,* 468–483.

51. Binkley, F., Nakamura, K. (1948). Metabolism of glutathione: Hydrolysis by tissues of the rat. *Journal of Biological Chemistry, 173,* 411–421.

52. Hanigan, M.H. (1995). Expression of γ-glutamyl transpeptidase provides tumor cells with a selective growth advantage at physiologic concentrations of cyst(e)ine. *Carcinogenesis, 16,* 181–185.

53. Karp, D.R., Shimooku, K., Lipsky, P.E. (2001). Expression of γ-glutamyl transpeptidase protects ramos B cells from oxidation-induced cell death. *Journal of Biological Chemistry, 276,* 3798–3804.

54. Lieberman, M.W., Wiseman, A.L., Shi, Z.Z., Carter, B.Z., Barrios, R., Ou, C.N., Chevez-Barrios, P., Wang, Y., Habib, G.M., Goodman, J.C., Huang, S.L., Lebovitz, R.M., Matzuk, M.M. (1996). Growth retardation and cysteine deficiency in γ-glutamyl transpeptidase-deficient mice. *Proceedings of the National Academy of Sciences USA, 93,* 7923–7926.

55. Barrios, R., Shi, Z.Z., Kala, S.V., Wiseman, A.L., Welty, S.E., Kala, G., Bahler, A.A., Ou, C.N., Lieberman, M.W. (2001). Oxygen-induced pulmonary injury in γ-glutamyl transpeptidase-deficient mice. *Lung, 179*, 319–330.

56. Pankiv, S., Moller, S., Bjorkoy, G., Moens, U., Huseby, N.E. (2006). Radiation-induced upregulation of γ-glutamyltransferase in colon carcinoma cells is mediated through the Ras signal transduction pathway. *Biochimica et Biophysica Acta, 1760*, 151–157.

57. Zhang, H., Liu, H., Dickinson, D.A., Liu, R.M., Postlethwait, E.M., Laperche, Y., Forman, H.J. (2006). γ-glutamyl transpeptidase is induced by 4-hydroxynonenal via EpRE/Nrf2 signaling in rat epithelial type II cells. *Free Radical Biology Medicine, 40*, 1281–1292.

58. Stipanuk, M.H., Dominy, J.E., Lee, J.I., Coloso, R.M. (2006). Mammalian cysteine metabolism: New insights into regulation of cysteine metabolism. *The Journal of Nutrition, 136*, 1652S–1659S.

59. Hanigan, M.H., Ricketts, W.A. (1993). Extracellular glutathione is a source of cysteine for cells that express γ-glutamyl transpeptidase. *Biochemistry, 32*, 6302–6306.

60. Griffith, O.W., Meister, A. (1979). Glutathione: Interorgan translocation, turnover, and metabolism. *Proceedings of the National Academy of Sciences USA, 76*, 5606–5610.

61. Garcia, R.A., Stipanuk, M.H. (1992). The splanchnic organs, liver and kidney have unique roles in the metabolism of sulfur amino acids and their metabolites in rats. *Journal of Nutrition, 122*, 1693–1701.

62. Jones, D.P. (2006). Extracellular redox state: Refining the definition of oxidative stress in aging. *Rejuvenation Research, 9*, 169–181.

63. Jones, D.P., Go, Y.M., Anderson, C.L., Ziegler, T.R., Kinkade, J.M., Kirlin, W.G. (2004). Cysteine/cystine couple is a newly recognized node in the circuitry for biologic redox signaling and control. *FASEB Journal, 18*, 1246–1248.

64. Anderson, C.L., Iyer, S.S., Ziegler, T.R., Jones, D.P. (2007). Control of extracellular cysteine/cystine redox state by HT-29 cells is independent of cellular glutathione. *American Journal of Physiology. Regulatory, Integrative and Comparative Physiology, 293*, R1069–R1075.

65. Banjac, A., Perisic, T., Sato, H., Seiler, A., Bannai, S., Weiss, N., Kolle, P., Tschoep, K., Issels, R.D., Daniel, P.T., Conrad, M., Bornkamm, G.W. (2008). The cystine/cysteine cycle: A redox cycle regulating susceptibility versus resistance to cell death. *Oncogene, 27*, 1618–1628.

66. Winyard, P.G., Moody, C.J., Jacob, C. (2005). Oxidative activation of antioxidant defence. *Trends in Biochemical Sciences. 30*, 453–461.

67. Halvey, P.J., Watson, W.H., Hansen, J.M., Go, Y.M., Samali, A., Jones, D.P. (2005). Compartmental oxidation of thiol-disulphide redox couples during epidermal growth factor signaling. *Biochemical Journal, 386*, 215–219.

68. Go, Y.M., Ziegler, T.R., Johnson, J.M., Gu, L., Hansen, J.M., Jones, D.P. (2007). Selective protection of nuclear thioredoxin-1 and glutathione redox systems against oxidation during glucose and glutamine deficiency in human colonic epithelial cells. *Free Radical Biology and Medicine, 42*, 363–370.

69. Sies, H., Cadenas, E. (1985). Oxidative stress: Damage to intact cells and organs. *Philosophical Transactions of the Royal Society of London. Series B, Biological Sciences, 311*, 617–631.

70. Jones, D.P. (2006). Redefining oxidative stress. *Antioxidants & Redox Signaling, 8,* 1865–1879.

71. Klaassen, C.D. (2001). *Casarett & Doull's Toxicology: The Basic Science of Poisons.* New York: McGraw-Hill.

72. Zamek-Gliszczynski, M.J., Hoffmaster, K.A., Nezasa, K., Tallman, M.N., Brouwer, K.L. (2006). Integration of hepatic drug transporters and phase II metabolizing enzymes: Mechanisms of hepatic excretion of sulfate, glucuronide, and glutathione metabolites. *European Journal of Pharmaceutical Sciences, 27,* 447–486.

73. Hayes, J.D., Flanagan, J.U., Jowsey, I.R. (2005). Glutathione transferases. *Annual Review of Pharmacology and Toxicology, 45,* 51–88.

74. Frova, C. (2006). Glutathione transferases in the genomics era: New insights and perspectives. *Biomolecular Engineering, 23,* 149–169.

75. Townsend, D.M., Tew, K.D. (2003). The role of glutathione-S-transferase in anti-cancer drug resistance. *Oncogene, 22,* 7369–7375.

76. Higgins, C.F. (1992). ABC transporters: From microorganisms to man. *Annual Review of Cell Biology, 8,* 67–113.

77. Cole, S.P., Deeley, R.G. (2006). Transport of glutathione and glutathione conjugates by MRP1. *Trends in Pharmacological Sciences, 27,* 438–446.

78. Deeley, R.G., Westlake, C., Cole, S.P. (2006). Transmembrane transport of endo- and xenobiotics by mammalian ATP-binding cassette multidrug resistance proteins. *Physiological Reviews, 86,* 849–899.

79. Yadav, S., Zajac, E., Singhal, S.S., Awasthi, S. (2007). Linking stress-signaling, glutathione metabolism, signaling pathways and xenobiotic transporters. *Cancer Metastasis Reviews, 26,* 59–69.

80. Stone, J.R., Yang, S. (2006). Hydrogen peroxide: A signaling messenger. *Antioxidants & Redox Signaling, 8,* 243–270.

81. Salmeen, A., Barford, D. (2005). Functions and mechanisms of redox regulation of cysteine-based phosphatases. *Antioxidants & Redox Signaling, 7,* 560–577.

82. Maher, P. (2006). Redox control of neural function: Background, mechanisms, and significance. *Antioxidants & Redox Signaling, 8,* 1941–1970.

83. Iles, K.E., Liu, R.M. (2005). Mechanisms of glutamate cysteine ligase (GCL) induction by 4-hydroxynonenal. *Free Radical Biology and Medicine, 38,* 547–556.

84. Dickinson, D.A., Levonen, A.L., Moellering, D.R., Arnold, E.K., Zhang, H., Darley-Usmar, V.M., Forman, H.J. (2004). Human glutamate cysteine ligase gene regulation through the electrophile response element. *Free Radical Biology and Medicine, 37,* 1152–1159.

85. Volkel, W., Sicilia, T., Pahler, A., Gsell, W., Tatschner, T., Jellinger, K., Leblhuber, F., Riederer, P., Lutz, W.K., Gotz, M.E. (2006). Increased brain levels of 4-hydroxy-2-nonenal glutathione conjugates in severe Alzheimer's disease. *Neurochemistry International, 48,* 679–686.

86. Denu, J.M., Tanner, K.G. (1998). Specific and reversible inactivation of protein tyrosine phosphatases by hydrogen peroxide: Evidence for a sulfenic acid intermediate and implications for redox regulation. *Biochemistry, 37,* 5633–5642.

87. Rahman, I., Biswas, S.K., Jimenez, L.A., Torres, M., Forman, H.J. (2005). Glutathione, stress responses, and redox signaling in lung inflammation. *Antioxidants & Redox Signaling, 7,* 42–59.

88. Benhar, M., Engelberg, D., Levitzki, A. (2002). ROS, stress-activated kinases and stress signaling in cancer. *EMBO Reports*, *3*, 420–425.

89. Fruehauf, J.P., Meyskens, F.L. (2007). Reactive oxygen species: A breath of life or death? *Clinical Cancer Research*, *13*, 789–794.

90. Cho, S.H., Lee, C.H., Ahn, Y., Kim, H., Ahn, C.Y., Yang, K.S., Lee, S.R. (2004). Redox regulation of PTEN and protein tyrosine phosphatases in H(2)O(2) mediated cell signaling. *FEBS Letters*, *560*, 7–13.

91. Walters, D.M., Cho, H.Y., Kleeberger, S.R. (2008). Oxidative stress and antioxidants in the pathogenesis of pulmonary fibrosis: A potential role for Nrf2. *Antioxidants & Redox Signaling*, *10*, 321–332.

92. Motohashi, H., Yamamoto, M. (2004). Nrf2-Keap1 defines a physiologically important stress response mechanism. *Trends in Molecular Medicine*, *10*, 549–557.

93. Cho, H.Y., Reddy, S.P., Kleeberger, S.R. (2006). Nrf2 defends the lung from oxidative stress. *Antioxidants & Redox Signaling*, *8*, 76–87.

94. Feng, R., Lu, Y., Bowman, L.L., Qian, Y., Castranova, V., Ding, M. (2005). Inhibition of activator protein-1, NF-kappaB, and MAPKs and induction of phase 2 detoxifying enzyme activity by chlorogenic acid. *Journal of Biological Chemistry*, *280*, 27888–27895.

95. Papaiahgari, S., Zhang, Q., Kleeberger, S.R., Cho, H.Y., Reddy, S.P. (2006). Hyperoxia stimulates an Nrf2-ARE transcriptional response via ROS-EGFR-PI3K-Akt/ERK MAP kinase signaling in pulmonary epithelial cells. *Antioxidants & Redox Signaling*, *8*, 43–52.

96. Folkerts, G., Kloek, J., Muijsers, R.B., Nijkamp, F.P. (2001). Reactive nitrogen and oxygen species in airway inflammation. *European Journal of Pharmacology*, *429*, 251–262.

97. Rahman, I., Yang, S.R., Biswas, S.K. (2006). Current concepts of redox signaling in the lungs. *Antioxidants & Redox Signaling*, *8*, 681–689.

98. Cantin, A.M., North, S.L., Hubbard, R.C., Crystal, R.G. (1987). Normal alveolar epithelial lining fluid contains high levels of glutathione. *Journal of Applied Physiology*, *63*, 152–157.

99. Cantin, A.M., White, T.B., Cross, C.E., Forman, H.J., Sokol, R.J., Borowitz, D. (2007). Antioxidants in cystic fibrosis. Conclusions from the CF antioxidant workshop, Bethesda, Maryland. *Free Radical Biology and Medicine*, *42*, 15–31.

100. Sultana, R., Butterfield, D.A. (2004). Oxidatively modified GST and MRP1 in Alzheimer's disease brain: Implications for accumulation of reactive lipid peroxidation products. *Neurochemical Research*, *29*, 2215–2220.

101. Ansari, M.A., Joshi, G., Huang, Q., Opii, W.O., Abdul, H.M., Sultana, R., Butterfield, D.A. (2006). In vivo administration of D609 leads to protection of subsequently isolated gerbil brain mitochondria subjected to in vitro oxidative stress induced by amyloid beta--peptide and other oxidative stressors: Relevance to Alzheimer's disease and other oxidative stress-related neurodegenerative disorders. *Free Radical Biology and Medicine*, *41*, 1694–1703.

102. Bharath, S., Andersen, J.K. (2005). Glutathione depletion in a midbrain-derived immortalized dopaminergic cell line results in limited tyrosine nitration of mitochondrial complex I subunits: Implications for Parkinson's disease. *Antioxidants & Redox Signaling*, *7*, 900–910.

103. Ray, G., Batra, S., Shukla, N.K., Deo, S., Raina, V., Ashok, S., Husain, S.A. (2000). Lipid peroxidation, free radical production and antioxidant status in breast cancer. *Breast Cancer Research and Treatment*, *59*, 163–170.

104. Sander, C.S., Chang, H., Hamm, F., Elsner, P., Thiele, J.J. (2004). Role of oxidative stress and the antioxidant network in cutaneous carcinogenesis. *International Journal of dermatology*, *43*, 326–335.

105. Hecht, S.S. (1999). Tobacco smoke carcinogens and lung cancer. *Journal of the National Cancer Institute*, *91*, 1194–1210.

106. Poschl, G., Seitz, H.K. (2004). Alcohol and cancer. *Alcohol and Alcoholism*, *39*, 155–165.

107. Droge, W. (2003). Oxidative stress and aging. *Advances in Experimental Medicine and Biology*, *543*, 191–200.

108. Locigno, R., Castronovo, V. (2001). Reduced glutathione system: Role in cancer development, prevention and treatment (review). *International Journal of Oncology*, *19*, 221–236.

109. Sies, H. (1999). Glutathione and its role in cellular functions. *Free Radical Biology and Medicine*, *27*, 916–921.

110. Flagg, E.W., Coates, R.J., Jones, D.P., Byers, T.E., Greenberg, R.S., Gridley, G., McLaughlin, J.K., Blot, W.J., Haber, M., Preston-Martin, S., Schoenberg, J.B., Austin, D.F., Fraumeni, J.F., Jr. (1994). Dietary glutathione intake and the risk of oral and pharyngeal cancer. *American Journal of Epidemiology*, *139*, 453–465.

111. Ripple, M.O., Henry, W.F., Rago, R.P., Wilding, G. (1997). Prooxidant-antioxidant shift induced by androgen treatment of human prostate carcinoma cells. *Journal of the National Cancer Institute*, *89*, 40–48.

112. Estrela, J.M., Obrador, E., Navarro, J., Lasso De la Vega, M.C., Pellicer, J.A. (1995). Elimination of Ehrlich tumours by ATP-induced growth inhibition, glutathione depletion and X-rays. *Nature Medicine*, *1*, 84–88.

113. Carretero, J., Obrador, E., Anasagasti, M.J., Martin, J.J., Vidal-Vanaclocha, F., Estrela, J.M. (1999). Growth-associated changes in glutathione content correlate with liver metastatic activity of B16 melanoma cells. *Clinical & Experimental Metastasis*, *17*, 567–574.

114. Honda, T., Coppola, S., Ghibelli, L., Cho, S.H., Kagawa, S., Spurgers, K.B., Brisbay, S.M., Roth, J.A., Meyn, R.E., Fang, B., McDonnell, T.J. (2004). GSH depletion enhances adenoviral bax-induced apoptosis in lung cancer cells. *Cancer Gene Therapy*, *11*, 249–255.

115. Berger, S.J., Gosky, D., Zborowska, E., Willson, J.K., Berger, N.A. (1994). Sensitive enzymatic cycling assay for glutathione: Measurements of glutathione content and its modulation by buthionine sulfoximine in vivo and in vitro in human colon cancer. *Cancer Research*, *54*, 4077–4083.

116. Perry, R.R., Mazetta, J.A., Levin, M., Barranco, S.C. (1993). Glutathione levels and variability in breast tumors and normal tissue. *Cancer*, *72*, 783–787.

117. Andreassen, K., Mortensen, B., Winberg, J.O., Huseby, N.E. (2002). Increased resistance towards oxidative stress accompanies enhancement of metastatic potential obtained by repeated in vivo passage of colon carcinoma cells in syngeneic rats. *Clinical & Experimental Metastasis*, *19*, 623–629.

CHAPTER 7

GLUTAREDOXIN AND THIOREDOXIN ENZYME SYSTEMS: CATALYTIC MECHANISMS AND PHYSIOLOGICAL FUNCTIONS

ELIZABETH A. SABENS and JOHN J. MIEYAL

7.1 INTRODUCTION

Antioxidant defense inside cells is dependent in large part on sulfur-containing amino acids in proteins and nonprotein cofactors. Prominent in this role is the nonprotein tripeptide glutathione (GSH) which is abundant within the cellular milieu. The sulfhydryl chemistry of both GSH and protein cysteine residues is critical for many cellular functions, including cell growth, cell death, cell survival, and cell signaling. Since sulfhydryl redox status plays such an important role in the regulation of cell function, it is easy to perceive how perturbations of the antioxidant system, including GSH and sulfur amino acids, can be linked to abnormal cell functioning, aging, and many diseases, among them neurodegenerative diseases, arthritis, diabetes, cardiovascular disorders, AIDS, and cancer [1]. Oxidative stimuli, either through normal cell signaling or overt oxidative stress associated with many disease conditions, are associated with modifications of the sulfur-containing amino acids, Cysteine (Cys) and Methionine (Met), with subsequent effects on protein function and intracellular homeostasis (Fig. 7.1). Within cells, oxidants alter free cysteine residues in either a reversible or irreversible fashion. Irreversible oxidations include sulfinic (RSO_2H) and sulfonic (RSO_3H) acid formation, usually leading to increased protein degradation. In contrast, reversible thiol modifications, mainly through formation of protein mixed disulfides with GSH, that is, protein-glutathionylation, as well as other reversible thiol modifications including intramolecular disulfides, intermolecular disulfides, and protein sulfenic acids, are thought to protect proteins from degradation allowing for a return to normal function after the oxidant challenge has subsided (Fig. 7.2).

Glutathione and Sulfur Amino Acids in Human Health and Disease. Edited by R. Masella and G. Mazza
Copyright © 2009 John Wiley & Sons, Inc.

Cellular Signaling and Oxidative Stress Modify Cysteine Residues of Proteins Affecting Signal Transduction Pathways in Cells

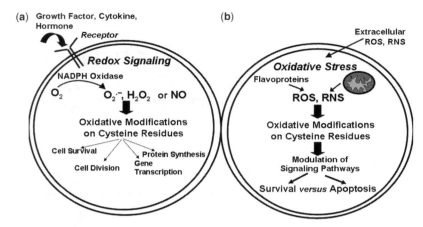

Figure 7.1 (a) Sulfhydryl modifications on cysteine residues initiated by physiological stimuli such as growth factors or hormones lead to the production of reactive oxygen species (ROS, e.g., superoxide and hydrogen peroxide) or reactive nitrogen species (RNS, e.g., nitric oxide) and propagate cell signaling cascades. (b) Sulfhydryl modification in response to oxidative stress either provided extracellularly via ROS or RNS, or intracellularly from the mitochondrial electron transport chain or from cytosolic or endoplasmic reticular flavoproteins, or nitric oxide synthase. Perturbation of redox homeostasis can shift the cell from survival to programmed cell death (apoptosis).

Sulfhydryl Homeostasis and Regulation: Oxidation & Regeneration of Vital Proteins

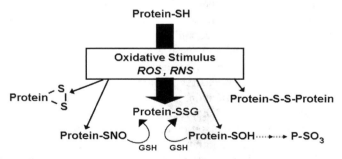

Figure 7.2 Oxidative stimulus leads to multiple types of sulfyhydryl modifications, including intramolecular disulfides, intermolecular disulfides, glutathionyl-protein mixed disulfides, protein sulfenic acids, and nitrosylated proteins. The latter two readily form protein-SSG mixed disulfides upon interaction with glutathione. Protein sulfenic acids also can be further oxidized to the irreversible protein sulfinic and sulfonic acids.

Oxidative modifications of Cys sulfhydryl moieties must be reduced to restore protein function, and this homeostatic process is catalyzed by enzymes. An important class of enzymes called thiol-disulfide oxidoreductases (TDORs) is involved in catalyzing thiol-disulfide exchange reactions occurring on the cysteine-thiol groups. The two principal TDORs that are involved in sulfhydryl homeostasis within cellular systems are thioredoxin (Trx) and glutaredoxin (Grx), which catalyze the reduction of disulfide bonds in both protein and nonprotein substrates [2, 3]. Each of these TDOR enzyme types has displayed substrate selectivities and redox potentials indicative of distinct physiological functions. Thioredoxin effectively reduces intramolecular and intermolecular disulfides bonds as well as sulfenic acids [4]. Glutaredoxin specifically reduces protein-glutathione mixed disulfides (Protein-SSG) [3]. Figure 7.3 illustrates the catalytic cycles for both Grx and Trx which are discussed below in their respective sections on mechanism of action. The special characteristics of the thioredoxin and glutaredoxin enzyme systems suggest different but complimentary functions for them, likely acting synergistically to maintain the thiol status in various types of cells.

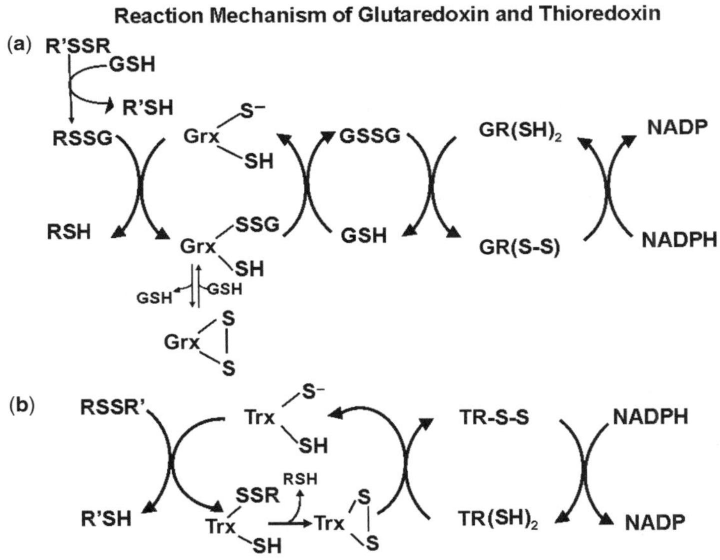

Figure 7.3 (a) Monothiol mechanism of glutaredoxin (Grx), showing specificity for glutathionylated substrates. Efficient catalysis cycles around intermediate formation of a covalent enzyme-glutathione mixed disulfide intermediate (Grx-SSG) not involving the second cys residue at the active site. Nonglutathione-containing disulfides must first react with GSH to form the actual substrate for Grx (upper left). Grx can form an intramolecular disulfide, but this detracts from catalysis and must react with GSH to return to the effective catalytic cycle. Grx-SSG is reduced by GSH, forming the dimeric disulfide, GSSG. GSSG is subsequently reduced by GSSG reductase (GR) and NADPH. (b) Thioredoxin (Trx) dithiol mechanism shows preference for reduction of inter- or intramolecular disulfides. The intramolecular disulfide form of Trx is reduced by thioredoxin reductase (TR) and NADPH.

Ribbon Diagrams of Thioredoxin And Glutaredoxin

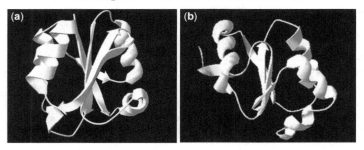

Figure 7.4 Ribbon diagrams of thioredoxin (Trx) and glutaredoxin (Grx) showing similar three-dimensional protein structures, namely the so-called thioredoxin fold. (a) Structure of reduced Trx. (b) Structure of reduced Grx. (a) From [159]. Used with permission. (b) From [160]. Used with permission.

TDORs have a characteristic active site motif of four amino acids, Cys-Xaa-Xaa-Cys, and they exhibit a similar three-dimensional structure referred to as the "thioredoxin fold," which is comprised of five β sheets enfolded within four α helices (Fig. 7.4). The TDORs featured in this chapter, Grx and Trx, are small (approximately 12 kDa), heat-stable proteins. Mechanistically, Grx and Trx function differently in their primary catalytic reactions, with Grx utilizing only one of the active site cysteines to effect specific reduction of glutathione-containing mixed disulfides (i.e., a monothiol mechanism) [5, 6], whereas Trx uses both cysteines in the active site to reduce intramolecular disulfides (i.e., a dithiol mechanism) [7]. Grx and Trx are recycled from their oxidized forms by separate enzyme systems dependent on the common cofactor NADPH (Fig. 7.3).

Protein disulfide isomerase (PDI), another member of the TDOR family, is an abundant enzyme, present at millimolar levels in the endoplasmic reticulum. Its key function is to promote the correct pairing of cysteine residues on proteins with multiple structural disulfide bonds and thereby ensure proper folding of the proteins. Containing two catalytic sites with CXXC motifs, one near the N-terminus and the other near the C-terminus, PDI mediates both oxidant and reductant catalysis in the formation and isomerization of intramolecular disulfide bonds [8, 9]. The remainder of this chapter is devoted to the two major types of TDORs involved in cysteine homeostasis and cell signaling regulation, namely glutaredoxin and thioredoxin.

7.2 GENERAL CHARACTERISTICS OF GLUTAREDOXINS

The family of enzymes called glutaredoxins (Grx), also known as *thioltransferases* according to the reactions that they catalyze, are part of the broader TDOR family. As indicated above, the distinguishing reaction catalyzed by the Grx enzymes is reduction of protein-glutathione mixed disulfides or protein-SSG via thiol-disulfide exchange (i.e., thiol transfer). *S*-glutathionylation of specific Cys residues on particular proteins occurs as a normal physiological response to extracellular effectors (hormones, cytokines, etc.). This modification allows propagation of cell signaling cascades initiated by reactive oxygen species (ROS) or reactive nitrogen species (RNS) acting as second messengers. Protein-SSG formation also serves as a homeostatic response under oxidative stress conditions to prevent irreversible oxidation of the thiol moieties of cysteine residues on proteins (Fig. 7.2). Analogous to kinase signaling pathways where the extent of phosphorylation is regulated by phosphatases (enzymes that remove a phosphate group from phosphorylated serine, threonine, or tyrosine residues on proteins) glutaredoxins deglutathionylate proteins, specifically and efficiently removing the glutathione and restoring the reduced Cys-SH residue [3, 5, 10, 11].

There are two forms of Grx that have been characterized in mammals, Grx1 and Grx2. However, five forms of Grx (Grx1-5) have been identified in *Escherichia coli* and yeast, and the gene for a mammalian form of Grx5 has been reported. Grx1 was discovered first in mutants of *E. coli* where the thioredoxin gene had been ablated, apparently providing a redundant or compensatory mechanism for electron donation to ribonucleotide reductase [12]. Grx1 contains a CXXC motif at its active site with the specific sequence of CPYC [13]. The Grx1 isoform is the better characterized isoform in mammalian systems, present in micromolar levels in mammalian cells [14]. Grx1 is primarily localized to the cytosol, and it has also recently being shown to exist in the intermembrane space of mitochondria [15, 16]; however, the specific functions of Grx1 in the mitochondria have yet to be elucidated. Localization of Grx1 in the nucleus of particular types of cells has been reported previously in immunocytochemical studies, specifically in the nuclei of calf cells [17], and within the stromal and epithelial cells of the human cervix [18–20]. In overexpression studies, Grx1 in HEK293 cells was evident in both the cytosol and the nucleus [21]. Despite these reports, neither confocal microscopy of immunostained cells nor isolation of Grx1 from purified nuclei has been performed to ensure that Grx1 does indeed exist in the nucleus. These studies will need to be extended to include analysis of endogenous Grx1 to determine if Grx1 exists normally in the nucleus, or if it translocates there under certain stimuli.

A second mammalian glutaredoxin (Grx2), containing 164 amino acids with a molecular weight of 18 kDa was discovered by an unusual database search which focused on particular domains rather than overall sequence similarity. Grx2 displays only about 30% sequence homology to Grx1 [10, 22, 23]. Among the differences in amino acid sequences is a change in the active site motif from CPYC to CSYC. To date, two human clones of Grx2 have been discovered, named Grx2a and Grx2b because of their distinct N-terminal sequences. Sequence analysis also identified a mitochondrial localization sequence in Grx2a which is cleaved upon entry into the mitochondrion altering its size to 16 kDa. Confirmation of mitochondrial localization was performed with a GFP fusion protein [22], and via analysis of isolated mitochondria in which matrix localization of Grx2 was documented [15]. Within the mitochondria, Grx2a is reported to exist as a dimer associated with a 2Fe-2S cluster [24] involving coordination by four Cys residues, two from the active sites of each Grx2 enzyme, and two from coordinated GSH molecules [25]. The second splice variant, referred to as Grx2b, was also tagged with GFP showing localization

Cellular Localization of Glutaredoxin, Thioredoxin, GSSG Reductase, and Thioredoxin Reducatase

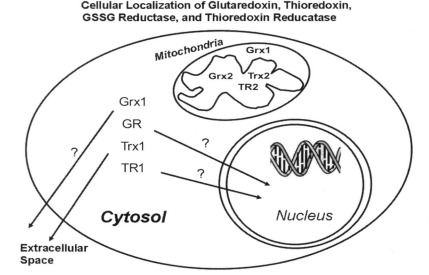

Figure 7.5 Diagram depicting the localization of thioredoxin (Trx) and glutaredoxin (Grx) isoforms as well as their corresponding reductases. Question marks indicate need for further study to document the proposed translocations. GR, GSSG reductase; TR, thioredoxin reductase.

to the perinuclear region; however, no putative nuclear localization sequence has been identified [23]. Despite lacking a nuclear localization sequence, Grx2b appears in the nucleus of certain reproductive cell types [10]. Localization of Grx2b to the nucleus would have multiple functional consequences, including regulation of transcription factors. However localization studies have yet to be conclusive, and functional studies have yet to be performed on isolated nuclei confirming localization and activity within the nucleus. Subcellular localization of Grx isoforms is depicted in Fig. 7.5.

A Grx5 homolog has been discovered in the mammalian genome, and is expressed during embryonic development in the mouse. However, its catalytic activity and functional roles have not yet been characterized, although it has been implicated in heme synthesis [16, 26, 27]. As indicated above, other isoforms of Grx exist in yeast, including Grx3, Grx4, and Grx5. At 16 kDa, Grx5 has been implicated in the formation of Fe-S clusters in mitochondrial biosynthesis in yeast where loss of Grx5 results in mitochondrial Fe accumulation and increased production of reactive oxygen species [27]. Grx5-deficient yeast mutants have also been shown to have impaired growth [26].

7.3 GENERAL CHARACTERISTICS OF THIOREDOXINS

Thioredoxin enzymes are characterized by a thioredoxin fold as well as the CXXC motif at the active site, specifically CGPC, and they are reported to selectively catalyze the reduction of intra- and intermolecular disulfides as well as protein sulfenic acids

[28, 29]. There are many members of the Trx family in all of biology; however, only two, Trx1 and Trx2, have been characterized in mammals. As shown in Fig. 7.5, Trx1 and Trx2 are localized in different compartments within the cell, namely, the cytosol and the mitochondria, along with the corresponding reductases, TR1 and TR2. The well-studied Trx1 system has been linked to cell signaling, cell growth, promotion of cell survival, and initiation of an immune response [30, 31].

Thioredoxin1, a 12 kDa protein, was initially discovered in *E. coli* as an electron donor to ribonucleotide reductases [32]. Human Trx1, which like Grx is ubiquitously expressed, was initially identified under multiple names, including adult T cell leukemia-derived factor, early pregnancy factor, and interleukin-2 receptor inducing factor, as a 105 amino acid protein with a molecular weight of 13 kDa [33]. Mammalian Trx1 contains three nonactive site cysteines (Cys 62, Cys 69, and Cys 73) which are not found in bacterial Trx [9, 30]. Upon oxidation of these Cys residues, Trx undergoes protein aggregation and loss of activity [7].

Trx1 is mainly a cytosolic enzyme, playing critical roles in redox homeostasis as well as in cellular signaling. It has been shown to translocate to the nucleus under overexpression conditions or be exported from the cell under certain stimuli including UV irradiation as demonstrated by immunocytochemistry [10, 34].

The Trx1 knockout mouse is embryonic lethal, illustrating its importance for mammalian development and its necessity to ribonucleotide reductases [35]. In contrast, the Grx1 knockout mouse is not embryonic lethal. Grx1 knockout does not impair development of the normal mouse [36], neither does the depletion of GSH interfere with DNA synthesis and ribonucleotide reductase activity in cell culture models [36, 37]. This strongly implicates Trx1 as the more important hydrogen donor to ribonucleotide reductase, distinguishing it from Grx1, which is more strongly implicated in other physiological functions (described below).

A second form of thioredoxin, Trx2, is localized to the mitochondria and contains an active site CGPC motif like Trx1. Unlike Trx1, Trx2 lacks any peripheral cysteine residues, and it contains a mitochondrial localization sequence, accounting for its larger initial size of 18 kDa [38]. However, Trx2 isolated from mitochondria lacks the 60 amino acid mitochondrial import sequence, reflecting an intramitochondrial size of 12 kDa, similar to that of Trx1 [38].

Other isoforms of thioredoxin were discovered through database searches of the human testis cDNA library. Each was identified by its CXXC motifs, and these include $p32^{TrxL}$, Sp-Trx-1, Sp-Trx-2, and Sp-Trx-3. Having a mass of 32 kDa, $p32^{TrxL}$ possesses high sequence homology to Trx1 in its 105 amino acid N-terminal region. However, neither the full length protein nor the truncated N-terminal portion were able to be reduced by thioredoxin reductase (TR) and NADPH, therefore actual Trx-like function has yet to be confirmed [39]. The three Sp-Trx isoforms are proposed to play roles in the regulation of spermatogenesis [40]. Sp-Trx-1, a 53 kDa protein, has two domains, the C-terminal domain resembles the typical Trx domain and the N-terminal domain contains 23 repeats of a 15 residue motif. Sp-Trx-1 was discovered to have Trx-like activity through reduction of the disulfide bonds in insulin, a common assay substrate for Trx, albeit with very little efficiency [41]. Sp-Trx-2, slightly larger than Sp-Trx-1 at 67 kDa, contains an N-terminal domain identical to Trx1. However, unlike Sp-Trx-1, Sp-Trx-2 failed to show Trx-like activity.

Sp-Trx-3, the least studied of the three isoforms, has one Trx domain [42]; however, Trx-like activity was not seen [42].

Migratory inhibitory factor (MIF) is secreted under oxidative stress conditions by T lymphocytes and macrophages to regulate macrophage migration as an inflammatory cytokine and endocrine factor [43]. Involved in both innate and acquired immunity, MIF, a 12.5 kDa protein, has TDOR-like catalytic activity with an atypical catalytic CXXC motif, namely CALC. MIF has no structural similarity to Trx; however, MIF must undergo a conformational change to become active and successfully reduce its substrates. Another potential member of the Trx family is glycosylation inhibitory factor (GIF), which has high sequence homology and three-dimensional structural similarity to MIF, and it may indeed be the same protein [43].

Nucleoredoxin, a 69 kDa protein, is another member of the Trx family containing a CXXC motif as its active site consisting of WCPPC. It has similar efficiency to that of bacterial Trx in the insulin reduction assay [44]. It was first isolated from mice utilizing a yeast artificial chromosome and was later shown to be conserved in the DNA in mammalian species. Nucleoredoxin is expressed in all tissues with highest expression in testis and skin. Nuclear localization when it is overexpressed in Cos-7 and NIH 3T3 cells is the basis for the name. However, localization of endogenous nucleoredoxin may be different since overexpression may promote accumulation in non-natural locales. In developing embryos, the expression of nucleoredoxin is restricted to the developing limbs, suggesting a role in regional patterning during development [45]. If nucleoredoxin is localized to the nucleus naturally, this would implicate it in the regulation of transcription factors, altering their redox status and potentially their activity.

Another apparent member of the Trx family is the TGF-β responsive gene product, transmembrane thioredoxin-like protein (TMX), which is shown to localize to the endoplasmic reticulum. TMX has a molecular weight of 31.8 kDa and it contains an atypical CXXC motif, CPAC, as well as a transmembrane domain. It is thought that the N-terminal sequence of TMX protrudes into the luminal face of the ER; however, the normal retention signal for the ER, typically the amino acid sequence KDEL, does not exist on TMX. Overexpression of active TMX inhibits apoptosis by brefeldin A, an inducer of ER stress by interfering with trafficking to the Golgi complex. TMX does exhibit TDOR-like activity; however, its activity has not been compared to that of Trx1 [46].

7.4 GLUTAREDOXIN MECHANISM OF ACTION

Grx functions with GSH as the cosubstrate to reduce protein-SSG mixed disulfides, as shown in Fig. 7.3. Grx works via a monothiol mechanism through a selective double displacement reaction in which the nucleophilic attack is performed by the N-terminal active site Cys of the CPYC motif, which exists as a thiolate anion due to its unusually low pKa of 3.5 [47]. The glutathionylated sulfur moiety of the protein-SSG is attacked by the thiolate anion of the enzyme (Grx-S$^-$), forming the covalent enzyme intermediate (Grx-SSG) and releasing the reduced protein-SH as the first product.

The second, rate-determining step involves reduction of the Grx-SSG by GSH to produce glutathione disulfide (GSSG) as the second product, and recycle the reduced enzyme (Grx-S$^-$) [48, 49]. GSSG is subsequently reduced to GSH by GSSG reductase (GR) and NADPH. Also, in systemic kinetics studies Grx (thioltransferase) was shown to be specific for glutathione-containing disulfides as the first substrate [6, 48, 50, 51], and GSH is the preferred second substrate [52] for the two-step reaction (details reviewed in Reference 3).

Both a monothiol mechanism, that is, requiring only one active site Cys, and a dithiol mechanism, that is, requiring both active site Cys, have been proposed for Grx activity. However, the monothiol mechanism is prevalent. Mutagenesis studies that replace the second Cys at the active site (distal from the C-terminus) have supported the monothiol mechanism. When this Cys is replaced (e.g., by serine, C25S mutation of human Grx1), Grx1 retains its normal catalytic function, and in fact becomes a better catalyst than the natural enzyme with both Cys residues at the active site [6]. This observation documents that the side reaction involving formation of the intramolecular disulfide form of the enzyme (C22-SS-C25) detracts from catalysis (Fig. 7.3). Nevertheless, others have proposed an alternative dithiol mechanism for Grx-mediated thiol-disulfide exchange analogous to the catalytic scheme proposed for Trx (Fig. 7.3). For example, a dithiol mechanism has been proposed for Grx1 catalysis of reduction of ribonucleotide reductase; however, specific kinetic data or other documentation were not provided [53]. In fact, Grx is likely to play a subordinate role, if any role at all, in the reduction of ribonucleotide reductase in mammalian cells, because knockout of the enzyme is not embryonic lethal in mice [37], contrasting with the lethal effect of Trx knockout, nor does knocking out Grx in cell lines alter DNA synthesis [38, 54]. Similarly, it was proposed previously that Grx operates through a dithiol mechanism in reducing dehydroascorbic acid (DHA, i.e., oxidized vitamin C) [47]. However, Grx more likely utilizes the monothiol mechanism in this context also [3, 47, 55]. Indeed, mutant Grx (C25S) with only the one active site cysteine catalyzes reduction of DHA to ascorbic acid with greater efficiency than the wild-type enzyme [47]. Although Grx catalysis may contribute to DHA reduction, most likely multiple other ascorbate reductases in cells contribute more importantly to maintaining the reduced form of vitamin C.

A third example where Grx is proposed to act via a dithiol mechanism involves ArsC, an enzyme that mediates the reduction of arsenate [56, 57]. However, further studies have supported the conclusion that catalysis of arsenate reduction involves an ArsC-SSG intermediate that is turned over by Grx via the typical monothiol mechanism [57]. Accordingly, arsenate reduction by ArsC can be supported by mutants of *E. coli* Grx1, 2, or 3 which have only one Cys at the active site [58]. Thus, studies with multiple substrates for both mammalian and bacterial Grx support the concept that the monothiol mechanism is the major mode of catalysis by Grx for reduction of glutathione-containing mixed disulfides (RSSG) and other glutathione-containing intermediates (Fig. 7.6).

The catalytic cycle for Grx-mediated reactions (Fig. 7.3) represents a nucleophilic double displacement mechanism in which Grx acts on a glutathionylated substrate to form the Grx-SSG intermediate, which is subsequently recycled by

Thiol Disulfide Exchange Reactions Catalyzed by Glutaredoxin:

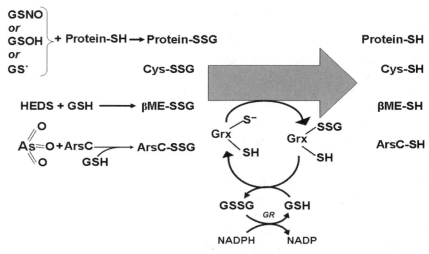

Figure 7.6   Illustrations depicting the common formation of glutathionyl mixed disulfides as substrates in various reactions catalyzed by glutaredoxin (Grx). Protein-SSG may be formed by multiple reactions as depicted. The prototype substrate cys-SSG represents the common feature of all protein-SSG substrates. β-mercaptoethanol glutathione disulfide (βME-SSG) is the product of the reaction of GSH with hydroxyethyl disulfide (HEDS). ArsC-SSG is the intermediate form of the arsenate reductase C enzyme which catalyzes reduction of arsenate. In each the glutathione mixed disulfide is reduced by Grx via the typical monothiol mechanism, coupled to GSSG disulfide reductase (GR) and NADPH.

reaction with GSH. This reaction scheme is documented by so-called *ping-pong* kinetics, which gives a characteristic parallel line pattern for the $1/V$ versus $1/S$ plots at several fixed concentrations of the cosubstrate (Fig. 7.7). This kinetic behavior has been documented for both isozymes of mammalian glutaredoxin (Grx1 and Grx2) [3, 29]. If a nonglutathionylated precursor is tested as the first substrate, then the two-substrate kinetics pattern changes to an ordered mechanism with a double reciprocal plot displaying converging lines at the same point on the x-axis (i.e., identical apparent Km values), reflecting the requirement of the initial reaction of the precursor with GSH to form the actual glutathionylated substrate for the enzyme, as depicted in the top of Fig. 7.3 [3].

Analogous to Grx1, Grx2 exhibits deglutathionylating activity for peptide and protein substrates, but its activity is approximately 10-fold lower than that of Grx1 [25, 48]. Mutating the active site of Grx2 (CSYC) to mimic that of Grx1 (CPYC) partially enhances the Grx2 activity but still remains less active than Grx1 [48], indicating that other features of the two proteins contribute the distinction in activity. Remarkably, Grx2 has been reported to be an enzyme with "high affinity" for the glutathione moiety, but this interpretation is problematic, because it was based on limited kinetic analysis [48]. Instead, comparison of Grx1 and Grx2 with the prototype substrate Cys-SSG, which represents the common feature of all protein-SSG substrates

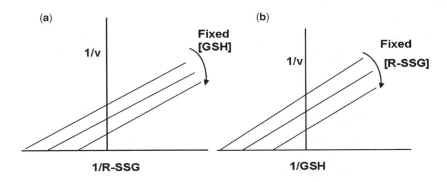

**Diagrammatic Double
Reciprocal Plots of Kinetics of
Deglutathionylation by Glutaredoxin**

Ping-Pong Kinetics reflect Nucleophilic Double Displacement Reaction

Figure 7.7   The ping-pong kinetics patterns characteristic of glutaredoxin 1 (Grx1) catalysis are obtained by using double reciprocal plots (Lineweaver-Burk, $1/V$ vs. $1/S$ plots) to represent the data for two-substrate kinetics experiments in which one substrate is varied while the other substrate is tested at several fixed concentrations (actual data is reported in Reference 28). (a) RSSG concentration is continuously varied, while GSH concentration is fixed for each set of experiments represented by one of the lines. (b) GSH is the variable substrate, and RSSG is kept constant.

and avoids steric constraints, shows essentially no difference in apparent Km for Cys-SSG for the two isoforms under the same assay conditions with a fixed concentration of GSH. Furthermore, two-substrate kinetic analysis of Grx2 indicates a ping-pong mechanism analogous to Grx1, whereby rapid covalent reactions supersede reversible binding of the protein-SSG or GSH substrates [59]. Hence, the usual interpretation of "substrate affinity" does not apply to the Grx enzymes. Another enzyme that displays this type of ping-pong kinetic behavior is glutathione peroxidase, which is highly selective for hydrogen peroxide and GSH as cosubstrates. However, neither substrate has "high affinity" for the enzyme in the traditional sense. Therefore, despite the specificity for the glutathionyl moiety, Grx and GPx enzymes are not inhibited by analogs of GSH, in contrast to the glutathione-*S*-transferase (GST) enzymes that bind GSH reversibly.

Grx2 activity within the cell may be further limited due to sequestration as dimers with a bridging Fe-S cluster masking the active site [24]. It has recently been reported that *S*-nitroglutathione treatment causes the release of Grx2 from these Fe-S clusters in vitro allowing for activity to be reestablished [60]. Hence, oxidative stimuli may lead to release of Grx2 from Fe-S clusters as a protective response to oxidative stress, thereby providing for thiol-disulfide homeostasis within the mitochondria.

Turnover of the Grx-SSG intermediate by GSH results in formation of GSSG, as shown in Fig. 7.6. GSSG reductase (GR) is the enzyme responsible for reducing

GSSG to replenish GSH. GR is a ubiquitously distributed protein whose primary function is to maintain a high GSH to GSSG ratio. GR consists of two identical subunits as well as two bound FAD molecules. Each subunit contains four domains, which include the FAD binding domain containing the redox active thiols, the NADPH binding domain, the interface domain, and the central domain [61]. The kinetic mechanism of GR implicates a ping-pong mechanism although a different ternary mechanism has been proposed for high GSSG concentrations [62]. GR in the mitochondria allows for the reduction of GSSG to GSH maintaining the mitochondria in a reduced state.

7.5 THIOREDOXIN MECHANISM OF ACTION

Thioredoxin, containing the active site CGPC, catalyzes reduction of inter- and intramolecular disulfides, as well as protein sulfenic acids via a two-step mechanism involving intermediate formation of the intramolecular disulfide form of thioredoxin. This oxidized form of Trx is recycled by thioredoxin reductase (TR) and NADPH, without the participation of glutathione. Thus, the catalytic mechanisms for Trx and Grx are quite distinct, although both involve nucleophilic double displacement reactions where thiols act as the nucleophiles (Fig. 7.3). Trx acts on oxidized sulfhydryls effectively due to the lower pKa (6.8–7.0) of its N-terminal active site Cys compared to the typical pKa of Cys (~8.5), which makes it more nucleophilic. Stabilization of the Cys-thiolate anion is attributed to the surrounding basic amino acids in the active site [7, 63]. The best studied substrates for Trx are intramolecular disulfides such as the oxidized form of the ribonucleotide reductase enzyme, and accordingly, the best characterized assay for Trx involves reduction of the prototype intramolecular disulfide substrate insulin [64]. Trx requires both active site Cys residues to effect reduction of disulfide bonds (dithiol mechanism), whereas Grx only requires the C-terminal Cys to be functional (monothiol mechanism, described above). Besides reversal of particular oxidized cysteine modifications, Trx also supports the reduction of methionine sulfoxides (oxidized methionine residues) (Fig. 7.8). The methionine sulfoxides are acted upon directly by methionine sulfoxide reductase (Msr), forming the intermediate Msr-intramolecular disulfide, which is a typical substrate for Trx. Trx coupled to TR recycles this intermediate back to its reduced, functional form, allowing for the continual reduction of methionine sulfoxides back to methionine [65]. Various examples of protein intramolecular disulfide subtrates for the thioredoxin system are depicted in Fig. 7.8. Multiple reviews report Trx working through a ping-pong mechanism in the reduction of disulfides. Although this is a reasonable assumption, two substrate kinetics studies documenting this mechanism were not included in the original cited studies [66]. Accordingly, oxidized Trx, with its active site as an intramolecular disulfide, is reverted back to the reduced dithiol form by TR (Fig. 7.3b) [9].

Besides serving as the coupling enzyme for turnover of Trx-disulfide, TR also is able to reduce small molecules, including selenite [67], GS-Se-SG [67], alloxan [68], and vitamin K [7]. TR is a FAD-containing enzyme of two linked subunits held nonconvalently together. Currently three mammalian TR enzymes are known, TR1, the cytosolic form, TR2, the mitochondrial form, and TGR, a testis-specific isoenzyme. Mammalian TRs are large selenoproteins consisting of two 55 kDa subunits

Thiol Disulfide Exchange Reactions Catalyzed by Thioredoxin:

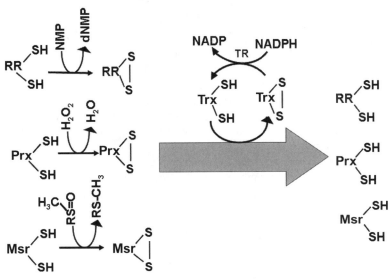

Figure 7.8 Illustrations depicting the common formation of protein-intramolecular disulfides as substrates for the thioredoxin (Trx) system. Ribonucleotide reductase (RR) is shown catalyzing formation of deoxynucleotide monophosphates (dNMP). Peroxiredoxin (Prx) is shown scavenging hydrogen peroxide, and methionine sulfoxide reductase (Msr) is shown mediating the reduction of methionine sulfoxides. Each enzyme-dithiol is oxidized to an intramolecular disulfide intermediate which serves as the substrate for reduction by Trx. Oxidized Trx is reduced by thioredoxin reductase (TR) and NADPH.

[34] containing a penultimate selenocysteine on the C-terminus allowing for substrate specificity not seen in the bacterial system [10]. Comparatively, in the bacterial system, each subunit comprising TR is approximately 35 kDa, forming a complete complex weighing 70 kDa, with each subunit containing an FAD molecule and redox active sulfhydryl in its active site [7].

7.6 CONTROL OF GRX EXPRESSION

Various natural and synthetic compounds, including oxidatively labile diphenols and organic hydroperoxides, are known to protect cells against chemical and radiation-induced carcinogenesis by elevating phase II detoxification enzymes. The induced enzymes include the *antioxidant defense enzymes* γ-glutamylcysteine synthetase (GSH synthetase), glutathione-*S*-transferase, and glutathione peroxidase [69, 70]. These inducers are believed to trigger cellular signals that activate gene transcription through an antioxidant response element (ARE) or electrophile response element (EpRE). In the mouse, the critical DNA regions that respond to antioxidant inducers have been likened to AP-1 sites and thus linked to the c-Fos and c-Jun transduction pathways [71]. Radical scavengers like *tert*-butylated hydroxyanisole

(BHA) are among the agents characterized as inducers of the antioxidant response. Increased longevity in mice treated with antioxidants (BHA, vitamin E, propylgallate) was attributed to induction of GSSG reductase levels and increase of the GSH to GSSG ratio in liver and brain [72]. BHA has also been reported to induce gluta-thione-S-transferase and glutaredoxin in mice [73]. In the mammalian system, the human *grx* gene has been cloned and reported to have an AP-1 site in its promoter region, implying regulation by oxidants as well as other factors that induce at AP-1 sites, including epidermal growth factor, TGF-β, cyclic AMP, and retinoic acid [74]. Thus, in some situations induction of glutaredoxin may be part of a pleiotropic response to stimulation of the antioxidant response element. Changes in expression of glutaredoxin in response to oxidative stress have been characterized in both pro-karyotic and eurkaryotic organisms. For example, in *E. coli*, Grx1 is upregulated upon hydrogen peroxide treatment via the induction of OxyR, a transcription factor involved in the regulation of the response of oxidative stress resulting from the production of hydrogen peroxide and superoxide anion [75]. Also, Grx levels were reported to be elevated in cells resistant to the anticancer agent adriamycin, which is a generator of oxyradicals [76]. In addition, Grx content is elevated in rat brain in response to oxidative stress injury [77]. In particular, H_2O_2 stimulated expression of Grx in a time- and dose-dependent manner in cultured human coronary artery smooth muscle cells [78]. Grx content has been reported to increase in various other oxidative stress contexts, both in well-characterized bacterial systems [75, 79] and in mammalian cells [80, 81]. It was recently proposed that 17β-estradiol protects H9c2 cardiomyocytes from oxidant-induced cell death via transcriptional upregulation of both Grx and GSH [3, 82]. Evidence implicating estradiol in the regulation of Grx1 was provided by the observation that pretreatment of bovine aortic endothelial cells with 17β-estradiol results in an increased Grx protein content as well as resistance to oxidative stress [81]. A potential mechanism by which estrogen may regulate Grx1 expression is via selective binding to an EpRE-1 site contained within the *grx* gene promoter [82]. UVB radiation is another oxidative stimulant to cause upregulation of transcription of Grx in rat keratinocytes potentially through activation of the AP-1 site [83]. Understanding of transcriptional regulation of Grx is still rudimentary, leaving much to be discovered. Also, there is evidence that in some situations glutaredoxin activity may be enhanced in response to an oxidative stimulus without an increase in Grx protein expression [84]; however, the mechanism of such Grx activation remains to be discovered.

7.7 CONTROL OF TRX EXPRESSION IN MAMMALIAN SYSTEMS

Trx expression is controlled transcriptionally by the elements associated with the promoter region of the *trx* gene, including an antioxidant response element (ARE), specific transcription factor 1 (SP-1), and a cyclic AMP response element (CRE). In addition, the *trx* gene contains an oxidative response element (ORE), which responds to oxidative stress caused by hydrogen peroxide, diamide, or menadione resulting in the upregulation of Trx [85]. Consistent with Trx being a cellular antioxidant, the *trx* gene can be stimulated for upregulation of Trx protein expression by a variety of cellular stresses, including viral infection, ultraviolet and x-irradiation, hydrogen peroxide, ischemia-reperfusion, and mitogen treatment [86]. Many studies have reported upregulation of the *trx* gene by numerous compounds, including retinol, estradiol, sulforaphane, and the antiulcer drug geranylgeranylacetone (GGA). *Tert*-butylhydroquinone, an electrophile, has been shown to elicit upregulation of the *trx* gene via the ARE element [87]. In rats, treatment with paraquat, an inducer of oxidative stress, resulted in the upregulation of Trx expression [88]. In newborn primates, breathing 100% oxygen upon birth caused an acute upregulation of Trx and TR; however, chronic elevation occurs in premature primates who develop chronic lung disease. Thus, upregulation of Trx is thought to be a response to hyperoxia [89]. Nuclear factor E2-related factor 2 (Nrf-2) is a known transcription factor that binds to ARE sites. Upon treatment of rat retinal cells with 4-hydroxynonehal, Trx was upregulated via the increased nuclear translocation and DNA binding of Nrf-2 to the ARE site in the trx promoter [90]. Overall, upregulation of the Trx system could be viewed as a protective measure utilized by the cell to combat oxidative stress [40].

7.8 CELLULAR FUNCTIONS OF GRX

Protein glutathionylation is a reversible posttranslational modification on cysteine residues that occurs under oxidative stress or in response to an oxidative stimulus and it may result in alteration in protein function. For example, *S*-glutathionylation leads to inhibition of protein tyrosine phosphatase-1B (PTP1B) [91, 92], but formation of hRas-SSG leads to activation [93]. Such regulation of cellular functions via reversible *S*-glutathionylation of Cys residues on specific proteins has evolved recently as an area of intense scientific investigation (see Chapter 8 and review articles) [5, 11, 94]. Although studies of isolated proteins and proteomic approaches have identified a large number of proteins as potentially being regulated via *S*-glutathionylation, only a few protein-SSG adducts have been documented as regulatory intermediates in a cellular context. As a guide to studying the literature on reversible glutathionylation as a regulatory mechanism in redox signal transduction, a series of five criteria have been proposed [5]. Namely, *S*-glutathionylation in a regulatory context has the following characteristics: (1) it alters the function of the modified protein, (2) it occurs in intact cells as a response to a physiological stimulus and elicits a physiological response, (3) it occurs at normal GSH to GSSG ratios, (4) it occurs in a rapid and efficient manner, and (5) it is reversed in a rapid and efficient manner. Criterion (5) is the focus of this section and chapter. Namely, the chief function of Grx is to catalyze deglutathionylation, and manipulation of its content in cells has been used effectively to document regulatory pathways that involve *S*-glutathionylated intermediates. Studies of three proteins, hRas, actin, and PTP1B, best illustrate the criteria, as discussed below.

S-glutathionylation has been shown to be a signaling mechanism within cells despite little if any change in the redox status (GSH to GSSG ratio) of the cell.

Such signaling events include cell proliferation [95], cytoskeletal organization [96], transcription [97–99], and protein synthesis [100]. Changes in the S-glutathionylation status of proteins has been implicated also in many diseases, including cancer, cardiovascular disease, diabetic retinopathy, and neurodegenerative diseases [98, 101, 102]. A few examples where Grx plays an instrumental role in the regulation of protein function are discussed below.

7.8.1 Grx-Mediated Regulation of Cytosolic Proteins

hRas belongs to the family of GTPases involved in cell survival, growth, and differentiation. Treatment of vascular smooth muscle cells with angiotensin II leads to S-glutathionylation of hRas on Cys118, documented by mass spectrometry. This activating modification initiates a signaling cascade involving phosphorylation of Akt and p38 leading to increased protein synthesis and cell proliferation. This modification is reversed by Grx overexpression, resulting in the cessation of the signal [100]. Analogous events involving hRas-SSG formation were also documented in cardiomyocytes in response to mechanical strain-induced redox signaling through the RAF/MEK/ERK growth pathway. These studies implicate Grx in the vital role of controlling cell proliferation and hypertrophy in various contexts [93].

Actin is part of the cellular cytoskeleton responsible for regulation of cytoskeletal homeostasis allowing for growth, division, remodeling, and motility of various types of cells. The Cys 374 residue of actin exists as the glutathionylated disulfide in unstimulated human epithelial cells (A431) [96] and mouse embryonic fibroblast cells (NIH 3T3) [107], despite the intracellular reducing environment. Since G-Actin-SSG polymerizes more slowly than G-Actin-SH to form actin fibrils (F-Actin), this glutathionylation inhibits the ability of actin to polymerize and migrate to the periphery of the cell. Upon stimulation of the A431 cells with epidermal growth factor (EGF), or NIH 3T3 cells with fibroblast growth factor (FGF), deglutathionylation of actin occurred in both types of cells. This change from actin-SSG to actin-SH, as well as the associated polymerization of actin and movement to the cell periphery with membrane ruffling, was prevented in NIH 3T3 cells in which Grx was depleted [103]. Paradoxically, actin deglutathionylation (a reductive event) occurred concurrently with an increase in ROS (an oxidative event) in both cell types, suggesting unusual molecular events, yet to be understood, that modulate Grx activity and/ or actin-SSG accessibility to Grx in these contexts. Nevertheless, these studies implicate Grx in regulation of cellular growth and division via deglutathionylation of actin.

Protein tyrosine phosphatase 1B (PTP1B) is a human enzyme specific for removing phosphates on tyrosine residues of proteins such as the insulin receptor [104]. EGF stimulation of A431 cells leads to the inactivation of PTP1B via glutathionylation at the active site Cys 215 [92], and this can be reversed (with coincident reactivation of PTP1B) upon the removal of the glutathionyl moiety by Grx [92]. In addition, Grx was shown to protect PTP1B inactivation by superoxide, an oxidative stimulus, in a concentration-dependent fashion, whereas Trx was shown to be ineffective [5, 91]. In related studies, Grx was shown to modulate platelet-derived growth factor (PDGF)-dependent cell signaling by regulating the redox status of low molecular weight protein tyrosine phosphatases (PTPs). Analogous to the previous studies of PTP1B, increased activation of the PDGF receptor in the situation where Grx1 was knocked down within the cells is likely due to decreased deglutathionylation of low molecular weight PTP-SSG, resulting in greater deactivation of PTP [95]. Thus, regulation of the activities of PTPs via reversible glutathionylation serves as another example of the role of glutaredoxin in modulation of the cellular responses to physiological stimuli (growth factors).

7.8.2 Grx Regulation of Transcription Factors

Nuclear factor-I (NF-I) is a DNA-binding protein involved in transcription of cellular and viral genes, including those regulating cell differentiation and development. Oxidation of Cys residues on NF-1 through S-glutathionylation leads to inhibition of DNA binding activity [105]. This inactivation was reversed by Grx in vitro, restoring DNA binding activity. The activity of NF-I within HeLa cells was also shown to be dependent on the status of GSH, suggesting a function for Grx in regulating the activity of NF-1 and its role in cell differentiation.

Nuclear factor kappa B (NF-κB) is a transcription factor linked to cell survival through its action on its target genes, including Bcl-xL, Bcl-2, and X chromosome-linked inhibitor of apoptosis. The NF-κB pathway can be redox-regulated on multiple levels [87], including upstream activating proteins such as IκB kinase (IKK) [99] as well as NF-κB itself [97, 98]. NF-κB is glutathionylated at Cys 62 on the p50 subunit under oxidizing conditions in vitro, resulting in inhibition of its DNA binding [98]. Perturbations in Grx content within retinal glial cells alter the activity of the NF-κB pathway [97], inducing S-glutathionylation of the upstream activating protein, IκB kinase (IKK) [106]. In another context, upstream regulation of the NF-κB pathway in lung cells appears to occur via glutathionylation of IκB kinase (IKK), thereby inactivating the kinase and preventing phosphorylation of IκB, ultimately limiting nuclear translocation of the NF-κB subunits [99].

While the above observations suggest that Grx generally acts as a deglutathionylase towards proteins in the NF-κB signaling pathway, there is an exceptional example where Grx appears to act in reverse, that is, by promoting glutathionylation of NF-κB [107]. In this case, pancreatic cancer cells exposed to hypoxic conditions and N-acetyl cysteine (NAC) were more susceptible to apoptosis. Under these conditions, NF-κB became glutathionylated as demonstrated by diminution in DNA binding that could be reversed by Grx treatment in vitro. However, when Grx was knocked down in the cells under the same hypoxic conditions with NAC they were less susceptible to apoptosis, and DNA binding activity of NF-κB was not diminished. These observations illustrate a potential role for Grx in mediating thiyl radical-dependent protein-SSG formation in cells [107], as demonstrated previously in model studies [108].

7.8.3 Grx-Mediated Inhibition of Apoptosis

Protein kinase B, or Akt, is a serine threonine kinase involved in cell survival pathways and protein manufacturing. Akt has been shown to prevent hydrogen peroxide-induced death of cardiac myocytes [109]. Akt is redox sensitive, the isolated protein being shown to become inactivated by formation of an intramolecular disulfide bond between Cys 297 and Cys 311 in the absence of GSH. Since the Akt intramolecular disulfide intermediate could react with cellular GSH to form Akt-SSG, Akt under oxidizing conditions might be a substrate for Grx1. Consistent with this interpretation, overexpression of Grx1 protected H9c2 cells from hydrogen peroxide-induced apoptosis, implicating Grx1 in the functional regulation of Akt [110]. An important limitation of this study, however, is that the yeast isoform of Grx was used for overexpression; this fact complicates the interpretation because yeast Grx displays glutathione peroxidase activity and could have protected the cells by scavenging hydrogen peroxide.

Grx has been shown to bind to the C-terminus of apoptosis signaling kinase 1 (ASK1) in an analogous fashion to Trx, which binds to the N-terminus of ASK1 (see Section 9.9.5). Release of Grx from ASK1 under oxidative conditions leads to activation of ASK1 and initiation of the apoptotic cascade through the JNK pathway [111]. In MCF-7 breast cancer cells dissociation of Grx from ASK1 was observed following oxidative stress via glucose deprivation. Depletion of GSH prevented the dissociation of Grx from ASK1 and inhibited apoptosis, illustrating a role for GSH in dissociation of the Grx-ASK1 complex. This example of ASK1 regulation by protein-protein interaction with Grx represents another mechanism of Grx regulation of cell survival that may be independent of the deglutathionylase activity of Grx.

The transcription factor AP-1, a heterodimer of Fos and c-Jun, is responsible for induction of apoptosis, cell proliferation, and cell differentiation. c-Jun, in particular, is associated with cell proliferation and is often dysregulated in cancer [112]. In vitro studies show that upon glutathionylation of c-Jun, DNA binding is inhibited, leading to impaired gene expression [113]. However, Grx's ability to regulate c-Jun has yet to be established in a physiological system.

7.8.4   New Frontiers of Regulation by Grx

Mitochondrial complex I is an NADH-ubiquinone oxidoreductase involved in proton pumping across the inner mitochondrial membrane, and catalyzing the initial step in the electron transport chain [114]. Inhibition of complex I results in decreases in ATP production, increased ROS production, and ultimately, cell death [115, 116]. Complex I has been shown to be inhibited by glutathionylation, causing an increase in the production of superoxide. Both mammalian Grx isoforms have been implicated in regulation of complex I via reversible glutathionylation. Recently, complex I was shown to be glutathionylated in isolated mitochondria treated with hydrogen peroxide. Glutathionylation occurred on the 75 kDa subunit only [117]. In the case of Grx1, knock-down of the enzyme in mice was accompanied by a decrease in complex I activity, suggesting Grx1 plays a role in maintenance of complex I activity [118, 119]. The situation for Grx2 is less straightforward, because the enzyme was reported to catalyze both deglutathionylation and glutathionylation of complex I under different conditions. This is consistent with the Grx catalytic mechanism, which is bidirectional depending on the relative concentrations of protein-SSG, protein-SH, GSH, and GSSG (Fig. 7.3). However, the deglutathionylase activity of Grx2 in situ may be limited by the amount of enzyme that exists as active monomer rather than inactive dimer [24]. Whether Grx2-mediated glutathionylation of complex I by GSSG is physiologically meaningful is also called into question, because the high concentrations of GSSG that were used may not be representative of the mitochondrial milieu [120]. Therefore, while both Grx1 and Grx2 have been implicated as potential regulators of complex I activity under oxidative stress conditions, additional studies are necessary to determine if changes in complex I activity within cells or tissues fulfill the criteria that characterize the reversible glutathionylation mechanism, as outlined above (Section 7.8).

HIV-1 protease, an aspartyl protease, is required for viral maturation essential for virus reproduction. HIV-1 protease contains two Cys residues that are highly conserved among samples isolated from patients with HIV. These two Cys residues can undergo glutathionylation under oxidizing conditions, resulting in alterations of HIV-1 protease function. Glutathionylation on Cys 95 or on both Cys 95 and Cys 67 inactivates the protease, whereas glutathionylation on Cys 67 alone is activating. Remarkably, Grx preferentially deglutathionylates Cys 95-SSG on the diglutathionylated enzyme, thereby converting the inactive enzyme to a supra-active enzyme [121]. HIV-1 virions were also shown to be capable of packaging human Grx, further supporting a potential role of host Grx in virus propagation via regulation of HIV-1 protease activity [122]. However, further studies will have to be performed in an in vivo context to evaluate the physiological significance of Grx-mediated regulation of the HIV-1 protease.

p53 mediates cell cycle regulation, DNA repair, and the cell's response to various stresses, including oxidative stress, DNA damage, and chemotherapeutics. Recently, exposure of human cancer cell lines to oxidative stress via chemotherapeutic agents or hydrogen peroxide resulted in glutathionylation of p53 and subsequent inhibition of DNA binding. Glutathionylation of p53 is also implicated in the inhibition of oligomerization, thus preventing transcriptional activation. Three Cys residues of p53, Cys 124, Cys 141, and Cys 182, have the potential to be glutathionylated as determined by mass spectrometry [123].

7.9 CELLULAR FUNCTIONS OF TRX

Trx has many roles within the cellular environment, including acting as a cofactor, a general antioxidant, an antiapoptotic factor, and as a regulator of transcription factors. Since knowledge of Trx preceded Grx, and the extent of study of Trx exceeds that of Grx, many redox events have been interpreted to be regulated by Trx that may also or instead be regulated by Grx. Additionally, as a cellular safeguard there may be redundancy of regulation of various targets by Grx and Trx, each acting by distinct mechanisms.

7.9.1 Trx as a Cofactor

In general, Trx catalyzes thiol-disulfide exchange reactions, specifically involving reduction of intramolecular disulfides and sulfenic acids. As discussed previously (Section 7.3), E. coli Trx was first discovered due to its ability, along with NADPH and TR, to mediate reduction of the intramolecular disulfide form of ribonucleotide reductase, which catalyzes conversion of nucleotides to deoxynucleotides. To date, observations that support such a role in mammalian cells include (1) knockout of Trx in mouse is embryonic lethal [35] and (2) inhibition of TR, the coupling enzyme for turnover of oxidized Trx, results in a decrease in ribonucleotide reductase activity [31]. However, the ability of Trx to act as a cofactor for mammalian ribonucleotide reductase has not been completely elucidated.

7.9.2   Trx as an Antioxidant

Trx, along with TR, functions in an antioxidant role by mediating the reduction of proteins involved in scavenging ROS. Trx may also be involved in the reduction of vitamin K epoxide reductase, an enzyme required for the manufacture of clotting factors [9]. Trx facilitates turnover of peroxiredoxins (Prxs), antioxidant enzymes that scavenge H_2O_2 and lipid peroxides. Thus, Trx coupled with TR reduces the peroxiredoxin-SOH intermediate more efficiently than dithioltreitol, and the Trx system is proposed to be the physiological reduction system for some Prxs [124, 125]. For example, Trx along with sulfiredoxin has been implicated in the reduction of 2 Cys Prx linking the Trx system to the reduction of sulfinic acids by 2 Cys Prx [126, 127]. Similarly, GSH functions as a cofactor for a subset of peroxiredoxins referred to as 1-Cys peroxiredoxins. In this case GSH is delivered to the 1-Cys Prx-SOH intermediate by glutathione-*S*-transferase resulting in 1-Cys Prx-SSG formation and its reduction to 1-Cys Prx-SH to complete the enzymatic cycle that scavenges peroxides [128].

Trx has also been reported to act as an electron donor for plasma glutathione peroxidase (GPx), an enzyme involved in the detoxification of hydrogen peroxide and lipid peroxides. Typically, the GPx enzymes are specific for GSH; however, plasma GPx has a higher affinity for Trx than for GSH. This relationship and the low micromolar levels of GSH in the plasma allows for the Trx system to become the main electron donor to GPx extracellularly. However, the opposite is true intracellularly where high levels and higher affinity of GSH for the GPx make Trx simply a back up electron donor system [129].

7.9.3   Trx as a Growth Factor

Trx1 has been shown to exist with an export sequence that explains its ability to be secreted from cells; however, the actual secretory pathway has not been completely established [130]. Trx1 secretion occurs after oxidative stimulus and has been shown to be independent of the typical endoplasmic reticulum-Golgi route. The secretion pathway is most similar to that of interleukin-1β (IL-1β). However, unlike IL-1β Trx1 has yet to be found in intracellular vessels [131]. Extracellular Trx1 has multiple possible functions, including acting as a growth factor, initiating an inflammatory response, or supporting reduction of oxidized protein thiols in the extracellular environment. Trx can stimulate growth of lymphocytes, normal fibroblasts, and multiple tumor cell lines. However, Trx1 has not been shown to bind to any specific growth factor according to ^{125}I-labeled-Trx binding studies, so it may simply act as a cofactor aiding other growth factors to bind to their respective receptors. Trx has been shown to amplify the growth signaling from IL-2 and FGF, but not insulin or EGF in MCF-7 cells, a breast cancer cell line [31].

7.9.4 Trx-Mediated Regulation of Transcription Factors

Trx has been implicated in the regulation of several transcription factors. Its ability to translocate to the nucleus upon oxidative stimulus makes it a good candidate for regulation within the nucleus [132, 133]; however, it is thought that most of the regulation occurs prior to nuclear translocation. Trx regulates glucocorticoid receptor [134], reducing a critical Cys to enhance DNA binding, and an analogous reduction is seen with p53 [135]. Trx has been implicated also in the regulation of AP-1, which exhibits increased DNA binding after reduction of a conserved Cys residue involved in an intramolecular disulfide bond. This reduction occurs through Ref-1, a DNA repair enzyme [136]. NF-κB has also been reported in many reviews as a transcription factor that is regulated by Trx [31, 38, 137, 138]. Also, a role for reduction mediated by Grx is supported by numerous studies in various cell lines implicating Grx regulation at multiple loci of the NF-κB pathway, as discussed previously (see Section 7.8.2) [97, 99].

7.9.5 Trx-Mediated Inhibition of Apoptosis

Studies have suggested a role for Trx in sequestering the apoptotic factor, ASK1, in an inactive conformation within the cytosol by binding to its N-terminus [139]. Trx requires its active CXXC motif to bind to ASK1, and only upon oxidation to its intramolecular disulfide form is the Trx released, enabling ASK1 to activate proteins that initiate apoptotic signaling, including c-Jun-N-terminal kinase (JNK) and members of the p38 MAPK pathway [9]. As discussed earlier, Grx can bind to the C-terminus of ASK1 apparently contributing also to sequestering the protein to the cytosol [140]. Binding to opposite ends of ASK1 suggests that Trx and Grx may independently regulate ASK1 under different conditions.

Trx has also been implicated in the cellular defense against apoptosis induced by a variety of agents, including dexamethasone, staurosporine, and etoposide. The ability of Trx to protect the cell from apoptosis from these harsh chemicals makes it an attractive target in the design of cancer chemotherapeutic agents. Multiple types of cancers have elevated levels of the Trx protein, and Trx overexpression is associated with cell growth and evasion of apoptosis, rendering cancer cells resistant to common chemotherapeutic agents. Importantly, the antiapoptotic function of Trx was documented in studies where it was overexpressed in the cells, so caution is warranted in assuming physiological relevance. Furthermore, these findings may reflect a general antioxidant function of Trx rather than a specific mode of inhibition of apoptosis since no molecular mechanism is described [9].

7.10 REVERSIBLE SULFHYDRYL OXIDATION AND DISEASE

Sulfhydryl modification occurs when cells are subjected to oxidative stress creating an oxidizing environment. However, only severe oxidative challenges would alter the GSH to GSSG ratio sufficiently so that GSSG concentration would be high enough to promote glutathionylation by thiol-disulfide exchange (i.e., not thermodynamically favored). Thus, alternative mechanisms of protein-SSG formation are more likely [16]. Also included in the redox system of the cell is the cysteine : cystine (Cys : CySS) redox couple. This system appears to be independently regulated with ratios shifting more towards an oxidizing system (i.e., more cystine (CySSCys)) at lower oxidant stress than the corresponding formation of GSSG [141].

Oxidation of protein-Cys sulfhydryl moieties via glutathionylation is thought to be a protective mechanism preventing irreversible sulfur oxidation on proteins, including sulfinic and sulfonic acid formation. Maintenance of an active sulfhydryl repair system, mainly through the TDORS, Grx and Trx, is critical to prevent irreversible damage. However, in many disease states alterations in activity of either of these enzymes (by downregulation or direct inhibition of active site sulfhydryl modification) can lead to deleterious outcomes, including enzyme inhibition, protein aggregation, and commitment to apoptosis through inhibition of transcription factors or alterations in signaling pathways. Protein modification via sulfhydryl oxidation has been associated with numerous diseases that involve oxidative stress, including AIDS, Freidrich's ataxia, type I and type II diabetes, and ischemia-reperfusion [102]. The emerging roles of Grx and Trx in numerous disease processes are described further below.

7.10.1 Glutaredoxin and Disease

The investigation of the roles of Grx in human disease is an evolving field with new discoveries of Grx in multiple diseases being published frequently. The potential role of Grx in various diseases has been studied primarily in the context of cell culture models, with some animal disease models utilized to address its function in the progression or inhibition of disease.

7.10.1.1 Diabetic Retinopathy   Diabetes is a disease characterized by oxidative stress in various organ systems linked to excess blood glucose, that is, hyperglycemia. Diabetic retinopathy, which may lead to blindness, is an inflammatory condition characterized by increased leukocyte adhesion, vascular permeability, and cell death. In a mouse model of diabetic retinopathy, retinas show increased abundance and activity of Grx, likely representing a response to the excessive oxidative stress caused by hyperglycemia. Although Grx normally functions as a protective mechanism towards protein sulfhydryl homeostasis, in this case the increased Grx in response to high glucose levels leads to increased activation of the transcription factor NF-κB, resulting in increased expression of intracellular adhesion molecule-1 (ICAM-1), a characteristic mediator of inflammation [97]. In this case, Grx upregulation appears to contribute a detrimental effect to the disease state rather than a protective one.

7.10.1.2 Chronic Obstructive Pulmonary Disease (COPD) COPD is a progressive disorder characterized by airflow limitation and increased oxidative stress. Grx1 expression was decreased in alveolar macrophages with the progression of COPD. In contrast, Grx1 content increased in sputum with disease progression, suggesting a secretory pathway for Grx1, possibly in response to the oxidative stress condition of COPD [142]. A basis for the dichotomy of Grx expression with decreased expression in the macrophage and increased expression in the sputum is currently unresolved.

7.10.1.3 Cardiovascular Disease Cardiovascular disease and heart failure are both associated with increased oxidative stress. It was reported that atherosclerotic lesions contain a significantly higher amount of Grx compared to nonlesioned endothelium. In this study oxidative stress simulated by hydrogen peroxide treatment of human coronary artery smooth muscle cells in culture induced the expression of Grx, suggesting a role for Grx1 in the antioxidant response of human coronary arteries [78]. An analogous antioxidant role for Grx1 in ischemic disease of the brain has also been suggested [143]. In addition Grx1 levels are elevated in the plasma during cardiopulmonary bypass surgery; however, this change correlates with increased hemolysis, suggesting release of Grx1 from ruptured red blood cells [144].

7.10.1.4 Parkinson's Disease Oxidative stress has been implicated in the onset and progression of Parkinson's disease (PD) [145]. One of the major proteins shown to be inhibited in PD is mitochondrial complex I, which displays decreased activity in postmortem brain and peripheral tissue samples. In mitochondria isolated from synapses, inhibition of complex I by only 25% shows impairment of oxidative phosphorylation to the same extent as that seen in PD. A potential role for Grx in PD specifically via deglutathionylation of complex I is suggested in several studies. First, in a mouse model, downregulation of Grx leads to inhibition of complex I [118]. Second, chemical inhibition of complex I with 1-methyl 4-phenyl 1,2,3,6-tetrahydropyridine resulted in increased Grx transcription and enzymatic activity concomitant with restoration of complex I function [118]. Third, Grx 2 has been shown in vitro to cause deglutathionylation of complex I under oxidative conditions [120]. And fourth, Grx2 from *E. coli* has been shown to be protective in isolated granule neurons treated with excess dopamine [146]. Despite these various model studies, alterations in Grx levels have yet to be determined in patients. Nevertheless, the above findings suggest that Grx may provide a potential antioxidant, protective role in neurons affected by PD.

7.10.1.5 Alzheimer's Disease Oxidative stress has been implicated in the pathogenesis and possible etiology of Alzheimer's disease (AD). Accordingly, expression levels of Grx in normal brain and those affected by AD have been compared. In postmortem patient samples increased expression of Grx was observed in the frontal cortex and the hippocampus of AD samples, while Trx levels were decreased. Treatment of SH-SY5Y cells with Aβ, a cell culture model for AD, led to oxidation of Grx and Trx, which was correlated to apoptotic death of the neurons.

Overexpression of Grx abated the Aβ-induced apoptosis [147]. Based on this report, upregulation of Grx in AD patients may not be protective if Aβ is produced in higher amounts in the disease state, so as to cause oxidation and inactivation of the Grx. However, upregulation of Grx in the diseased state may prove to be consequential as more is learned from further investigation of patient samples.

7.10.2 Thioredoxin and Disease

Trx1 is a ubiquitously expressed protein in mammalian tissues. Plasma levels of thioredoxin have been reported to vary over a range of 10 to 80 ng/mL (0.8 to 6.6 nM) with higher levels seen in patients with cancers or HIV [9]. Changes in Trx expression have been observed in numerous disease states, and an increase in cellular Trx is associated with protection from oxidative stress. It appears that Trx expression must be highly regulated in order to keep a balance between its positive and negative effects. For example, Trx levels are upregulated in sun-exposed skin, where reactive species are formed, presumably as a protective response [148]. Also in the developing embryo, elevation in Trx is thought to provide immune protection [9]. On the other hand, enhanced expression of Trx and TR has been associated with negative affects in diseases, including cancer, AIDS, rheumatoid arthritis, and atherosclerosis [9, 33]. Because of these links to disease progression, Trx is currently being targeted for development of inhibitory therapeutics [30, 31].

7.10.2.1 Cancer   Lung, colon, and pancreatic tumors have been shown to over-express Trx compared to normal tissue [9]. Trx overexpression in tumors might be a response to overt oxidative stress, boosting antioxidant capacity, and eventually aiding in the growth and malignancy potential of the tumor. Potential mechanisms of the prosurvival effects of Trx include (1) Trx may serve as an antiapoptotic factor through its inhibition of ASK1 and p53; (2) Trx may promote neovascularization by activating hypoxia inducing factor 1α (HIF-1α), leading to increased vascular endothelial growth factor; (3) Trx may inhibit tumor suppressing proteins such as phosphatase and tensin homolog (PTEN). In cancer, therefore, Trx may represent a potential target for inhibition which would result in a weakened defense against chemotherapeutics by tumor cells [30, 31].

7.10.2.2 Acquired Immune Deficiency Syndrome (AIDS)   Altered levels of Trx have been correlated with AIDS. In early stages of the disease, tissue levels of Trx are decreased, possibly reflecting depleted sulfur stores resulting from immune deficiency. In later stages of the disease, cellular Trx levels are elevated, with potential beneficial effects on viral replication via redox changes in CD4, the primary receptor for AIDS [30]. Despite the potential protective effect of increased intracellular Trx, increased plasma Trx levels are correlated with a poor prognosis; that is, Trx plasma levels in AIDS patients with the poorest prognosis were three times as high as compared to normal control subjects, 30 ng/mL compared to 11 ng/mL [149]. Understanding the basis for the opposite correlation between intracellular and plasma Trx content and severity of disease requires further study.

7.10.2.3 Inflammation Trx1 upregulation in inflammatory diseases, such as rheumatoid arthritis, implies a function of Trx1 in mediating or responding to inflammation [38]. Trx1 has been shown to act as a chemotaxic agent, signaling to immune cells: neutrophils, monocytes, and T cells [130]. However, a similar study found that Trx-overexpressing mice experience decreased neutrophil recruitment under inflammatory conditions (air pouch model) [149]. Similarly, in a cell culture model, Trx causes inhibition of chemotaxis via L-selectin which is required for neutrophil migration, and neutrophil adhesion. This inhibition by Trx is dependent on a functional active site [149, 150]. A definitive role of Trx in chemotaxis, either aiding in recruiting immune cells or inhibiting immune cell migration, remains to be elucidated.

7.10.2.4 Cardiovascular Disease Trx1 is ubiquitously expressed in vascular smooth muscle cells and fibroblasts. It has been implicated in both the protection of the heart, as in ischemia-reperfusion injury [151], and in the demise of the heart, as in age-related myocarditis [152]. In ischemia-reperfusion injury, upregulation of Trx protects the heart from significant damage. Specifically, treatment of mice with Trx via intraperitoneal injection during ischemia decreased infarct size as well as the amount of myocardial apoptosis [153]. While Trx appears to be cardioprotective during ischemia-reperfusion injury, it has been associated with atherosclerosis, with elevated levels observed in atherosclerotic plaques of human coronary arteries examined upon autopsy [33]. In atherosclerosis, Trx may contribute to the disease or be a part of a protective response. The increase in Trx is thought to reflect infiltration of macrophages, which express high levels of Trx to combat the excess oxidative insult of the atherosclerotic state [78]. Trx may be considered a marker for cardiovascular disease as it is also elevated in endothelial cells in patients with acute coronary syndrome, dilated cardiomyopathy, and chronic heart failure [154].

7.10.2.5 Neurodegenerative Disease Trx has been shown to have neuroprotective effects in the nervous system. Overexpression of Trx in murine brain leads to increased life span [155], resistance to focal ischemia [143], and resistance to excitotoxic stress as compared to wild type littermates [156]. Trx1 protein and mRNA are upregulated in PC12 cells treated with nerve growth factor (NGF), and are associated with neurite formation [157]. Trx may be decreased in Alzheimer's disease; however, this interpretation is tentative due to a limited sample size [158]. Playing a general role as an antioxidant (as described in Section 9.9.2) could represent the importance of Trx to various oxidant stress diseases of the brain, including Alzheimer's disease and Parkinson's disease.

7.11 CONCLUSIONS

Sulfhydryl homeostasis within cellular systems is highly regulated in order to maintain the redox status of the cell. Perturbations of the redox homeostasis either as a consequence of cellular signaling or overt oxidative stress alter protein function within cells. Multiple antioxidant homeostatic mechanisms are established to maintain proper functioning of cellular proteins and to aid in cell survival. One main antioxidant repair system is the TDOR enzymes, specifically thioredoxin and glutaredoxin. Trx and Grx both facilitate reduction of oxidatively modified cysteine-sulfhydryls on cellular proteins; however, unique substrate specificities reflect their distinct functions. Trx selectively reduces intramolecular disulfides, intermolecular disulfides, and protein sulfenic acids while Grx specifically and efficiently reduces protein mixed disulfides (protein-SSG). Since GSH is an abundant antioxidant within the cellular milieu, protein-SSG formation is likely the dominant modification in response to oxidative stimuli. Perturbations in the cell's antioxidant defenses specifically through alteration in activity or content of Trx or Grx can lead to aberrant signaling, alterations in protein functions, and ultimately cell death. With this in mind, it becomes understandable that Trx and Grx could have a substantial role in multiple disease processes. Learning the unique properties of Trx and Grx will deepen the understanding of their individual roles as well as their synergistic roles in cellular function and disease.

REFERENCES

1. Hirota, K., Nakamura, H., Masutani, H., Yodoi, J. (2002). Thioredoxin superfamily and thioredoxin-inducing agents. *Annals of the New York Academy of Sciences, 957*, 189–199.

2. Ziegler, D.M. (1985). Role of reversible oxidation-reduction of enzyme thiols-disulfides in metabolic regulation. *Annual Review of Biochemistry, 54*, 305–329.

3. Mieyal, J.J., Srinivasan, U., Starke, D.W., Gravina, S.A, Mieyal, P.A. (1995). Glutathionyl specificity of the thioltransferases: Mechanistic and physiological implications. In Packer, L., and Cadenas, E., Eds., *Biothiols in Health and Disease*, pp. 305–372. New York: Marcel Dekker.

4. Jacob, C., Knight, I., Winyard, P.G. (2006). Aspects of the biological redox chemistry of cysteine: From simple redox responses to sophisticated signaling pathways. *Biological Chemistry, 387*, 1385–1397.

5. Shelton, M.D., Chock, P.B., Mieyal, J.J. (2005). Glutaredoxin: Role in reversible protein S-glutathionylation and regulation of redox signal transduction and protein translocation. *Antioxidants and Redox Signaling, 7*, 348–366.

6. Yang, Y., Jao, S., Nanduri, S., Starke, D.W., Mieyal, J.J., Qin, J. (1998). Reactivity of the human thioltransferase (glutaredoxin) C7S, C25S, C78S, C82S mutant and NMR solution structure of its glutathionyl mixed disulfide intermediate reflect catalytic specificity. *Biochemistry, 37*, 17145–17156.

7. Holmgren, A. (1985) Thioredoxin. *Annual Review of Biochemistry, 54*, 237–271.

8. Wilkinson, B., Gilbert, H.F. (2004). Protein disulfide isomerase. *Biochimica et Biophysica Acta, 1699*, 35–44.

9. Powis, G., Montfort, W.R. (2001). Properties and biological activities of thioredoxins. *Annual Review of Pharmacology and Toxicology, 41*, 261–295.

10. Lillig, C.H., Holmgren, A. (2007). Thioredoxin and related molecules: From biology to health and disease. *Antioxidants and Redox Signaling, 9*, 25–47.

11. Klatt, P., Lamas, S. (2000). Regulation of protein function by S-glutathiolation in response to oxidative and nitrosative stress. *European Journal of Biochemistry, 267*, 4928–4944.

12. Berndt, C., Lillig, C.H., Holmgren, A. (2007). Thiol-based mechanisms of the thioredoxin and glutaredoxin systems: Implications for diseases in the cardiovascular system. *American Journal of Physiology. Heart and Circulatory Physiology, 292*, H1227–H1236.

13. Mieyal, J.J., Starke, D.W., Gravina, S.A., Hocevar, B.A. (1991). Thioltransferase in human red blood cells: Kinetics and equilibrium. *Biochemistry, 30*, 8883–8891.

14. Starke, D.W., Chen, Y., Bapna, C.P., Lesnefsky, E.J., Mieyal, J.J. (1997). Sensitivity of protein sulfhydryl repair enzymes to oxidative stress. *Free Radical Biology and Medicine, 23*, 373–384.

15. Pai, H.V., Starke, D.W., Lesnefsky, E.J., Hoppel, C.L., Mieyal, J.J. (2007). What is the functional significance of the unique localization of glutaredoxin 1 (Grx1) in the inter-membrane space of mitochondria? *Antioxidants and Redox Signaling, 9*(11), 2027–2033.

16. Gallogly, M.M., Mieyal, J.J. (2007). Mechanisms of reversible protein glutathionylation in redox signaling and oxidative stress. *Current Opinion in Pharmacology, 7*(4), 381–391.

17. Rozell, B., Barcena, J.A., Martinez-Galisteo, E., Padilla, C.A., Holmgren, A. (1993). Immunochemical characterization and tissue distribution of glutaredoxin (thioltransfer-ase) from calf. *European Journal of Cell Biology, 62*, 314–323.

18. Lysell, J., Stjernholm, V.Y., Ciarlo, N., Holmgren, A., Sahlin, L. (2003). Immuno-histochemical determination of thioredoxin and glutaredoxin distribution in the human cervix, and possible relation to cervical ripening. *Gynecological Endocrinology, 17*, 303–310.

19. Sahlin, L., Wang, H., Stjernholm, Y., Lundberg, M., Ekman, G., Holmgren, A., Eriksson, H. (2000). The expression of glutaredoxin is increased in the human cervix in term pregnancy and immediately post-partum, particularly after prostaglandin-induced delivery. *Molecular Human Reproduction, 6*, 1147–1153.

20. Stavreus-Evers, A., Masironi, B., Landgren, B.M., Holmgren, A., Eriksson, H., Sahlin, L. (2002). Immunohistochemical localization of glutaredoxin and thioredoxin in human endometrium: A possible association with pinopodes. *Molecular Human Reproduction, 8*, 546–551.

21. Hirota, K., Matsui, M., Murata, M., Takashima, Y., Cheng, F.S., Itoh, T., Fukuda, K., Yodoi, J. (2000). Nucleoredoxin, glutaredoxin, and thioredoxin differentially regulate NF-kappaB, AP-1, and CREB activation in HEK293 cells. *Biochemical and Biophysical Research Communications, 274*, 177–182.

22. Gladyshev, V.N., Liu, A., Novoselov, S.V., Krysan, K., Sun, Q.A., Kryukov, V.M., Kryukov, G.V., Lou, M.F. (2001). Identification and characterization of a new mammalian glutaredoxin (thioltransferase), Grx2. *Journal of Biological Chemistry, 276*, 30374–30380.

23. Lundberg, M., Johansson, C., Chandra, J., Enoksson, M., Jacobsson, G., Ljung, J., Johansson, M., Holmgren, A. (2001). Cloning and expression of a novel human glutare-doxin (Grx2) with mitochondrial and nuclear isoforms. *Journal of Biological Chemistry, 276*, 26269–26275.

24. Lillig, C.H., Berndt, C., Vergnolle, O., Lonn, M.E., Hudemann, C., Bill, E., Holmgren, A. (2005). Characterization of human glutaredoxin 2 as iron-sulfur protein: A possible role as redox sensor. *Proceedings of the National Academy of Sciences USA, 102*, 8168–8173.

25. Johansson, C., Kavanagh, K.L., Gileadi, O., Oppermann, U. (2007). Reversible sequestration of active site cysteines in a 2Fe-2S-bridged dimer provides a mechanism for glutaredoxin 2 regulation in human mitochondria. *Journal of Biological Chemistry, 282*, 3077–3082.

26. Rodriguez-Manzaneque, M.T., Ros, J., Cabiscol, E., Sorribas, A., Herrero, E. (1999). Grx5 glutaredoxin plays a central role in protection against protein oxidative damage in *Saccharomyces cerevisiae*. *Molecular and Cellular Biology*, *19*, 8180–8190.

27. Wingert, R.A., Galloway, J.L., Barut, B., Foott, H., Fraenkel, P., Axe, J.L., Weber, G.J., Dooley, K., Davidson, A.J., Schmid, B., Paw, B.H., Shaw, G.C., Kingsley, P., Palis, J., Schubert, H., Chen, O., Kaplan, J., Zon, L.I. (2005). Deficiency of glutaredoxin 5 reveals Fe-S clusters are required for vertebrate haem synthesis. *Nature*, *436*, 1035–1039.

28. Gravina, S.A., Mieyal, J.J. (1993). Thioltransferase is a specific glutathionyl mixed disulfide oxidoreductase. *Biochemistry*, *32*, 3368–3376.

29. Mannervik, B., Axelsson, K., Sundewall, A.C., Holmgren, A. (1983). Relative contributions of thioltransferase- and thioredoxin-dependent systems in reduction of low-molecular-mass and protein disulphides. *Biochemical Journal*, *213*, 519–523.

30. Burke-Gaffney, A., Callister, M.E., Nakamura, H. (2005). Thioredoxin: Friend or foe in human disease? *Trends in Pharmacological Sciences*, *26*, 398–404.

31. Powis, G., Mustacich, D., Coon, A. (2000). The role of the redox protein thioredoxin in cell growth and cancer. *Free Radical Biology and Medicine*, *29*, 312–322.

32. Laurent, T.C., Moore, E.C., Reichard, P. (1964). Enzymatic synthesis of deoxyribonucleotides. IV. Isolation and characterization of thioredoxin, the hydrogen donor from *Escherichia coli B. Journal of Biological Chemistry*, *239*, 3436–3444.

33. Gromer, S., Urig, S., Becker, K. (2004). The thioredoxin system: From science to clinic. *Molecular and Cellular Biology*, *24*, 40–89.

34. Masutani, H., Hirota, K., Sasada, T., Ueda-Taniguchi, Y., Taniguchi, Y., Sono, H., Yodoi, J. (1996). Transactivation of an inducible anti-oxidative stress protein, human thioredoxin by HTLV-I Tax. *Immunology Letters*, *54*, 67–71.

35. Matsui, M., Oshima, M., Oshima, H., Takaku, K., Maruyama, T., Yodoi, J., Taketo, M.M. (1996). Early embryonic lethality caused by targeted disruption of the mouse thioredoxin gene. *Developmental Biology*, *178*, 179–185.

36. Ho, Y.S., Xiong, Y., Ho, D.S., Gao, J., Chua, B.H., Pai, H., Mieyal, J.J. (2007). Targeted disruption of the glutaredoxin 1 gene does not sensitize adult mice to tissue injury induced by ischemia/reperfusion and hyperoxia. *Free Radical Biology and Medicine*, *43*(9), 1299–1312.

37. Spyrou, G., Holmgren, A. (1996). Deoxyribonucleoside triphosphate pools and growth of glutathione-depleted 3T6 mouse fibroblasts. *Biochemical and Biophysical Research Communications*, *220*, 42–46.

38. Watson, W.H., Yang, X., Choi, Y.E., Jones, D.P., Kehrer, J.P. (2004). Thioredoxin and its role in toxicology. *Toxicological Sciences*, *78*, 3–14.

39. Miranda-Vizuete, A., Gustafsson, J.A., Spyrou, G. (1998). Molecular cloning and expression of a cDNA encoding a human thioredoxin-like protein. *Biochemical and Biophysical Research Communications*, *243*, 284–288.

40. Kondo, N., Nakamura, H., Masutani, H., Yodoi, J. (2006). Redox regulation of human thioredoxin network. *Antioxidants and Redox Signaling*, *8*, 1881–1890.

41. Miranda-Vizuete, A., Ljung, J., Damdimopoulos, A.E., Gustafsson, J.A., Oko, R., Pelto-Huikko, M., Spyrou, G. (2001). Characterization of Sptrx, a novel member of the thioredoxin family specifically expressed in human spermatozoa. *Journal of Biological Chemistry*, *276*, 31567–31574.

42. Jimenez, A., Zu, W., Rawe, V.Y., Pelto-Huikko, M., Flickinger, C.J., Sutovsky, P., Gustafsson, J.A., Oko, R., Miranda-Vizuete, A. (2004). Spermatocyte/spermatid-specific thioredoxin-3, a novel Golgi apparatus-associated thioredoxin, is a specific marker of aberrant spermatogenesis. *Journal of Biological Chemistry*, *279*, 34971–34982.

43. Thiele, M., Bernhagen, J. (2005). Link between macrophage migration inhibitory factor and cellular redox regulation. *Antioxidants and Redox Signaling*, *7*, 1234–1248.

44. Laughner, B.J., Sehnke, P.C., Ferl, R.J. (1998). A novel nuclear member of the thioredoxin superfamily. *Plant Physiology*, *118*, 987–996.

45. Kurooka, H., Kato, K., Minoguchi, S., Takahashi, Y., Ikeda, J., Habu, S., Osawa, N., Buchberg, A.M., Moriwaki, K., Shisa, H., Honjo, T. (1997). Cloning and characterization of the nucleoredoxin gene that encodes a novel nuclear protein related to thioredoxin. *Genomics*, *39*, 331–339.

46. Matsuo, Y., Akiyama, N., Nakamura, H., Yodoi, J., Noda, M., Kizaka-Kondoh, S. (2001). Identification of a novel thioredoxin-related transmembrane protein. *Journal of Biological Chemistry*, *276*, 10032–10038.

47. Washburn, M.P., Wells, W.W. (1999). The catalytic mechanism of the glutathione-dependent dehydroascorbate reductase activity of thioltransferase (glutaredoxin). *Biochemistry*, *38*, 268–274.

48. Johansson, C., Lillig, C.H., Holmgren, A. (2004). Human mitochondrial glutaredoxin reduces S-glutathionylated proteins with high affinity accepting electrons from either glutathione or thioredoxin reductase. *Journal of Biological Chemistry*, *279*, 7537–7543.

49. Holmgren, A., Johansson, C., Berndt, C., Lonn, M.E., Hudemann, C., Lillig, C.H. (2005). Thiol redox control via thioredoxin and glutaredoxin systems. *Biochemical Society Transactions*, *33*, 1375–1377.

50. Jao, S.C., English Ospina, S.M., Berdis, A.J., Starke, D.W., Post, C.B., Mieyal, J.J. (2006). Computational and mutational analysis of human glutaredoxin (thioltransferase): Probing the molecular basis of the low pKa of cysteine 22 and its role in catalysis. *Biochemistry*, *45*, 4785–4796.

51. Chrestensen, C.A., Starke, D.W., Mieyal, J.J. (2000). Acute cadmium exposure inactivates thioltransferase (glutaredoxin), inhibits intracellular reduction of protein-glutathionyl-mixed disulfides, and initiates apoptosis. *Journal of Biological Chemistry*, *275*, 26556–26565.

52. Srinivasan, U., Mieyal, P.A., Mieyal, J.J. (1997). pH profiles indicative of rate-limiting nucleophilic displacement in thioltransferase catalysis. *Biochemistry*, *36*, 3199–3206.

53. Holmgren, A. (1979). Glutathione-dependent synthesis of deoxyribonucleotides. Characterization of the enzymatic mechanism of Escherichia coli glutaredoxin. *Journal of Biological Chemistry*, *254*, 3672–3678.

54. Fernandes, A.P., Holmgren, A. (2004). Glutaredoxins: Glutathione-dependent redox enzymes with functions far beyond a simple thioredoxin backup system. *Antioxidants and Redox Signaling*, *6*, 63–74.

55. Wells, W.W., Yang, Y., Deits, T.L., Gan, Z.R. (1993). Thioltransferases. *Advances in Enzymology and Related Areas of Molecular Biology*, *66*, 149–201.

56. Gladysheva, T.B., Oden, K.L., Rosen, B.P. (1994). Properties of the arsenate reductase of plasmid R773. *Biochemistry*, *33*, 7288–7293.

57. Rosen, B.P. (2002). Biochemistry of arsenic detoxification. *FEBS Letters*, *529*, 86–92.

58. Shi, J., Vlamis-Gardikas, A., Aslund, F., Holmgren, A., Rosen, B.P. (1999). Reactivity of glutaredoxins 1, 2, and 3 from Escherichia coli shows that glutaredoxin 2 is the primary hydrogen donor to ArsC-catalyzed arsenate reduction. *Journal of Biological Chemistry*, *274*, 36039–36042.

59. Gallogly, M.M., Starke, D.W., Leonberg, A.K., Ospina, S.M., Mieyal, J.J. (2008). Kinetic and mechanistic characterization and versatile catalytic properties of mammalian glutaredoxin 2: implications for intracellular roles. *Biochemistry*, *47*, 11144–11157.

60. Hashemy, S.I., Johansson, C., Berndt, C., Lillig, C.H., Holmgren, A. (2007). Oxidation and S-nitrosylation of cysteines in human cytosolic and mitochondrial glutaredoxins: Effects on structure and activity. *Journal of Biological Chemistry*, *282*, 14428–14436.

61. Untucht-Grau, R., Schirmer, R.H., Schirmer, I., Krauth-Siegel, R.L. (1981). Glutathione reductase from human erythrocytes: Amino-acid sequence of the structurally known FAD-binding domain. *European Journal of Biochemistry*, *120*, 407–419.

62. Vanoni, M.A., Wong, K.K., Ballou, D.P., Blanchard, J.S. (1990). Glutathione reductase: Comparison of steady-state and rapid reaction primary kinetic isotope effects exhibited by the yeast, spinach, and Escherichia coli enzymes. *Biochemistry*, *29*, 5790–5796.

63. Kallis, G.B., Holmgren, A. (1980). Differential reactivity of the functional sulfhydryl groups of cysteine-32 and cysteine-35 present in the reduced form of thioredoxin from Escherichia coli. *Journal of Biological Chemistry*, *255*, 10261–10265.

64. Luthman, M., Holmgren, A. (1982). Glutaredoxin from calf thymus: Purification to homogeneity. *Journal of Biological Chemistry*, *257*, 6686–6690.

65. Antoine, M., Boschi-Muller, S., Branlant, G. (2003). Kinetic characterization of the chemical steps involved in the catalytic mechanism of methionine sulfoxide reductase A from *Neisseria meningitidis*. *Journal of Biological Chemistry*, *278*, 45352–45357.

66. Holmgren, A. (1979). Thioredoxin catalyzes the reduction of insulin disulfides by dithiothreitol and dihydrolipoamide. *Journal of Biological Chemistry*, *254*, 9627–9632.

67. Bjornstedt, M., Kumar, S., Holmgren, A. (1995). Selenite and selenodiglutathione: Reactions with thioredoxin systems. *Methods in Enzymology*, *252*, 209–219.

68. Holmgren, A., Lyckeborg, C. (1980). Enzymatic reduction of alloxan by thioredoxin and NADPH-thioredoxin reductase. *Proceedings of the National Academy of Sciences USA*, *77*, 5149–5152.

69. Prestera, T., Zhang, Y., Spencer, S.R., Wilczak, C.A., Talalay, P. (1993). The electrophile counterattack response: Protection against neoplasia and toxicity. *Advances in Enzyme Regulation*, *33*, 281–296.

70. Buetler, T.M., Gallagher, E.P., Wang, C., Stahl, D.L., Hayes, J.D., Eaton, D.L. (1995). Induction of phase I and phase II drug-metabolizing enzyme mRNA, protein, and activity by BHA, ethoxyquin, and oltipraz. *Toxicology and Applied Pharmacology*, *135*, 45–57.

71. Friling, R.S., Bergelson, S., Daniel, V. (1992). Two adjacent AP-1-like binding sites form the electrophile-responsive element of the murine glutathione S-transferase Ya subunit gene. *Proceedings of the National Academy of Sciences USA*, *89*, 668–672.

72. Khanna, S.C., Garg, S.K., Sharma, S.P. (1992). Antioxidant-influenced alterations in glutathione reductase activity in different age groups of male mice. *Gerontology*, *38*, 9–12.

73. Di Simplicio, P., Jensson, H., Mannervik, B. (1989). Effects of inducers of drug metabolism on basic hepatic forms of mouse glutathione transferase. *Biochemical Journal*, *263*, 679–685.

74. Park, J.B., Levine, M. (1997). The human glutaredoxin gene: Determination of its organization, transcription start point, and promoter analysis. *Gene, 197,* 189–193.

75. Prieto-Alamo, M.J., Jurado, J., Gallardo-Madueno, R., Monje-Casas, F., Holmgren, A., Pueyo, C. (2000). Transcriptional regulation of glutaredoxin and thioredoxin pathways and related enzymes in response to oxidative stress. *Journal of Biological Chemistry, 275,* 13398–13405.

76. Wells, W.W., Rocque, P.A., Xu, D.P., Meyer, E.B., Charamella, L.J., Dimitrov, N.V. (1995). Ascorbic acid and cell survival of adriamycin resistant and sensitive MCF-7 breast tumor cells. *Free Radical Biology and Medicine, 18,* 699–708.

77. Kenchappa, R.S., Diwakar, L., Boyd, M.R., Ravindranath, V. (2002). Thioltransferase (glutaredoxin) mediates recovery of motor neurons from excitotoxic mitochondrial injury. *Journal of Neurosciences, 22,* 8402–8410.

78. Okuda, M., Inoue, N., Azumi, H., Seno, T., Sumi, Y., Hirata, K., Kawashima, S., Hayashi, Y., Itoh, H., Yodoi, J., Yokoyama, M. (2001). Expression of glutaredoxin in human coronary arteries: Its potential role in antioxidant protection against atherosclerosis. *Arteriosclerosis, Thrombosis and Vascular Biology, 21,* 1483–1487.

79. Tao, K. (1997). oxyR-dependent induction of Escherichia coli grx gene expression by peroxide stress. *Journal of Bacteriology, 179,* 5967–5970.

80. Kumar, S., Holmgren, A. (1999). Induction of thioredoxin, thioredoxin reductase and glutaredoxin activity in mouse skin by TPA, a calcium ionophore and other tumor promoters. *Carcinogenesis, 20,* 1761–1767.

81. Ejima, K., Nanri, H., Araki, M., Uchida, K., Kashimura, M., Ikeda, M. (1999). 17beta-estradiol induces protein thiol/disulfide oxidoreductases and protects cultured bovine aortic endothelial cells from oxidative stress. *European Journal of Endocrinology, 140,* 608–613.

82. Urata, Y., Ihara, Y., Murata, H., Goto, S., Koji, T., Yodoi, J., Inoue, S., Kondo, T. (2006). 17Beta-estradiol protects against oxidative stress-induced cell death through the glutathione/glutaredoxin-dependent redox regulation of Akt in myocardiac H9c2 cells. *Journal of Biological Chemistry, 281,* 13092–13102.

83. Rosen, C.F., Poon, R., Drucker, D.J. (1995). UVB radiation-activated genes induced by transcriptional and posttranscriptional mechanisms in rat keratinocytes. *American Journal of Physiology, 268,* C846–C855.

84. Pan, S., Berk, B.C. (2007). Glutathiolation regulates tumor necrosis factor-alpha-induced caspase-3 cleavage and apoptosis: Key role for glutaredoxin in the death pathway. *Circulation Research, 100,* 213–219.

85. Taniguchi, Y., Taniguchi-Ueda, Y., Mori, K., Yodoi, J. (1996). A novel promoter sequence is involved in the oxidative stress-induced expression of the adult T-cell leukemia-derived factor (ADF)/human thioredoxin (Trx) gene. *Nucleic Acids Research, 24,* 2746–2752.

86. Nakamura, H., Nakamura, K., Yodoi, J. (1997). Redox regulation of cellular activation. *Annual Review of Immunology, 15,* 351–369.

87. Osborne, S.A., Hawkes, H.J., Baldwin, B.L., Alexander, K.A., Svingen, T., Clarke, F.M., Tonissen, K.F. (2006). The tert-butylhydroquinone-mediated activation of the human thioredoxin gene reveals a novel promoter structure. *Biochemical Journal, 398,* 269–277.

88. Tomita, M., Okuyama, T., Katsuyama, H., Hidaka, K., Otsuki, T., Ishikawa, T. (2006). Gene expression in rat lungs during early response to paraquat-induced oxidative stress. *International Journal of Molecular Medicine, 17*, 37–44.

89. Das, K.C., Guo, X.L., White, C.W. (1999). Induction of thioredoxin and thioredoxin reductase gene expression in lungs of newborn primates by oxygen. *American Journal of Physiology, 276*, L530–L539.

90. Tanito, M., Agbaga, M.P., Anderson, R.E. (2007). Upregulation of thioredoxin system via Nrf2-antioxidant responsive element pathway in adaptive-retinal neuroprotection in vivo and in vitro. *Free Radical Biology and Medicine, 42*, 1838–1850.

91. Barrett, W.C., DeGnore, J.P., Keng, Y.F., Zhang, Z.Y., Yim, M.B., Chock, P.B. (1999). Roles of superoxide radical anion in signal transduction mediated by reversible regulation of protein-tyrosine phosphatase 1B. *Journal of Biological Chemistry, 274*, 34543–34546.

92. Barrett, W.C., DeGnore, J.P., Konig, S., Fales, H.M., Keng, Y.F., Zhang, Z.Y., Yim, M.B., Chock, P.B. (1999). Regulation of PTP1B via glutathionylation of the active site cysteine 215. *Biochemistry, 38*, 6699–6705.

93. Pimentel, D.R., Adachi, T., Ido, Y., Heibeck, T., Jiang, B., Lee, Y., Melendez, J.A., Cohen, R.A., Colucci, W.S. (2006). Strain-stimulated hypertrophy in cardiac myocytes is mediated by reactive oxygen species-dependent Ras S-glutathiolation. *Journal of Molecular and Cellular Cardiology, 41*, 613–622.

94. Ghezzi, P. (2005). Regulation of protein function by glutathionylation. *Free Radical Research, 39*, 573–580.

95. Kanda, M., Ihara, Y., Murata, H., Urata, Y., Kono, T., Yodoi, J., Seto, S., Yano, K., Kondo, T. (2006). Glutaredoxin modulates platelet-derived growth factor-dependent cell signaling by regulating the redox status of low molecular weight protein-tyrosine phosphatase. *Journal of Biological Chemistry, 281*, 8518–28528.

96. Wang, J., Boja, E.S., Tan, W., Tekle, E., Fales, H.M., English, S., Mieyal, J.J., Chock, P.B. (2001). Reversible glutathionylation regulates actin polymerization in A431 cells. *Journal of Biological Chemistry, 276*, 47763–47766.

97. Shelton, M.D., Kern, T.S., Mieyal, J.J. (2007). Glutaredoxin regulates nuclear factor kappa-B and intercellular adhesion molecule in Muller cells: Model of diabetic retinopathy. *Journal of Biological Chemistry, 282*(17), 12467–12474.

98. Pineda-Molina, E., Klatt, P., Vazquez, J., Marina, A., Garcia, D.L., Perez-Sala, D., Lamas, S. (2001). Glutathionylation of the p50 subunit of NF-kappaB: A mechanism for redox-induced inhibition of DNA binding. *Biochemistry, 40*, 14134–14142.

99. Reynaert, N.L., van der Vliet, A., Guala, A.S., McGovern, T., Hristova, M., Pantano, C., Heintz, N.H., Heim, J., Ho, Y.S., Matthews, D.E., Wouters, E.F., Janssen-Heininger, Y.M. (2006). Dynamic redox control of NF-kappaB through glutaredoxin-regulated *S*-glutathionylation of inhibitory kappaB kinase beta. *Proceedings of the National Academy of Sciences USA, 103*, 13086–13091.

100. Adachi, T., Pimentel, D.R., Heibeck, T., Hou, X., Lee, Y.J., Jiang, B., Ido, Y., Cohen, R.A. (2004). S-glutathiolation of Ras mediates redox-sensitive signaling by angiotensin II in vascular smooth muscle cells. *Journal of Biological Chemistry, 279*, 29857–29862.

101. Kenchappa, R.S., Diwakar, L., Annepu, J., Ravindranath, V. (2004). Estrogen and neuroprotection: Higher constitutive expression of glutaredoxin in female mice offers protection against MPTP-mediated neurodegeneration. *FASEB Journal, 18*, 1102–1104.

102. Giustarini, D., Rossi, R., Milzani, A., Colombo, R., Dalle-Donne, I. (2004). S-glutathionylation: From redox regulation of protein functions to human diseases. *Journal of Cellular and Molecular Medicine*, 8, 201–212.

103. Wang, J., Tekle, E., Oubrahim, H., Mieyal, J.J., Stadtman, E.R., Chock, P.B. (2003). Stable and controllable RNA interference: Investigating the physiological function of glutathionylated actin. *Proceedings of the National Academy of Sciences USA*, 100, 5103–5106.

104. Zhang, S., Zhang, Z.Y. (2007). PTP1B as a drug target: Recent developments in PTP1B inhibitor discovery. *Drug Discovery Today*, 12, 373–381.

105. Bandyopadhyay, S., Starke, D.W., Mieyal, J.J., Gronostajski, R.M. (1998). Thioltransferase (glutaredoxin) reactivates the DNA-binding activity of oxidation-inactivated nuclear factor I. *Journal of Biological Chemistry*, 273, 392–397.

106. Shelton, M.D., Distler, A.M., Kern, T.S., Mieyal, J.J. (2009). Glutaredoxin regulates autocrine and paracrine proinflammatory responses in retinal glial (Müller) cells. *Journal of Biological Chemistry*, 284, 4760–4766.

107. Qanungo, S., Starke, D.W., Pai, H.V., Mieyal, J.J., Nieminen, A.L. (2007). Glutathione supplementation potentiates hypoxic apoptosis by S-glutathionylation of p65-NFκB. *Journal of Biological Chemistry*, 282, 18427–18436.

108. Starke, D.W., Chock, P.B., Mieyal, J.J. (2003). Glutathione-thiyl radical scavenging and transferase properties of human glutaredoxin (thioltransferase): Potential role in redox signal transduction. *Journal of Biological Chemistry*, 278, 14607–14613.

109. Pham, F.H., Sugden, P.H., Clerk, A. (2000). Regulation of protein kinase B and 4E-BP1 by oxidative stress in cardiac myocytes. *Circulation Research*, 86, 1252–1258.

110. Murata, H., Ihara, Y., Nakamura, H., Yodoi, J., Sumikawa, K., Kondo, T. (2003). Glutaredoxin exerts an antiapoptotic effect by regulating the redox state of Akt. *Journal of Biological Chemistry*, 278, 50226–50233.

111. Song, J.J., Rhee, J.G., Suntharalingam, M., Walsh, S.A., Spitz, D.R., Lee, Y.J. (2002). Role of glutaredoxin in metabolic oxidative stress. Glutaredoxin as a sensor of oxidative stress mediated by H_2O_2. *Journal of Biological Chemistry*, 277, 6566–46575.

112. Shaulian, E., Karin, M. (2002). AP-1 as a regulator of cell life and death. *Nature Cell Biology*, 4, E131–E136.

113. Klatt, P., Molina, E.P., De Lacoba, M.G., Padilla, C.A., Martinez-Galesteo, E., Barcena, J.A., Lamas, S. (1999). Redox regulation of c-Jun DNA binding by reversible S-glutathiolation. *FASEB Journal*, 13, 1481–1490.

114. Hurd, T.R., Costa, N.J., Dahm, C.C., Beer, S.M., Brown, S.E., Filipovska, A., Murphy, M.P. (2005). Glutathionylation of mitochondrial proteins. *Antioxidants and Redox Signaling*, 7, 999–1010.

115. Tretter, L., Sipos, I., Adam-Vizi, V. (2004). Initiation of neuronal damage by complex I deficiency and oxidative stress in Parkinson's disease. *Neurochemical Research*, 29, 569–577.

116. Gandhi, S., Wood, N.W. (2005). Molecular pathogenesis of Parkinson's disease. *Human Molecular Genetics*, 14(Spec No. 2), 2749–2755.

117. Hurd, T.R., Requejo, R., Filipovska, A., Brown, S., Prime, T.A., Robinson, A.J., Fearnley, I.M., Murphy, M.P. (2008). Complex I within oxidatively stressed bovine heart mitochondria is glutathionylated on Cys 531 and Cys 704 of the 75 kDa subunit: potential role of

CYS residues in decreasing oxidative damage. *Journal of Biological Chemistry, 283,* 24801–24815.

118. Kenchappa, R.S., Ravindranath, V. (2003). Glutaredoxin is essential for maintenance of brain mitochondrial complex I: Studies with MPTP. *FASEB Journal, 17,* 717–719.

119. Diwakar, L., Kenchappa, R.S., Annepu, J., Ravindranath, V. (2007), Downregulation of glutaredoxin but not glutathione loss leads to mitochondrial dysfunction in female mice CNS: Implications in excitotoxicity. *Neurochemistry International, 51,* 37–46.

120. Beer, S.M., Taylor, E.R., Brown, S.E., Dahm, C.C., Costa, N.J., Runswick, M.J., Murphy, M.P. (2004). Glutaredoxin 2 catalyzes the reversible oxidation and glutathionylation of mitochondrial membrane thiol proteins: Implications for mitochondrial redox regulation and antioxidant defense. *Journal of Biological Chemistry, 279,* 47939–47951.

121. Davis, D.A., Dorsey, K., Wingfield, P.T., Stahl, S.J., Kaufman, J., Fales, H.M., Levine, R.L. (1996). Regulation of HIV-1 protease activity through cysteine modification. *Biochemistry, 35,* 2482–2488.

122. Davis, D.A., Newcomb, F.M., Starke, D.W., Ott, D.E., Mieyal, J.J., Yarchoan, R. (1997). Thioltransferase (glutaredoxin) is detected within HIV-1 and can regulate the activity of glutathionylated HIV-1 protease in vitro. *Journal of Biological Chemistry, 272,* 25935–25940.

123. Velu, C.S., Niture, S.K., Doneanu, C.E., Pattabiraman, N., Srivenugopal, K.S. (2007). Human p53 is inhibited by glutathionylation of cysteines present in the proximal DNA-binding domain during oxidative stress. *Biochemistry, 46,* 7765–7780.

124. Rhee, S.G., Chae, H.Z., Kim, K. (2005). Peroxiredoxins: A historical overview and speculative preview of novel mechanisms and emerging concepts in cell signaling. *Free Radical Biology and Medicine, 38,* 1543–1552.

125. Chae, H.Z., Chung, S.J., Rhee, S.G. (1994). Thioredoxin-dependent peroxide reductase from yeast. *Journal of Biological Chemistry, 269,* 27670–27678.

126. Biteau, B., Labarre, J., Toledano, M.B. (2003). ATP-dependent reduction of cysteine-sulphinic acid by *S. cerevisiae* sulphiredoxin. *Nature, 425,* 980–984.

127. Woo, H.A., Jeong, W., Chang, T.S., Park, K.J., Park, S.J., Yang, J.S., Rhee, S.G. (2005). Reduction of cysteine sulfinic acid by sulfiredoxin is specific to 2-cys peroxiredoxins. *Journal of Biological Chemistry, 280,* 3125–3128.

128. Manevich, Y., Feinstein, S.I., Fisher, A.B. (2004). Activation of the antioxidant enzyme 1-CYS peroxiredoxin requires glutathionylation mediated by heterodimerization with pi GST. *Proceedings of the National Academy of Sciences USA, 101,* 3780–3785.

129. Bjornstedt, M., Xue, J., Huang, W., Akesson, B., Holmgren, A. (1994). The thioredoxin and glutaredoxin systems are efficient electron donors to human plasma glutathione peroxidase. *Journal of Biological Chemistry, 269,* 29382–29384.

130. Bertini, R., Howard, O.M., Dong, H.F., Oppenheim, J.J., Bizzarri, C., Sergi, R., Caselli, G., Pagliei, S., Romines, B., Wilshire, J.A., Mengozzi, M., Nakamura, H., Yodoi, J., Pekkari, K., Gurunath, R., Holmgren, A., Herzenberg, L.A., Herzenberg, L.A., Ghezzi, P. (1999). Thioredoxin, a redox enzyme released in infection and inflammation, is a unique chemo-attractant for neutrophils, monocytes, and T cells. *Journal of Experimental Medicine, 189,* 1783–1789.

131. Nickel, W. (2003). The mystery of nonclassical protein secretion. A current view on cargo proteins and potential export routes. *European Journal of Biochemistry, 270,* 2109–2119.

132. Arai, R.J., Masutani, H., Yodoi, J., Debbas, V., Laurindo, F.R., Stern, A., Monteiro, H.P. (2006). Nitric oxide induces thioredoxin-1 nuclear translocation: Possible association with the p21Ras survival pathway. *Biochemical and Biophysical Research Communications*, *348*, 1254–1260.

133. Malik, G., Gorbounov, N., Das, S., Gurusamy, N., Otani, H., Maulik, N., Goswami, S., Das, D.K. (2006). Ischemic preconditioning triggers nuclear translocation of thioredoxin and its interaction with Ref-1 potentiating a survival signal through the PI-3-kinase-Akt pathway. *Antioxidants and Redox Signaling*, *8*, 2101–2109.

134. Makino, Y., Yoshikawa, N., Okamoto, K., Hirota, K., Yodoi, J., Makino, I., Tanaka, H. (1999). Direct association with thioredoxin allows redox regulation of glucocorticoid receptor function. *Journal of Biological Chemistry*, *274*, 3182–3188.

135. Ravi, D., Muniyappa, H., Das, K.C. (2005). Endogenous thioredoxin is required for redox cycling of anthracyclines and p53-dependent apoptosis in cancer cells. *Journal of Biological Chemistry*, *280*, 40084–40096.

136. Wei, S.J., Botero, A., Hirota, K., Bradbury, C.M., Markovina, S., Laszlo, A., Spitz, D.R., Goswami, P.C., Yodoi, J., Gius, D. (2000). Thioredoxin nuclear translocation and interaction with redox factor-1 activates the activator protein-1 transcription factor in response to ionizing radiation. *Cancer Research*, *60*, 6688–6695.

137. Nakamura, H., Nakamura, K., Yodoi, J. (1997). Redox regulation of cellular activation. *Annual Review of Immunology*, *15*, 351–369.

138. Nordberg, J., Arner, E.S. (2001). Reactive oxygen species, antioxidants, and the mammalian thioredoxin system. *Free Radical Biology and Medicine*, *31*, 1287–1312.

139. Saitoh, M., Nishitoh, H., Fujii, M., Takeda, K., Tobiume, K., Sawada, Y., Kawabata, M., Miyazono, K., Ichijo, H. (1998). Mammalian thioredoxin is a direct inhibitor of apoptosis signal-regulating kinase (ASK) 1. *EMBO Journal*, *17*, 2596–2606.

140. Song, J.J., Lee, Y.J. (2003). Differential role of glutaredoxin and thioredoxin in metabolic oxidative stress-induced activation of apoptosis signal-regulating kinase 1. *Biochemistry Journal*, *373*, 845–853.

141. Jones, D.P. (2006). Redefining oxidative stress. *Antioxidants and Redox Signaling*, *8*, 1865–1879.

142. Peltoniemi, M.J., Rytila, P.H., Harju, T.H., Soini, Y.M., Salmenkivi, K.M., Ruddock, L.W., Kinnula, V.L. (2006). Modulation of glutaredoxin in the lung and sputum of cigarette smokers and chronic obstructive pulmonary disease. *Respiration Research*, *7*, 133.

143. Takagi, Y., Mitsui, A., Nishiyama, A., Nozaki, K., Sono, H., Gon, Y., Hashimoto, N., Yodoi, J. (1999). Overexpression of thioredoxin in transgenic mice attenuates focal ischemic brain damage. *Proceedings of the National Academy of Sciences USA*, *96*, 4131–4136.

144. Lundberg, M., Fernandes, A.P., Kumar, S., Holmgren, A. (2004). Cellular and plasma levels of human glutaredoxin 1 and 2 detected by sensitive ELISA systems. *Biochemical and Biophysical Research Communications*, *319*, 801–809.

145. Olanow, C.W., Tatton, W.G. (1999). Etiology and pathogenesis of Parkinson's disease. *Annual Review of Neuroscience*, *22*, 123–144.

146. Daily, D., Vlamis-Gardikas, A., Offen, D., Mittelman, L., Melamed, E., Holmgren, A., Barzilai, A. (2001). Glutaredoxin protects cerebellar granule neurons from dopamine-induced apoptosis by dual activation of the ras-phosphoinositide 3-kinase and jun N-terminal kinase pathways. *Journal of Biological Chemistry*, *276*, 21618–21626.

147. Akterin, S., Cowburn, R.F., Miranda-Vizuete, A., Jimenez, A., Bogdanovic, N., Winblad, B., Cedazo-Minguez, A. (2006). Involvement of glutaredoxin-1 and thioredoxin-1 in beta-amyloid toxicity and Alzheimer's disease. *Cell Death and Differentiation, 13*, 1454–1465.

148. Sachi, Y., Hirota, K., Masutani, H., Toda, K., Okamoto, T., Takigawa, M., Yodoi, J. (1995). Induction of ADF/TRX by oxidative stress in keratinocytes and lymphoid cells. *Immunology Letters, 44*, 89–193.

149. Nakamura, H., De Rosa, S.C., Yodoi, J., Holmgren, A., Ghezzi, P., Herzenberg, L.A., Herzenberg, L.A. (2001). Chronic elevation of plasma thioredoxin: Inhibition of chemotaxis and curtailment of life expectancy in AIDS. *Proceedings of the National Academy of Sciences USA, 98*, 2688–2693.

150. Nakamura, H., Herzenberg, L.A., Bai, J., Araya, S., Kondo, N., Nishinaka, Y., Herzenberg, L.A., Yodoi, J. (2001). Circulating thioredoxin suppresses lipopolysaccharide-induced neutrophil chemotaxis. *Proceedings of the National Academy of Sciences USA, 98*, 15143–15148.

151. Aota, M., Matsuda, K., Isow, N., Wada, H., Yodoi, J., Ban, T. (1996). Protection against reperfusion-induced arrhythmias by human thioredoxin. *Journal of Cardiovascular Pharmacology, 27*, 727–732.

152. Miyamoto, M., Kishimoto, C., Nimata, M., Nakamura, H., Yodoi, J. (2004). Thioredoxin, a redox-regulating protein, is expressed in spontaneous myocarditis in inbred strains of mice. *International Journal of Cardiology, 95*, 315–319.

153. Tao, L., Gao, E., Hu, A., Coletti, C., Wang, Y., Christopher, T.A., Lopez, B.L., Koch, W., Ma, X.L. (2006). Thioredoxin reduces post-ischemic myocardial apoptosis by reducing oxidative/nitrative stress. *British Journal of Pharmacology, 149*, 311–318.

154. Kobayashi-Miura, M., Shioji, K., Hoshino, Y., Masutani, H., Nakamura, H., Yodoi, J. (2007). Oxygen sensing and redox signaling: The role of thioredoxin in embryonic development and cardiac diseases. *American Journal of Physiology. Heart and Circulatory Physiology, 292*, H2040–H2050.

155. Mitsui, A., Hamuro, J., Nakamura, H., Kondo, N., Hirabayashi, Y., Ishizaki-Koizumi, S., Hirakawa, T., Inoue, T., Yodoi, J. (2002). Overexpression of human thioredoxin in transgenic mice controls oxidative stress and life span. *Antioxidants and Redox Signaling, 4*, 693–696.

156. Takagi, Y., Hattori, I., Nozaki, K., Mitsui, A., Ishikawa, M., Hashimoto, N., Yodoi, J. (2000). Excitotoxic hippocampal injury is attenuated in thioredoxin transgenic mice. *Journal of Cerebral Blood Flow and Metabolism, 20*, 829–833.

157. Masutani, H., Bai, J., Kim, Y.C., Yodoi, J. (2004). Thioredoxin as a neurotrophic cofactor and an important regulator of neuroprotection. *Molecular Neurobiology, 29*, 229–242.

158. Asahina, M., Yamada, T., Yoshiyama, Y., Yodoi, J. (1998). Expression of adult T cell leukemia-derived factor in human brain and peripheral nerve tissues. *Dementia and Geriatric Cognitive Disorders, 9*, 181–185.

159. Weichsel, A., Gasdaska, J.R., Powis, G., Montfort, W.R. (1996). Crystal structures of reduced, oxidized, and mutated human thioredoxins: Evidence for a regulatory homodimer. *Structure, 4*, 735–751.

160. Sun, C., Berardi, M.J., Bushweller, J.H. (1998). The NMR solution structure of human glutaredoxin in the fully reduced form. *Journal of Molecular Biology, 280*, 687–701.

CHAPTER 8

METHIONINE SULFOXIDE REDUCTASES: A PROTECTIVE SYSTEM AGAINST OXIDATIVE DAMAGE

HERBERT WEISSBACH and NATHAN BROT

8.1 INTRODUCTION

It has become increasingly clear that oxidative damage plays a significant, if not major, role in the age-related physiological changes that occur in animals, including man. As will be discussed elsewhere in this chapter, many of the genetic experiments in animals resulting in extended life span involve decreasing the amount of reactive oxygen species (ROS) in cells, produced primarily by mitochondria, or enhancing the cellular systems used to protect against oxidative damage. In some of the experiments in which life extension has been observed there is also clear evidence that the onset of most, if not all, of the age-related physiological changes can be delayed. Thus, life extension has been obtained with a high quality of life in these older animals. This important observation suggests that a common factor, such as oxidative damage, may be involved in the wide array of age-related diseases and understanding the etiology of the aging process may have important ramifications for extending life in humans while maintaining good health.

If one assumes that oxidative damage is a major factor in the aging process, modulation of the normal defense mechanisms cells use to protect against oxidative damage could lead to new therapeutic approaches to many of the age-related diseases. The two basic mechanisms used by cells to protect against oxidative damage involve destruction of the ROS by enzymes such as superoxide dismutase (SOD), catalase, peroxidases, etc., and/or repair of the oxidative damage to macromolecules, including nucleic acids, lipids, and proteins. The DNA repair systems are an example of a repair mechanism that has been thoroughly studied [1]. In the case of proteins it is known that at least six of the amino acids are easily oxidized (Table 8.1), and most of these oxidations are not reversible. However, oxidation of cysteine (Cys) and

Glutathione and Sulfur Amino Acids in Human Health and Disease. Edited by R. Masella and G. Mazza
Copyright © 2009 John Wiley & Sons, Inc.

TABLE 8.1   Amino Acids Sensitive to Oxidation
by Reactive Oxygen Species

Amino Acid	Oxidation Product
Cysteine	Cystine
Histidine	Imidazole oxidation
Lysine	Carbonyl derivative
Methionine	Met sulfoxide
Tyrosine	Ring oxidation
Tryptophan	Oxyindole

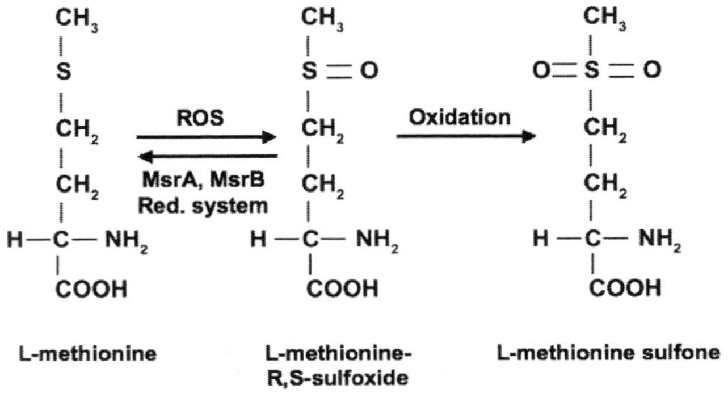

Figure 8.1   Oxidation of methionine. Oxidation of methionine (Met) by ROS to methionine sulfoxide Met(o) results in the formation of two epimers of Met(o) called Met-R-(o) and Met-S-(o). Further oxidation of Met(o) yields methionine sulfone. Msr, methionine sulfoxide reductase.

methionine (Met) residues are reversible. Met is one of the most sensitive amino acids to ROS damage, being converted to methionine sulfoxide (Met(o)), as seen in Fig. 8.1. Since the sulfur atom of Met(o) is a chiral center, oxidation of Met by ROS results in an equal mixture of both the R and S epimers of Met(o) as indicated in Fig. 8.1. Further oxidation yields methionine sulfone, which has been detected in tissues, although the mechanism by which it is formed or its relevance remains unknown. One of the recently discovered systems that cells use to protect against oxidative damage is the methionine sulfoxide reductase system (Msr), which can reduce Met(o) in proteins back to Met. This chapter will focus on the biochemistry and genetics of the Msr system and the possible role of this system in aging and age-related diseases.

8.2   HISTORY OF THE MSR SYSTEM

Although the reduction of free Met(o) back to Met was first demonstrated in yeast more than 40 years ago [2], the reduction of protein bound Met(o) was first reported in 1981 [3]. In these experiments it was observed that *Escherichia coli* ribosomal protein L12 was readily inactivated by hydrogen peroxide and that the loss of activity was due to the oxidation of one or more of the three Met residues in the protein. L12 is normally a dimer and oxidation caused monomerization of the protein and subsequent loss of binding of the protein to the large ribosomal subunit. As a follow up to these studies two Met(o) reducing enzymes were purified from soluble extracts of *E. coli*, one that reduced free Met(o) and a second enzyme that could reduce Met(o) residues in protein L12 and restore its activity [3–5]. The latter enzyme was initially called peptide methionine sulfoxide reductase but is currently referred to as MsrA. Subsequent studies on alpha-1-proteinase inhibitor showed that inactivation of this protein by specific oxidation of a Met residue at position 358 could be reversed, in part, by MsrA [6, 7]. By the early 1990s it was apparent that a large number of proteins and peptides were affected by Met oxidation, suggesting a more important role for MsrA in protecting cells against oxidative damage. A few examples of proteins and peptides whose activities are altered by Met oxidation, that have been studied in detail, are shown in Table 8.2. In order to do biochemical, structural, and genetic studies on MsrA it was clear that the gene for MsrA had to be identified and large amounts of the protein produced by rDNA technology. The *E. coli* msrA gene was cloned in the early 1990s [8] and soon after the bovine msrA gene was also cloned [9]. The msrA gene is essentially ubiquitous in nature and highly conserved [10]. After it was demonstrated that MsrA is stereospecific [11] and only reduces the S-epimer (Met-S-(o)) it was obvious to look for a comparable enzyme that was specific for Met-R-(o). Initial experiments in *E. coli* did not show detectable levels of such an activity, but Grimaud and coworkers [12] cloned an *E. coli* gene (yeaA) that had homology to the carboxyl terminal region of the PilB protein from *Neisseria gonorrhoeae*, a protein that had been shown to possess MsrA activity [10]. However, PilB is unique in that it has a mass of 57 KDa, more than twice that of other MsrA proteins. The MsrA domain was located closer to the N-terminus of the PilB protein. The *E. coli* YeaA protein had Msr activity and was shown to reduce the R epimer of Met(o) in proteins, and this protein was called MsrB [12]. The carboxyl portion of the PilB protein was also shown to possess MsrB activity, in addition to MsrA activity [13]. Thus, in *N. gonorrhoeae*, and a few other select organisms, the MsrA and MsrB activities are located on the same protein (Table 8.3), with the MsrA and MsrB activities located at the N- and C-terminals, respectively. In *E. coli* and most other microorganisms, and in animals, the genes for MsrA and MsrB are distinct. Table 8.3 also shows that the

TABLE 8.2 Some Proteins and Peptides Affected by Methionine Oxidation

E. coli ribosomal protein L12
α-1-Proteinase inhibitor
Calmodulin
Thrombomodulin
Drosophila Shaker K+ channel
β-Amyloid peptide
Cytochrome C

TABLE 8.3   PilB Msr Domain Structure and Msr Reductase Activity

	S-S oxid. red.		MsrA	MsrB	Specific Activity	
					Met-R-(o)	Met-R-(o)
PilB					4.5	5.0
PilB					0.7	9.0
PilB					6.8	0.0
CBS-1					5.5	0.0
yeaA					5.1	0.0

The activity of various PilB constructs, as well as human (CBS-1) and *E. coli* MsrB (YeaA) homologues, toward epimeric forms of Met(o) is shown.

Source: From Lowther et al. [13]. With permission.

TABLE 8.4   Mammalian Methionine Sulfoxide Reductases

Enzyme	Substrate	Location
MsrA	Met-S-(o)	Cytoplasm, mitochondria
MsrB1	Met-R-(o)	Cytoplasm
MsrB2	Met-R-(o)	Mitochondria
MsrB3	Met-R-(o)	Mitochondria, ER

E. coli MsrB (Yea A) [12] and a human gene called CBS-1 [14], which had been identified based on its homology to PilB, also specifically reduce Met-R-(o). In principle the reduction of R and S epimers of Met(o) in proteins, formed by oxidation of the Met residues by reactive oxygen species (ROS), could be accomplished by the action of both MsrA and MsrB.

Bacteria have a single copy of the MsrA and MsrB genes but mammalian cells have a more complex situation. As shown in Table 8.4, there is one gene for MsrA which through alternative splicing can yield mitochondrial and cytosolic forms [15, 16], whereas with MsrB there are three coding genes, referred to as msrB1, msrB2, and msrB3. As summarized in Table 8.4, MsrB1 is localized primarily in the cytosol, MsrB2 in the mitochondria, and MsrB3 in the endoplasmic reticulum and in the mitochondria [17]. It should be noted that all three MsrB proteins contain zinc and MsrB1 is also a selenoprotein [18].

8.3   MSRA AND MSRB PROTEIN STRUCTURE AND MECHANISM OF ACTION

The cloning of the MsrA gene made it possible to produce large amounts of the protein for structure/activity studies. The bovine, *E. coli*, and *Mycobacterium tuberculosis* MsrA proteins have been crystallized [19–21]. In the bovine MsrA there are three cysteine residues (Cys72, Cys218, and Cys 227) located in the vicinity of the active site. Conformational changes in the carboxyl terminal of the enzyme allow the three cysteines to participate in the catalytic reaction. The Cys at position 72 is directly involved in the catalysis and the mechanism involves a thiol-disulfide exchange, as shown in Fig. 8.2. In the initial step the Cys72 attacks the Met(o) with the release of Met and the formation of a sulfenic acid derivative (intermediate 3) on the enzyme, as first shown in studies on the *E. coli* enzyme [19]. The loss of water results in disulfide bond formation between Cys72 and Cys 218. Following a shift of the disulfide bond to Cys 218 and Cys 227 the oxidized protein is reduced by thioredoxin (Trx) to regenerate the reduced, active protein.

The crystal structure of the MsrB domain of the PilB protein from *N. gonorrhoeae* and the MsrB from *N. meningitidis* have also been elucidated [13, 22]. Although the crystal structure does not resemble the structure of MsrA the active sites show a mirror symmetry. Once again a Cys or selenocysteine (SeC) on the MsrB is involved in the catalytic reaction, and a sulfenic acid intermediate is formed. As discussed below there is still uncertainty as to how the sulfenic acid intermediate on the MsrB enzymes is reduced when there is not another Cys (resolving Cys) on the protein available to form a disulfide bond.

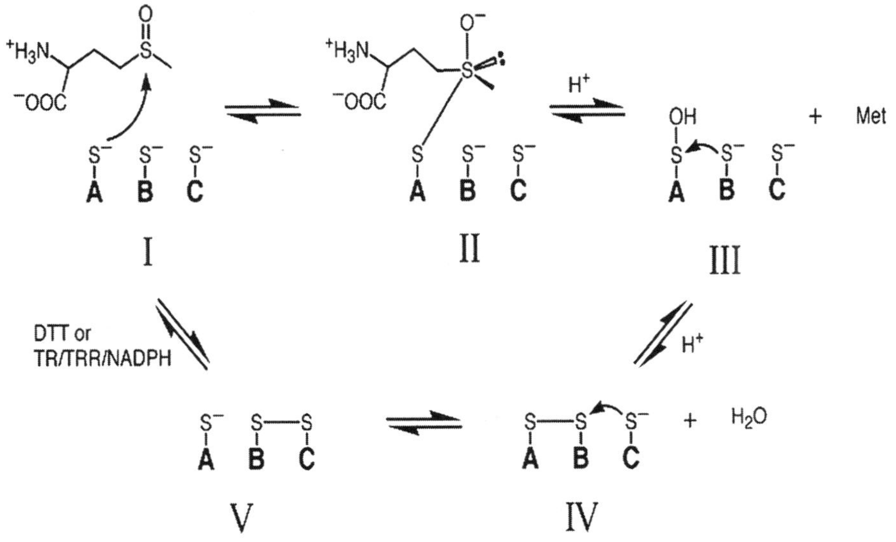

Figure 8.2 MsrA catalytic mechanism using the bovine methionine sulfoxide reductase (MsrA) as a model. (A) Cys 72; (B) Cys 218; (C) Cys 228. Proposed reaction mechanism for MsrA catalysis. Protonation of Met(o) (I) leads to the formation of a sulfonium ion (II). Possibly concomitant with sulfoxide protonation, cysteine 72 attacks the sulfur atom of the sulfonium ion, leading to the formation of a sulfenic acid intermediate (III). Breakdown of the complex is facilitated by proton transfer and the attack on cysteine 72 by cysteine 218 (IV). Return to a fully reduced state (I) is facilitated by thiol-disulfide exchange using either dithiothreitol (DTT) or reduced thioredoxin (V). Abbreviations: TR, thioredoxin; TRR, thioredoxin reductase. From Weissbach et al. [65]. Used with permission. See References 19 to 21 for more details.

8.4 MSR REDUCING REQUIREMENT

Dithiothreitol (DTT) is an excellent chemical reducing agent for the Msr proteins and is used routinely in the enzymatic reactions [23]. It was initially assumed that Trx is the natural reducing system for the Msr enzymes, based on studies on MsrA, in which Trx was a very efficient reducing agent for both *E. coli* and bovine MsrA and *E. coli* MsrB [3, 24, 25]. It was thus surprising to find that human MsrB2 and MsrB3 (hMsrB2, hMsrB3) do not function well with Trx from either *E. coli* or mammalian cells under the conditions used [25]. It should be noted that hMsrB2 and hMsrB3 differ from MsrA and *E. coli* MsrB, since they contain only the catalytic Cys with no resolving Cys residues [26].

A typical experiment, in which the activity of various Msr proteins is compared, with either DTT or Trx as the reducing agent, is shown in Table 8.5. Although *E. coli* MsrA, bovine MsrA, and *E. coli* MsrB readily use Trx as the reducing agent, human MsrB2 and MsrB3 do not. These latter enzymes, as noted above, have a Cys at the catalytic site but no resolving Cys residues, unlike MsrA and the bacterial MsrB proteins.

Of interest was the recent finding that thionein, the metal free apoprotein of metallothionein, can function as a reducing system for hMsrB2 and hMsrB3 [25]. Thionein can efficiently be generated from zinc metallothionein (Zn-MT) by treatment of the Zn-MT with EDTA. Thionein is a small protein of about 60 amino acids and contains 20 Cys residues, which accounts for its high reducing capability [27]. As seen in Table 8.6, thionein is not as efficient as DTT with MsrA and *E. coli* MsrB, but is a much better reducing agent than Trx with hMsrB3, since the activity of hMsrB3 with thionein is one-third that seen with DTT. Surprisingly thionein was not active with hMsrB2. There is no in vivo evidence to support the view that thionein is the natural reductant for hMsrB3. However, these results do raise the possibility that thionein, whose sole function in the past was thought to be the binding of metals and regulation of zinc metabolism [28], may have a physiological role as a reducing agent.

In a search for other agents that could supply the reducing power for MsrB1 and MsrB2 it was also observed that certain selenium compounds, such as

TABLE 8.5 Trx and DTT as Reducing Agents with Various Msr Proteins

Msr Proteins	DABS-met Formed (nmol)		Ratio Trx : DTT
	Trx	DTT	
eMsrA	46.8	46.2	1.0
eMsrB	60.3	11.1	5.4
bMsrA	15.8	30.0	0.53
hMrsB2	0.8	31.3	0.03
hMsrB3	1.7	53.8	0.03

DABS-met-S-(o) was used as substrate with MsrA proteins and DABS-met-R-(o) was used as substrate with MsrB proteins, EMsrA, *E. coli* MsrA : eMsrB, *E. coli* MsrB; bMsrA, bovine MsrA; hMsrB, human MsrB2; hMsrB3, human MsrB3.

Source: From Sagher et al. [25]. With permission.

**TABLE 8.6   Comparison of the Activity of Msr
Proteins in the Presence of Zn-MT or DTT**

Msr Proteins	nmoles DABS-met	
	Zn-MT	DTT
eMsrA	33.9	45.7
eMsrB	8.3	27.8
bMsrA	14.1	38.9
bMsrB2	0.9	27.1
hMsrB3	18.0	53.7

Incubations with zinc metallothionein (Zn-MT) routinely contained
5 nM EDTA to convert the Zn-MT to thionein. No significant activity
was detected in the absence of EDTA. See Table 8.5 and Sagher et al.
[25] for further details.

selenocysteamine and selenocystine, the reduced products of selenocystamine and
selenocysteine (Fig. 8.3), were powerful reducing agents [29]. A typical experiment
using selenocystamine in the presence of a reducing system is shown in Table 8.7.
Trx was used to reduce the selenocystamine to selenocysteamine in these experiments,
but it was also shown that thionein could function as a reducing agent for the selenium
compounds. The selenium compounds used do not appear to be in sufficient quantities
in tissues to have physiological relevance and a major unanswered question at this time
is the nature of the natural reducing system for MsrB2 and MsrB3. The above studies
on the reducing requirement for the Msr enzymes are summarized in Fig. 8.4. The
Msr enzymes, like MsrA and *E. coli* MsrB that have a resolving Cys, in addition to
the Cys at the active site, have a catalytic mechanism that involves the formation of

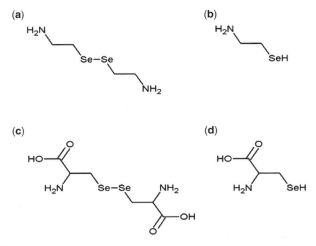

Figure 8.3   Structure of selenium compounds. (a) Selenocystamine; (b) selenocysteamine;
(c) selenocystine; (d) selenocysteine.

**TABLE 8.7   Effect of Selenocystamine on the Activity
of Msr Proteins Using the Trx Reducing System**

Enzyme	nmoles DABS-met Formed		
	No Addition	Trx	Trx + SeCm
eMsrA	1.9	15.3	18.6
eMsrB	<1	22.5	24.2
bMsrA	<1	13.1	45.9
hMsrB2	<1	2.3	65.3
hMrsB3	<1	1.0	55.7

All of the incubations that contained Trx also contained Trx reductase and
NADPH. Where indicated, SeCm (50 µM) was added. For other details
see Sagher et al. [29].

a sulfenic acid intermediate followed by formation of a disulfide bond on the enzyme.
The latter can be reduced by the Trx system (Fig. 8.4a). In contrast MsrB enzymes,
such as MsrB2 and MsrB3, which do not have a resolving cysteine, form a sulfenic
acid intermediate that is not efficiently reduced by cytosolic Trx, *E. coli* Trx, or mitochondrial Trx (Trx2) (Fig. 8.4b). However, thionein and certain selenium compounds

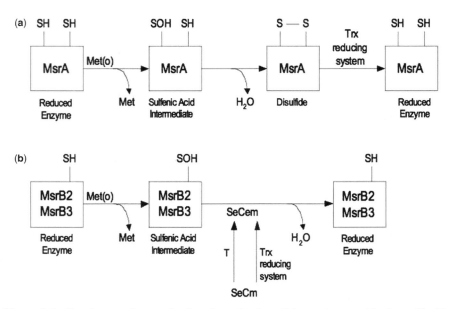

Figure 8.4   Putative reaction mechanism for reduction of the various methionine sulfoxide
reductase (Msr) enzymes by thioredoxin (Trx), thionein (T), and selenocysteamine (SeCem).
(a) MsrA or other Msr enzymes that contain a second cysteine, in addition to the catalytic
cysteine, that is capable of forming a disulfide bond on the enzyme. (b) MsrB2 and MsrB3,
examples of enzymes that do not contain a resolving cysteine. SeCm, selenocystamine. From
Sagher et al. [29]. Used with permission.

are able to reduce a sulfenic acid intermediate on these enzymes. We cannot eliminate the possibility that mammalian cells contain another Trx-like protein that could function as the reducing agent for MsrB2 and MsrB3. There is preliminary data that a drought-induced stress protein (CDSP32) from chloroplasts, whose structure is composed of two Trx modules with only one active site in the C-terminal domain in tandem, can function as a reducing agent for a chloroplast MsrB (called MsrB1) that cannot use Trx as the reducing agent [30], similar to human hMsrB2 and hMsrB3. Preliminary results have shown that CDSP32 can function with human MsrB2 and MsrB3 (unpublished data), but since there is no mammalian homologue of CDSP32, the question remains as to what is the natural reductant for human hMsrB2 and hMsrB3.

The reducing agent for MsrB1, which contains SeC at the active site and a resolving Cys residue, has not been extensively studied, but based on the available data this protein should be able to use Trx as the reducing agent.

8.5 OTHER MEMBERS OF THE MSR FAMILY

As noted above MsrA and MsrB appear to be the major proteins involved in repairing oxidative damage to Met residues in proteins. When MsrA was first purified from *E. coli* another Msr activity was identified in soluble *E. coli* extracts that could reduce free Met(o) [4]. In addition, there appeared to be significant Met(o) reducing activity in the membrane (insoluble) fraction obtained after low speed centrifugation [4]. The soluble Msr protein(s) that reduced free Met(o) was purified, but never characterized thoroughly. In more recent studies employing an MsrA/MsrB double mutant of *E. coli* it has been possible to obtain further information on the nature of these Met(o) reducing activities in *E. coli* [31, 32]. The results are summarized in Table 8.8. In addition to MsrA and MsrB there are Msr activities (fRMsr and fSMsr) in *E. coli* that can reduce free Met-R-(o) and Met-S-(o), respectively. There is another weak MsrA-like activity (MsrA1) that has not been further characterized and a very active membrane associated activity (mem-R,S-Msr) that can reduce the R and S epimers of Met(o), both free and peptide bound. The nature of this activity(s)

TABLE 8.8 Methionine Sulfoxide Reductases in *E.coli*

Msr	Free-R-(o)	Free-S-(o)	Peptide-R-(o)	Peptide-S-(o)
		Substrates		
MsrA		+		+
MsrB	(+)		+	
fRMsr	+			
fSMsr		+		
MsrA1				+
Mem-R,S-Msr	+	+	+	+

Summary of studies from Etienne et al. [31] and Spector et al. [32].

has also not been elucidated. Although detailed substrate specificity studies have not been done on all of the Msr members described in Table 8.8, it appears that MsrA, from *E. coli* or bovine liver, has the broadest specificity in that it can reduce free and peptide bound Met(o) as well as other compounds that have a methyl sulfoxide moiety such as dimethyl sulfoxide [9]. As will be discussed below a nonsteroidal anti-inflammatory prodrug, sulindac, is also a substrate for MsrA, converting it to sulindac sulfide, a cyclooxygenase inhibitor. In contrast, *E. coli* MsrB can reduce peptide bound Met(o), but has very weak activity towards free Met(o) and there is no evidence that MsrB can efficiently reduce compounds that do not contain a Met(o) structure. As noted in Table 8.8 the mem-*R,S*-Msr can reduce both the free and bound R and S epimers of Met(o) and there is preliminary evidence that other methyl sulfoxide compounds can also be reduced.

The free Met-R-(o) activity (fRMsr) in Table 8.8 appears to be quite specific for Met-R-(o). This protein has been purified and during the sequence analysis it was discovered that the crystal structure of the protein had been determined previously by the Structural genomiX bacterial genomics project, although no function had been assigned to this protein at that time. This protein is of interest since it belongs to the GAF family of signal transduction proteins [33]. The fRMsr appears to have three Cys residues that participate in the reaction mechanism, which involves the formation of a disulfide bond that covers a small active site region, and could explain its substrate specificity. Other GAF domain proteins, which specifically bind cyclic nucleotides, chromophores, and other ligands involved in the signal transduction process do not contain these Cys residues [34]. The fRMsr is the only known GAF protein to have catalytic activity [33]. It is possible that Met-R-(o) may be a signaling molecule in response to oxidative stress in *E. coli* and other organisms. A homologous mammalian gene to the *E. coli* fRmsr gene has not been detected. The free Met-S-(o) reducing activity in the soluble *E. coli* extracts (fSMsr) has not been studied in detail with regard to its substrate specificity.

8.6 THE MSR SYSTEM: BOTH A REPAIR ENZYME AND A SCAVENGER OF ROS

The initial studies on *E. coli* ribosomal protein L12 showed that the Msr system could function as a repair enzyme and reverse the damage due to Met oxidation by ROS [3]. As noted above (Table 8.2) there are now dozens of proteins and peptides whose function is affected specifically by Met oxidation. The broad specificity of both MsrA and MsrB toward protein bound Met(o) makes it likely that the activities of these enzymes are the primary mechanism responsible for the repair of Met oxidation in proteins. However, Levine et al. [35], in studies on glutamine synthetase, suggested that the Msr system could also be involved in scavenging ROS. They pointed out that all exposed Met residues in proteins have the potential to be oxidized by ROS, which would destroy the ROS leaving a Met(o) residue on the protein. Reduction of the Met(o) by the Msr system would regenerate the Met, with the net result that each round of Met oxidation and reduction would destroy one equivalent of ROS. Thus,

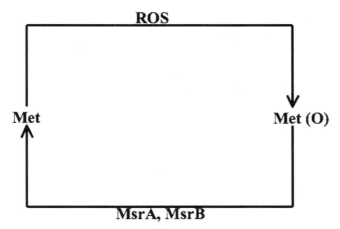

Figure 8.5   Roles of the methionine sulfoxide reductase (Msr) system. The Msr system is both a protein repair system and part of an ROS scavenger system. In the latter mechanism the Msr system permits Met residues in proteins to function as catalytic antioxidants since each round of Met oxidation and reduction by Msr enzymes will destroy a reactive oxygen species.

the Met residues in proteins could function as catalytic antioxidants, because of the activity of the Msr system. This ROS scavenger role of Met based on the Msr system is depicted in Fig. 8.5. There is now convincing data in cell culture experiments to support the role of the Msr system in scavenging ROS, as will be discussed below [36, 37].

8.7 GENETIC STUDIES ON THE ROLE OF THE MSR SYSTEM IN PROTECTING CELLS AGAINST OXIDATIVE DAMAGE

Once the MsrA gene was cloned it was possible to address the question as to whether the Msr system played a role, in vivo, in protecting cells against oxidative damage. All of the early studies on Met oxidation in proteins and reversal by the Msr enzymes were in vitro. The initial experiments were done using a mutant strain of *E. coli* lacking the MsrA gene [38]. Using a filter disc semiquantitative assay it was shown that the MsrA mutant was much more sensitive to oxidative stress than the wild type organism and that the mutant could regain the wild type phenotype after transformation with the MsrA gene. A more quantitative study in *E. coli* was later performed [39] and the results are summarized in Fig. 8.6. In these experiments four *E. coli* strains were used, wild type, MsrA mutant, MsrA mutant transformed with wild type MsrA, and Msr mutant transformed with a mutant gene that would express an inactive MsrA (Cys 58 to Ser). The viability (Y axis) is a log scale and shows that in the absence of peroxide all of the strains grow well. However, in the presence of peroxide there is a >90% loss of viability in the MsrA mutant and the MsrA mutant transformed with the mutant msrA gene. However, the wild type strain and the MsrA mutant

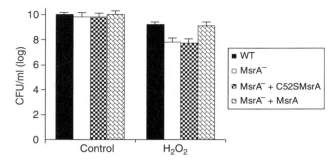

Figure 8.6   Methionine sulfoxide reductase (Msr) A can protect *E. coli* against oxidative damage. Four *E. coli* strains were grown in the absence or presence of hydrogen peroxide and cell viability determined. See text for details. From St. John et al. [39]. Used with permission.

strain transformed with the wild type msrA gene are much more resistant to the oxidative stress. These initial studies in *E. coli* were the first clear demonstration that MsrA might play an important role in protecting cells against oxidative damage. It should be noted that preliminary experiments (unpublished results) in which MsrB has been knocked out in *E. coli* have not shown increased sensitivity to oxidative stress, which is an unexpected result.

Table 8.9 summarizes some of the genetic experiments on the role of MsrA in protecting cells against oxidative damage. A similar effect of knocking out MsrA in *E. coli* has now been demonstrated in other bacterial strains [40–43], animal cells such as lens and retinal cells [37, 44], and in a MsrA knockout mouse [45]. In the latter case the MsrA knockout mice died earlier, were sensitive to high oxygen pressure, and had a neurological lesion (see Chapter 11). On the other hand overexpression of MsrA has been shown to protect yeast and animal cells, including thymocytes, PC12 cells, and lens cells against oxidative damage and extend the life span of flies [36, 46–49].

Studies using PC12 cells have demonstrated that overexpression of MsrA can protect these cells against oxidative damage caused by hypoxia and reoxygenation, and lower the level of ROS [36]. It was observed that the level of ROS drops by about 30% in cells that overexpress MsrA and these cells are protected against apoptotic cell death. These results support the role of the Msr system as part of a scavenger mechanism for ROS by permitting Met residues in proteins to act as

TABLE 8.9   Summary of Genetic Studies on the Role of MsrA

1. Knockout
   A. Bacteria, yeast, and animal cells are more sensitive to ROS
   B. Mice have shortened life span, are oxygen sensitive and have a neurological lesion
2. Transgenic (Overexpress MsrA)
   A. Animal cells in culture have increased resistance to ROS
   B. Flies are resistant to oxidative stress and have extended life span

catalytic antioxidants [35]. In these experiments MsrA also protected cells against hypoxia-induced depolarization of the mitochondrial membrane potential [36] and the results suggested that the Msr system may have a therapeutic potential in other diseases where there is damage due to hypoxia/reoxygenation, such as ischemic heart disease and stroke.

There is considerable evidence suggesting that both lens and retina are sensitive to oxidative damage. Lens crystalline proteins do not turnover and with age accumulate high levels of Met(o) [50]. In addition, retinal pigmented epithelial cells (RPE) are also sensitive to oxidation [51]. Thus, these eye cells seemed ideal tissues to look at the protective role of the Msr system. As seen in Fig. 8.7, human lens cells are protected against oxidative damage by overexpression of MsrA [47]. Also, siRNA silencing of MsrA in lens cells causes a loss of viability and increased ROS levels [37], once again supporting the view that the Msr system may be involved in scavenging

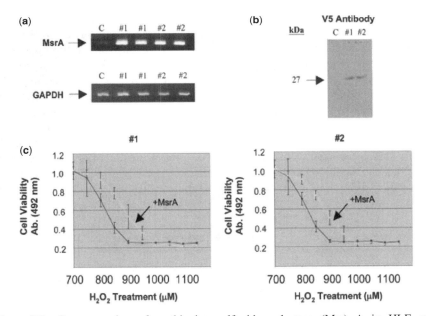

Figure 8.7 Overexpression of methionine sulfoxide reductase (Msr) A in HLE cells (SRA01/04). (a) Ethidium bromide-stained gels showing the relative levels of MsrA detected between two separately constructed overexpressing cell lines (#1 and #2) compared with control (C) cells. (b) Immunoblotting of 15 μg of protein extracts from control (C) cells and the two MsrA-overexpressing cell lines (#1 and #2) with a mouse monoclonal antibody raised against the 14-aa V5-epitope fused to the C-terminal end of the recombinant MsrA protein. (c) Representative graphs depicting increased resistance to H_2O_2 stress treatments of the two MsrA-overexpressing cell lines relative to control cells, using MTS cell viability assays. H_2O_2 treatments were conducted for 24 h in serum-free media. The absorbance readings and H_2O_2 concentrations used starting at 700 μM are indicated. Error bars represent standard deviations of eight separate cell viability assays. From Kantorow et al. [47]. Used with permission.

ROS [35]. In addition, primate retinal RPE cells, in which MsrA expression is inhibited using siRNA, are also significantly more sensitive to oxidative stress [44]. In these experiments control and siRNA transfected lens and retinal cells were exposed to varying concentrations of an oxidant and their viability measured. The results in both tissues clearly showed that cells lacking MsrA are more sensitive to oxidative stress than control cells. The retinal studies [44] also looked at the nature of the MsrA in this tissue. MsrA has been typically found as a monomer but evidence for an MsrA dimer and higher aggregates was found in the retina [44]. These multimeric forms were not dissociated in the presence of DTT and SDS and their nature remains unknown.

8.8 EVIDENCE THAT OXIDATIVE DAMAGE IS A MAJOR FACTOR IN AGING: ROLE OF MITOCHONDRIA AND THE MSR SYSTEM

Understanding the aging problem has medical, economic, and social implications. As we enter into the twenty-first century, age-related diseases and quality of life will become the major health issues in this country. Survival data support this conclusion as premature death from other causes decreases. As shown in Fig. 8.8 the median life span in humans (age at which 50% of the population survive) is approaching what some have called a theoretical value of about 80 to 85 years, whereas the maximum life span is about 110 years, with only rare exceptions. For someone born only 100 years ago the values would have been 60 years for the median life span with the maximum life span value remaining about the same as today. This large increase in the median life expectancy during the twentieth century is due primarily to the discovery of antibiotics that significantly reduced premature deaths due to infectious diseases. Unless there is a significant conceptual breakthrough on the aging problem one

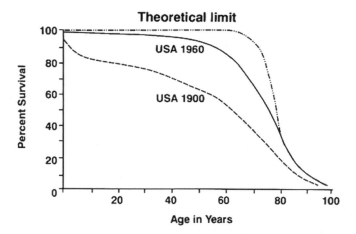

Figure 8.8 Survival curves in human populations. Data for populations in the United States during the past century. Adapted from Walford [52]. Used with permission.

does not expect the survival curves to change dramatically. There are two obvious approaches to the aging problem. One approach is to find a treatment or cure for the dozens of age-related diseases and other changes that affect the quality of life. The second approach is to try to delay the aging process. The latter approach would be possible if there were a common cause or etiology for most, or all, of the age-related changes that occur. In animals it has now become quite clear that this may be the case since there are several examples where it is possible to delay the aging process and significantly extend life span.

The first experiments go back to around 1960 and were done by Roy Walford, who showed that animals on a calorie-restricted diet with adequate nutrition lived longer and had a delay in the aging process [52]. Caloric restriction is the only well-accepted method that can increase maximum life span in all animal species tested without involving genetic manipulations. An example from the early work of Weindruch et al. [53] is shown in Fig. 8.9. A 50% increase in the median life span and maximum life span of mice was obtained on a diet in which calories were restricted by 50%, but otherwise provided adequate nutrition. The complex biochemical and physiological changes that occur in an organism on calorie restriction has made it difficult to understand the underlying mechanism of life extension in these animals. Several major theories have been put forth, including increased resistance to stress and less oxidative damage in animals on a calorie-restricted diet. There is evidence from yeast studies that the Sir2 gene (a histone deacetylase), and from other organisms, that the FOXO transcription family may be involved [54–56]. It is known that animals on a calorie-restricted diet have lower levels of the biochemical markers for oxidative damage, such as lower levels of protein oxidation, lipid oxidation, and mitochondrial DNA mutations [57, 58]. The oxidative damage theory has received the most attention since there are clear genetic experiments, unrelated to calorie restriction, that show if you can decrease oxidative damage in an organism it will live longer.

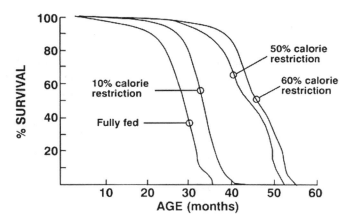

Figure 8.9 Life extension in mice on calorie-restricted diets. Adapted from Weindruch et al. [53]. Used with permission.

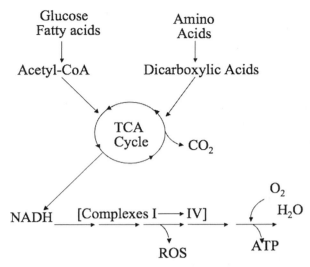

Figure 8.10   Mitochondrial production of ROS. Role of the tricarboxylic acid cycle (TCA) and the respiratory chain in ROS production. See text for details.

The bulk of the ROS produced in the cells arises from the mitochondrial respiratory chain and mitochondrial dysfunction has been implicated in the major neurodegenerative diseases [59]. Metabolism of nutrients from glycolysis, fatty acid oxidation, and amino acid metabolism results in the formation of NADH, primarily from the tricarboxylic acid cycle, that can enter the mitochondrial respiratory chain where the hydrogens and electrons are transferred through complexes and eventually reduce molecular oxygen to water (Fig. 8.10). This process is fundamental for providing the chemical energy in the form of ATP that is required for cells to survive. Although it has been estimated that 97% to >99% of the electrons that enter the respiratory chain are used to reduce oxygen to water, there is some leakage of electrons from the intermediary respiratory complexes. These electrons can react with oxygen to yield a partially reduced oxygen species, especially superoxide anion, that can be converted to other ROS (Table 8.10). It is clear that the efficiency of this process is crucial to the survival of the cell. In calorie-restricted animals the respiratory chain is more efficient and there is less leakage of electrons from Complex 1 [60]. In contrast, as the respiratory chain

TABLE 8.10   Major Reactive Oxygen Species Produced in Cells

- Superoxide anion
- Hydrogen peroxide
- Hypochlorous acid
- Hydroxyl radical
- Peroxynitrite

TABLE 8.11   Genetic Studies Linking Oxidative Damage to Life Span

Gene	Species	Life Span Extension (%)
SOD	Flies	40
Catalase	Mice	20
MsrA	Flies	70
INDY	Flies	80

For details see References 49, 61–64.

loses efficiency more ROS are formed causing more damage to the mitochondria. Since mitochondria play an important role in cell death by apoptosis, extensive damage will lead to apoptotic cell death.

Many of the genetic experiments on life extension involve mitochondria, in that the genes involved play a role in decreasing oxidative damage by lowering the level of ROS or increasing the repair mechanisms present in the cell (Table 8.11). These include the overexpression of SOD in flies, both the cytoplasmic form in motor neurons and the mitochondrial enzyme [61, 62], and the overexpression of catalase, specifically in the mitochondria of mice [63]. Some of these genetic manipulations would directly reduce the level of ROS in mitochondria. The third example is the overexpression of MsrA in flies. In these experiments the MsrA gene, which is found in the cytoplasm and mitochondria, was fused to GFP so that it was possible to detect the location of the expressed gene. Using the gal-4 expression system and various driver strains it was possible to show a marked extension of life span when the MsrA gene was expressed primarily in the nervous system [49]. A typical experiment is shown in Fig. 8.11. With both male and female flies the median life

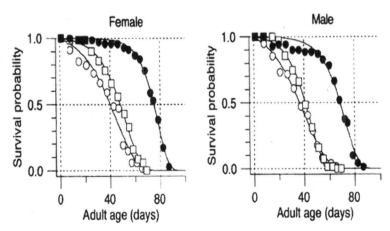

Figure 8.11   Life span of flies overexpressing methionine sulfoxide reductase (Msr) A in neural tissues. Closed circles, MsrA overexpressing flies; open symbols, control flies. From Ruan et al. [49]. Used with permission.

span is increased from about 40 to 45 days in the control flies to about 70 to 75 days in the MsrA transgenic flies. In addition, the maximum life span increases from 60 days in the control flies to >80 days in the transgenic flies.

It was also shown that the MsrA transgenic flies are more resistant to oxidative stress caused by paraquat [49]. The final example in Table 8.11 is knocking out of the INDY gene in flies [64]. This gene codes for a dicarboxylic transporter that brings these tricarboxylic acid intermediates into the cell and the mitochondria, a situation that might mimic calorie restriction in animals, where there is a reduced level of ROS in cells, resulting from an increase in the efficiency of the respiratory chain [60]. All of the above results strongly support the hypothesis that enhancing the systems that cells use to protect against oxidative stress can extend life span.

8.9   HOW CAN THE MSR SYSTEM BE UTILIZED FOR DRUG DEVELOPMENT?

The results described above suggest that enhancing the activity of the Msr system could have important therapeutic effects in protecting cells against oxidative damage. One approach would involve identifying compounds that are substrates for MsrA and/or MsrB that could act as catalytic antioxidants similar to Met in proteins

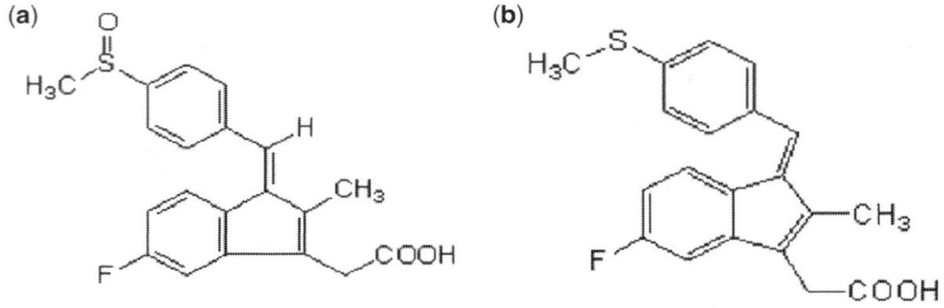

Figure 8.12   Structure of sulindac and sulindac sulfide: (a) sulindac and (b) sulindac sulfide.

TABLE 8.12   Activity of *E.coli* Msr Enzymes Using Sulindac as a Substrate

Enzyme	Units of Activity
MsrA	11.3
MsrB	0
fRMsr	0
fSMsr	0
MsrA1	<0.9
Mem-R,S-Msr	5.1

Unit of activity is defined as nmol of sulindac sulfide formed per hour. See Table 8.8 and text for further details on the *E. coli* enzymes.

Source: From Etienne et al. [65]. With permission.

TABLE 8.13   Subcellular Distribution in Calf Liver of Sulindac Reductase Activity

Liver Fractions	Specific Activity
S-10	4.39
S-100	6.20
Mitochondria	2.44
Microsomes	1.31

Specific activity is given as nmoles of sulindac sulfide synthesized per hour per mg of protein.

Source: From Etienne et al. [65]. With permission.

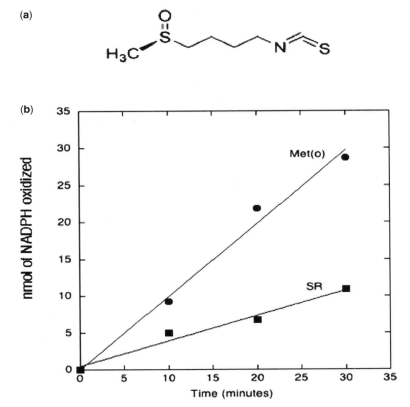

Figure 8.13   Sulforaphane is a substrate for methionine sulfoxide reductase (Msr) A. (a) Structure of sulforaphane and (b) time course of sulforaphane (SR) and Met(o) reduction by MsrA. The assay was based on NADPH oxidation. From Weissbach et al. [67]. Used with permission.

as described above. In the course of examining the substrate specificity of bovine MsrA, preliminary results indicated that the NSAID prodrug sulindac (Fig. 8.12), that is converted in vivo to sulindac sulfide, a known COX inhibitor, was a substrate for this enzyme [9]. More recently a simple spectrophotometric assay was developed to measure the reduction of sulindac to sulindac sulfide and this reaction was studied in more detail [65]. It should be noted that sulindac also has a chiral center and is composed of a mixture of the R and S epimers. As shown in Table 8.12, MsrA and the membrane Msr are the only *E. coli* Msr members that can reduce sulindac. MsrA reduces the S epimer of sulindac, whereas the *E. coli* membrane Msr reduces primarily the R epimer. The reduction of sulindac was also observed in animal cells. Extracts of calf liver kidney and brain showed reductase activity and subcellular studies using liver extracts showed that sulindac could be reduced by enzymes in the cytosol, mitochondria, and microsomes (Table 8.13). Other studies showed that the S epimer was preferentially reduced in the cytosol and mitochondria but the R epimer was mainly reduced by the ER [65]. The available evidence indicates that reduction of the S epimer is catalyzed by MsrA, but the enzyme in mammalian tissues responsible for reduction of the R epimer of sulindac is unknown. Experiments are in progress to test whether sulindac can function to protect cells against oxidative damage. It has also been shown that sulforaphane (Fig. 8.13), a natural product, containing a methyl sulfoxide moiety, that has been reported to possess both anticancer and antioxidant activity [66], can also be reduced by MsrA [67].

A second approach to use the Msr system to develop novel therapeutics would be to employ high throughput screening to identify compounds that could enhance the activity of the Msr enzymes.

8.10 METHIONINE SULFOXIDE AND DISEASE

Over more than three decades there has been an accumulation of evidence showing that in a number of diseases there is a significant oxidation of methionine residues in proteins, which in many cases results in a loss of biological activity. Many of these diseases appear to be age related. Some of these diseases are enumerated below.

8.10.1 Cataracts

Proteins of the lens are thought to be especially susceptible to oxidation because of constant exposure to the damaging effects of light and the long half-life of these proteins. In spite of this there are only very low amounts of Met(o) found in the proteins of normal lens. In contrast, with the development of cataracts, as much as two-thirds of the methionine content of lens proteins has been oxidized to Met(o) [68, 69]. It is also to be noted that the increase in Met(o) appears to be related to the severity of the cataract. Whether this is a result or cause of the cataract is not known. Other studies have shown that the increase in Met(o) is not due to differences in the level of Msr activity [70] between normal and cataractous lens.

8.10.2 Adult Respiratory Distress Syndrome, Smoker's Emphysema, and Rheumatoid Arthritis

One common feature of the above diseases is the involvement of a protein called alpha-1-proteinase inhibitor (α-1-PI). This protein is the major inhibitor of serum elastase and its inactivation by oxidation has been implicated in the pathology of these diseases. A decreased activity of α-1-PI in tissues, which would result in an elevated elastase activity, has been associated with pulmonary emphysema. Additionally, patients with a deficiency of this protein due to a genetic mutation develop precocious emphysema. This has led to the suggestion that pulmonary emphysema may be due to an imbalance between elastase and α1-P-I in lung tissue.

α-1-PI contains nine methionine residues and it has been shown that four of these residues are oxidized to Met(o) when the protein was isolated from the bronchoalveolar lavage (BAL) fluid of smokers [71], rats exposed to cigarette smoke [72], or the synovial fluid of patients with rheumatoid arthritis [73]. In addition the protein had a reduced ability to inhibit elastase, which is due to the oxidation of an essential methionine residue. There was no Met(o) present in the protein when isolated from normal patients.

A very similar situation appears to exist in patients with adult respiratory distress syndrome (ARDS). Cochrane and coworkers [74] showed that BAL from these patients also contained inactive α-1-PI. Although the amount of protein available was insufficient to allow a direct assay for the presence of Met(o) residues, these authors found that when the inactive protein was incubated with MsrA and dithiothreitol the ability of the protein to inhibit elastase was significantly increased. These results strongly support the idea that the α-1-PI from these patients was inactive due to the oxidation of one or more methionine residues. In vitro experiments, using purified components, have corroborated the relationship between the oxidation of methionine in α-1-PI and its inability to bind elastase. Thus, it was shown that when the protein was oxidized with chloramine-T, it completely lost its ability to bind elastase. However, when the oxidized protein was incubated with MsrA its activity was restored, which was dependent on the presence of DTT or thioredoxin [6]. Taken together the data suggests that the oxidative inactivation of α-1-PI is due to the oxidation of one or more methionine residues, which renders the protein unable to form a binary complex with elastase. In the lung this could result in alveolar connective tissue becoming more susceptible to the destructive action of leukocyte proteases. Conceivably the Msr system could play a therapeutic role in reversing the effects of oxidized α-1-PI in these various diseases.

Another protein that is involved in ARDS and in which the oxidation of Met may play a role in the disease is the soluble Fas ligand (sFasL). Fas is a membrane receptor protein that induces apoptosis after interaction with its cognate ligand (FasL). FasL exists in a membrane bound form as well as a soluble form and it has been shown that the bioactivity of sFasL is related to the formation oxygen induced multimerization of sFasL. Hagimoto et al. [75] found that only the BAL fluid from patients with ARDS, and not patients at risk for the disease, induced apoptosis in lung epithelial cells. It is known that the BAL fluid from patients with ARDS contains an increased number of neutrophils as well as myeloperoxidase (MPO) activity. Preliminary evidence suggests that the sFasL in the BAL from the ARDS patients is multimeric. In addition, incubating monomeric, recombinant sFasL with ARDS BAL or MPO-derived oxidants resulted in the multimerization of the protein, oxidation of Met to Met(o), concomitant with an increase in apoptotic activity. Furthermore when the oxidized protein was incubated in the presence of MsrA and MsrB (PilB) the sFasL was converted to a monomeric form and had a reduced apoptotic activity. These authors suggested that the oxidation of Met residues in sFasL promotes its multimerization, which leads to an increase in the apoptotic activity in the lungs of patients with injury.

The data suggests that in ARDS, the oxidation of methionine residues in two different proteins leads to a deleterious situation, which can result in epithelial destruction in the lungs either through increased elastase activity or by increased apoptosis. It would be interesting to speculate based on the in vitro ability of the Msr system to reverse these effects, that if the BAL fluid could be supplemented with MsrA and B and an appropriate reducing system, it might have a therapeutic effect.

8.10.3 Atherosclerosis

High density lipoproteins (HDL) remove cholesterol from cells of the artery wall thus protecting against atherosclerosis [76, 77]. Apolipoprotein A-1 (apoA-1) is the major protein of HDL and constitutes >70% of the total protein. It promotes cholesterol and phospholipid efflux mostly by a transport system mediated by the ABCA1 transporter. It is known that oxidation of apo-1 severely decreases cholesterol efflux by he ABCA1 pathway [78–80] and that HDL is chlorinated in human atherosclerotic lesions and in the blood obtained from patients with coronary artery disease [78]. This suggests that apoA-1 oxidation might be involved in atherogenesis. One of the major sources for apoA-1 oxidation is hypochlorous acid generated by the MPO system, which is present in macrophages in human atherosclerotic tissue. In addition to the chlorination of HDL, the presence of Met(o) has also been found in circulating HDL [81]. In vitro studies have shown that when ApoA-1 is exposed to the MPO system, only tyrosine 192 was converted to 3-chlorotyrosine, which resulted in a loss of the ability of the protein to remove cholesterol from BHK cells [82]. However, when the tyrosine was mutated to phenylalanine (which was not chlorinated) there was still a loss (although less) of activity, suggesting another oxidizable amino acid. ApoA-1 contains three methionine residues and LC-ESI-MS/MS analysis showed that all three Met residues had been oxidized to Met(o) when incubated with MPO. When wild type ApoA-1 was oxidized and incubated with MsrA/MsrB(PilB), all three Met(o) residues were reduced and partial reactivation of its activity was observed [82]. However, when the phenylalanine mutant was oxidized and incubated with MsrA/MsrB, the ability of the protein to cause efflux of cholesterol was restored to wild type levels. These results suggest that methionine oxidation as well as tyrosine chlorination are involved in the loss of the ability of ApoA-1 to remove cholesterol from cells. One might expect that oxidation-resistant forms of ApoA-1 could be anti-artherogenic in vivo.

8.10.4 Alzheimer's Disease

Alzheimer's disease (AD) is the most common form of dementia, affecting almost four million adults in the United States [83, 84]. It is most prevalent in the elderly, with an incidence of about 19% and 47% for those 75 to 84 and over 85 years old, respectively. It is one of the five leading causes of death in the United States. As the age of the population increases, and if no cure is found, it is estimated that about nine million people could develop AD by the year 2040 [85]. Its main pathological features are the presence of senile plaques, synapse loss, and neurofibrillar tangles (NFT), which are associated with cognitive decline [83]. The senile plaque contains a core of the amyloid beta protein (Aβ), which is generated from the proteolysis of the amyloid precursor protein. There are two main forms of Aβ (1-40) and (1-42) with the latter being the major component of the plaques. Genetic evidence suggests that the metabolism of Aβ is linked to AD and that deposition of Aβ in the brain is important for the pathology of the disease. A number of studies have shown an association of brain tissue oxidative damage with AD [86–88]. One of the mechanisms proposed for the oxidation is the synthesis of ROS directly from Aβ [89, 90]. This generation of ROS usually requires the reaction of O_2 with Cu^{2+} or Fe^{3+} or other redox ions. When Aβ binds either of these two metals redox reactions occur reducing the oxidation state of the metal and producing H_2O_2 from O_2 in a catalytic manner [91, 92]. It has been shown that the reduction of the metal is coupled with the oxidation of the single Met residue to Met(o) of Aβ at position 35. In AD brains the oxidized form of the peptide was estimated to comprise between 10% and 50% of the total brain Aβ [90].

Methionine 35 has been shown to play an important role in the pathology associated with the neurotoxicity, aggregation, and ROS generation of Aβ [89, 90]. Several observations have led to this conclusion. It was found that the substitution of the methionine residue by norleucine or cysteine abolishes the neurotoxicity and oxidative stress of Aβ (1-42), but does not affect the morphology of the fibrils [93]. Also, in vivo experiments, in which Met 35 was replaced by cysteine and expressed in *Caenorhabditis elegans*, resulted in no protein oxidation even though the deposition of the peptide was the same as the native peptide. Finally, it has been shown that a truncated Aβ (1-28), which lacks Met, does not induce neurotoxicity. Although the exact mechanism of toxicity of the Aβ is still not clear a number of studies have shown that both the native form and the oxidized form of the peptide bind metals, produce ROS, and are toxic. The evidence suggests that the toxicity occurs via the same mechanism of metal-dependent ROS formation and Aβ aggregation. It is to be noted that there are two methods of inducing aggregation of Aβ, metal-induced cross linking, which yields amorphous aggregates, and fibril formation. Oxidation of the methionine residue inhibits fibril aggregation, but not the metal-mediated aggregation, suggesting that fibrils are not the toxic species. The oxidized Aβ would be expected to be more hydrophilic than the native, which would alter the peptide interaction with membranes and make it more soluble. In concert with this observation it has been reported that synaptic damage and cognitive impairment in AD patients is associated with the soluble forms of Aβ [90]. As stated above, Met(o)Aβ has been found in high concentration in AD brains, is soluble and toxic, and is less likely to be associated with lipids. The solubility of Met(o)Aβ, as compared to the native form, would allow it to be transported to the synapse where it could bind to synaptic Cu^{2+} released upon neurotransmission and increase the toxicity of the peptide. It is interesting to note that Msr has been reported to be decreased in the brains of AD patients [94], which could result in increased levels of Met(o)Aβ. Since it appears that the oxidized peptide is more toxic than the native peptide, if there were a drug that would increase the activity of the Msr it might have a beneficial effect in AD patients.

8.10.5   Parkinson's Disease

There have been a number of studies that have suggested that oxidative damage may be involved in Parkinson's disease (PD) due to the degeneration of dopaminergic neurons [95–97]. Although the brain constitutes about 5% of body weight it consumes about 25% of respired oxygen. During the course of mitochondria respiration, appreciable amounts of ROS are formed as described above. The dopaminergic neurons in the substantia nigra are particularly sensitive to oxidation due probably to the large amounts of dopamine and ferrous ion [98, 99]. In patients with PD the dopaminergic neurons contain inclusion bodies known as Lewy bodies and Lewy neuritis in which the major component is α-synuclein. Although it was previously thought that the inclusion bodies might be the cause of the disease recent evidence has suggested that the fibrils are not cytotoxic but rather some precursor oligomeric species.

The finding that a mutation in the synuclein gene was associated with autosomal inherited PD and an accumulation of aggregates focused attention on the role of this protein in this disease. Synuclein is a 140 amino acid protein containing four methionine (Met) residues and when these Mets are oxidized the protein has a slightly more disordered conformation due possibly to its decreased hydrophobicity [100]. Using a fluorescence assay to detect fibrillation, it was shown that while native synuclein readily formed fibrils, the Met oxidized protein was resistant to fibril formation. Furthermore, it was shown that while the native protein elutes from a size exclusion gel as a monomer the Met oxidized protein elutes as an oligomer [100]. Other studies [101] have shown that when the Met residues are mutated to leucines and then subjected to oxidation, the amount of inhibition of fibrillation by the synuclein containing Met(o) is proportional to the number of Mets oxidized. Each Met residue appears to have an equal effect on the inhibition of fibrillation.

As mentioned above the toxic species of synuclein may be the oligomeric form, which is present when the Met residues are oxidized. It appears likely that some fraction of the Met residues in synuclein will be oxidized in the dopaminergic neurons. The large amounts of synuclein in the brain, each containing four equivalents of Met, could act as a sink for any oxidants in the brain. It is not known whether these Met(o) residues would be substrates for the Msr system, but if they are the Msr system could play an important role in controlling the fibrillation state of synuclein and be an important component of PD.

ACKNOWLEDGMENT

This article is contribution #P200704 of the Center of Excellence in Biomedical and Marine Biotechnology of Florida Atlantic University from the State of Florida, which funded part of these studies.

REFERENCES

1. *Trends in Biochemical Sciences*, 20 (10, October) 1995. Volume dedicated on DNA Repair. pp. 381–440.

2. Black, S., Harte, E.M., Hudson, B., Wartofsky, L. (1960). A specific enzymatic reduction of L(-) methionine sulfoxide and a related nonspecific reduction of disulfides. *Journal of Biological Chemistry*, 235, 2910–2916.

3. Brot, N., Weissbach, L., Werth, J., Weissbach, H. (1981). Enzymatic reduction of protein-bound methionine sulfoxide. *Proceedings of the National Academy of Sciences USA*, 78, 2155–2158.

4. Ejiri, S.-I., Weissbach, H., Brot, N. (1979). The reduction of methionine sulfoxide to methionine by *Escherichia coli*. *Journal of Bacteriology*, 139, 161–164.

5. Ejiri, S.-I., Weissbach, H., Brot, N. (1980). The purification of methionine sulfoxide reductase from *Escherichia coli*. *Analytical Biochemistry*, 102, 393–398.

6. Abrams, W.R., Weinbaum, G., Weissbach, L., Weissbach, H., Brot, N. (1981). Enzymatic reduction of oxidized a-1-proteinase inhibitor restores biological activity. *Proceedings of the National Academy of Sciences USA*, 78, 7483–7486.

7. Carp, H., Janoff, A., Abrams, W., Weinbaum, G., Drew, R.T., Weissbach, H., Brot, N. (1983). Human methionine sulfoxide-peptide reductase, an enzyme capable of reactivating oxidized a-1-proteinase inhibitor in vitro. *American Review of Respiratory Diseases*, 127, 301–305.

8. Rahman, M.A., Nelson, H., Weissbach, H., Brot, N. (1992). Cloning, sequencing, and expression of the *Escherichia coli* peptide methionine sulfoxide reductase gene. *Journal of Biological Chemistry*, 267, 15549–15551.

9. Moskovitz, J., Weissbach, H., Brot, N. (1996). Cloning and expression of a mammalian gene involved in the reduction of methionine sulfoxide residues in proteins. *Proceedings of the National Academy of Sciences USA*, 93, 2095–2099.

10. Lowther, W.T., Brot, N., Weissbach, H., Honek, J., Matthews, B. (2000). Thiol-disulfide exchange is involved in the catalytic mechanism of peptide methionine sulfoxide reductase. *Proceedings of the National Academy of Sciences USA*, 97, 6463–6468.

11. Moskovitz, J., Singh, V.K., Requena, J., Wilkinson, B.J., Jayaswal, R.K., Stadtman, E.R. (2002). Purification and characterization of methionine sulfoxide reductases from mouse and *Staphylococcus aureus* and their substrate specificity. *Biochemical and Biophysical Research Communications*, 290, 62–65.

12. Grimaud, R., Ezraty, B., Mitchell, J.K., Lafitte, D., Briand, C., Derrick, P.J., Barras, F.J. (2001). Repair of oxidized proteins: Identification of a new methionine sulfoxide reductase. *Journal of Biological Chemistry*, 276, 48915–48920.

13. Lowther, W.T., Weissbach, H., Etienne, F., Brot, N., Matthews, B.W. (2002). The "mirrored" methionine sulfoxide reductases of *Neisseria gonorrhoeae* pilB. *Nature Structural Biology*, 9(5), 348–352.

14. Huang, W., Escribano, J., Sarfarazi, M., Coca-Prados, M. (1999). Identification, expression and chromosomal localization of a human gene encoding a novel protein with similarity to the pilB family of transcriptional factors (pilin) and to bacterial peptide methionine sulfoxide reductase. *Gene*, 233, 233–240.

15. Hansel, A., Kuschel, L., Hehl, S., Lemke, C., Agricola, H.J., Hoshi, T., Heinemann, S.H. (2002). Mitochondrial targeting of the human peptide methionine sulfoxide reductase A

(MSRA), an enzyme involved in the repair of oxidized proteins. *FASEB Journal, 16,* 911–913.

16. Vougier, S., Mary, J., Friguet, B. (2003). Subcellular localization of methionine sulfoxide reductase A (MsrA): Evidence for mitochondrial and cytosolic isoforms in rat liver cells. *Biochemical Journal, 373,* 531–537.

17. Kim, H.Y., Gladyshev, V.N. (2004). Methionine sulfoxide reduction in mammals: Characterization of methionine-R-sulfoxide reductases. *Molecular Biology of the Cell, 15,* 1055–1064.

18. Kryukov, G.V., Kumara, A., Koc, A., Sun, Z., Gladyshev, V.N. (2002). Selenoprotein R is a zinc-containing stereospecific methionine sulfoxide reductase. *Proceedings of the National Academy of Sciences USA, 99,* 4245–4250.

19. Tete-Favier, F., Cobessi, D., Azza, S., Boschi-Muller, S., Branlant, G., Aubry, A. (2000). Crystal structure of the *Escherichia coli* peptide met sulphoxide reductase at 1.9 Å resolution. *Structure, Folding & Design, 15,* 1167–1178.

20. Lowther, W.T., Brot, N., Weissbach, H., Matthews, B.W. (2000). Structure and mechanism of peptide methionine sulfoxide reductase, an "anti-oxidation" enzyme. *Biochemistry, 39,* 13307–13312.

21. Taylor, A.B., Benglis, D.M., Jr., Dhandayuthapani, S., Hart, J.P. (2003). Structure of *Mycobacterium tuberculosis* methionine sulfoxide reductase A in complex with protein-bound methionine. *Journal of Bacteriology, 185,* 4119–4126.

22. Kauffmann, B., Favier, B.F., Olry, A., Boschi-Muller, S., Carpentier, P., Branlant, G., Aubry, A. (2002). Crystallization and preliminary X-ray diffraction studies of *Neisseria meningitidis* PILB. *Acta Crystallographica. Section D, Biological Crystallography, 58,* 1467–1469.

23. Brot, N., Werth, J., Koster, D., Weissbach, H. (1982). Reduction of N-Acetyl methionine sulfoxide: A simple assay for peptide methionine sulfoxide reductase. *Analytical Biochemistry, 122,* 291–294.

24. Brot, N., Weissbach, H. (1982). The biochemistry of methionine sulfoxide residues in proteins. *Trends in Biochemical Sciences, 7,* 137–139.

25. Sagher, D., Brunell, D., Hejtmancik, J.F., Kantorow, M., Brot, N., Weissbach, H. (2006). Thionein can serve as a reducing agent for the methionine sulfoxide reductases. *Proceedings of the National Academy of Sciences USA, 103*(23), 8656–8661.

26. Kim, H.Y., Gladyshev, V.N. (2005). Different catalytic mechanisms in mammalian selenocysteine- and cysteine-containing methionine-R-sulfoxide reductases. *PLoS Biology, 3,* e375.

27. Robbins, A.H., McRee, D.E., Williamson, M., Collet, S.A., Xuong, N.H., Furey, W.F., Wang, B.C., Stout, C.D. (1991). Refined crystal structure of Cd, Zn metallothionein at 2.0 angstrom resolution. *Journal of Molecular Biology, 221,* 1269–1293.

28. Vallee, B.L. (1995). The function of metallothionein. *Neurochemistry International, 27,* 23–33.

29. Sagher, D., Brunell D., Brot, N., Vallee, B.L., Weissbach, H. (2006). Selenocompounds can serve as oxido-reductants with the methionine sulfoxide reductase enzymes. *Journal of Biological Chemistry, 281*(42), 31184–31187.

30. Rey, P., Cuiné, S., Eymery, F., Garin, J., Court, M., Jacquot, J.-P., Rouhier, N., Broin, M. (2005). Analysis of the proteins targeted by CDSP32, a plastidic thioredoxin participating in oxidative stress responses. *Plant Journal, 41,* 31–42.

31. Etienne, F., Spector, D., Brot, N., Weissbach, H. (2003). A methionine sulfoxide reductase in *Escherichia coli* that reduces the R enantiomer of methionine sulfoxide. *Biochemical and Biophysical Research Communications, 300*, 378–382.

32. Spector, D., Etienne, F., Brot, N., Weissbach, H. (2003). New membrane associated and soluble peptide methionine sulfoxide reductases in *Escherichia coli*. *Biochemical and Biophysical Research Communications, 302*, 284–289.

33. Lin, Z., Johnson, L.C., Weissbach, H., Brot, N., Lively, M.O., Lowther, W.T. (2007). The free methionine-*R*-sulfoxide reductase from *Escherichia coli* reveals a new GAF domain function. *Proceedings of the National Academy of Sciences USA, 104*(23), 9597–9602.

34. Aravind, L., Ponting, C.P., (1997). The GAF domain: An evolutionary link between diverse phototransducing proteins. *Trends in Biochemical Science, 22*, 458–459.

35. Levine, R.L., Mosoni, L., Bertlett, B.S., Stadtman, E.R. (1996). Methionine residues as endogenous antioxidants in proteins. *Proceedings of the National Academy of Sciences USA, 96*, 15036–15040.

36. Yermolaieva, O., Xu, R., Schinstock, C., Brot, N., Weissbach, H., Heinemann, S., Hoshi, T. (2004). Methionine sulfoxide reductase A (MSRA) protects neuronal cells against brief hypoxia-reoxygenation. *Proceedings of the National Academy of Sciences USA, 101*, 1159–1164.

37. Marchetti, M., Lee, W., Cowell, T., Wells, T., Weissbach, H., Kantorow, M. (2006). Silencing of the methionine sulfoxide reductase A gene results in loss of mitochondrial membrane potential and increased ROS production in human lens cells. *Journal of Experimental Eye Research, 83*(5), 1281–1286.

38. Moskovitz, J., Rahman, A., Strassman, J., Yancey, S.O., Kushner, S.R., Brot, N., Weissbach, H. (1995). *Escherichia coli* peptide methionine sulfoxide reductase gene: Regulation of expression and role in protecting against oxidative damage. *Journal of Bacteriology, 177*, 502–507.

39. St. John, G., Brot, N., Ruan, J., Erdjument-Bromage, H., Tempst, P., Weissbach, H., Nathan, C. (2001). Peptide methionine sulfoxide reductase from *Escherichia coli* and *Mycobacterium tuberculosis* protects bacteria against oxidative damage from reactive nitrogen intermediates. *Proceedings of the National Academy of Sciences USA, 98*, 9901–9906.

40. Hassouni, M.E., Chambost, J.P., Expert, D., Van Gijsegem, F., Barras, F. (1999). The minimal gene set member msrA, encoding peptide methionine sulfoxide reductase, is a virulence determinant of the plant pathogen *Erwinia chrysanthemi*. *Proceedings of the National Academy of Sciences USA, 96*, 887–892.

41. Skaar, E.P., Tobiason, D.M., Quick, J., Judd, R.C., Weissbach, H., Etienne F., Brot, N., Seifert, H.S. (2002). The outer membrane localization of the *Neisseria gonorrhoeae* MsrA/B is involved in survival against reactive oxygen species. *Proceedings of the National Academy of Sciences USA, 99*, 10108–10113.

42. Dhandayuthapani, S., Blaylock, M.W., Bebear, C.M., Rasmussen, W.G., Baseman, J.B. (2001). Peptide methionine sulfoxide reductase (MsrA) is a virulence determinant in *Mycoplasma genitalium*. *Journal of Bacteriology, 183*, 5645–5650.

43. Alamuri, P., Maier, R.J. (2006). Methionine sulfoxide reductase in *Helicobacter pylori*: Interaction with methionine-rich proteins and stress-induced expression. *Journal of Bacteriology, 188*(16), 5839–5850.

44. Lee, J., Gordiyenko, N., Marchetti, M., Tserentsoodol, N., Sagher, D., Alam, S., Weissbach, H., Kantorow, M., Rodriguez, I. (2006). Gene structure, localization and role in oxidative stress of methionine sulfoxide reductase A (msrA) in the monkey retina. *Journal of Experimental Eye Research, 82*(5), 816–827.

45. Moskovitz, J., Bar-Noy, S., Williams, W.M., Requena, J., Bertlett, B.S., Stadtman, E.R. (2001). Methionine sulfoxide reductase (MsrA) is a regulator of antioxidant defense and lifespan in mammals. *Proceedings of the National Academy of Sciences USA, 98*, 12920–12925.

46. Moskovitz, J., Flescher, E., Bertlett, B.S., Azare, J., Poston, J.M., Stadtman, E.R. (1998). Overexpression of peptide-methionine sulfoxide reductase in *Saccharomyces cerevisiae* and human T cells provides them with high resistance to oxidative stress. *Proceedings of the National Academy of Sciences USA, 95*, 14071–14075.

47. Kantorow, M., Hawse, J.R., Cowell, T.L., Benhamed, S., Pizarro, G.O., Reddy, V.N., Hejtmancik, J.F. (2004). Methionine sulfoxide reductase A is important for lens cell viability and resistance to oxidative stress. *Proceedings of the National Academy of Sciences USA, 101*, 9654–9659.

48. Marchetti, M., Pizarro, G.O., Sagher, D., DeAmicis, C., Brot, N., Hejtmancik, J.F., Weissbach, H., Kantorow, M. (2005). Methionine sulfoxide reductases B1, B2, and B3 are present in the human lens and confer oxidative stress resistance to lens cells. *Investigative Ophthalmology and Visual Science, 46*, 2107–2112.

49. Ruan, H., Tang, X.D., Chen, M.-L., Joiner, M.A., Sun, G., Brot, N., Weissbach, H., Heinemann, S.H., Iverson, L., Wu, C.-F., Hoshi, T. (2002). High-quality life extension by the enzyme peptide methionine sulfoxide reductase. *Proceedings of the National Academy of Sciences USA, 99*, 2748–2753.

50. Smith, J.B., Jiang, X., Abraham, E.C. (1997). Identification of hydrogen peroxide oxidation sites of alpha A- and alpha B-crystallins. *Free Radical Research, 26*, 103–111.

51. Bonnel, S., Mohand-Said, S., Sahel, J.-A. (2003). The aging of the retina. *Experimental Gerontology, 38* (Review), 825–831.

52. Walford, R.L. (1983). *Maximum Life Span*. New York: W.W. Norton & Co.

53. Weindruch, R., Walford, R.L., Fligiel, S., Guthrie, D. (1986). The retardation of aging in mice by dietary restriction: longevity, cancer, immunity and lifetime energy intake. *Journal of Nutrition, 116*, 641–654.

54. Kaeberlein, M., McVey, M., Guarente, L. (1999). The SIR2/3/4 complex and SIR2 alone promote longevity in *Saccharomyces cerevisiae* by two different mechanisms. *Genes & Development, 13*, 2570–2580.

55. Kimura, K.D., Tissenbaum, H.A., Liu, Y., Ruvkun, G. (1997). *daf-2*, an insulin receptor-like gene that regulates longevity and diapause in *Caenorhabditis elegans*. *Science, 277*, 942–946.

56. Brunet, A., Park, J., Tran, H., Hu, L.S., Hemmings, B.A., Greenberg, M.E. (2001). Protein kinase SGK mediates survival signals by phosphorylating the forkhead transcription factor FKHRL1 (FOXO3a). *Molecular and Cellular Biology, 21*, 952–965.

57. Youngman, L.D., Park, J.Y., Ames, B.N. (1992). Protein oxidation associated with aging is reduced by dietary restriction of protein or calories. *Proceedings of the National Academy of Sciences USA, 89*, 9112–9116.

58. Ward, W.F., Qi, W., Van Remmen, H., Zackert, W.E., Roberts, L.J. II., Richardson, A. (2005). Effects of age and caloric restriction on lipid peroxidation: Measurement of

oxidative stress by F2-isoprostane levels. *Journals of Gerontology. Series A, Biological Sciences and Medical Sciences, 60,* 847–851.

59. Lin, M.T., Beal, M.F. (2006). Mitochondrial dysfunction and oxidative stress in neuro-degenerative diseases. *Nature, 443,* 787–795.

60. Sanz, A., Caro, P., Ibanez, J., Gomez, J., Gredilla, R., Barja, G. (2005). Dietary restriction at old age lowers mitochondrial oxygen radical production and leak at complex I and oxidative DNA damage in rat brain. *Journal of Bioenergetics and Biomembranes, 37,* 83–90.

61. Parkes, T.L., Elia, A.J., Dickinson, D., Hilliker, A.J., Phillips, J.P., Boulianne, G.L. (1998). Extension of *Drosophila* lifespan by overexpression of human SOD1 in motor-neurons. *Nature Genetics, 19,* 171–174.

62. Sun, J., Folk, D., Bradley, T.J., Tower, J. (2002). Induced overexpression of mitochondrial Mn-superoxide dismutase extends the life span of adult *Drosophila melanogaster. Genetics, 161,* 661–672.

63. Shriner, S.E., Linford, N.J., Martin, G.M., Treuting, P., Ogburn, C.E., Emond, M., Coskun, P.E., Ladiges, W., Wolf, N., Van Remmen, H., Wallace, D.C., Rabinovitch, P.S. (2005). Extension of murine life span by overexpression of catalase targeted to mito-chondria. *Science, 308,* 1909–1911.

64. Rogina, B., Reenan, R.A., Nilsen, S.P., Helfand, S.L. (2000). Extended life-span con-ferred by cotransporter gene mutations in *Drosophila. Science, 290,* 2137–2140.

65. Etienne, F., Resnick, L., Sagher, D., Brot, N., Weissbach, H. (2003). Reduction of sulindac to its active metabolite, sulindac sulfide: Assay and role of the methionine sulfoxide reductase system. *Biochemical and Biophysical Research Communications, 312,* 1005–1010.

66. Zhang, Y., Talalay, P., Cho, C.C., Posner, G.H. (1992). A major inducer of anticarcino-genic protective enzymes from broccoli, isolation and elucidation of structure. *Proceedings of the National Academy of Sciences USA, 89,* 2399–2405.

67. Weissbach, H., Resnick, L., Brot, N. (2005). Methionine sulfoxide reductases: History and cellular role in protecting against oxidative damage. *Biochimica et Biophysica Acta, 1703,* 203–212.

68. Truscott, R.J.W., Augusteyn, R.C. (1977). Oxidative changes in human lens proteins during senile nuclear cataract formation. *Biochimica et Biophysica Acta, 492,* 43–52.

69. Garner, M.H., Spector, A. (1980). Selective oxidation of cysteine and methionine in normal and senile cataractous lenses. *Proceedings of the National Academy of Sciences USA, 77,* 1274–1277.

70. Spector, A., Scotto, R., Weissbach, H., Brot, N. (1982). Lens methionine sulfoxide reductase. *Biochemical and Biophysical Research Communications, 108,* 429–434.

71. Carp, H., Miller, F., Hoidal, J.R., Janoff, A. (1982). Potential mechanism of emphysema: Alpha-1 proteinase inhibitor recovered from lungs of cigarette smokers contains oxidized methionine and has decreased elastase inhibitory capacity. *Proceedings of the National Academy of Sciences USA, 79,* 2041–2045.

72. Janoff, A., Carp, H., Lee, D.K., Drew, R.T. (1979). Cigarette smoke inhalation decreases alpha-1-antitrypsin activity in the lung. *Science, 206,* 1313–1314.

73. Wong, P.S., Travis, J. (1980). Isolation and properties of oxidized alpha-1-proteinase inhibitor from human rheumatoid synovial fluid. *Biochemical and Biophysical Research Communications, 96,* 1449–1454.

74. Cochrane, C.G., Spragg, R., Revak, S.B. (1983). Pathogenesis of the adult respiratory distress syndrome. Evidence of oxidant activity in bronchalveolar lavage fluid. *Journal of Clinical Investigation, 71,* 754–761.

75. Hagimoto, N., Matute-Bello, G., Kajikawa, O., Park, D.R., Goodman, R.B., Fu, X., Martin, T.R. (2006). Biological activity of soluble Fas ligand in patients with ARDS is regulated by oxidation-induced multimerization. *Proceedings of the American Thoracic Society, 3,* A206.

76. Oram, J.F. (2003). HDL apolipoprotein and ABCA1: Partners in the removal of excess cellular cholesterol. *Arteriosclerosis, Thrombosis and Vascular Biology, 23,* 720–727.

77. Wang, N., Tall, A.R. (2003). Regulation and mechanisms of ATP-binding cassette transporter A1-mediated cellular cholesterol efflux. *Arteriosclerosis, Thrombosis and Vascular Biology, 23,* 1178–1184.

78. Bergt, C., Pennathur, S., Fu, X., Byun, J., Obrien, K., McDonald, T.O., Singh, P., Anantharamaia, G.M., Chait, A., Brunzell, J., Geary, R.L., Oram, J.F., Heinicke, J.W. (2004). The myeloperoxidase product hypochlorous acid oxidizes HDL in the human artery wall and impairs ABCA1-dependent cholesterol transport. *Proceedings of the National Academy of Sciences USA, 101,* 13032–13037.

79. Pennathur, S., Bergt, C., Shao, B., Byun, J., Kassim, S.Y., Singh, P., McDonald, T.O., Brunzell, J., Chait, A., Oram, J.F., Obrien, K., Geary, R.I., Heinicke, J.W. (2004). Human atherosclerotic intima and blood of patients with established coronary artery disease contain high density lipoprotein damaged by reactive nitrogen species. *Journal of Biological Chemistry, 279,* 42977–42983.

80. Zheng, I., Nakuna, B., Brennan, M.L., Sun, M., Goornastic, M., Settle, M., Schmitt, D., Fu, X., Thomson, L., Fox, P.L., Ischiropoulos, H., Smith, J.D., Kinter, M., Hazen, S.L. (2004). Apolipoprotein A-1 is a selective target for myeloperoxidase catalyzed oxidation and functional impairment in subjects with cardiovascular disease. *Journal of Clinical Investigation, 11,* 529–541.

81. Pankhurst, G., Wang, X.L., Wilcken, D.E., Baernthaler, G., Panzenbock, U., Raftery, M., Stocker, R. (2003). Characterization of specifically oxidized apolipoproteins in mildly oxidized high density lipoprotein. *Journal of Lipid Research, 44,* 349–355.

82. Shao, B., Oda, M.N., Bergt, C., Fu, X., Green, P.S., Brot, N., Oram, J.F., Heinicke, J.W. (2006). Myeloperoxidase impairs ABCA1-dependent cholesterol efflux through methionine oxidation and site specific tyrosine chlorination of apolipoprotein A-1. *Journal of Biological Chemistry, 282,* 9001–9004.

83. Katzman, R., Saitoh, T. (1991). Advances in Alzheimer's disease. *FASEB Journal, 5,* 278–286.

84. Evans, D.A., Funkenstein, H.H., Albert, M.S., Scherr, P.A., Cook, N.R., Chown, M.J., Hebert, L.E., Hennekens, C.H., Taylor, J.O. (1989). Prevalence of Alzheimer's disease in a community population of older people. *JAMA, 262,* 2551–2556.

85. Katzman, R. (1976). The prevalence and malignancy of Alzheimer's disease: A major killer. *Archives of Neurology, 33,* 217–218.

86. Hensley, K., Hall, N., Subramaniam, R., Cole, P., Harris, M., Aksenov, M., Aksenova, M., Gabbita, P., Wu, J.F., Carney, J.M., Lovell, M., Markesbery, W., Butterfield, D.A. (1995). Brain regional correspondence between Alzheimer's disease histopathology and biomarkers of protein oxidation. *Journal of Neurochemistry, 65,* 2146–2156.

87. Subbarao, K.V., Richardson, J.S., Ang, L.C. (1990). Autopsy samples of Alzheimer's cortex show increased peroxidation in vitro. *Journal of Neurochemistry, 55,* 342–345.

88. Butterfield, D.A., Lauderback, C.M. (2002). Lipid peroxidation and protein oxidation in Alzheimer's disease brain: Potential causes and consequences involving beta-peptide-associated free radical oxidative stress. *Free Radical Biology and Medicine, 32,* 1050–1060.

89. Schoneich, C. (2005). Redox processes of methionine relevant to β-amyloid oxidation and Alzheimer's disease. *Archives of Biochemistry and Biophysics, 397,* 370–376.

90. Butterfield, D.A., Boyd-Kimball, D. (2005). The critical role of methionine 35 in Alzheimer's amyloid β-peptide (1-42)-induced oxidative stress and neurotoxicity. *Biochimica et Biophysica Acta, 1703,* 149–156.

91. Huang, X., Atwood, C.S., Hartshorn, M.A., Multhaup, G., Goldstein, L.E., Scarpa, R.C., Cuajungco, M.P., Gray, D.N., Lim, J., Moir, R.D., Tanzi, R.E., Bush, A.I. (1999). The Aβ peptide of Alzheimer's disease directly produces hydrogen peroxide through metal ion reduction. *Biochemistry, 38,* 7609–7616.

92. Opazo, C., Huang, X., Chemy, R.A., Moir, R.D., Roher, A.E., White, A.R., Cappai, R., Masters, C.L., Tanzi, R.E., Inestrosa, N.C., Bush, A.I. (2002). Metalloenzyme-like activity of Alzheimer's disease β-amyloid. *Journal of Biological Chemistry, 277,* 40302–40308.

93. Yatin, S.M., Varadarajan, C.D., Link, D.A., Butterfield, D.A. (1999). In vitro and in vivo oxidative stress associated with Alzheimer's amyloid β-peptide (1-42). *Neurobiology of Aging, 20,* 325–330.

94. Gabbita, S.P., Aksenov, M.Y., Lovell, M.A., Markesbery, W.R. (1999). Decrease in peptide methionine sulfoxide reductase in Alzheimer's disease brain. *Journal of Neurochemistry, 73,* 1660–1666.

95. Beal, M.F. (2003). Mitochondria oxidative damage and inflammation in Parkinson's disease. *Annals of the New York Academy of Sciences, 991,* 120–131.

96. Ischiropoulos, H., Beckman, J.S. (2003). Oxidative stress and nitration in neurodegeneration: Effect or association? *Journal of Clinical Investigation, 111,* 163–169.

97. Dawson, T.M., Dawson, V.L. (2003). Molecular pathways of neurodegeneration in Parkinson's disease. *Science, 302,* 819–822.

98. Cohen, G. (2000). Oxidative stress, mitochondria respiration and Parkinson's disease. *Annals of the New York Academy of Sciences, 899,* 112–120.

99. Moos, T., Morgan, E.H. (2004). The metabolism of neuronal iron and its pathological role in neurological disease. *Annals of the New York Academy of Sciences, 1012,* 14–26.

100. Uversky, V.N., Yamin, G., Soulillac, P.O., Goers, J., Glaser, C.B., Fink, A.L. (2002). Methionine oxidation inhibits fibrillation of human alpha-synuclein in vitro. *FEBS Letters, 517,* 239–244.

101. Hokenson, M.J., Uversky, V.N., Goers, J., Yamin, G., Munishkina, L.A., Fink, A.L. (2004). Role of individual methionines in the fibrillation of methionine oxidized alpha-synuclein. *Biochemistry, 43,* 4621–4633.

PART IV

BIOACTIVITY OF GSH AND SULFUR AMINO ACIDS AS REGULATORS OF CELLULAR PROCESSES

CHAPTER 9

REGULATION OF PROTEIN FUNCTION BY GLUTATHIONYLATION

PIETRO GHEZZI and PAOLO DI SIMPLICIO

9.1 INTRODUCTION

Glutathione (GSH) is a major antioxidant acting as a free radical scavenger that protects the cell from reactive oxygen species (ROS). An impressive literature shows that GSH depletion is associated with oxidative stress in a variety of pathological conditions and after administration of toxicants. In several experimental models, in vivo or in vitro, a protective effect against a variety of insults was reported by administration of GSH, cell-permeable GSH derivatives (e.g., GSH methyl ester) or GSH synthesis precursors (e.g., *N*-acetylcysteine, NAC; L-2-oxo-4-thiazolidinecarboxylic acid, OTC). Likewise, depletion of cellular GSH, which can be achieved with inhibitors of GSH synthesis such as D,L-buthionine-*S*,*R*-sulfoximine (BSO), or chemicals that react with GSH (e.g., diethylmaleate, DEM; phorone) has worsening effects in many models of diseases or of toxic insult.

The chemical basis of the protective effect of GSH is in the simplest interpretation, GSH action as a scavenger, where GSH reacts with ROS so that they will not hit proteins or other vital macromolecules instead. In one of the most important of these reactions, GSH can react with peroxides (including H_2O_2) producing glutathione disulfide (GSSG):

$$2GSH + ROOH \longrightarrow GSSG + ROH + H_2O$$

All thiols can undergo this reaction and thus act as scavengers but the role of GSH is predominant in terms of cell concentration and enzymes (e.g., glutathione peroxidase, GPx) that accelerate this reaction. This detoxifying action of GSH is also exerted versus many electrophiles by conjugation reactions that in turn are fortified in vivo by isoenzymes of GSH-S-transferases.

Glutathione and Sulfur Amino Acids in Human Health and Disease. Edited by R. Masella and G. Mazza
Copyright © 2009 John Wiley & Sons, Inc.

Despite this evidence of GSH protective effects, most of the data have not resulted in a step from laboratory animals to patients' bedside and the results of many clinical trials have not provided convincing evidence to the regulatory agencies for the registration of GSH, GSH-repleting agents, or even other thiol antioxidants. Most of them (e.g., N-acetylcysteine, NAC and sodium 2-sulfanylethanesulfonate) are approved, as thiol antioxidants, only as chemoprotectants either to prevent the toxic side effects of anticancer drugs or as antidotes against paracetamol overdose) although thiol antioxidants are often used off-label as nutritional supplements in "alternative medicines" for many diseases. While this is common to most antioxidants, and not only thiol compounds, we believe that the difficulty of establishing a role for GSH metabolism in many diseases is due to the fact that GSH is not only an antioxidant or scavenger of electrophilic agents but also a signaling molecule.

This chapter introduces one mechanism by which GSH can exert its regulatory role, namely protein glutathionylation, or simply glutathionylation (the formation of glutathione-protein mixed disulfides, PSSG), GSH being a fundamental element of the signaling cascade evoked by ROS and reactive nitrogen species (RNS). We will first give a historical introduction to the concept of redox regulation and the signaling role of GSH that emerged in the field of innate immunity and inflammation, stemming from research on oxidative stress. Recent interest has been aimed at studying the redox state of the thiol group of protein cysteines, with particular interest in pKa values of protein SH groups (PSH), the mechanisms of protein glutathionylation/ deglutathionylation, the methods used to identify glutathionylated proteins, and the functional consequences of this modification.

9.2 GLUTATHIONE AND REDOX REGULATION IN IMMUNITY

The mid-1980s saw the identification, purification, and cloning of several molecules that would later be shown to be key ones in the inflammatory response, including the cytokines tumor necrosis factor (TNF) [1, 2] and interleukin-1 (IL-1) [3, 4], and the transcription factor (nuclear factor-kappa B; NF-κB) [5]. In the next years several papers appeared reporting that GSH can regulate the "cytokine system" at various steps. In particular, it was shown that oxidants participate in the activation of NF-κB and thiol antioxidants, including glutathione and NAC, inhibit it [6, 7]; that antioxidants, including GSH and NAC, inhibit the production and the action of TNF [8, 9]; and that TNF augments, and GSH or NAC inhibit, HIV proliferation [10–12].

The papers reporting these findings, including those from our group, were still focused on the "simple" concept that oxidative stress was implicated in inflammatory and infective diseases, and that it could participate in triggering cytokine production and NF-κB activation or in augmenting the sensitivity to their actions. All these data introduced the notion, in the title of a seminal paper from the group of Baeuerle, that ROS could serve as "messengers" [6]. Despite the fact that the interpretation was often the simple one, that ROS are bad and antioxidants are good, buried in some of those works are some observations that may have anticipated some of the current concepts on the role of protein thiol modification in redox regulation. In particular, Dröge and associates provided evidence that oxidized glutathione (GSSG) is required for optimal activation of NF-κB in T cells [13]. This aspect is not yet fully understood in terms of mechanism of NF-κB activation, but it was hypothesized that GSSG could stabilize phosphotyrosine by inhibiting protein phosphatases, which have a cysteine in the active site that must be maintained reduced for them to be active.

It was also shown that ROS are not only produced under pathological conditions. For instance epidermal growth factor induces production of hydrogen peroxide [14]. The fact that ROS do not act only as pathogenic mediators but also as intracellular messengers is now established in the literature.

Therefore, our current hypothesis, far less established, is that, under physiological conditions, or in any case in conditions not associated with oxidative stress, GSH and other thiols may act in various ways as reducing agents, and not only as simple free radical scavengers, this notion being intrinsically linked to the various actions displayed by SH groups.

9.3 PROTEIN CYSTEINE OXIDATION

If one looks at a classical textbook of biochemistry, the structure of many proteins is well defined, or highly stable, with some cysteines as free SH and others engaged in disulfide bonds. A typical example is serum albumin, with 17 cysteines, of which 16 are engaged in 8 disulfide bonds and one is free. However, in some proteins, thiols and disulfides can undergo oxidoreduction under physiological conditions, or at least under conditions not associated with cellular dysfunctions or death. This is, in our opinion, what really identifies proteins undergoing redox regulation, whether they are the ultimate target or the "redox sensor" upstream in the signaling cascade.

Thus, the challenge is first to identify proteins whose thiol-disulfides can be oxidoreduced, and then understand mechanisms of glutathionylation-deglutathionylation processes, a more complicated problem than the identification of "structural" disulfide bonds.

Several oxidation states of cysteines have been described. These include formation of intra- and interchain disulfide bonds (PSSP), but also oxidation to sulfinic (PSO$_2$H) and sulfenic acids (PSO$_3$H), and formation of mixed disulfides with small molecular weight thiols, including cysteine (cysteinylation, PSSC) and glutathione (glutathionylation, PSSG). The latter modification has gained particular attention as a means of redox regulation because its reversibility by thiol/disulfide exchange is regulated by glutaredoxin (Grx) [15, 16]. If we consider glutathionylation as a regulatory posttranslational modification analogous with phosphorylation, then the point made above that thiol antioxidants do not just act as free radical scavengers is strengthened. In this double perspective of GSH as a detoxifying agent (as scavenger of electrophiles and free radicals) and signaling molecule, GSH depletion by oxidation to GSSG, or depletion of total glutathione levels, such as that achieved with the widely used inhibitor of protein synthesis buthionine sulfoximine, will modulate or remove an essential signaling molecule (somewhat like depleting cells of phosphate would not only deplete energy, ATP levels, but also prevent signaling mediated by protein kinases).

TABLE 9.1   Redox States of Protein Cysteines

Species	Reversibility
Free thiol (SH)	
Intraprotein disulfides (SS)	Thioredoxin
Mixed disulfides: glutathionylation (PSSG); cysteinylation (PSSC)	Glutaredoxin, thioredoxin, GSH
S-nitrosothiols (SNO)	Glutaredoxin, thioredoxin, ascorbate
Sulfenic acids (SOH)	Easily reduced by GSH or Trx
Sulfinic acids (SO$_2$H)	Can be reduced by thioredoxin, but this is debated and it was suggested that only sulfiredoxin does it
Sulfonic acids (SO$_3$H)	Irreversible

Protein can undergo different types of thiol oxidation, some reversible and some irreversible, as outlined in Table 9.1.

9.3.1   Disulfides

Disulfide bonds are formed in the endoplasmic reticulum and this is important for the stability and folding of the protein [17], and the state of the cysteine is viewed as part of the tertiary structure of the protein. Since the intracellular environment is highly reducing, free cysteines are normally prevalent in the cytoplasm where GSH is at its maximum levels. A possible exception is hyperthermophilic bacteria, where intracellular proteins are rich in disulfide bonds, probably a key factor in stabilizing thermostable proteins [18]. Secreted proteins are known to be rich in disulfide bonds and the extracellular environment, under aerobic conditions, is predisposed to be more oxidant than the cytoplasmic one, a condition that guarantees the maintenance of preexisting protein disulfides (PSSP) in secreted proteins. It may be not obvious to the reader of a textbook that, under physiological conditions, a cysteine normally listed as "free thiol" may be present as a (reversible) disulfide; and vice versa.

Consequently, in the framework of redox regulation, some cysteines are normally fluctuating between two different oxidoreduction states and this condition is regulated by many oxidoreducing enzymes that participate in protein folding in ER as well as in redox signaling [19–23]. In this intriguing and complex context, a number of proteins can form reversible disulfide bonds, changing their properties of state redox regulators, for example, the transcription factor OxyR and the chaperonin Hsp33 [24, 25]. The notion that PSH and PSSP are not stable but flexible molecular entities is reinforced by the fact that using proteomic techniques, a great PSSP variety is formed in the cytoplasm upon exposure of cells to oxidative stress [26, 27].

9.3.2   Protein Glutathionylation and Cysteinylation

PSH can form mixed disulfides with small molecular weight thiols (PSSX) and in living organisms those at GSH, and to a lesser extent at cysteine, are the most abundant ones. The fact that GSH can form PSSG has been known since the late 1960s [28–30], whereas successive studies by Brigelius et al. [31, 32] indicated more reliable values.

Usually, up to 20% of total glutathione is considered present in the form of protein-bound mixed disulfide, but this value might be overestimated by likely occurrence of artifacts; however, this amount can increase up to 50% or more under oxidative stress [33, 34]. The amount of PSSG may vary dependent on cell type and richness of more accessible PSH. The phenomenon is rapidly reversible provided that active reducing enzyme (Grx) and substrate (GSH) are available [35]. Excessive glutathionylation may cause irreversible protein thiolation by lack of substrate (GSH) [33] even though the enzyme (Grx) necessary to deglutathionylate protein remains active [36]. This is an important issue that has never been investigated adequately. For example, it is unknown why the enzyme (Grx) necessary to deglutathionylate proteins is subjected to loss of efficiency for lack of substrate (GSH) that has been used to glutathionylate proteins. At the moment we can only speculate that an excess of PSSG formation with respect to GSH, for an overexposure to oxidative events, may serve to regenerate GSH by PSSP formation by the reaction: PSSG + PSH → PSSP + GSH. This speculation is supported by the fact that PSSG of Grx is able to transfer GSH to other PSH [37]. Since in the deglutathionylation process by Grx, PSSG of Grx is formed and GSH is the obligatory substrate [35] and PSSG of Grx are in turn involved in glutathionylation of PSH, generating PSSP [37], it remains to be established under what conditions Grx is used to deglutathionylate or glutathionylate.

Cysteinylation has attracted far less attention than glutathionylation. The intracellular concentrations of cysteine are lower than those of GSH; a recent study on human cell lines reported 5 to 10 times lower concentrations [38], even though cysteine may be found at much higher concentrations in tumors [33, 39]. Extracellular cysteine is more abundant than GSH: it was recently estimated that 99.5% of GSH in human blood was in erythrocytes and 97% of cysteine (Cys) was in plasma [33, 40]. Thus, extracellular proteins may be predominantly cysteinylated. In fact, while hemoglobin in red blood cells is glutathionylated [41], plasma proteins such as albumin [42] and transthyretin [43] are mainly cysteinylated. Cysteinylation has also been reported for many proteins including secreted cytokines, such as MIF/GIF [44] and the extracellular domain of cytokine receptors such as the high affinity interleukin-6 (IL-6) receptor and its gp130 signal transducer [45, 46]. The common finding of cysteinylation is reflected by the fact that reduction of cysteinylated peptides by specific thioltransferases, particularly by a protein disulfide oxidoreductase known as gamma interferon-inducible lysosomal thiol reductase (GILT) [47, 48], is a key step in antigen processing and presentation [49–51]. Although in theory all PSH may be glutathionylated or cysteinylated, in that the process is not enzymatically governed, the relative proportion of PSSG and PSSC would depend on the accessibility to PSH of thiols and disulfides (that is their relative mass and charge) and on the enzyme activity causing deglutathionylation. As compared with GSH, cysteine has a higher reactivity, due to its smaller size and a more neutral charge than GSH [52, 53].

9.3.3 Higher Oxidation States

Cysteines can form other oxidation products, including sulfenic (Cys-SOH), sulfinic (Cys-SO$_2$H), and sulfonic acids (Cys-SO$_3$H). While the latter are considered irreversible forms of oxidation, sulfenic acids are not, and react with GSH to give a glutathionylated protein [54].

9.4 MECHANISMS FOR PSSG FORMATION AND THE COMPLEX SCENARIO OF PROTEIN GLUTATHIONYLATION

Depending on the nature of the PSH (essential versus nonessential), PSSG may express a regulatory event (cell signaling), or a buffering action towards toxic compounds. When oxidative stress is excessive to uncontrolled the onset of detrimental effects can occur, and excessive glutathionylation and GSH depletion has been associated with apoptosis and necrosis [36].

Although oxidative stress by ROS is the fundamental requisite for PSSG formation, increased PSSG is not always strictly linked to oxidation, as in the case of diamide [33], Kathon[36], and nitrosocompounds [55, 56] that cannot be considered classical oxidants. Several mechanisms, schematically distinguishable in sulfhydryl/disulfide (SH/SS) exchange reactions of low and high molecular weight thiols and disulfides, in formation of sulfenic acids (PSOH), nitrosoproteins (PSNO), and nitrosoglutathione (GSNO) are involved in PSSG formation, but transformation to higher oxidation grades than disulfides (oxidation grades of disulfides, symmetrical, XSSX, or asymmetrical, RSSX of low or high molecular weight is -1) may occur, such as sulfenic (oxidation grade 0), sulfinic (oxidation grade $+2$), or sulfonic (oxidation grade $+4$) acids. In living organisms even severe oxidations do not usually exceed the state of disulfides or that of sulfenic acids, that in turn is an obligatory intermediate of disulfide generation.

Kathon and diamide are compounds that react with thiols (PSH and GSH) forming adducts as intermediate and then GSSG, PSSG, or GSSG + PSSG dependent on the cell model [57].

The following reactions of PSSG formation via ROS and RNS are theoretically possible [57], even if other more complex mechanisms have been described:

Reaction 1: $PSH + GSSG \longrightarrow PSSG + GSH$

(SH/SS exchange reactions with small disulfides)

Reaction 2: $PSSG + P*SH \longrightarrow P*SSG + PSH$

(SH/SS exchange reactions between protein disulfides)

Reaction 3: $PSSG + P*SH \longrightarrow P*SSP + GSH$

(SH/SS exchange reactions between protein disulfides where pKa of PSH, is higher than that of GSH)

Reaction 4: $PSOH + GSH \longrightarrow PSSG + H_2O$ (reactions with sulfenic acid)

Reaction 5: $PSNO + GSH \longrightarrow PSSG + HNO$ (exchange with PSNO)

Reaction 6: $PSH + GSNO \longrightarrow PSSG + HNO$ (exchange with GSNO)

The equilibria of reactions 1 to 6 regulating PSSG concentrations are governed by thermodynamic parameters, as well as by mass and charge characteristics of each component and by protein accessibility (conformation).

The PSSG concentration varies in a dose-response manner dependent on the stimulus entity, and PSSG obtained by oxidative stress (ROS) is normally much higher than that obtained by nitrosative stress (RNS) because the former is biologically more relevant than the latter. In this context, in both cases, it remains undefined how "minute" amounts of ROS and RNS are able to evoke physiological messages, such as those of cell signaling. At the same time, since glutathionylation has been considered a molecular event implicated in cell signaling, it remains also to be established why and how "excessive" glutathionylation becomes associated with detrimental effects. These difficult issues are still unresolved in terms of important targets and mechanisms, though little some progress has been made, for example, analyzing the PSH role. In this connection it is now sufficiently clear the reason why an important portion of essential PSH are usually characterized by pKa values much lower than that of endogenous thiols (e.g., GSH, cysteine, homocysteine and so on) that have a pKa range above 8.0. We think that these differences between PSH and small thiols may serve to accelerate dethiolation process rates of essential PSH as explained in Section 9.5 below. In fact, thiolated PSH are favored as leaving group in SH/SS exchange reactions (reverse of reaction 1) when the pKa value of PSH in mixed disulfide is lower than that of the other thiol linked as disulfide. Using thiolated albumin as a model of PSSX involved in SH/SS exchange reactions, we have confirmed that the difference in pKa values between sulfur atoms engaged in PSSX is an important requisite to observe dethiolations, such as the reverse of reaction 1, or the thiol substitution on the protein with another thiol (RSH) by a reaction called protein substitution: PSSX + RSH → PSSR + XSH [58]. In fact, when Cys34 of albumin, whose lone thiol (Cys34) is scarcely accessible to the solvent and characterized by low pKa (pKa about 5 to 6), is linked to thiols of lower pKa (of about 4.0), the attack of whatever thiol with pKa higher than Cys34 was accompanied by thiol substitution, because the thiol with the lowest pKa (4.0) is destined to abandon the mixed disulfide. On the contrary, when mixed disulfides of albumin are characterized by compounds (e.g., GSH, CSH, Hcy whose pKa is above 8.0) with pKa higher than albumin, SH/SS exchange reactions of albumin with these thiols are only accompanied by dethiolation because the protein leaves the system as albumin thiolated anion (reverse of reaction 1) [58]. Applying these simple rules and considering mass and charge characteristics of each compound, it is easy to explain why plasma mixed disulfides at Hcy of normal and pathological subjects are preferentially and proportionally bound to albumin with respect to all other endogenous thiols [58]. In exchange reactions between PSH of albumin and whatever plasma asymmetrical disulfide of low molecular weight:

$$PSH + XSSR \longrightarrow PSSX + RSH$$
$$PSH + XSSR \longrightarrow PSSR + XSH$$

it is the thiol at higher pKa (Hcy) that is favored to produce a mixed disulfide with albumin.

The PSSG generation by reactions 1 to 6 is a simplified aspect of a more complex scenario probably occurring in in vivo situations. In fact, since in all cells the PSH concentration is much higher than GSH per se, we cannot exclude that initial PSSG targets, caused by oxidative stress events, may be transformed in other PSSG targets. These events are supported by a recent study in which the mixed disulfide at GSH of Grx1 (Grx1 is a type of glutaredoxin) is able to transfer the bound GSH to other PSH with new formation of PSSG [37]. In other words this is the first example in which Grx is not only able to deglutathionylate but also to glutathionylate proteins. During SH/SS exchange reactions involving the GSH/Grx1 mixed disulfide, the new PSSG (from PSSG to P * SSG, reaction 2) can occur because the pKa value of Grx1 (pKa = 3.5) [59, 60] is lower than GSH (pKa = 8.7) [61]. Subsequent transfer of GSH from PSSG to another P * SH is possible if the pKa of PSH bound to GSH is lower than that of GSH. So, this process may take place several times, provided that appropriate favorable conformational conditions of the P * SH approaching PSSG exist. The existence of a great potential of proteins that can exchange GSH bound as mixed disulfides is suggested by the estimate of pKa range of PSH, whose order of magnitude seems to be 10^6 [62]. By similar considerations, we can explain PSSP formations (reaction 3, where GSH is a leaving group), that were recently shown to be formed abundantly under oxidative stress [26, 27].

Obviously, the PSSG formation by the reactions described above cannot ignore the intrinsic characteristics of each component. For example, although GSSG (via reaction 1) has been considered an important factor to glutathionylate proteins dependent on a great variety of in vitro studies [33, 63], its real contribution must be considered more limited in comparison with other smaller and less charged disulfides, such as cystine and homocystine [58]. At the same time, the known PSSG formation via nitrosoproteins or via GSNO probably occurs via reactions 5 and 6 dependent on the electronegativity difference between S and N in PSNO and GSNO.

H_2O_2 or organic hydroperoxides are formed during oxidative stress. Since hydroperoxides are more lipophilic and less charged than GSSG their possibility to form PSSG via sulfenic acid (reaction 4) is higher than that via GSSG (reaction 1). The peroxide first attacks PSH forming sulfenic acid (PSOH) (e.g., H_2O_2 + PSH → PSOH + H_2O), which in turn reacts with thiols forming PSSG by reaction 4.

The appropriate physiological amount of PSSG formed by hydroperoxides via ROS and/or RNS might be regulated by modulation of glutathione peroxidase (GPx) and glutathione reductase (GR) activities.

Evidence for the occurrence of the majority of all the reactions described above (1–6) have been published. While most studies invoke the first two reactions as the most important ones, it should be noted that thiol/disulfide exchange is probably a viable method only for easily accessible thiols, whereby for less accessible thiols the steric hindrance of GSSG may become a problem. It should be noted that, although we and others used GSSG to glutathionylate some proteins in vitro (e.g., thioredoxin and cyclophilin A) [64, 65], this may take place only at GSSG concentration unlikely to be observed in the cell and protein glutathionylation in cells has been observed in the absence of any change in the GSH:GSSG ratio [33, 66, 67].

9.5 DEGLUTATHIONYLATION

Reversibility is an obvious prerequisite for a posttranslational modification to have a regulatory function, and protein glutathionylation is reversible. The protein-glutathione disulfide bond can be reduced by any thiol reductant, both small molecular weight thiols such as GSH or cysteine [68, 69] and protein thiols [70] through a reaction of thiol/disulfide exchange (reverse of reaction 1 above).

Deglutathionylation is catalyzed by enzymes in the family of the protein disulfide oxidoreductase. These enzymes are often characterized by a CXXC redox active site and include thioredoxin (Trx), glutaredoxin (Grx), protein disulfide isomerase (PDI), all of which can reduce glutathionylated proteins through thiol/disulfide exchange with GSH [15, 69, 71]. Glutaredoxins, some of which lack the CXXC motif and can act through a monothiol mechanism, are thought to be the most important enzyme to carry out deglutathionylation [16, 72, 73]. This is demonstrated by the fact that inhibiting Grx with siRNA increases protein glutathionylation [74].

Although mechanisms of deglutathionylation of specific proteins have not been investigated extensively, they can be predicted adequately on the basis of differences in pKa values of thiols involved in mixed disulfides. In fact, as explained above, it is known that the attack of any thiolate anion to the disulfides in SH/SS exchange reactions is more likely to occur on the more positive sulfur atom. These simple notions may serve to predict the metabolism of a protein-thiol mixed disulfide (PSSX) when subjected to successive attacks by thiols.

For example, if in PSSX the PSH pKa is higher than XSH, the attack of whatever thiolated anion will preferentially target the protein sulfur (the more positive sulfur) and consequently XS^- will be the leaving group. In this case, if the entering group (the nucleophilic group attacking the disulfide) belongs to a P'SH, the end product will be a protein disulfide, for example, of PSSX where pKa (PSH) $\rightarrow$ pKa (XSH):

$$PSSX + P'SH \longrightarrow PSSP' + XSH \text{ (reaction 7)}$$

(dethiolation with protein disulfideformation)

whereas if the entering group is a small thiol of low molecular weight (RSH), RSH will substitute XSH forming a different mixed disulfide (protein substitution):

$$PSSX + RSH \longrightarrow PSSR + XSH \text{ (reaction 8)}$$

(protein substitution, no change in protein-thiol mixed disulfide concentration)

If the entering group is a protein P'SH and PSH of PSSX has a pKa (PSH) $<$ pKa (XSH), we have a dethiolation of PSSX and a new thiol-protein mixed disulfide

$$PSSX + P'SH \longrightarrow PSH + P'SSX \text{ (reaction 9)}$$

(new thiol-protein mixeddisulfide; no change in protein-thiol mixed disulfide concentration)

If the entering group is a small thiol (RSH) and PSH of PSSX has a pKa (PSH) $<$ pKa (XSH), we will have a simple dethiolation:

$$PSSX + RSH \longrightarrow PSH + XSSR \text{ (reaction 10)}$$

(protein dethiolation)

All these possibilities of PSSX metabolism introduce a further complexity inherent to the dethiolation process and may be the origin of further activity modulation. Moreover, dependent on the mass and charge characteristics of disulfides, symmetrical XSSX or asymmetrical XSSR, of small molecular weight new SH/SS exchange reactions (new thiolation) can be observed according to reaction 1.

When PSSP are obtained as end products of oxidative and nitrosative stress, the return to normal levels of original PSH should be achieved (via the reactions above) depending on the accessibility of the protein disulfides to every thiol. On the contrary when we try to apply these mechanisms to the reduction of PSSP of known proteins such as DsbA [75], we do not find any confirmation of the theoretical mechanisms explained by reactions 7 to 9. This might indicate that the process reversibility of PSSP after oxidative or nitrosative stress must be even more complex than described here on the basis of the pKa difference of thiols engaged in PSSP.

Glutathionylation of PSSP can be carried out by Trx as well as by some forms of Grx (Grx1) [37]. Grx1 has been involved in both glutathionylation (PSSG formation from PSSP) as well as in deglutathionylation (PSSP formation from PSSG). The regulation of this dual role of Grx remains unknown. Nevertheless, Grx remains the most important protein to deglutathionylate PSSG, with formation of PSH and GSSG [35, 69].

9.6 IDENTIFICATION OF PROTEINS UNDERGOING GLUTATHIONYLATION

Some proteins, such as actin or GAPDH, have long been known as targets of glutathionylation, but only recently proteomics technologies have been used in an attempt to identify glutathionylated proteins [76–79]. This led to the identification of many proteins undergoing glutathionylation, about 100 of which are listed in Table 9.2.

Identification of proteins undergoing glutathionylation has been done using a variety of techniques. We adapted a technique originally developed in the laboratory of R.B. Johnston, Jr. [80] using ^{35}S-cysteine to radiolabel intracellular GSH so that proteins undergoing glutathionylation (i.e., that incorporate radioactivity when exposed, for instance, to H_2O_2 or diamide) could be observed. Using this method we were able to detect about 40 proteins in human T lymphocytes [76]. Radiolabeled proteins identified on two-dimensional gels can then be identified by peptide mapping after tryptic digestion. Others have successfully used biotynylated GSH, with obvious advantages over radioactive labeling [79]. The bias of these methods is that they cannot be employed to study the glutathionylation state of proteins but rather the turnover of glutathionylation or, in general, allow the identification of "proteins susceptible to glutathionylation," not "glutathionylated proteins." In theory, if a protein is present

TABLE 9.2   Proteins Undergoing Glutathionylation

Actin capping protein	Malate dehydrogenase
Actin beta	My032 protein
Adenylate kinase 2	Myosin
Aldolase A	Neuropolypeptide h3
Aldose reductase	Nicotinamide N-methyltransferase
Annexin A2	Nucleophosmin
Ash protein	Nucleosidediphosphate kinase A
Aspartyl-tRNA synthetase	Nudix-type motif 6
ATP synthase beta subunit	PDI
c-Jun	NF-κB p50 subunit
Caspase 3	Peptidylprolyl isomerase (cyclophilin A)
Chaperonin	Peroxiredoxin 1
Cofilin	Peroxiredoxin 2
Creatine kinase	Peroxiredoxin 4
CRK-like protein	Peroxiredoxin 5
Crystallin, alpha	Peroxiredoxin 6
Cytochrome c oxidase Va	Phosphoglycerate kinase
Cytochrome c oxidase Vb	6-Phosphogluconolactonase
DUTP pyrophosphatase	Profilin
Elongation factor 2	Prohibitin
Enolase-alpha	Prolyl 4-hydroxylase
Endoplasmic reticulum protein	Protein disulfide isomerase
ERP60	Phospholipase C gamma
ERP72	20S proteasome subunit
Glutaredoxin	Protein tyrosine phosphatase1B
GRP94	Pyruvate kinase. M2 Isozyme 57
EnoyI CoA hydratase	Ran specific GTPase activating protein
Eukaryotic translation initiation factor 6	h-Ras
Fatty acid binding protein	40S ribosomal protein S12
Beta galactoside soluble lectin (galectin 1)	RNA-binding protein regulatory subunit
Glucosidase II precursor	SFR1 splicing factor
Glutathione-S-transferase	Stress-induced phosphoprotein 1
Glycogen phosphorylase	T complex protein 1
GRP78	Thioredoxin
Heat shock cognate 70	Thioredoxin reductase
HSP10	Transgelin, SM22 homolog calponin-Iike
Hemoglobin	Translation elongation factor
Hepatoma derived growth factor	Triosephosphate isomerase
Histamine releasing factor	Tubulin
Histidine triad nucleotide binding protein 2	Tropomyosin
3-Hydroxyacyl-CoA-dehydrogenase If	Ubiquitin carboxyl-terminal hydrolase
Ig lambda chain	isozyme L3
Inosine 5′-monophosphate dehydrogenase 2	Ubiquitin conjugating enzyme E2N
Laminin (p40)	Vimentin
L-lactate dehydrogenase	14-3-3 Protein sigma
Lymphocyte specific protein 1	14-3-3 Protein zeta

Main sources are from References 76 to 79.

as maximally glutathionylated, it will not incorporate further (labeled) GSH and will not show up with these techniques.

Clearly, the optimal way would be to have antibodies specific to glutathionylated proteins (as we have for phosphospecific antibodies to phosphotyrosine or specific phosphorylated proteins). Although they are not directed to specific proteins, a number of "anti-GSH" antibodies are commercially available and have been used to identify glutathionylated proteins in proteomics studies [78]. Another approach is based on the use of enzymes that specifically recognize (and bind) GSH or glutathionylated proteins. A protein overlay technique using biotinylated GST has also been used [81, 82]. Last but not least, Grx, which specifically recognizes glutathionylated proteins, has been used to allow tag glutathionylated proteins using sequential alkylation-reduction steps and their proteomics identification [83].

9.7 FUNCTIONAL CONSEQUENCES OF PROTEIN GLUTATHIONYLATION

Protein glutathionylation has been suggested to have various functions and was shown to have different consequences on its targets.

In terms of functional significance glutathionylation has been suggested to:

1. Have a regulatory role through modification of protein function (similar to phosphorylation).
2. Protect sensitive protein thiols from other, sometimes irreversible, forms of oxidation.
3. Avoid loss of GSH during oxidative stress, by keeping it bound to protein in a form that can easily release it when the stress condition is overcome.

In terms of consequences, glutathionylation has been shown to:

1. Inhibit functional activities of proteins. This is probably the most commonly described consequence of glutathionylation. Most of the enzymes susceptible to glutathionylation are inhibited by this posttranslational modification; glutathionylation inhibits DNA binding of p53 [84] and of transcription factors NF-κB and AP-1 by modification of p50 and c-Jun subunits, respectively [85, 86]; actin glutathionylation decreases its polymerization rate [87] and decreases dimerization of HIV protease [88].
2. Increasing functional activities of protein. There are quite a few examples of glutathionylation-induced activation of proteins (or gain of function). Some enzymes are activated by glutathionylation achieved by thiol/disulfide exchange with GSSG, although they are less numerous than those inhibited by glutathionylation. HIV protease glutathionylation of Cys67 increases its activity, whereas the same modification at cysteine 95 leads to inhibition of activity [89]; Cys67-glutathionylated HIV protease is more stable [89]. Glutathionylation increases calcium-binding activity of S100A1 [90], enhances calcium channel activity of ryanodine receptors [91], and activates sarco/endoplasmic reticulum calcium ATPase (SERCA) [92].

9.8 STRUCTURAL CHANGES INDUCED BY PROTEIN GLUTATHIONYLATION

The above effects can be explained by different structural changes induced by glutathionylation. Inhibition of enzymes by glutathionylation of an essential cysteine is easily explained in terms of molecular mechanism. However, we must keep in mind that adding a GSH molecule to a protein not only blocks a free cysteine but attaches to the protein an amino acid or a tripeptide with different steric hindrance and isoelectric point (due to the addition of the glutamic acid moiety of GSH most proteins will become more acidic upon glutathionylation). Therefore, the consequences on protein functions are not (necessarily) the same as alkylating, or mutating, a cysteine. For the same reasons, glutathionylation and cysteinylation (formation of mixed disulfides with free Cys) can affect protein functions differently. This has clearly been shown with protein kinase C where different forms of S-thiolations may have different effects [93, 94].

Direct evidences that glutathionylation alters protein structure has been obtained, using circular dichroism, for human cyclophilin A [95] and *Escherichia coli* cobalamin-independent methionine synthase [96].

9.9 CONCLUSIONS

We hope to have conveyed to the reader the notion that regulation of protein function via protein glutathionylation is a growing field and is likely at the basis of the also popular concept of redox regulation. In this review we underlined the complexity of this biochemical process and the many open questions. In particular, the reader will note that we think that the chemical reactions by which protein glutathionylation and deglutathionylation occur in living organisms, as well as the determinant of the susceptibility of specific cysteines to this modification, are largely unknown. Their definition will likely require not only further studies but also technological advances to study glutathionylation of proteins.

REFERENCES

1. Beutler, B., Greenwald, D., Hulmes, J.D., Chang, M., Pan, Y.C., Mathison, J., Ulevitch, R., Cerami, A. (1985). Identity of tumour necrosis factor and the macrophage-secreted factor cachectin. *Nature*, *316*, 552–554.

2. Pennica, D., Nedwin, G.E., Hayflick, J.S., Seeburg, P.H., Derynck, R., Palladino, M.A., Kohr, W.J., Aggarwal, B.B., Goeddel, D.V. (1984). Human tumour necrosis factor: Precursor structure, expression and homology to lymphotoxin. *Nature*, *312*, 724–729.

3. Auron, P.E., Webb, A.C., Rosenwasser, L.J., Mucci, S.F., Rich, A., Wolff, S.M., Dinarello, C.A. (1984). Nucleotide sequence of human monocyte interleukin 1 precursor cDNA. *Proceedings of the National Academy of Sciences USA*, *81*, 7907–7911.

4. Lomedico, P.T., Gubler, U., Hellmann, C.P., Dukovich, M., Giri, J.G., Pan, Y.C., Collier, K., Semionow, R., Chua, A.O., Mizel, S.B. (1984) Cloning and expression of murine interleukin-1 cDNA in *Escherichia coli*. *Nature*, *312*, 458–462.

5. Sen, R., Baltimore, D. (1986). Inducibility of kappa immunoglobulin enhancer-binding protein Nf-kappa B by a posttranslational mechanism. *Cell*, *47*, 921–928.

6. Schreck, R., Rieber, P., Baeuerle, P.A. (1991). Reactive oxygen intermediates as apparently widely used messengers in the activation of the NF-kappa B transcription factor and HIV-1. *EMBO Journal*, *10*, 2247–2258.

7. Staal, F.J., Roederer, M., Herzenberg, L.A. (1990). Intracellular thiols regulate activation of nuclear factor kappa B and transcription of human immunodeficiency virus. *Proceedings of the National Academy of Sciences USA*, *87*, 9943–9947.

8. Peristeris, P., Clark, B.D., Gatti, S., Faggioni, R., Mantovani, A., Mengozzi, M., Orencole, S.F., Sironi, M., Ghezzi, P. (1992). N-acetylcysteine and glutathione as inhibitors of tumor necrosis factor production. *Cellular Immunology*, *140*, 390–399.

9. Zimmerman, R.J., Marafino, B.J., Jr., Chan, A., Landre, P., Winkelhake, J.L. (1989). The role of oxidant injury in tumor cell sensitivity to recombinant human tumor necrosis factor in vivo. Implications for mechanisms of action. *Journal of Immunology*, *142*, 1405–1409.

10. Kalebic, T., Kinter, A., Poli, G., Anderson, M.E., Meister, A., Fauci, A.S. (1991). Suppression of human immunodeficiency virus expression in chronically infected monocytic cells by glutathione, glutathione ester, and N-acetylcysteine. *Proceedings of the National Academy of Sciences USA*, *88*, 986–990.

11. Mihm, S., Ennen, J., Pessara, U., Kurth, R., Droge, W. (1991). Inhibition of HIV-1 replication and NF-kappa B activity by cysteine and cysteine derivatives. *AIDS*, *5*, 497–503.

12. Roederer, M., Staal, F.J., Raju, P.A., Ela, S.W., Herzenberg, L.A. (1990). Cytokine-stimulated human immunodeficiency virus replication is inhibited by N-acetyl-L-cysteine. *Proceedings of the National Academy of Sciences USA*, *87*, 4884–4888.

13. Dröge, W., Schulze-Osthoff, K., Mihm, S., Galter, D., Schenk, H., Eck, H.P., Roth, S., Gmunder, H. (1994). Functions of glutathione and glutathione disulfide in immunology and immunopathology. *FASEB Journal*, *8*, 1131–1138.

14. Bae, Y.S., Kang, S.W., Seo, M.S., Baines, I.C., Tekle, E., Chock, P.B., Rhee, S.G. (1997). Epidermal growth factor (EGF)-induced generation of hydrogen peroxide. Role in EGF receptor-mediated tyrosine phosphorylation. *Journal of Biological Chemistry*, *272*, 217–221.

15. Holmgren, A. (1989). Thioredoxin and glutaredoxin systems. *Journal of Biological Chemistry*, *264*, 13963–13966.

16. Holmgren, A., Aslund, F. (1995). Glutaredoxin. *Methods in Enzymology*, *252*, 283–292.

17. Sevier, C.S., Kaiser, C.A. (2002). Formation and transfer of disulphide bonds in living cells. *Nature Reviews. Molecular Cell Biology*, *3*, 836–847.

18. Mallick, P., Boutz, D.R., Eisenberg, D., Yeates, T.O. (2002). Genomic evidence that the intracellular proteins of archaeal microbes contain disulfide bonds. *Proceedings of the National Academy of Sciences USA*, *99*, 9679–9684.

19. Arner, E.S., Holmgren, A. (2000). Physiological functions of thioredoxin and thioredoxin reductase. *European Journal of Biochemistry*, *267*, 6102–6109.

20. Mannervik, B., Axelsson, K., Sundewall, A.C., Holmgren, A. (1983). Relative contributions of thioltransferase- and thioredoxin-dependent systems in reduction of low-molecular-mass and protein disulphides. *Biochemical Journal*, *213*, 519–523.

21. Rietsch, A., Beckwith, J. (1998). The genetics of disulfide bond metabolism. *Annual Review of Genetics*, *32*, 163–184.

22. Molinari, M., Helenius, A. (1999). Glycoproteins form mixed disulphides with oxidoreductases during folding in living cells. *Nature*, *402*, 90–93.

23. Prinz, W.A., Aslund, F., Holmgren, A., Beckwith, J. (1997). The role of the thioredoxin and glutaredoxin pathways in reducing protein disulfide bonds in the *Escherichia coli* cytoplasm. *Journal of Biological Chemistry, 272,* 15661–15667.

24. Choi, H., Kim, S., Mukhopadhyay, P., Cho, S., Woo, J., Storz, G., Ryu, S. (2001). Structural basis of the redox switch in the OxyR transcription factor. *Cell, 105,* 103–113.

25. Jakob, U., Muse, W., Eser, M., Bardwell, J.C. (1999). Chaperone activity with a redox switch. *Cell, 96,* 341–352.

26. Brennan, J.P., Wait, R., Begum, S., Bell, J.R., Dunn, M.J., Eaton, P. (2004). Detection and mapping of widespread intermolecular protein disulfide formation during cardiac oxidative stress using proteomics with diagonal electrophoresis. *Journal of Biological Chemistry, 279,* 41352–41360.

27. Cumming, R.C., Andon, N.L., Haynes, P.A., Park, M., Fischer, W.H., Schubert, D. (2004). Protein disulfide bond formation in the cytoplasm during oxidative stress. *Journal of Biological Chemistry, 279,* 21749–21758.

28. Harding, J.J. (1969). Glutathione-protein mixed disulphides in human lens. *Biochemical Journal, 114,* 88P–89P.

29. Harrap, K.R., Jackson, R.C., Riches, P.G., Smith, C.A., Hill, B.T. (1973). The occurrence of protein-bound mixed disulfides in rat tissues. *Biochimica et Biophysica Acta, 310,* 104–110.

30. Modig, H. (1968). Cellular mixed disulphides between thiols and proteins, and their possible implication for radiation protection. *Biochemical Pharmacology, 17,* 177–186.

31. Brigelius, R., Lenzen, R., Sies, H. (1982). Increase in hepatic mixed disulphide and glutathione disulphide levels elicited by paraquat. *Biochemical Pharmacology, 31,* 1637–1641.

32. Brigelius, R., Muckel, C., Akerboom, T.P., Sies, H. (1983). Identification and quantitation of glutathione in hepatic protein mixed disulfides and its relationship to glutathione disulfide. *Biochemical Pharmacology, 32,* 2529–2534.

33. Di Simplicio, P., Cacace, M.G., Lusini, L., Giannerini, F., Giustarini, D., Rossi, R. (1998). Role of protein-SH groups in redox homeostasis: The erythrocyte as a model system. *Archives of Biochemistry and Biophysics, 355,* 145–152.

34. Gilbert, H.F. (1984). Redox control of enzyme activities by thiol/disulfide exchange. *Methods in Enzymology, 107,* 330–351.

35. Gravina, S.A., Mieyal, J.J. (1993). Thioltransferase is a specific glutathionyl mixed disulfide oxidoreductase. *Biochemistry, 32,* 3368–3376.

36. Di Stefano, A., Frosali, S., Leonini, A., Ettorre, A., Priora, R., Di Simplicio, F.C., Di Simplicio, P. (2006). GSH depletion, protein S-glutathionylation and mitochondrial transmembrane potential hyperpolarization are early events in initiation of cell death induced by a mixture of isothiazolinones in HL60 cells. *Biochimica et Biophysica Acta, 1763,* 214–225.

37. Xiao, R., Lundstrom-Ljung, J., Holmgren, A., Gilbert, H.F. (2005). Catalysis of thiol/disulfide exchange. Glutaredoxin 1 and protein-disulfide isomerase use different mechanisms to enhance oxidase and reductase activities. *Journal of Biological Chemistry, 280,* 21099–21106.

38. Hultberg, B., Hultberg, M. (2004). High glutathione turnover in human cell lines revealed by acivicin inhibition of γ-glutamyltranspeptidase and the effects of thiol-reactive metals during acivicin inhibition. *Clinica Chimica Acta, 349,* 45–52.

39. Koch, C.J., Evans, S.M. (1996). Cysteine concentrations in rodent tumors: Unexpectedly high values may cause therapy resistance. *International Journal of Cancer, 67,* 661–667.

40. Mills, B.J., Lang, C.A. (1996). Differential distribution of free and bound glutathione and cyst(e)ine in human blood. *Biochemical Pharmacology*, *52*, 401–406.

41. Mawatari, S., Murakami, K. (2004). Different types of glutathionylation of hemoglobin can exist in intact erythrocytes. *Archives of Biochemistry and Biophysics*, *421*, 108–114.

42. Brennan, S.O., Fellowes, A.P., George, P.M. (1999). Albumin banks peninsula: A new termination variant characterised by electrospray mass spectrometry. *Biochimica et Biophysica Acta*, *1433*, 321–326.

43. Terazaki, H., Ando, Y., Suhr, O., Ohlsson, P.I., Obayashi, K., Yamashita, T., Yoshimatsu, S., Suga, M., Uchino, M., Ando, M. (1998). Post-translational modification of transthyretin in plasma. *Biochemical & Biophysical Research Communications*, *249*, 26–30.

44. Watarai, H., Nozawa, R., Tokunaga, A., Yuyama, N., Tomas, M., Hinohara, A., Ishizaka, K., Ishii, Y. (2000). Posttranslational modification of the glycosylation inhibiting factor (GIF) gene product generates bioactive GIF. *Proceedings of the National Academy of Sciences USA*, *97*, 13251–13256.

45. Cole, A.R., Hall, N.E., Treutlein, H.R., Eddes, J.S., Reid, G.E., Moritz, R.L., Simpson, R.J. (1999). Disulfide bond structure and N-glycosylation sites of the extracellular domain of the human interleukin-6 receptor. *Journal of Biological Chemistry*, *274*, 7207–7215.

46. Moritz, R.L., Hall, N.E., Connolly, L.M., Simpson, R.J. (2001). Determination of the disulfide structure and N-glycosylation sites of the extracellular domain of the human signal transducer gp130. *Journal of Biological Chemistry*, *276*, 8244–8253.

47. Arunachalam, B., Phan, U.T., Geuze, H.J., Cresswell, P. (2000). Enzymatic reduction of disulfide bonds in lysosomes: Characterization of a γ-interferon-inducible lysosomal thiol reductase (GILT). *Proceedings of the National Academy of Sciences USA*, *97*, 745–750.

48. Maric, M., Arunachalam, B., Phan, U.T., Dong, C., Garrett, W.S., Cannon, K.S., Alfonso, C., Karlsson, L., Flavell, R.A., Cresswell, P. (2001). Defective antigen processing in GILT-free mice. *Science*, *294*, 1361–1365.

49. Chen, W., Yewdell, J.W., Levine, R.L., Bennink, J.R. (1999). Modification of cysteine residues in vitro and in vivo affects the immunogenicity and antigenicity of major histocompatibility complex class I-restricted viral determinants. *Journal of Experimental Medicine*, *189*, 1757–1764.

50. Collins, D.S., Unanue, E.R., Harding, C.V. (1991). Reduction of disulfide bonds within lysosomes is a key step in antigen processing. *Journal of Immunology*, *147*, 4054–4059.

51. Haque, M.A., Hawes, J.W., Blum, J.S. (2001). Cysteinylation of MHC class II ligands: Peptide endocytosis and reduction within APC influences T cell recognition. *Journal of Immunology*, *166*, 4543–4551.

52. Bump, E.A., Cerce, B.A., al-Sarraf, R., Pierce, S.M., Koch, C.J. (1992). Radioprotection of DNA in isolated nuclei by naturally occurring thiols at intermediate oxygen tension. *Radiation Research*, *132*, 94–104.

53. Ruoso, P., Hedley, D.W. (2004). Inhibition of γ-glutamyl transpeptidase activity decreases intracellular cysteine levels in cervical carcinoma. *Cancer Chemotherapeutic Pharmacology*, *54*, 49–56.

54. Barrett, W.C., DeGnore, J.P., Keng, Y.F., Zhang, Z.Y., Yim, M.B., Chock, P.B. (1999). Roles of superoxide radical anion in signal transduction mediated by reversible regulation of protein-tyrosine phosphatase 1B. *Journal of Biological Chemistry*, *274*, 34543–34546.

55. Konorev, E.A., Kalyanaraman, B., Hogg, N. (2000). Modification of creatine kinase by S-nitrosothiols: S-nitrosation vs. S-thiolation. *Free Radical Biology and Medicine*, 28, 1671–1678.

56. Xian, M., Chen, X., Liu, Z., Wang, K., Wang, P.G. (2000). Inhibition of papain by S-nitrosothiols. Formation of mixed disulfides. *Journal of Biological Chemistry*, 275, 20467–20473.

57. Ghezzi, P., Di Simplicio, P. (2007). Glutathionylation pathways in drug response. *Current Opinion Pharmacology*, 7, 398–403.

58. Summa, D., Spiga, O., Bernini, A., Venditti, V., Priora, R., Frosali, S., Margaritis, A., Giuseppe, D.D., Niccolai, N., Simplicio, P.D. (2007). Protein-thiol substitution or protein dethiolation by thiol/disulfide exchange reactions: The albumin model. *Proteins*, 62, 369–378.

59. Gan, Z.R., Sardana, M.K., Jacobs, J.W., Polokoff, M.A. (1990). Yeast thioltransferase: The active site cysteines display differential reactivity. *Archives of Biochemistry and Biophysics*, 282, 110–115.

60. Yang, Y.F., Wells, W.W. (1991). Catalytic mechanism of thioltransferase. *Journal of Biological Chemistry*, 266, 12766–12771.

61. Szajewski, R.P., Whitesides, G.M. (1980). Rate constants and equilibrium constants for thiol-disulfide interchange reactions involving oxidized glutathione. *Journal of the American Chemical Society*, 102, 2011–2026.

62. Snyder, G.H., Cennerazzo, M.J., Karalis, A.J., Field, D. (1981). Electrostatic influence of local cysteine environments on disulfide exchange kinetics. *Biochemistry*, 20, 6509–6519.

63. Ziegler, D.M. (1985). Role of reversible oxidation-reduction of enzyme thiols-disulfides in metabolic regulation. *Annual Review of Biochemistry*, 54, 305–329.

64. Casagrande, S., Bonetto, V., Fratelli, M., Gianazza, E., Eberini, I., Massignan, T., Salmona, M., Chang, G., Holmgren, A., Ghezzi, P. (2002). Glutathionylation of human thioredoxin: A possible crosstalk between the glutathione and thioredoxin systems. *Proceedings of the National Academy of Sciences USA*, 99, 9745–9749.

65. Ghezzi, P., Casagrande, S., Massignan, T., Basso, M., Bellacchio, E., Mollica, L., Biasini, E., Tonelli, R., Eberini, I., Gianazza, E., Dai, W.W., Fratelli, M., Salmona, M., Sherry, B., Bonetto, V. (2005). Redox regulation of cyclophilin A by glutathionylation. *Proteomics*, 6, 817–825.

66. Chai, Y.C., Ashraf, S.S., Rokutan, K., Johnston, R.B., Jr., Thomas, J.A. (1994). S-thiolation of individual human neutrophil proteins including actin by stimulation of the respiratory burst: Evidence against a role for glutathione disulfide. *Archives of Biochemistry and Biophysics*, 310, 273–281.

67. Dalle-Donne, I., Rossi, R., Giustarini, D., Colombo, R., Milzani, A. (2003). Actin S-glutathionylation: Evidence against a thiol-disulphide exchange mechanism. *Free Radical Biology and Medicine*, 35, 1185–1193.

68. Di Simplicio, P., Giannerini, F., Giustarini, D., Lusini, L., Rossi, R. (1998). The role of cysteine in the regulation of blood glutathione-protein mixed disulfides in rats treated with diamide. *Toxicology and Applied Pharmacology*, 148, 56–64.

69. Jung, C.H., Thomas, J.A. (1996). S-glutathiolated hepatocyte proteins and insulin disulfides as substrates for reduction by glutaredoxin, thioredoxin, protein disulfide isomerase, and glutathione. *Archives of Biochemistry and Biophysics*, 335, 61–72.

70. Rossi, R., Cardaioli, E., Scaloni, A., Amiconi, G., Di Simplicio, P. (1995). Thiol groups in proteins as endogenous reductants to determine glutathione-protein mixed disulphides in biological systems. *Biochimica et Biophysica Acta, 1243,* 230–238.

71. Hayano, T., Inaka, K., Otsu, M., Taniyama, Y., Miki, K., Matsushima, M., Kikuchi, M. (1993). PDI and glutathione-mediated reduction of the glutathionylated variant of human lysozyme. *FEBS Letters, 328,* 203–208.

72. Lundstrom-Ljung, J., Vlamis-Gardikas, A., Aslund, F., Holmgren, A. (1999). Reactivity of glutaredoxins 1, 2 and 3 from *Escherichia coli* and protein disulfide isomerase towards glutathionyl-mixed disulfides in ribonuclease A. *FEBS Letters, 443,* 85–88.

73. Herrero, E., de la Torre-Ruiz, M.A. (2007). Monothiol glutaredoxins: A common domain for multiple functions. *Cellular and Molecular Life Sciences, 64,* 1518–1530.

74. Wang, J., Tekle, E., Oubrahim, H., Mieyal, J.J., Stadtman, E.R., Chock, P.B. (2003). Stable and controllable RNA interference: Investigating the physiological function of glutathionylated actin. *Proceedings of the National Academy of Sciences USA, 100,* 5103–5106.

75. Zapun, A., Cooper, L., Creighton, T.E. (1994). Replacement of the active-site cysteine residues of DsbA, a protein required for disulfide bond formation in vivo. *Biochemistry, 33,* 1907–1914.

76. Fratelli, M., Demol, H., Puype, M., Casagrande, S., Eberini, I., Salmona, M., Bonetto, V., Mengozzi, M., Duffieux, F., Miclet, E., Bachi, A., Vandekerckhove, J., Gianazza, E., Ghezzi, P. (2002). Identification by redox proteomics of glutathionylated proteins in oxidatively stressed human T lymphocytes. *Proceedings of the National Academy of Sciences USA, 99,* 3505–3510.

77. Lind, C., Gerdes, R., Hamnell, Y., Schuppe-Koistinen, I., von Lowenhielm, H.B., Holmgren, A., Cotgreave, I.A. (2002). Identification of S-glutathionylated cellular proteins during oxidative stress and constitutive metabolism by affinity purification and proteomic analysis. *Archives of Biochemistry and Biophysics, 406,* 229–240.

78. Townsend, D.M., Findlay, V.J., Fazilev, F., Ogle, M., Fraser, J., Saavedra, J.E., Ji, X., Keefer, L.K., Tew, K.D. (2006). A glutathione S-transferase pi-activated prodrug causes kinase activation concurrent with S-glutathionylation of proteins. *Molecular Pharmacology, 69,* 501–508.

79. Brennan, J.P., Miller, J.I., Fuller, W., Wait, R., Begum, S., Dunn, M.J., Eaton, P. (2006). The utility of N,N-biotinyl glutathione disulfide in the study of protein S-glutathiolation. *Molecular and Cellular Proteomics, 5,* 215–225.

80. Rokutan, K., Thomas, J.A., Johnston, R.B., Jr., (1991). Phagocytosis and stimulation of the respiratory burst by phorbol diester initiate S-thiolation of specific proteins in macrophages. *Journal of Immunology, 147,* 260–264.

81. Cheng, G., Ikeda, Y., Iuchi, Y., Fujii, J. (2005). Detection of S-glutathionylated proteins by glutathione S-transferase overlay. *Archives of Biochemistry and Biophysics, 435,* 42–49.

82. Nonaka, K., Kume, N., Urata, Y., Seto, S., Kohno, T., Honda, S., Ikeda, S., Muroya, T., Ikeda, Y., Ihara, Y., Kita, T., Kondo, T. (2007). Serum levels of S-glutathionylated proteins as a risk-marker for arteriosclerosis obliterans. *Circulation Journal, 71,* 100–105.

83. Hamnell-Pamment, Y., Lind, C., Palmberg, C., Bergman, T., Cotgreave, I.A. (2005). Determination of site-specificity of S-glutathionylated cellular proteins. *Biochemical and Biophysical Research Communications, 332,* 362–369.

84. Velu, C.S., Niture, S.K., Doneanu, C.E., Pattabiraman, N., Srivenugopal, K.S. (2007). Human p53 is inhibited by glutathionylation of cysteines present in the proximal DNA-binding domain during oxidative stress. *Biochemistry, 46*, 7765–7780.

85. Klatt, P., Molina, E.P., De Lacoba, M.G., Padilla, C.A., Martinez-Galesteo, E., Barcena, J.A., Lamas, S. (1999). Redox regulation of c-Jun DNA binding by reversible S-glutathiolation. *FASEB Journal, 13*, 1481–1490.

86. Pineda-Molina, E., Klatt, P., Vazquez, J., Marina, A., Garcia de Lacoba, M., Perez-Sala, D., Lamas, S. (2001). Glutathionylation of the p50 subunit of NF-kappaB: A mechanism for redox-induced inhibition of DNA binding. *Biochemistry, 40*, 14134–14142.

87. Wang, J., Boja, E.S., Tan, W., Tekle, E., Fales, H.M., English, S., Mieyal, J.J., Chock, P.B. (2001). Reversible glutathionylation regulates actin polymerization in A431 cells. *Journal of Biological Chemistry, 276*, 47763–47766.

88. Davis, D.A., Brown, C.A., Newcomb, F.M., Boja, E.S., Fales, H.M., Kaufman, J., Stahl, S.J., Wingfield, P., Yarchoan, R. (2003). Reversible oxidative modification as a mechanism for regulating retroviral protease dimerization and activation. *Journal of Virology, 77*, 3319–3325.

89. Davis, D.A., Dorsey, K., Wingfield, P.T., Stahl, S.J., Kaufman, J., Fales, H.M., Levine, R.L. (1996). Regulation of HIV-1 protease activity through cysteine modification. *Biochemistry, 35*, 2482–2488.

90. Goch, G., Vdovenko, S., Kozlowska, H., Bierzynski, A. (2005). Affinity of S100A1 protein for calcium increases dramatically upon glutathionylation. *FEBS Journal, 272*, 2557–2565.

91. Hidalgo, C., Donoso, P., Carrasco, M.A. (2005). The ryanodine receptors Ca^{2+} release channels: Cellular redox sensors? *IUBMB Life, 57*, 315–322.

92. Adachi, T., Weisbrod, R.M., Pimentel, D.R., Ying, J., Sharov, V.S., Schoneich, C., Cohen, R.A. (2004). S-Glutathiolation by peroxynitrite activates SERCA during arterial relaxation by nitric oxide. *Nature Medicine, 10*, 1200–1207.

93. Chu, F., Chen, L.H., O'Brian, C.A. (2004). Cellular protein kinase C isozyme regulation by exogenously delivered physiological disulfides: Implications of oxidative protein kinase C regulation to cancer prevention. *Carcinogenesis, 25*, 585–596.

94. Chu, F., Ward, N.E., O'Brian, C.A. (2001). Potent inactivation of representative members of each PKC isozyme subfamily and PKD via S-thiolation by the tumor-promotion/ progression antagonist glutathione but not by its precursor cysteine. *Carcinogenesis, 22*, 1221–1229.

95. Ghezzi, P., Casagrande, S., Massignan, T., Basso, M., Bellacchio, E., Mollica, L., Biasini, E., Tonelli, R., Eberini, I., Gianazza, E., Dai, W.W., Fratelli, M., Salmona, M., Sherry, B., Bonetto, V. (2006). Redox regulation of cyclophilin A by glutathionylation. *Proteomics, 6*, 817–825.

96. Hondorp, E.R., Matthews, R.G. (2004). Oxidative stress inactivates cobalamin-independent methionine synthase (MetE) in *Escherichia coli*. *PLoS Biology, 2*, e336.

CHAPTER 10

GSH, SULFUR AMINO ACIDS, AND APOPTOSIS

GIUSEPPE FILOMENI, KATIA AQUILANO, and MARIA ROSA CIRIOLO

10.1 INTRODUCTION

Cysteine, homocysteine, methionine, and taurine are the four common sulfur-containing amino acids. In animal cells methionine represents the essential amino acid from which cysteine is synthesized, while homocysteine is on the route of methionine/cysteine synthesis and its increase constitutes a risk factor for neurodegeneration and cardiovascular diseases. Taurine, which is derived from cysteine, is found in millimolar concentrations in most mammalian tissues and appears to have multiple functions in many physiological processes, such as osmoregulation, immunomodulation, and bile salts formation. Therefore, cysteine could be considered the core of the system that controls the concentrations of the free sulfur-containing amino acids. Moreover, besides being incorporated into proteins it is a fundamental precursor of glutathione (γ-glutamyl-cysteinylglycine), which represents the most abundant low molecular weight thiol currently present as reduced (GSH) or disulfide forms (GSSG; GSSR, where R is a free or a thiol-protein). The synthesis of GSH from glutamate, cysteine, and glycine is cytosolic and catalyzed sequentially by two enzymes, γ-glutamylcysteine synthetase (γ-GCS) and GSH synthetase; moreover, compelling evidence demonstrates that the synthesis depends on γ-GCS activity, cysteine availability, and GSH feedback regulation. The elucidation of the physiological roles played by GSH has advanced greatly over the past decades, as a consequence of research on free radicals, oxidative stress, and, more recently, redox signaling. In particular, GSH is involved in nutrient metabolism, antioxidant defense and regulation of cellular metabolic functions ranging from gene expression, DNA and protein synthesis to signal transduction, cell proliferation and apoptosis. This chapter will start with an overview of the biochemistry of GSH and sulfur amino acids with particular emphasis

Glutathione and Sulfur Amino Acids in Human Health and Disease. Edited by R. Masella and G. Mazza
Copyright © 2009 John Wiley & Sons, Inc.

on the role of the tripeptide in buffering redox changes; the text will then focus on the role of GSH in cell signaling and regulation of the apoptotic process.

Sulfur is present in four amino acids: methionine, an essential amino acid; the nonessential cysteine that can be made by methionine; homocysteine that is on the pathway of cysteine/methionine synthesis; and taurine, an ubiquitous amino acid abundant in mammalian tissues with different cell protecting and neuromodulatory functions [1] (Fig. 10.1). Among these only methionine and cysteine are incorporated into proteins and the latter plays a central role in the metabolism of the sulfur-containing amino acids. Indeed, cysteine not only is an essential constituent of proteins but also lies on the major route of incorporation of inorganic sulfur into organic compounds. It is formed in plants and in bacteria from sulfide and serine by the catalysis of cysteine synthase. Subsequently, it can be converted to methionine; on the contrary, in animals, the converse process is responsible for the synthesis of cysteine. In fact, due to the inability of animal cells to incorporate sulfide directly into cysteine, this amino acid must be either provided in the diet or formed from dietary methionine [2] (Fig. 10.1). Cysteine and its disulfide form cystine are relatively insoluble and are toxic in excess; therefore, their excretion is usually controlled carefully. An important cysteine catabolic pathway in animals is its oxidation to cysteine sulfinate, a two step process requiring O_2, NAD(P)H, and Fe^{2+}. Cysteine sulfinate can be further oxidized to cysteine sulfonate, which can be decarboxylated to taurine [3] (Fig. 10.1). Taurine is a component of bile salts [4] and one of the most abundant amino acid in human tissues, with several functions ranging from regulator of osmotic pressure to neurotransmitter [5–7]. Another pathway of degradation of cysteine sulfinate is transamination to 3-sulfinylpyruvate, a compound that undergoes loss of SO_2. The latter compound needs to be transformed in sulfate before being excreted either free or esterified with oligosaccharides and phenolic compounds [3].

Although sulfur belongs to the same group as oxygen in the periodic table it is much less electronegative. This characteristic confers unique properties on sulfur-containing

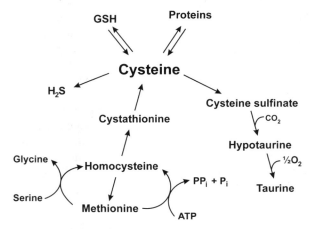

Figure 10.1   Major pathways of sulfur amino acid metabolism.

amino acids. For instance, methionine is the sole initiating amino acid in the synthesis of almost all eukaryotic proteins; and cysteine, due to its capacity to form disulfide bonds, plays a crucial role in protein structure and folding. Moreover, the redox state of some cysteine residues influences the activity of sensitive proteins implicated in various cellular processes, including signal transduction [8]. In particular, it has been suggested that the intermolecular disulfide bridge formation could lead to protein arrangement in dimers and/or multimers influencing the association between different cellular proteins implicated in regulatory pathways [9, 10]. Cysteine is also essential for the synthesis of glutathione (GSH), a low molecular weight antioxidant which under some circumstances can be considered a reservoir of cysteine [11].

GSH synthesis occurs in virtually all cells, but the liver plays a particular role in that it is the tissue where the bulk of dietary-derived cysteine is metabolized, mainly by converting it to GSH, which is then released into the plasma. However, protein synthesis had a higher priority for cysteine than GSH synthesis does; indeed GSH depletion occurs under sulfur amino acid intakes marginal but adequate for protein synthesis [3]. Under physiological conditions GSH is easily oxidized and regenerated very rapidly by redox reactions either directly or by several enzymes (e.g., glutathione peroxidase, glutathione reductase), that are involved in maintaining the intracellular redox environment. This characteristic allows it to play an essential role in many biochemical and pharmacological reactions where GSH acts as a reducing and antioxidant agent. It is involved in the metabolism of different cell molecules and xenobiotics [12, 13]. Today the implication of GSH in many other cellular functions has been recognized [14]. In fact, GSH modulates immune responses and it has been discovered that it participates in gene expression and in the regulation of the activity of sulfhydryl-containing proteins either via thiol-disulfide exchange reactions or by the reduction of potentially toxic peroxides [9, 15]. Moreover, GSH is involved in the mitochondrial mechanisms that link opening of the permeability transition pore complex and activation of cell death by apoptosis [15]. The cross-talk between the phosphorylative cascade mediated by MAPKs and cell signaling involved in cell cycle regulation and apoptosis is also profoundly modulated by the GSH:GSSG ratio [10, 16]. However, to understand the potential relevance of GSH to apoptosis it is important first to briefly review the pathways involved in GSH metabolism.

10.2 SYNTHESIS AND FUNCTIONS OF GSH

GSH is a ubiquitous tripeptide synthesized intracellularly from the precursor amino acids cysteine, glutamate, and glycine. The chemical structure of this compound, γ-glutamylcysteinil-glycine, provides peculiar characteristics ranging from insusceptibility to proteolysis to redox thiols catalysis. These features, together with its high intracellular concentration (1 to 10 mM), make GSH the most important redox-active thiol [10, 12]. The available evidence indicates that the majority of the intracellular GSH pool derives from synthesis occurring in the cytoplasm while a small amount is synthesized in other organelles such as the mitochondria [17, 18]. Virtually all mammalian cells have the capacity to synthesize GSH by two sequential

ATP-dependent reactions catalyzed by γ-glutamylcysteine synthetase (γ-GCS), recently renamed glutamate-cysteine ligase, and GSH synthetase [19]. These enzymes catalyze, respectively, the following reactions:

(1)   L-glutamate + L-cysteine + ATP ⟷ L-γ-glutamyl-L-cysteine + ADP + Pi

(2)   L-γ-glutamyl-L-cysteine + glycine + ATP ⟷ GSH + ADP + Pi

γ-GCS functions as a homodimer of 118 kDa and is the rate-limiting enzyme involved in the two-step synthesis of GSH. It belongs to the class of proteins that "sense" oxidizing conditions as a regulatory mechanism because, through reversible disulfide bond formation, the enzyme undergoes a gain of function [20]. The holo-enzyme is formed by a 70 kDa catalytic subunit (γ-GCSc) and a 27 kDa regulatory/modulatory subunit (γ-GCSr/m) [21]. Although both subunits present several cysteine residues, only two disulfide bonds and a thiol cysteine residue at the active site are required for optimal enzyme activity. One disulfide bond is intermolecular and it is necessary to link the two subunits; the other is intramolecular and does not affect the active site [22]. The synthesis of GSH from its amino acids occurs constitutively, but can also be upregulated in response to stress. However, the intracellular concentrations of the two subunits are not equimolar, but rather γ-GCSc is far in excess allowing constitutive synthesis of the tripeptide, whereas association with γ-GCSr/m is necessary to increase the rate of synthesis such as is required under oxidative stress [23, 24]. In several cases the increase in γ-GCS activity requires an up-modulation of gene expression of one or both subunits. Oxidative stress conditions that result in GSH depletion promote formation of the intermolecular disulfide. This produces a conformational change that increases the affinity and the specificity of the glutamate binding site [25]. On the other hand, physiological GSH concentration reduces the intermolecular disulfide, thus producing changes in conformation that favor GSH feedback inhibition. Sustained increases in GSH content are controlled primarily through induction of two genes, γ-GCSc and γ-GCSr/m, leading to the transcription of the two subunits of the γ-GCS [26, 27]. Additional to these genes is GS, encoding for the second enzyme, the GSH synthase. Each of the three genes is encoded by a single copy gene in the haploid human genome. While no information is available for potential regulatory elements of GS, for the other two genes, sequence analysis and studies with reporter constructs have revealed that the human γ-GCSc promoter contains many potential cis-acting elements, including consensus recognition sites for binding of electrophile response element (EpRE), nuclear factor κB (NF-κB), Sp-1, activator protein-2 (AP-2), and TRE-like [28]. The γ-GCSr/m promoter contains many of the same elements with the exception of the κB element [28]. Therefore, even though the GSH synthesis seems to be regulated at several levels, the majority of studies support the notion of redox-dependent signaling pathways controlling the expression of the GSH biosynthetic genes γ-GCSc and γ-GCSr/m. In humans these genes are characterized as phase II genes regulated in a nuclear erythroid factor 2-related factor 2 (Nrf2)-dependent manner [29]. Therefore, GSH synthesis is regulated mainly through modulation of γ-GCS expression and activity level and by the availability of precursor amino acids. Several oxidizing conditions (oxidative/nitrosative stress, inflammatory cytokines, ionizing radiation, heat shock, GSH depletion, heavy metals, chemotherapy) increase γ-GCS activity or expression level, whereas γ-GCS phosphorylation, hyperglycemia, and dietary protein deficiency inhibit the enzyme at the transcription or activity level [30]. Moreover, cysteine availability is also a rate limiting step in the synthesis of GSH particularly under conditions of malnutrition or dietary protein intake deficiency [31].

Glutathione is present as a reduced form (GSH) and two oxidized species: glutathione disulfide (GSSG) and glutathione mixed disulfide with protein thiols (GS-R). Under physiological conditions GSH is the major form with its concentration from 10- to 100-fold higher than GSSG and GS-R [19]. GSSG is predominantly produced by the catalysis of glutathione peroxidase, during the detoxification from hydrogen peroxide and other peroxides, as well as from the direct reactions of GSH with electrophilic compounds, such as radical species [32]. The production of GS-R, instead, requires for the protein-cysteinyl residue to be "reactive" at physiological pH and in the thiolate form; these residues, under oxidative stress, are prone to oxidation in sulfenic acid, which efficiently reacts with GSH leading to a glutathionylated-cysteine derivative (GS-R) [33–35]. Both GSSG and GS-R can be catalytically reduced back to GSH by the NADPH-dependent glutathione reductase and thioredoxin/glutaredoxin system, respectively. Moreover, the nonenzymatic interconversion between GSSG and GS-R can occur [19, 36].

Due to the high intracellular concentration of GSH the GSH/GSSG redox couple can readily interact with most of the physiologically relevant redox couples (NADPH/NADP$^+$), (thioredoxin-SH/thioredoxin-SS), undergoing reversible oxidation or reduction reactions, thereby maintaining the appropriate redox balance in the cell [36]. Experimental evidence, over the last decade, has demonstrated that changes in GSH/GSSG ratio may govern several cellular functions involved in signal transduction, cell cycle regulation, and other cellular processes [14, 36, 37]. Oxidative stimuli are fundamental for the fluctuation in the GSH : GSSG ratio, even under physiological conditions, where the value (usually >10) tends to decrease by either a raise in the concentration of GSSG or a decrease in the GSH content. The GSH redox state, under a burst of radical species, can be maintained also by other mechanisms such as induction of enzyme activities of glutathione reductase and γ-GCS or through active extrusion of GSSG. This species may, finally, be degraded by γ-glutamyl-transpeptidase, present on the external plasma membrane of specific cells, into glutamic acid and cysteinyl-glycine; this dipeptide is further hydrolyzed by cell surface dipeptidases and the resulting amino acids taken up by cells for regeneration of intracellular GSH [38]. However, when oxidative stress becomes prolonged and cellular systems are no longer able to counteract the oxidative-mediated insults, the amount of free GSH decreases leading to irreversible cell degeneration and death.

10.2.1 Cell Detoxification: An Old Story Related to Conjugation, Scavenging, and Antioxidant Function of GSH

The GSH and GSH-related enzymatic systems are efficient tools that cells have exploited in detoxification and, at the same time, this process represents the most ancient notice on the physiological role played by the tripeptide. GSH in fact is both a nucleophile and a reductant, and therefore can react with electrophilic or oxidizing species rendering the former molecules more soluble and excretable, and the latter unable to interact with more critical cellular constituents such as lipids, nucleic acids, and proteins. In this section, we will give an overview of the involvement of GSH in detoxification. Readers may refer to more detailed reviews (see Chapter 6 of this book and References 39 to 42).

GSH reacts with many electrophiles, physiological metabolites, and xenobiotics to form mercapturates. These reactions are catalyzed by glutathione transferases, a super-family of phase II detoxification enzymes that catalyze the conjugation of GSH with target compounds to form GSH conjugates; these compounds are then converted to mercapturic acids and excreted [43] (Fig. 10.2). The glutathione transferase (formerly known as glutathione-S-transferase, GSTs) catalyzes the conjugation of nonpolar compounds that contain an electrophilic carbon, nitrogen, or sulfur atom to GSH. In this way GSTs contribute to the metabolism of drugs, pesticides, peroxides, and other xenobiotics as well as physiological compounds. There are three types of GSTs: canonical or cytosolic, mitochondrial, and microsomal. GSTs from different organisms were divided into classes depending on structural homology greater than 40%; therefore, there are currently more than ten recognized classes, indicated with Greek letters. The enzymes are dimers of 25 kDa subunits. GST monomers of the same class can form heterodimers if multiple genes are present [44]. Moreover, from recent studies it is emerging that GSTs are a highly diverse family of enzymes, deriving from different progenitor isoenzymes, with functions ranging from detoxification to biosynthesis of leukotriene and prostaglandin [44, 45]. In fact, it has been proposed that the mitochondrial and the cytosolic GST families have diverged from a thioredoxin-like ancestor through a parallel mechanism: the mitochondrial (κ class) through a disulfide bond isomerase, DsbA-like ancestor and the cytosolic GST via a glutaredoxin-like ancestor [46]. Moreover, the microsomal GSTs are now known as "membrane-associated proteins in eicosanoid and glutathione metabolism" (MAPEGs) [47, 48]. From these findings new functions have been added to the former detoxification role of the GSH/GSTs system.

Nevertheless, even if most of the GSH conjugates are less toxic and more polar and can be excreted, GSTs convert dichloromethane and short-chain alkyl halides to unstable and mutagenic GSH-conjugates [49]. Moreover, conjugation and efflux of GSH can eventually result in its intracellular depletion leading to the impairment of cellular defense based on GSH conjugation. Electrophiles could then freely exert their damaging action through their interaction with biological macromolecular targets [50].

Later on, GSH has been related to the antioxidant cell systems [51]. In particular, the knowledge that the metabolic processes give rise to the production of ROS, even under physiological conditions, has opened up another branch of research focusing on the role of GSH as both antioxidant and radical scavenger. GSH effectively scavenges free radicals and other reactive oxygen (ROS) and nitrogen species (RNS) (e.g., hydroxyl radical, lipid peroxyl radical, superoxide anion, and hydrogen peroxide) directly and indirectly through enzymatic reactions. In such reactions, due to both

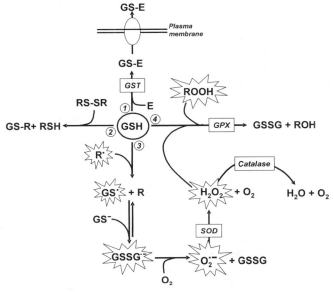

Figure 10.2 Antioxidant and detoxifying activity of GSH. GSH can react with several molecules, directly or via the catalysis of several enzymes. (1) The conjugation reaction with electrophiles, physiological metabolites, and xenobiotics (E) to form GSH conjugates (GS-E) is catalyzed by glutathione transferases (GST); GS-E are then converted to mercapturic acids and excreted. (2) The thiol-disulfide exchange is the result of a spontaneous reaction between GSH and mixed or intramolecular disulfides (RS-SR). In the case that R represents a protein, the process is referred as S-glutathionylation, and glutaredoxin or thioredoxin participate in ensuring the reduction back of the mixed disulfide. GSH is also a potent antioxidant and participates in scavenging radicals by one- or two-electron reduction reactions. (3) GSH can react with mono-electron radicals ($R^\bullet$) to generate the glutathione thiyl radical ($GS^\bullet$). Next, the high concentration of GSH (mainly of its thiolate form, GS^-) leads to the formation of the glutathione disulfide radical anion, $GSSG^{\bullet-}$, which, in the presence of oxygen, produces superoxide ($O_2^{\bullet-}$) and GSSG. In such a way, the one-electron reduction is kinetically driven in the forward direction, even though it would not be favorable. Superoxide dismutase (SOD) finally buffers $O_2^{\bullet-}$ reactivity by producing hydrogen peroxide (H_2O_2). (4) H_2O_2 and other peroxides (ROOH) are then totally reduced by glutathione peroxidase (GPx), which, by using two molecules of GSH as cofactor, forms the corresponding alcohol (ROH) and GSSG. Alternatively H_2O_2 is dismutated to H_2O by catalase.

its high intracellular concentrations and the thiol group of the cysteine residue, GSH is oxidized to form GSSG, which is then reduced back to GSH by glutathione reductase. Glutathione reductase is a flavoprotein catalyzing the NADPH-dependent reduction of GSSG to GSH, thus representing an essential molecular factor for the maintenance of intracellular GSH levels. Nevertheless, the principal role of GSH in ROS scavenging is linked to the activity of the selenium-containing enzyme glutathione peroxidase (GPx), which catalyzes the GSH-dependent reaction of hydroperoxides (ROOH), where R can be an aliphatic or aromatic group or, simply, hydrogen (Fig. 10.2).

The products of this reduction reaction are H_2O, or an alcohol (ROH), and GSSG, thus indicating that GSH behaves as a two-electron donor. Hence, to have a complete reduction of the substrate, two molecules of GSH are needed to finally generate GSSG [52]. The GSH-mediated one-electron reduction with radicals, instead, is not chemically favorable since it would generate the unstable thiyl radical GS$^{\bullet}$. However, the reaction is kinetically driven in the forward direction by the removal of GS$^{\bullet}$ through the following reactions with thiolate anion (GS^{-}) and then with oxygen. The first reaction leads to the generation of one of the most reductant molecules, GSSG$^{\bullet-}$, which in the presence of O_2, generates GSSG and superoxide ($O_2^{\bullet-}$) (Fig. 10.2). Eventually, the high catalytic efficiency of the antioxidant enzyme superoxide dismutase (SOD) in association with catalase or GPx, determines the complete free radicals scavenging [53] (Fig. 10.2). Therefore, the outcomes of radical scavenging by GSH are oxygen consumption and $O_2^{\bullet-}$ production. The sequence of reactions described above could be regarded as a generator system of oxidative stress; however, from another perspective, the mechanism enables GSH to act as an intermediary for "channelling" radicals to $O_2^{\bullet-}$. In such a way $O_2^{\bullet-}$ acts as a radical sink; therefore, due to the high concentration and high catalytic constant of Cu, Zn SOD, the sequence of reactions starting from GSH and ending with SOD provides an elegant mechanism for a single enzyme to control the effects of the generation of a huge number of radicals [53] (Fig. 10.2).

10.2.2 Cell Detoxification: Newest Evidence for Antioxidant Functions of GSH

Additional roles for the antioxidant function of GSH have emerged in the last few years and are related to (1) the interaction of the tripeptide with nitric oxide (NO) or with RNS and (2) the involvement of GSH in the process of protein glutathionylation during redox signaling and oxidative stress.

NO is a gaseous free radical produced by the activity of nitric oxide synthases (NOSs). Its physiological concentration is in the nanomolar range, with micromolar concentrations being pathological [54, 55]. NO itself is generally unreactive at physiological concentrations and its reaction with thiols is essentially low in the absence of oxygen [56, 57]. However, direct NO reaction with thiol residues could occur in the presence of thiyl radical leading to the formation of S-nitrosothiols (SNO), which are far longer lived species than NO [56]. As GSH is present intracellularly at millimolar concentrations, the interaction of NO with the thiyl radical on its cysteine is plausible. This reaction may have a protective role in preventing thiyl or NO radicals from reacting with other species to form further harmful oxidation products. Moreover, in the presence of oxygen, NO intermediates directly react with GSH, whereas other pathways in which GSH or protein thiols can react with NO, to form S-nitrosoglutathione (GSNO), require electron acceptors, such as the transition metal ions Fe^{3+} or Cu^{2+} [58]. Therefore, besides representing a physiological store of NO, GSH by interacting with NO and RNS can contribute to scavenging their cytotoxic effects. In fact, it has been demonstrated that upon NO overproduction a prompt increase of GSH levels is induced intracellularly (observation from our

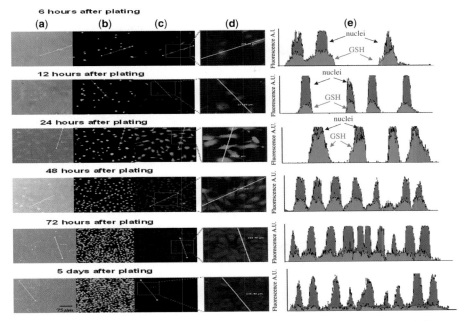

Figure 3.2 Confocal microscopic images of 3T3 fibroblasts during cell growth. Cells were plated in chamber slides 5 days, 72 h, 48 h, 24 h, 12 h, and 6 h before the experiment and were stained and analyzed the same day. Triple staining was performed on living cells: Hoechst 33342 to localize nuclei, CMFDA to mark GSH, and propidium iodide to exclude dead cells. During microscopic confocal analysis cells were maintained in the chamber provided with 5% CO_2 and at 37°C. Images were taken by light microscopy (panel A) and by confocal microscopy, to capture blue fluorescence of nuclei (panel B), green fluorescence that marks GSH (panel C), and red fluorescence of dead cells (results not shown). Maximum projection images were analyzed by profile of fluorescence, where a cross section white line of 200 $\pm$ 20 μm was drawn through a cell field (best shown on amplified detail on panel D) to compare distribution of green CMFDA fluorescence (levels of GSH) along the line (green area under the curves on E panels) with blue Hoechst fluorescence (nuclei localization) (blue area under the curve in E panels).

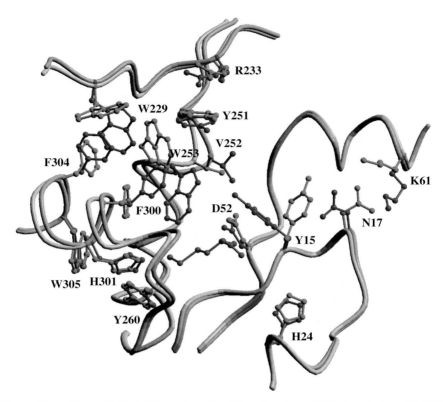

Figure 16.5 The synthetic/editing active site of *E. coli* methionyl-tRNA synthetase (MetRS). Hydrophobic and hydrogen bonding interactions provide specificity for the cognate substrate L-methionine. Superimposition of a-carbon chain backbones for the MetRS · Met complex (burly-wood) and free MetRS (light gray), solved at 1.8 Å resolution, shows movements of active site residues upon binding of methionine. Residue colors are red in the MetRS · Met complex and green in free MetRS, and L-methionine is magenta. Reprinted with permission from Reference 134.

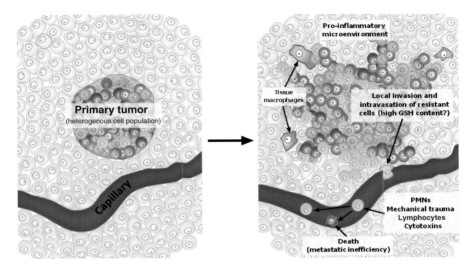

Figure 19.1 Malignant tumor spread. Tumor formation follows three steps: initiation (accumulation of nonlethal mutations), promotion (characteristic clonal expansion of preneoplastic cells, also known as benign tumor), and progression (changes at cellular and molecular levels leading to the typical genomic instability that characterizes the transition from preneoplastic to a neoplastic state). In these stages tumors are surrounded by a continuous basement membrane. Preneoplastic cells suffer metabolic adaptations during the transition to the invasive phenotype. These adaptations facilitate their escape from immune attacks, invasion of local normal tissue, intravasation, and colonization of distant organs. Most circulating cancer cells are eliminated by physiological mechanisms, a fact called "metastatic inefficiency." PMNs, polymorphonuclear cells.

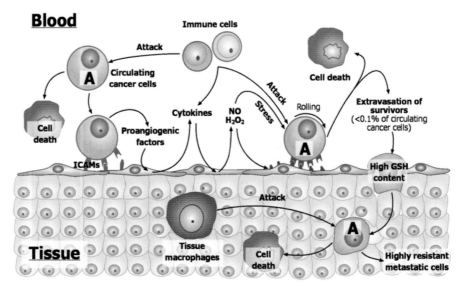

Figure 19.2 Interaction between metastatic cells and the vascular endothelium induce molecular mechanisms that lead to tumor cell death or invasion. In a first step, circulating cancer cells establish weak links with the endothelium. Metastatic growth factors induce endothelial cytokine release and, consequently, generation of cytotoxic NO and H_2O_2. Both reactive species, in cooperation with the immune system, contribute to cancer cell death. Nevertheless, some tumor cells adapted to the metastatic microenvironment survive and can colonize the extravascular tissue. Metastatic cell invaders, which will be further attacked by tissue macrophages, may follow more gene expression adaptations to enhance their resistance against stress/therapy. (A = key "adaptation" steps that may lead to a highly resistant phenotype).

laboratory and References 59 and 60). Moreover, the overload of NO is able to stimulate the activation of Nrf-2, a transcription factor that encodes protective antioxidant and detoxification genes, including those governing the GSH synthesis and GSTs [61]. As well as RSNO, GSNO generally has a longer lifetime than NO and it has been considered as a more persistent or buffered pool of NO that can be released when or where it is required for signaling [62]. Therefore, the decay of GSNO to release NO is performed by the intervention of an electron donor, particularly transition metal ions such as Cu^+. Also protein thiols such as that present in thioredoxin can donate an electron to release NO and a thiolate anion. Alternatively, RSNO/ GSNO by reaction with a thiolate group could displace the nitroxyl anion (NO^-), leaving a disulfide and NO_2, which is unstable and rapidly decays by a number of pathways, including reaction with O_2 to form $ONOO_2$ [56, 63]. RSNO/GSNO is known to arise in vivo, for example, after prolonged exposure to NO or when endogenous NO synthesis is stimulated [64–67]. In addition to acting as an NO store, the formation of RSNO on proteins may alter their function and is thought to be a significant posttranslational modification for reversibly regulating proteins, akin to phosphorylation [65, 68, 69].

Protein S-glutathionylation is an important posttranslation modification, providing protection of protein cysteines from irreversible oxidation and, at the same time, serving to transduce a redox signal. The process is observed either under massive increase of radical species or under physiological ROS flux. Actin, Ras, and the protein tyrosine phosphatases (PTPs) are the most established examples of proteins that underwent reversible process of S-glutathionylation during cell signaling [70–73]. The process of S-glutathionylation may proceed spontaneously by thiol-disulfide exchange. However, for the majority of proteins these reactions could occur only under conditions of a ratio of GSH to GSSG that are not physiological (i.e., 1 : 1). There is only the case of the nuclear transcription factor c-Jun, which due to an unusual redox potential could react with GSSG at a relatively high ratio of GSH to GSSG = 13 [74]. Therefore, likely mechanisms of protein glutathionylation within the cells involves reaction of the "critical cysteine" on protein or GSH with a corresponding oxidized derivative such as S-nitrosyl (S-NO), sulfenic acid (S-OH), thiyl radical (S•). Protein-sulfenic and glutathione sulfenic acids result from reaction with endogenously produced ROS or RNS but usually these species are rapidly transformed in prot-SSG or GSSG as more stable derivatives (Fig. 10.3). Evidence that a sulfenic acid intermediate is formed during redox regulation exists for c-Jun, Fos, nuclear factor 1, nuclear factor κB (NF-κB), GAPDH, and PTPs. The nitrosylation process is responsible for the formation of prot-SNO and GSNO under a variety of physiological and pathological conditions. Moreover, GSNO has an additional role to promote the formation of prot-SSG in vivo [37, 75, 76]. The thiyl radical could also be produced inside the cells under oxidative stress or redox signaling and these species can also give rise to prot-SSG [77, 78]. Currently, no enzyme catalysis has been involved in the process of glutathionylation, although potential examples are reported, including the π isoforms of GSTs and human glutaredoxin [79, 80].

On the contrary, the process of deglutathionylation is mediated by enzymes: the most thoroughly characterized is that of glutaredoxin (Grx). The cytosolic mammalian

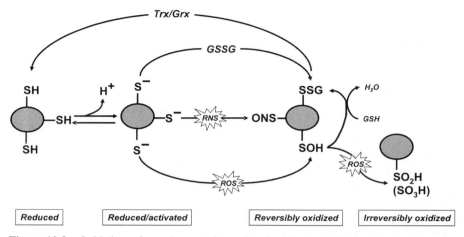

Figure 10.3 Oxidation of reactive cysteines. At physiological pH, reactive cysteines on protein surface (−SH) are normally present under thiolate form (−S⁻) and inclined to undergo S-nytrosylation (−SNO), by the reaction with nitric oxide and its derived reactive species (RNS); or S-hydroxylation (−SOH), by the reaction with reactive oxygen species (ROS); or S-glutathionylation (−SSG), directly by the reaction with GSSG. The occurrence of one modification with respect to the others relies on different characteristics, such as the steric hindrance, the surrounding charge as well as the concentration/reactivity of oxidants. The sulfenic derivative (−SOH) can be transformed in a mixed disulfide (−SSG), in the presence of GSH, or further oxidized to sulfinic (−SO₂H) or sulfonic (−SO₃H) that represent irreversibly oxidized derivatives. The reduction of the glutathionylate-derivative of cysteine is catalyzed by glutaredoxin (Grx) or thioredoxin (Trx).

form, Grx1, operates via a nucleophilic ping-pong mechanism and is highly specific for glutathionylated proteins with respect to other mixed disulfides, regulating diverse intracellular signaling pathways. Recently, other enzymes have been reported to exhibit deglutathionylating activity, but their contribution to intracellular protein deglutathionylation is uncertain. The importance of Grx1 in redox signaling under physiological and pathological states is supported by cellular studies implicating regulation by Grx1 in several pathways such as mitogenesis [81], protein synthesis [82], cytoskeletal organization [83], Ca^{2+} homeostasis [84], and cell outcome [85]. These pathways were modulated through the process of deglutathionylation of PTP1B, Ras, actin, SERCA, and IκB kinase, respectively. Recently, a second form of Grx (Grx2) was discovered, which exhibits deglutathionylation activity for peptides and proteins but with a catalytic activity 10-fold lower with respect to Grx1. The intracellular role of Grx2 is still uncertain; the enzyme is present in the mitochondrial matrix where it could favor the deglutathionylation of Complex I [86]. In overexpression and knockdown experiments Grx2 was demonstrated to protect cells from oxidant-induced death [87, 88]. Moreover, several isoforms of GST have been reported to catalyse protein deglutathionylation in in vitro systems, but the involvement of this process in vivo is not yet demonstrated [89, 90].

10.3 APOPTOSIS: A PROGRAMMED MODE TO DIE

Apoptosis is a morphologically distinct form of cell death that is designed to rapidly remove unwanted and potentially dangerous cells. During development, apoptosis plays a key role in removing surplus cells of the developing embryo. In addition, the inappropriate regulation of apoptosis is associated with a variety of diseases, including cancer, AIDS, neurodegenerative diseases, and ischemic stroke [91]. The existence of a cell-suicide program was originally proposed on the basis of the typical and common morphological changes characterizing apoptotic cell (plasma membrane blebs, cell shrinkage, chromatin condensation, protein aggregates, and apoptotic body formation). From these studies emerged the importance of an unusual class of proteases, termed caspases (cysteine proteases that specifically cleave at an aspartate residue) [92]. Caspases function in apoptosis and/or cytokine processing. Among the 14 different classes that have been discovered so far, caspase-3, -6, and -7 (*executioners*) are directly involved in proteolysis of cellular macromolecules leading to cell death, whereas caspase-2, -8, -9, and -10 (*initiators*) are fundamental in the commitment of apoptosis, as they activate executer caspases. The remaining classes are involved in inflammatory response. To date, at least three distinct pathways of induction of apoptosis have been characterized.

The first is that induced by T killer lymphocytes on tumoral or viral-infected cells. In this case, the apoptotic process is associated with perforin-mediated membrane alteration and granzyme B activation, which leads to direct activation of caspases [91]. The second apoptotic pathway is that mediated by the so-called "death receptors," including tumour necrosis factor (TNF), Fas (APO1/CD95), and TNF-related apoptosis inducing ligand (TRAIL) [93]. These receptors are transmembrane proteins that, upon extracellular ligand binding, are able to trimerize and to recruit adaptor proteins and caspases-8 in the intracellular domain. Pro-caspases-8 and the death effector domain of intermediate adaptor proteins form a complex at the receptor site called the death inducing signal complex (DISC), which finally leads to caspases-8 auto-cleavage and activation (Fig. 10.4).

The third pathway is the most important one since it represents the convergence point where many apoptotic stimuli (also those dependent on death receptors) get to. The apoptotic pathway activated by chemical or physical stresses such as ultraviolet and γ radiations, growth factor withdrawal, and prooxidant molecules has been defined as the "mitochondrial pathway" because these organelles are the place where well-characterized and crucial events for commitment of apoptosis occur. Particularly, cytochrome c released into the cytosol is the primary event for the recruitment of (d)ATP-bound apoptotic protease activated factor 1 (APAF1). Seven of the resulting cytochrome c/APAF1 dimers associate with numerous molecules of pro-caspase-9 to generate the so-called "apoptosome," a multimolecular complex in which pro-caspase-9 is cleaved and activated to caspase-9, which in turn leaves the apoptosome to proteolyse and activate the executioner downstream caspases [94, 95]. Cytochrome c is released from the intermembrane space into the cytosol through pores formed by specialized proteins such as Bax, a pro-apoptotic member of the Bcl-2 superfamily [96, 97]. A growing number of members have been found to belong to this class of

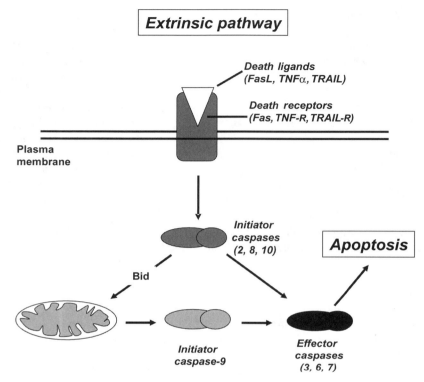

Figure 10.4   Apoptosis: the extrinsic receptor-mediated pathway. Upon binding of death ligands to their receptors, the initiator caspase-2, -8, and -10 are cleaved and activated in order to proteolyse the downstream effector cognates (caspase-3, -6, -7). These members of the caspase family finally cause the cleavage of a broad range of substrates and activate the execution phase of apoptosis. Concomitantly, caspase-8 cleaves the BH3-only member of the Bcl-2 family, Bid, which, in its truncated form (t-Bid), translocates onto the external mitochondrial membrane and induces cytochrome c release within the cytosol. This event is responsible for the occurrence of the intrinsic pathway of apoptosis, thus making Bid the trait d'union between the two routes.

proteins, the ancestor of which is Bcl-2 itself. The oncoprotein B cell lymphoma-2 (Bcl-2) is certainly the most known "guardian" of the mitochondrial integrity and inducers of cell survival; in fact, although widely present on organelle membranes, it has been characterized as the first negative regulator of apoptosis via the intrinsic mitochondrial pathway [98]. Upon apoptotic stimuli, pro-apoptotic members of the Bcl-2 superfamily, such as Bax, Bak, and Bid are overexpressed and stoichiometrically associate to Bcl-2 (or to the other anti-apoptotic equivalent Bcl-X_L) to sequester it, thus causing its selective degradation. Actually, due to their high homology of sequence, the members of this family of proteins can interact each other, and in line with this feature, the remaining pro-apoptotic members are able to create multimers that arrange in forming pores through which cytochrome c is released.

Moreover, other pro-apoptotic factors are resident in mitochondria. Smac (second mitochondria-derived activator of caspases) and its murine homolog DIABLO (direct IAP-binding protein with low pI) have been described to bind specific inhibitors of apoptotic proteins (IAPs) in order to induce programmed cell death [99]. The interactions between cytosolic (IAPs) and mitochondrial (Smac/DIABLO, cytochrome c) proteins modulate caspase activation, which in turn can induce or inhibit apoptosis (Fig. 10.5). Apoptosis-inducing factor (AIF), a flavoprotein with oxidoreductase function, and Endonuclease G (EndoG) can be released also in response to apoptotic stimuli, and upon translocation into the nucleus they can induce caspase-independent apoptotic cell death [100] (Fig. 10.5). Mitochondria are also the main source of ROS as by-product of oxygen consumption either under physiological conditions or as a secondary effect of apoptosis execution. In particular, several

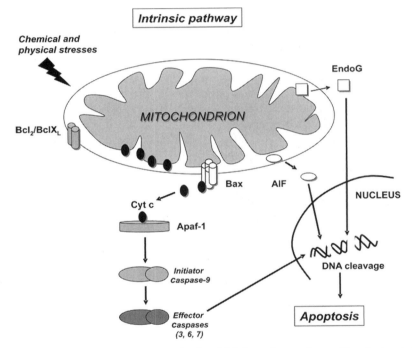

Figure 10.5 Apoptosis: the intrinsic mitochondrial-dependent pathway. Chemical and physical stresses normally result in the activation of the mitochondrial (intrinsic) pathway of apoptosis by inducing the generation of mitochondrial pores (formed by pro-apoptotic members of the Bcl-2 family, i.e., Bax and Bak) through which cytochrome c (Cyt c) is released from the intermembrane space into the cytosol. Once released cytochrome c binds to Apaf-1 and forms the apoptosome, a multi-molecular complex which activates caspase-9 and the downstream executioner caspases. Other proteins are released from mitochondria: AIF and EndoG, which translocate into the nuclear compartment and directly activate the DNAses. This event determines the cleavage of DNA and the occurrence of the so-called "caspase-independent apoptosis."

apoptotic inducers are prooxidant agents, and various proteins and apoptotic pathways are inhibited by antioxidants, as well as by overexpression of the anti-apoptotic protein Bcl-2 by way of the antioxidant pathway. Therefore, particularly concerning oxidative stress-induced apoptosis, mitochondria play a central role, since they hold the role of both source and target of oxidative conditions. This allows generalizing that the induction of apoptosis through the mitochondrial pathways represents a redox-dependent type of cell death. This assumption is in line with the huge amount of evidence indicating in ROS production and/or alteration of GSH status two phenomena always associated with apoptotic events downstream of the mitochondria.

10.4 ROLE OF GSH AND CYSTEINE IN APOPTOSIS

10.4.1 The First Evidence of the Involvement of GSH in Apoptosis

10.4.1.1 GSH: A New Character in Search of an Author Almost two decades ago, researchers began to point out that the intracellular amount of GSH could determine the capability of the cell to undergo apoptosis; in particular, we demonstrated that several pro-apoptotic stimuli induced an early extrusion of GSH from cells, leading to widespread mitochondrial damage and to cytochrome *c* release from the intermembrane space into the cytosol [101]. This event was accompanied neither by an increase of GSSG in dying cells nor its accumulation in the extracellular medium, demonstrating that GSH loss was not necessarily preceded by an operative oxidative stress. Later on, the finding that the extracellular release of GSH was mediated by specific carriers led to the understanding that this was an active process that cells carried out to decrease intracellular GSH levels and finally commit suicide [102]. In fact, we demonstrated that cells rescued by incubation with specific inhibitors of such carriers (e.g., methionine or cystathionine) remained viable even after the removal of the apoptogenic compounds and were able to replicate, indicating that a complete rescue of viability and not just a delay of apoptosis was achieved by forcing GSH to remain within the cells [102]. Moreover, the evidence that the inhibition of GSH extrusion failed to exert any anti-apoptotic activity in cells previously deprived of GSH finally highlighted that the protection against cell death did not rely on the blockage of GSH efflux per se, but was the result of the maintenance of the intracellular GSH levels further induced (Fig. 10.6).

On the basis of what had been reported, the idea that the active extrusion of GSH preceded and was responsible for irreversible morpho-functional changes of apoptosis started to take root. Nevertheless, this belief came into doubt when the decrease of GSH per se was demonstrated to be unable to trigger activation of the apoptotic machinery. In fact, in several experimental systems, cell viability was not affected when the depletion of the tripeptide was obtained by the chemical inhibition of its synthesis [103], such as upon incubation with the γ-GCS inhibitor, buthionine sulfoximine. Anyway, under these circumstances we observed a rapid and transient cytosolic release of cytochrome *c*, although it was not effective in inducing the further activation of the apoptosome and the execution of caspase-dependent cell death. In fact, the concomitant activation of heat shock (Hsp) and NF-κB systems, together

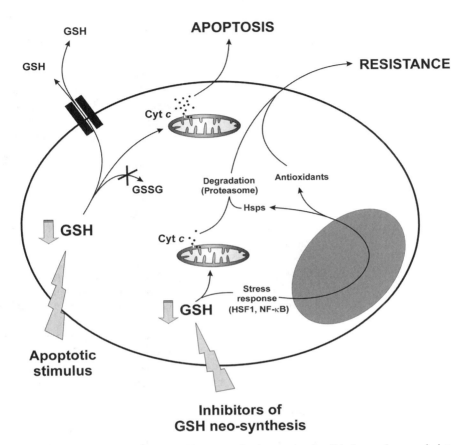

Figure 10.6   Role of GSH decrease in apoptosis. Apoptotic stimuli induce a decrease in intra-cellular GSH concentration. This phenomenon does not depend on oxidation processes (GSSG formation), but completely relies on the active extrusion of the tripeptide through specific car-riers. The resulting redox imbalance represents the key event for the release of cytochrome c within the cytosol and the following activation of apoptosis via the intrinsic pathway. Conversely, when GSH decrease is induced chemically by inhibiting its neosynthesis (i.e., by means of treatment with BSO), cytochrome c only transiently escapes from mitochondria with-out triggering any death event downstream. Actually, the resulting redox alteration activates the cellular stress response, mainly mediated by HSF1 and NF-κB. The former induces an increase of both Hsp27 and Hsp70, which mediates the degradation of cytochrome c via proteasome, whereas the latter determines the induction of several antioxidant enzymes (such as SOD2, γ-GCS). Altogether, these processes concur in enhancing anti-apoptotic response thus inducing a complete resistance to cell death.

with the following proteasome-dependent degradation of cytochrome *c* itself, led the apoptotic phenomenon to switch off rapidly without any further death event [104] (Fig. 10.6). It was, therefore, concluded that GSH levels were important for the decision between life and death but it was not the principal event underlying the mito-chondrial route of apoptosis. In particular it was reinforced that the process leading to cytochrome c release was strictly redox-dependent and not a mere consequence of mitochondrial membrane alteration. Moreover, GSH depletion was indicated as *necessary* to induce the first phases of the mitochondrial pathway but it was as much accepted that GSH decrease per se was not *sufficient* to reach the "point of no return" and trigger cell death, because the absence of any concomitant pro-apoptotic conditions allowed the cells to activate stress response and overcome the redox imbalance induced.

On the basis of the studies performed in the late 1990s, a general scheme connecting the intracellular GSH status and apoptosis seemed to be completely drawn and commonly accepted at last. Nevertheless, something was missing; in fact the role played by GSH in apoptosis became further complicated when, later on, it was demonstrated that a rapid decrease of intracellular GSH content, able to allow the cells to be completely voided of the tripeptide, protects lymphoid cells from Fas-induced apoptosis [105]. Under these circumstances, no activation of caspase-8 was in fact observed and any cleavage of apoptotic substrates was induced. Surprisingly, external GSH addition was able to turn on again the apoptotic signaling network, thus inducing the execution of cell death in a rapid and complete manner. These results made the scenario more intriguing since now the absence of GSH seemed even protective under certain conditions and the idea of the functional relationship between GSH and the events underlying apoptosis, correct once more. Apoptosis began to be considered a much more finely regulated process than before stated, being fulfilled only when the intracellular levels of GSH were within a well-defined range. Over a physiological millimolar range, the conditions were permissive for cell growth and survival, whereas under too low concentration the cell death program was completely blocked. As a result, it became clear that GSH was necessary not only for the maintenance of cell viability, but also for cell death induction.

10.4.1.2 GSH and Bcl-2: The Odd Couple

In the 1990s the biomedical research community was deeply involved in the characterization and dissection of apoptosis. From those studies it has emerged that the Bcl-2 family had a very important role in regulating cell fate under several conditions. Moreover, they began to guess that its anti-apoptotic role strictly correlated with an additional antioxidant function and, particularly, with GSH content. Initial insight into how Bcl-2 functions was elucidated by Hockenbery et al. [98] and Veis et al. [106], who demonstrated that Bcl-2 knockout mice suffered from pathologies resembling those associated with chronic oxidative stress or with defects in the antioxidant pathways, suggesting that Bcl-2 was involved in the maintenance of cellular redox potential in response to oxidative stress [98]. Moreover, other studies that examined brains from Bcl-2 knockout mice demonstrated an increased amount of oxidized proteins as well as a decrease in the total number of neural cells [107]. These studies led to investigation of the role of Bcl-2 in redox pathways in cellular models of oxidative stress, and it was demonstrated that the cytotoxic effects mediated by several compounds that generate ROS were efficiently buffered by enforced expression of Bcl-2, suggesting a model system in which the protein regulated the pathways where free radicals are generated [98, 108, 109]. Only a few years later new biological functions were ascribed to Bcl-2, due to the fact that the three-dimensional protein crystallographic structure was solved. Indeed results obtained showed a tight correlation between Bcl-2 structure and that of the pore-forming domains of bacterial toxins [110], indicating how this protein could be implicated in mitochondrial pore formation and in the release of cytochrome c in the cytosolic compartment (as previously described in Section 10.2, and References 96 and 97).

In the same years, studies from different groups indicated that increase in Bcl-2 expression, either spontaneous or isogenic, was associated with a raise in the intracellular content of GSH [111–113] and to a redistribution of the tripeptide into the cellular organelles, particularly within the nucleus [114]. The authors provided a model for Bcl-2-mediated resistance to apoptosis speculating that Bcl-2 could mediate GSH sequestration into the nucleus, thus altering the nuclear redox environment and inhibiting caspase activity. Several hypotheses have been suggested in order to explain the mechanisms underlying the direct relationship between the increase of GSH level and Bcl-2 content. Taking into account that, under steady-state conditions, GSH biosynthesis was not altered by Bcl-2 overexpression, it was hypothesized that the increased levels of the GSH was due to an inhibition of the methionine-dependent GSH efflux [115]. However, the functional correlation between GSH and Bcl-2 remained still unclear; rather, many other conflicting results were adding very quickly. For instance, experiments performed in other cell types indicated that, as previously demonstrated, the resistance to hydrogen peroxide mediated by Bcl-2 overexpression passed through a rise in GSH content, but conversely, it was also associated with a parallel increase in the expression level of γ-GCS. At the molecular level this effect was related to an increased constitutive NF-κB activation, which represents the upstream nuclear transcription factor of γ-GCS [116]. To partially solve this tangle of conflicting information, it was further reported that the impact of Bcl-2 on GSH metabolism was a cell line-dependent event [112]. Nevertheless, despite this huge amount of data, no fundamental step in the comprehension of a univocal molecular mechanism underlying the link between Bcl-2 and GSH was carried out.

On the basis of what has been reported, accumulating results strengthened the notion of the pivotal role of GSH in the occurrence of each step of the apoptotic program. However, no elucidation of the mechanisms had been provided; in fact, the molecular mechanism(s) through which GSH could modulate apoptosis even without any apparent interaction with ROS was still lacking.

10.4.2 GSH-Mediated Cell Signaling in Apoptosis: A New Perspective Based on Cysteine Reactivity

In the same years, biochemical studies on signal transduction were demonstrating the importance of a well-known redox reaction in propagating the signal throughout the cell: the redox modification of reactive cysteine residues (S-thiolation) on redox-sensitive proteins. As previously described, when a chemical environment causes a pKa decrease of a specific cysteine residue, it can undergo deprotonation. thus increasing, under thiolate form, its reactivity towards oxidant species. The steric hindrance, the surrounding charge as well as the concentration/reactivity of oxidants finally concur in determining the resulting adduct: sulfenic acid (S-OH); which can undergo further ROS-mediated oxidation to sulfinic (S-O$_2$H) and sulfonic (S-O$_3$H) derivatives; nitrosothiol (S-NO); mixed disulfide with GSH (S-SG) [117, 118]. The last adduct can result directly from the reaction between the cysteine sulfydryl group and GSSG; however, the low concentration of GSSG inside the cells, even under oxidative conditions, does not allow this reaction to proceed, if not with GSSG being in the millimolar range. Conversely, the occurrence of a GSH-mediated reduction of the hydroxyl-cysteine to form H$_2$O and the S-glutathionylated adduct is more plausible (Fig. 10.2). The principal feature of such modifications is their reversibility. Indeed, also for sulfinic acid derivative, which was previously believed to represent an irreversible form of thiol oxidation, a huge amount of data indicates the existence of an enzyme-dependent reduction back to the sulfydryl form [119]. Therefore, as consequence to what was emerging on the role of thiols in cell signaling, the functional relationship between GSH and apoptosis concomitantly changed: GSH was not only a simple measure of cell health, but also a direct mediator of the mechanisms governing life and death. Year by year, the number of proteins identified that could sense and, in turn, be regulated in their function by GSH-dependent reversible modifications on cysteine residues was growing. Among them, transcription factors; protein kinases; cytoskeleton proteins, which mediates the transduction of the signal from the cytosol within the nucleus; as well as those proteins located within mitochondria or on the plasma membrane, were found to belong to the class of proteins undergoing S-glutathionylation, and many of them were recognized to participate in the apoptotic cascade.

10.4.2.1 *Proteins Involved in Gene Transcription*   Thiol-dependent redox-modulation of protein activities was first evidenced for transcription factors in bacteria. To survive in adverse environments, bacteria have evolved different and sophisticated mechanisms in order to rapidly modulate gene transcription to counteract several insults. Moreover, the absence of a physical barrier that isolates DNA makes the intracellular medium more efficient in buffering alterations of the extracellular environment. OxyR is a well-known example of a redox-responsive prokaryotic transcription factor [120]. In particular, redox regulation of OxyR depends on the chemical status of specific cysteine residues and is responsive to H$_2$O$_2$, sulfydryl-reactive compounds (i.e., diamide) and RNS [121, 122]. Pioneering studies by Zheng et al. showed that, upon exposure to hydrogen peroxide, the activation of OxyR involves the formation of a disulfide bond between Cys-199 and Cys-208, two residues that are separated by 17 Å in the reduced—and inactive—form of the protein. The net outcome of this reaction is a change in DNA binding specificity, which occurs in a tetrameric conformation, and the recruitment of RNA polymerase [123]. Recent findings from the Stamler laboratory demonstrate that, besides this "on-off" modulation, a finer regulation for OxyR binding to DNA can occur [124]. Only one thiol residue (Cys-199) is critical for OxyR activity and this residue can be differently oxidized depending on the extent of redox unbalance and the nature of the oxidizing molecules. The results obtained show that the redox stimuli differently affect its DNA binding, which is dependent on cooperative effects between OxyR subunits. Therefore,

cysteine modification by *S*-nitrosylation, *S*-glutathionylation, intramolecular disulfide bond formation, or oxidation to sulfenic acid (*S*-hydroxylation) may be alternatively exploited to control gene expression [124]. OxyR is a model of *direct* and *highly inducible* regulation, being a quick response to cellular oxidative unbalance, which induces its binding to DNA in the oxidized form.

While the response of prokaryotes to oxidative stress depends essentially on the "duration" or "moment" of exposure, eukaryotes have evolved a *spatial* regulation of transcription factors activity. In multicellular organisms "environment" is also, in a wider meaning, the relationship among cell populations through specialized signaling molecules such as hormones and growth factors. In this context, oxidative stress, from being an external challenge to cell survival takes up a further role in the regulation of many physiological processes. In particular, cell death represents a necessary event for the integrity and survival of cell populations, which, once induced by environmental challenge, has to occur in a gene-programmed manner (apoptosis). Changes of intracellular redox state become an additional signaling event that, besides buffering external oxidative challenge like in bacteria and yeast, can regulate proliferation, cell cycle, and apoptosis. As a matter of fact, in multicellular eukaryotes, the activity of several transcription factors has been suggested to be modulated by redox changes of specific cysteines. Some of these redox-sensitive factors, such as p53, c-Jun/AP-1, NF-κB, and heat shock factor 1 (HSF1), are involved in the control of gene expression associated with cell cycle regulation and apoptosis. Many observations indicate that cells of different origin treated with oxidative stress-inducing agents, such as transition metals, oxyradicals, or thiol-reactive compounds, are efficiently activated for nuclear translocation [125]. On the other hand, binding of transcription factors to DNA is permitted only upon reduction. In fact, in vitro experiments demonstrated that oxidative modification of specific cysteine residues could inhibit DNA binding. In particular, it has been reported that Cys-62 of the p50 subunit of NF-κB must be in a reduced state in order to allow binding to promoter regions of its target genes [126]. Cys-269 of c-Jun, closed to the interface of AP-1 dimer, can undergo *S*-glutathionylation inhibiting AP-1 formation and DNA binding [74]. Oxidation of Cys-182 of p53 to a mixed disulfide with GSH may prevent proper helix-helix interaction within the DNA binding domain and contribute to tetramer dissociation [127]. These conclusions are supported by the evidence that the nucleus represents a very reducing compartment, in which GSH and thioredoxin (Trx) as well as redox sensitive factors such as Redox factor 1 (Ref-1), are present at high concentrations. In fact, Trx seems to translocate into the nucleus upon oxidative cell stimulation in order to modulate Ref-1, which, relying on a cysteine residue located at its N-terminal end, regulates the redox state of the above-mentioned transcription factors [128]. HSF1 is also regulated by the intracellular redox state: a prooxidant environment favors its nuclear translocation, while DNA binding is increased by the reduction of critical cysteine residues. It has been demonstrated that hydrogen peroxide upregulates Trx before HSF1 activation, indicating that Trx directly reduces HSF1 allowing its DNA binding during oxidative stress [128]. Such "double step" regulation (oxidation within the cytosol and reduction inside the nucleus) has two important consequences: (1) the nuclear compartment is sheltered from oxidative damage, which may have mutagenetic effects; and (2) gene transcription is activated only upon reversible oxidation of cysteine residues.

Another transcription factor for which a redox regulation has been recently demonstrated is Nrf2. However, differently from the other example of redox-regulated transcription factors reported above, Nrf2, although it possesses several reactive cysteines needed for DNA binding, does not respond to redox changes within the cytosol for its activation. Normally, Nrf2 is sequestered in the cytoplasm, particularly at the level of actin filaments, where it binds strongly to kelch-like ECH-associated protein 1 (Keap1), a microfilaments-associated protein [129]. Keap1 binding to Nrf2 maintains Nrf2 unable to pass the nuclear membrane and to recognize EpRE sequences. In fact, it is an oxidative stress-activated anti-apoptotic transcription factor that, in response to ROS production or alteration in GSH/GSSG ratio induces transcription of genes for antioxidant defense and detoxification. Keap1 represents the real redox switch for Nrf2 activation, since, upon oxidation of specific cysteines onto its surface, Keap1 changes its conformation leaving Nrf2 free to translocate into the nucleus and activate gene transcription [129, 130]. Therefore, although Nrf2 is the final effector, Keap1 represents the real inducer of antioxidant response, indicating for the Nrf2/Keap1 dimer a novel two-module redox-sensitive system. Nrf2 modulation could seem more complex with respect to a single component, such as p53 and AP-1, where the redox modification affected the transcription factor itself; however, it allows the system to be highly protected against irreversible oxidative insults. This can explain why this novel mode of signaling has been successfully exploited by redox-activated protein kinases, which mediate apoptotic response.

10.4.2.2 *Proteins Involved in Phosphorylative Cascades* Cross talk and/or sequential partnership between two different signaling mechanisms have been found to occur in some cases of cell regulation. Trx/ASK1 was the first system identified by Saitoh and coworkers where a redox switch resulted in a phosphorylative process [131]. Apoptosis signal-regulating kinase (ASK1) belongs to the stress-activated protein kinases (SAPK) family that regulates the activation of different mitogen activated protein (MAP) kinase kinases (MKK). ASK1 has been suggested to activate p38- and c-Jun-N-terminal kinase (JNK)-upstream kinases, MKK 3/6 and MKK 4/7, respectively [132], and can be activated by chemical and physical stress, as well as through stimulation of death receptors. Studies using the yeast two-hybrid system, led to the identification of Trx as an ASK1 interacting regulatory protein [131]. The association between Trx and ASK1 gives rise to a dimer Trx/ASK1, which inactivates the kinase activity of ASK1; moreover, this interaction was found only in nonstressed cells and seemed to be modulated by the intracellular redox state. In particular, a more oxidizing environment has been suggested to cause disulfide bridge formation on the Trx moiety, thus destabilizing the dimer. As a result, ASK1 can escape from Trx inhibition and undergo multimerization, which corresponds to the active form of the enzyme [133]. As already mentioned, Trx is a small protein implicated in a variety of cellular functions such as correct folding of proteins inside the endoplasmic reticulum, activation of T lymphocytes after the recognition of antigen presenting cells, and reduction of ribonucleotide reductase.

Trx possess two vicinal cysteines forming intra- or intermolecular disulfide bridges. The first characterization of this tightly regulated system was carried out in the presence of high concentrations of hydrogen peroxide, but later it was demonstrated that an increase in intracellular disulfide potential, in terms of mixed disulfides between GSH and protein thiols, could also induce the dissociation of Trx from ASK1 and downstream activate the phosphorylative cascade that ultimately induces transcription of several genes involved in the regulation of cell cycle and apoptosis [134].

The second system, for which a strict association between redox imbalance and phosphorylative events has been found, is represented by the GST/JNK complex [135]. JNK activity is physiologically maintained at low levels within the cell, even in the presence of high concentrations of growth factors and it seems to be inhibited in unstressed cells. Adler and coworkers purified the inhibitory component of JNK and identified it as GST [136]. They demonstrated that under resting conditions, JNK phosphorylation is inhibited by its association with GST, while under hydrogen peroxide or UV treatment, the GST/JNK complex dissociates leading to formation of GST dimer and/or multimers and phospho-activation of JNK [137]. The dissociation process seems to be highly affected by oxidative conditions able to induce a reversible dissociation between the two subunits [138].

The identification of Trx and GST proteins as modulators of ASK1 and JNK activities provides strong evidence for the mechanism through which a redox-mediated signaling event could be strictly connected to downstream processes mediated by stress kinases activation. In particular, increased disulfide potential (which corresponds to a decreased GSH : GSSG ratio) leads to the activation of protein kinases and, in some cases, to the induction of apoptosis.

Phosphorylative cascades are modulated by both protein kinases, which turn on the signal in order to be propagated, and protein phosphatases, which, conversely, try to counterbalance the hyperactivation of cell response by switching off phosphorylative reactions and restoring basal conditions. The extent of intracellular phosphodiester bound-modified proteins, which normally parallels the degree of activation of certain signaling networks, is therefore the result of two opposite reactions: phosphorylation and dephosphorylation. Hitherto, we have described how redox environment and GSH status affect the levels of phospho-active proteins involved in early phases of apoptosis induction by describing the redox-dependent modes of regulation of JNK and p38. Nevertheless, other protein kinases, such as the last members of the MAP kinases family, the extracellular signal-regulated kinase 1/2 (ERK1/2), are induced by alteration in GSH redox state, by means of the inhibition of their specific protein phosphatases. In particular, we previously demonstrated that prooxidant conditions, induced by chemical depletion of GSH, affect ERK1/2-mediated proliferation of adenocarcinoma gastric cells and induce apoptosis as a downstream event of a time-prolonged G2/M blockage of the cell cycle [138]. The discovery of the occurrence of redox regulation of the activity of ERK1/2 specific MAP kinase phosphatase-3 (MPK3) by means of the modulation of Cys-293 redox state has allowed a complete understanding of the dependence of ERK1/2 on GSH : GSSG ratio alteration [139]. Although this example has been of fundamental importance in order to generalize the existence of upstream redox-sensors as early inducers of the MAP kinases-mediated apoptotic signaling, the finest defined GSH-dependent regulation of phosphatase activity remains that of PTPs. PTPs activity is highly regulated by oxidation-reduction reactions involving the cysteine residue required for catalysis [73]. PTPases share a conserved 230 amino acid domain containing the cysteine residue that catalyzes the hydrolysis of phosphate from phospho-tyrosine residues by the formation of a cysteinyl-phosphate intermediate. PTPs are specifically involved in the regulation of reversible tyrosine phosphorylation in the insulin action pathway. Recently, it has been established that insulin stimulation generates a burst of intracellular hydrogen peroxide in insulin-sensitive cells, which is associated with reversible oxidative inhibition of overall cellular PTP activity, especially the PTP-1B family member [73]. Therefore, it can be concluded that oxidative alterations are able to function as positive regulators of phosphorylation-mediated apoptosis by activating protein kinases, such as JNK and ASK1, and, at the same time, by inducing a reversible loss of function of protein phosphatases (e.g., MPK3 and PTPs).

10.4.2.3 Cytoskeleton Proteins
Among proteins that have been recently indicated to be regulated in their function by GSH : GSSG ratio and undergo S-glutathionylation, actin and tubulin hold an important role, mainly regarding their contribution to growth and apoptotic signaling. Actin has been shown to possess several cysteine residues that undergo oxidation, thus forming S-glutathionylated adducts or disulfide bonds between actin monomers. These processes occur either on the globular (G) or on the filamentous (F) isoform of the protein, thus influencing actin polymerization and, in turn, affecting cell attachment to extracellular matrix [140–142]. It seems that a prominent decrease in GSH : GSSG ratio induces S-glutathionylation of actin which dissociates from myosin heavy chain (MHC) and leads to cytoskeleton reorganization [143]. Concomitantly, the formation of mixed disulfides between GSH and annexin II, a protein that mediates actin anchoring to plasma membrane, causes the loss of both the binding to cell membrane and the cell morphology. These GSH-mediated processes are fundamental for cell motility and division; however, if the GSH : GSSG ratio remains low for a long time, such as under oxidative stress, it could represent a signal for cell death induction. In fact, one of the characteristic phenotypes the cell shows during the execution phase of apoptosis is the detachment from the matrix, a phenomenon relying on alteration in actin framework homeostasis.

α- and β-tubulin represent two other redox-sensitive proteins implicated in maintenance of cell structure. In fact α- and β-tubulin contain 12 and 8 cysteine residues, respectively [144, 145]. Gupta et al. [146] recently demonstrated by a mutagenesis study using *Saccharomyces cerevisiae* that Cys-12β and Cys-354β residues play important roles in maintaining the structure and function of tubulin. Very recently it has been indicated that these residues are also the site where tubulin could be oxidized by several garlic-derived organo-sulfur compounds to form S-allyl derivatives. Such a modification has been indicated to be the crucial step for aberrant mitotic spindle formation, which, in turn, represents the key phenomenon underlying growth arrest and apoptosis induced by garlic-derived molecules in tumor cells [147]. S-glutathionylation of Cys-12β and Cys-354β has been proposed as the mechanism able to transform an irreversible (*S*-allyl) to a reversible (*S*-SG) modification, thus suggesting for it a protective role to prevent structure and function of tubulin and, in turn, microtubules network.

Other proteins involved in cyto-architecture maintenance such as plectin and Tau seem to be tightly regulated by redox modification in which GSH plays a pivotal role. Plectin interlinks intermediate filaments [148], connects them to actin and microtubule networks, and anchors them to the subplasma membrane skeleton and to the plasma membrane-cytoskeleton junctional complexes [149]. Very recently it has been demonstrated that plectin contains at least 13 cysteine residues, 5 of which at the C-terminal domain are strategic for protein function and can be redox regulated by undergoing modification both with NO and with GSH [150]. Tau is a microtubule associated protein (MAP), which has been recently strictly associated also with actin microfilaments [151]. Although no evidence for a direct redox modification in modulating its function has emerged, protein phosphatase 1 (PP1), which mediates the phosphorylation state of Tau, has been found to sense the oxidative condition [152]. As previously described for protein phosphatases, PP1 activity has been associated with the redox environment as well, being inhibited under oxidative stress conditions, such as over-production of ROS or decrease in the GSH : GSSG ratio. Since Tau phosphorylation state causes its hyperaggregation and the formation of unproteolyzed protein aggregates, it has been often linked to certain neurodegenerative syndromes (taupathies) due to the selective loss of specific neuronal populations by apoptosis.

10.4.2.4 *Mitochondrial Proteins*   As already reported protein *S*-glutathionylation is a modification both for defense against oxidative damage and for redox cell signaling. Since both processes occur in the mitochondria, *S*-glutathionylation in these bodies is of fundamental importance. Due to the higher content of protein sulfhydryls with respect to GSH, the process of protein oxidation at the mitochondrial level could represent a buffer system against ROS and, at the same time, could preserve the GSH : GSSG ratio, either under basal radical species production or under transitory bursts [58]. In fact, in the former case, ROS can directly oxidize reactive cysteine on proteins giving rise to the formation of thiyl radicals or sulfenic acid derivatives, which can be further oxidized to sulfonic or sulfinic acids by direct reaction with oxygen [68, 77]. The efficient reaction of GSH with thiyl radical or sulfenic acid forming mixed disulfides represents a strategy to avoid the formation of more oxidized thiol derivatives. GSSG produced under oxidizing conditions could also react with thiol on proteins leaving one or two GSH molecules depending on the formation of mixed or intramolecular disulfide, respectively. Mainly within mitochondria, these thiol/disulfide exchanges allow preservation of the ratio of GSH to GSSG under transient oxidative impairment. In fact, once the oxidative stress has subsided, mixed disulfides can be reduced back by GSH or enzymatically by Trx2 or Grx2 [58]. However, the occurrence of this process in in vivo systems is uncertain due to the high concentrations of protein thiols, which can directly react with ROS.

Exposure of mitochondria to oxidative stress leads to the oxidation of the mitochondrial GSH pool, which in turn causes the increase of persistently *S*-glutathionylated proteins and/or protein disulfides [153]. These redox changes, depending on the oxidative insult applied, are associated with alterations of oxidative phosphorylation and with the induction of the mitochondrial permeability transition [154, 155]. Several studies report that mitochondria exposed to low GSH : GSSG ratio decrease protein thiol content in association with the formation of intraprotein disulfides rather than GSH-mixed disulfides [84]. However, although we know little about the details of mitochondrial protein oxidation so far, several proteins have been identified to be modulated by the S-glutathionylation process. Complex I of the mitochondrial transport chain is the most deeply studied in this respect [156, 157]. It is persistently glutathionylated, under oxidative stress; however, its activity is not impaired by this process but, rather, it is affected by exhaustive prooxidant conditions in the presence of a very low GSH : GSSG ratio. It has been hypothesized that complex I is glutathionylated by Grx2 in response to slight oxidation of the mitochondrial GSH pool [158]; however, the real meaning of such oxidation is not yet identified. Recently, it has been reported that mitochondrial complex II also undergoes S-glutathionylation to address situations of oxidative stress and to regulate its enzymatic function [159]. Indeed, the major role for mitochondrial protein S-glutathionylation is to regulate the redox signal that occurs under oxidative stress, such as upon postischemic injury. Moreover, in vitro studies using isolated enzymes suggest that the glutathionylation protects the 70 kDa flavin protein of complex II from hypersensitivity to oxidative stress allowing the correct electron transfer efficiency to be maintained and avoiding electron leakage to molecular oxygen [160]. Other mitochondrial proteins have been identified as being glutathionylated: cytochrome c oxidase subunit Va in human T lymphocyte in response to diamide treatment [161], as well as subunit Vb in rat hepatocytes treated with menadione [158]. Alpha-ketoglutarate dehydrogenase is also reversibly inactivated upon oxidation of the GSH pool and, since the inactivation was preserved by Grx, it was hypothesized that the process is via S-glutathionylation [162]. There are also reports about the glutathionylation of pyruvate dehydrogenase during apoptosis in HeLa cells [163] and of aconitase during heart ischemia-reperfusion injury [164]. Nonetheless, although a growing number of publications are indicating the occurrence of S-glutathionylation processes on numerous mitochondrial-sited proteins, the physiological significance of these modifications is not clearly established.

One of the main events associated with apoptosis is the uncoupling of the mitochondrial oxidative phosphorylation that gives rise to the loss of transmembrane mitochondrial potential ($\Delta\Psi_m$), a decrease in ATP formation, and an increase in ROS production [97]. This has been often associated with the opening of mitochondrial permeability transition pore (MPTP) or megachannel [165]. MPTP is localized as a join multiprotein complex between the two mitochondrial membranes. The voltage-dependent anion channel (VDAC) and the adenine nucleotide translocator (ANT) represent the nucleus of the pore structure and are sited at the external and internal mitochondrial membranes, respectively. Both proteins have a fundamental role for cell survival: VDAC guarantees a free passage of low molecular weight compounds to the cytoplasm, whereas ANT transports ATP outside of the matrix exchanging it with cytosolic-produced ADP. Several proteins are associated with the nucleus of MPTP, but only a few have been identified; among which benzodiazepine receptor, creatin kinase, and hexokinase II are the most important [166]. The capability of cyclosporin A to inhibit MPTP opening through the binding with the mitochondrial protein cyclophilin-D has contributed to the finding of the molecular mechanism governing this phenomenon. In particular, Halestrap and coworkers proposed the formation of an intramolecular disulfide bridge in the ANT structure upon oxidative stress and suggested a putative interaction of cyclophilin-D with ANT [165]. Moreover, Chernyak and Bernardi have provided data suggesting that two distinct groups of cysteine residues are implicated in modulating the activity of MPTP [167]. One is sensitive to GSH oxidation, while the other is sensitive to the redox state of the mitochondrial matrix NAD(P)H. The latter group accounts for the well-documented stimulatory effect of the matrix NADH on MPT, perhaps through the mediation of Trx. ANT is known to have three distinct cysteine residues that show differential reactivity towards various thiol reagents and oxidizing agents. These cysteines may represent the thiol groups that regulate both cyclophilin-D binding and the inhibitory effects of ADP on the MPTP [168]. Recent data suggests that oxidative cross-linking of the two matrix facing cysteine residues on the ANT (Cys-56 and Cys-159) plays the key role in regulating the MPTP. Adenine nucleotide binding to the ANT is inhibited by Cys-159 modification while oxidation of Cys-56 increases cyclophilin-D binding to the ANT, probably at Pro-61 [15]. Moreover, the data in the literature indicates that thiol cross-linkers cause a covalent modification of ANT which, beyond any control by Bcl-2, leads to mitochondrial membrane permeabilization and cell death [169].

10.4.2.5 *Plasma Membrane-Associated Proteins*

The extracellular environment can dialogue with the intracellular compartments in a wide range of modalities. External molecules such as lipophilic hormones or estherified compounds can freely cross the plasma membrane owing to their chemical nature and act inside the cell without restrictions. On the other hand, hydrophilic molecules can enter the cell only through the action of specific channels or ATP-dependent pumps. There are also compounds that are totally membrane-impermeable but can stimulate a cell response by their binding to specific receptors that transduce the signal into the cytosol. Each molecule could then represent a specific marker of the extracellular environment and induce a stimulus to which the cell responds. Reducing or oxidizing molecules, such as Trx and hydrogen peroxide, can be present outside the cell, thus changing the extracellular redox milieu. Furthermore, hydrogen peroxide can cross the plasma membrane and enter the cell leading to changes in the intracellular redox environment. Many membrane proteins can produce hydrogen peroxide upon different stimuli. These include the NADPH oxidase expressed on neutrophil membrane, generating high levels of hydrogen peroxide as a defense mechanism in response to bacterial attack. Besides this "non-futile" generation of oxidant species, during an inflammatory response, cells produce low amounts of hydrogen peroxide at the plasma membrane level, by non-phagocyte NADPH-oxidase protein homolog, during binding of hormones to their receptors (e.g., insulin), or as a by-product of enzyme reactions, such as that catalyzed by the membrane-associated enzyme γ-glutamyl transpeptidase [170]. As a consequence of hydrogen peroxide generation, the intracellular redox environment shifts towards oxidative conditions, which is tightly associated with alteration in the GSH : GSSG ratio. It is interesting also that several death ligands, such as those belonging to the TNF superfamily, can produce hydrogen peroxide upon binding to their receptors, which in turn leads to protein *S*-glutathionylation [171] and protein-protein disulfide bond formation [136]. Taking into account that the *S*-glutathionylation process can affect either upstream protein kinases (such as SAPK, ERK1/2, JNK, and p38 [172]) or downstream transcription factors (such as AP-1 and NF-κB), the decision between life and death depends on the relative strength of the oxidative stress and on the type of cell involved.

The mechanisms by which redox-active permeable molecules alter the intracellular environment are well established; however, little data exists on the relevance of impermeable redox molecules. Up to few years ago, the sole suggested role for cysteine residues on the extracellular side of cell membrane-associated proteins regarded their structural function; hence, extracellular thiols were believed to be present only in oxidized (disulfide) form. However, results obtained in the last decade pointed out that several intrinsic membrane proteins have their exofacial sulfhydryls in the reduced form as needed residues for modulating protein function. One of the well-known examples of such regulated proteins is the glutamate (*N*-methyl-D-aspartate, NMDA) receptor, for which it has been indicated that reducing agents enhance, whereas oxidizing agents decrease, NMDA-evoked currents. Multiple cysteine residues located in different NMDA receptor subunits have been identified as molecular determinants underlying redox modulation [173]. The NMDA receptor is also regulated by NO-related species directly, not involving cyclic GMP, but the molecular mechanism of this action has heretofore not been entirely clear although an *S*-nitrosylation process has been proposed as main modulator of its activity [174, 175]. The confusion arose at least partly due to the fact that various redox forms of NO (NO$^+$, NO$^\bullet$, NO$^-$, each having an additional electron compared with the previous) have distinct mechanisms of action. Recently, a critical cysteine residue (Cys-399) on the NR2A subunit has been shown to react under physiological conditions with NO by *S*-nitrosylation (transfer of the NO$^+$ to cysteine thiol) or by reaction with NO$^-$ (nitroxyl anion) to underlie this form of modulation [175].

The idea of the presence of reactive cysteine residues on the surface of the cell membrane had been suggested also by results obtained from titration of sulfhydryls on living cell membranes, which evidenced the presence of reduced thiol groups [176, 177]. Moreover, other experiments revealed that treatment with impermeable redox molecules was able to alter the redox state of such cysteines, thus changing the intracellular redox environment without crossing the plasma membrane. In particular, experiments performed with ovary cell lines showed that oxidation of exofacial thiols resulted in a decrease of intracellular GSH concentration [178]. Conversely, the chemical inhibition of intracellular GSH neosynthesis was able to induce a decrease in extracellular amounts of reduced sulfhydryls [178].

Pioneering studies performed with isolated erythrocytes demonstrated that by adding increasing concentrations of the impermeable Ellmann's reagent to red blood cells, intracellular GSH levels decreased in a dose-dependent manner [179] due to the formation of intracellular mixed disulfides. Moreover, by adding GSH, which is impermeable to red blood cells, an increase in the intracellular GSH content previously engaged with protein thiols was obtained [180]. The mechanism underlying these phenomena was explained in terms of a thiol-disulfide exchange among cysteine residues of proteins spanning across the plasma membrane, thus indicating this process as a novel mode for transducing signals from the extracellular milieu to the intracellular environment.

Therefore, in the light of what has been described, some questions have arisen:

1. Can GSSG also affect the redox state of exofacial cysteines?
2. How much should extracellular GSSG be concentrated to mediate oxidation/thiolation of exofacial cysteines?

GSSG can be present outside the cells but it is a mild oxidant. Hence, assuming that it could affect the extracellular thiol redox state, it should be present in the millimolar range in order to produce a significant oxidation of cysteine residues. This is an extreme condition that could be reasonable only under an oxidative burst following the immune response. In fact, under these circumstances, macrophages themselves are subjected to a massive production of ROS downstream the induction of NADPH oxidase, mainly hydrogen peroxide which can freely cross cell membranes, such as those of phagosomes. This scenario allows one to assume that at least three consequent events could occur: (1) in macrophages the intracellular GSH is very rapidly oxidized to GSSG (directly or by the action of glutathione peroxidase); (2) GSSG is extruded by the cell to restore the GSH : GSSG ratio and prevent irreversible alteration of intracellular redox state; (3) the concentration of GSSG in the extracellular microenvironment surrounding activated macrophages could reach values close to the millimolar range.

Five years ago, in line with results previously obtained on purified erythrocytes, we mimicked these conditions by incubating promonocytic cells with pharmacologic doses of GSSG. Without crossing cell membranes, exogenous GSSG was able to produce a decrease of intracellular GSH concentration, together with a dramatic increase in the levels of S-glutathionylated proteins. These biochemical changes preceded the induction of apoptosis by means of the activation of the p38-mediated mitochondrial pathway [134]. The relevance of such results was that they indicated, for the first time, the oxidation of exofacial sulfydryls as the determinant process for cell death induction, suggesting a sequence of events where the oxidative stimulus was transduced within the cells by a likely thiol-disulfide exchange along a chain of cysteine residues of still unknown transmembrane proteins. Surprisingly, when the experiments were extended to other histotypes, we realized that this phenomenon was not of general application, but it relied on cell-type specific proteins; in fact, neuroblastoma and hepatoma cells, although they showed a significant amount of exofacial thiols, were completely resistant to GSSG-mediated toxicity [177]. This difference in cell sensitivity allowed hypothesizing a model in which extracellular GSSG could function as death inducer solely for macrophages, thus helping the removal of used up cells after immune response. At the same time its ineffectiveness in triggering apoptosis in surrounding tissues avoids any side effects of toxicity and protects organs from chronic oxidative conditions, which, conversely, could occur with other oxidants, such as hydrogen peroxide, directly generated by the same immune cells (Fig. 10.7).

Although they are still under investigation, putative protein targets of GSSG-mediated oxidation could be represented by the cysteine-rich TNF receptors that are particularly concentrated on the plasma membrane of immune cells. Even if interactions between redox-active molecules and these receptors are probably not as efficient as those mediated by binding of physiological effectors, the structure and the function of membrane receptors may be modified by reaction with these compounds in such a way as to start a signaling pathway. These results highlight a novel modality for the extracellular redox milieu in cell signaling and viability without the intervention of ROS. This is particularly evident in the mechanisms of signaling mediated by antigen-presenting cells (APC), specialized cells for T cell activation. In particular, we demonstrated that APC increase extracellular cysteine levels in order to stimulate the proliferation of activated T cells [181]. Under physiological conditions extracellular cysteine equivalents exist as the oxidized form, cystine, which T cells are unable to internalize; during immune response, antigen-presenting cells take up cystine and extrude cysteine into the extracellular space where it becomes available for T cells and necessary for their growth and activation [182].

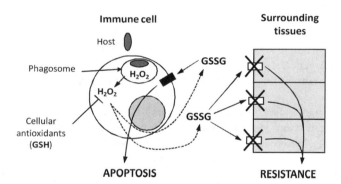

Figure 10.7 Scheme of the pro-apoptotic activity of GSSG towards immune cells. Upon of the activation of immune system by pathogens, immune cells, mainly machrophages, produce hydrogen peroxide (H_2O_2) to kill hosts. The high concentration of intracellular GSH leads machrophages to be protected by unwanted hydrogen peroxide-mediated oxidative damages. Concomitantly, new GSH is synthesized or formed by the reduction catalyzed by glutathione reductase; however, under massive oxidative bursts, a huge amount of GSSG is extruded in the surrounding environment in order to allow this protective system to be continuously operative. High extracellular concentrations of GSSG result in the selective induction of apoptosis of immune cells, by inducing signal transduction pathways through specific transmembrane proteins. This complex and still hypothetical system could represent a highly safe mechanism during immune response, since GSSG could function as death inducer solely for macrophages, thus helping the removal of used up cells after immune response. On the other hand, its ineffectiveness in triggering apoptosis in surrounding tissues, due to lack of GSSG-sensitive proteins in the extracellular compartment, avoids any side effects of toxicity and protects organs from chronic oxidative conditions, such as those occurring upon hydrogen peroxide treatment.

10.5 SULFUR AMINO ACIDS IN APOPTOSIS

Methionine, cysteine, taurine, and homocysteine are metabolically related sulfur amino acids [1]. However, methionine and cysteine may be considered to be the principal sulfur-containing amino acids because they are incorporated into proteins [2]. In particular, methionine by virtue of its high hydrophobicity is found in the interior hydrophobic core in globular proteins; in membrane-spanning protein domains and is often found to interact with the lipid bilayer. In some proteins a fraction of the methionine residues could be surface exposed thus undergoing oxidation giving raise to methionine S and R sulfoxide diastereoisomeric forms. It is believed that these oxidized methionine residues could function as endogenous antioxidants in proteins [183]. The oxidized methionine residues in proteins can be catalytically reversed by the peptide methionine sulfoxide reductase enzymes, MsrA and MsrB, respectively, allowing the recovery of the protein function. In eukaryotes, Msr are virtually localized in all cellular compartments, particularly in the cytosol, mitochondria, nuclei, and endoplasmic reticulum (ER). It is considered that the impaired activity of Msr and the subsequent accumulation of methionine sulfoxide residues are associated with oxidative stress-mediated neuronal apoptosis, age-related diseases, neurodegeneration, and shorter lifespan [184, 185]. Moreover, alterations in nutrient availability can modulate apoptosis; indeed, methionine deprivation in cultured cells may lead to the induction of cell death with the feature of apoptosis since caspases activation and DNA laddering is elicited [186]. Malignant cells fail to utilize homocysteine in place of methionine and they are dependent on exogenous methionine for growth. For this reason, methionine deficiency (also called methionine stress) has been proposed as a sensitization factor to chemotherapeutic agents alkylating DNA. Methionine stress has a wide spectrum of antiproliferative activities and has been shown to be effective against the majority of tumors. In particular, methionine deficiency always involves inhibition of cyclin-dependent kinase 1 (CDK1) and in most cases the upregulation of check-points kinases such as CDK1, p21, and p27 and commitment of apoptotic cell death via the TNFα and TRAIL pathways [187].

Together with methionine, cysteine is also highly susceptible to oxidative modification (disulfide bridges and cysteine sulfenic acids) [3], which can be reversed by dedicated enzymatic systems, including thioredoxin/thioredoxin reductase and glutaredoxin/glutathione/glutathione reductase. Also inadequate elimination of oxidized cysteines could be upstream of the processes leading to cell death by apoptosis especially in neurons, which are particularly vulnerable to oxidative stress. The role of cysteine in apoptosis is closely related to its function as a protein residue that can easily undergo oxidative modification following the reaction with ROS (S-hydroxylation), RNS (S-nitrosylation) and GSSG (S-glutathionylation). Moreover, considering the role of S-glutathionylation in apoptotic cell signaling and how cysteine is fundamental for GSH synthesis and function, its role in apoptosis cannot be separated from that played by GSH. Therefore, for an in-depth discussion of this topic, we refer to the previous sections in which it has been examined in detail (see 10.4.2).

Although not incorporated into proteins, taurine is considered to be an essential amino acid for mammals because of the relatively low abundance of cysteine sulfonic acid decarboxylase, the key enzyme responsible for its biosynthetic pathway [188]. In fact, taurine is physiologically provided not only by its uptake from external cells, but also by endogenous synthesis [3]. Particularly in the central nervous system, the taurine biosynthetic pathway essentially proceeds via three steps: (1) cysteine is converted to cysteine sulfinate, a reaction catalyzed by cysteine dioxygenase; (2) then cysteine sulfinate is converted to hypotaurine by cysteine sulfinate decarboxylase; (3) finally, hypotaurine is nonenzymatically converted to taurine (see Fig. 10.1). Taurine is a very important molecule in several essential biological processes: it represents a trophic factor in the development of the CNS, it is involved in the maintenance of the membrane structural integrity and in the regulation of calcium binding and transport; it acts as an osmolyte, neuromodulator, neurotransmitter, and neuroprotector against glutamate-induced neurotoxicity [5–7, 189]. Moreover, it has been suggested that taurine plays an antioxidant role through its ability to scavenge hypochlorous acid and ROS [190, 191]. Therefore, taurine may be an important regulator of oxidative stress and, in so doing, it may wield an antiapoptotic role. Taurine prevents high-glucose-mediated endothelial cell apoptosis by attenuating the high-glucose-mediated increase of ROS formation and elevated intracellular Ca^{2+} levels. Moreover, in endothelial cells taurine attenuates sodium arsenite and/or TNFα-induced apoptosis [192]. Taurine also has relevance in immune response; in fact it is responsible for downregulation of FasL protein expression, which was associated with decreased FasL mRNA expression and reduced NF-κB activation [193].

In view of the fact that osmotic stress, calcium overload, and oxidative stress adversely impact mitochondrial function [194], a beneficial effect on mitochondria function and an inhibitory action on mitochondrial/intrinsic-induced apoptosis has been postulated for taurine. Actually, it has been discovered that taurine loading in ischemic cardiomyocytes prevents mitochondrial apoptosis. However, taurine does not directly act on mitochondria as it is not able to inhibit collapse of transmembrane potential and release of cytochrome c, but it suppresses the formation of the Apaf-1/caspase-9 apoptosome and the interaction of caspase-9 with Apaf-1 [195]. These events are crucial in inhibiting ischemia-induced cleavage of caspase-9 and -3. More recently, it has been established that taurine also reduces caspase-8 and caspase-9 expression during brain ischemia [196]. The relevance of taurine in tissue and cell physiology is particularly evident in knockout mice for taurine transporter. These mice display several pathological features, among which the most prominent is represented by the severe and progressive retinal degeneration caused by apoptotic cell death of photoreceptors [197].

The increased level of homocysteine (hyperhomocysteinemia) has been recognized as a risk factor for a number of human diseases, including cardiovascular diseases [198] and stroke [199]. Elevated levels of homocysteine also play an important role in neural tube defects [200], dementia, and Alzheimer's disease [201]. Several potential mechanisms have been proposed to explain the molecular mechanisms underlying homocysteine toxicity; among those, increased formation of ROS is included. Indeed, homocysteine has prooxidant activity because it can undergo autooxidation, in the presence of molecular oxygen and transition metals. The products of autooxidation are homocystine, the disulfide dimer of homocysteine, and hydrogen peroxide [202].

Moreover, the generation of ROS seems to derive, also, from the homocysteine-induced activation of cyclooxygenases and lipoxygenases [203] or from its incorporation into proteins, via disulfide or amide linkages (S-homocysteinylation or N-homocysteinylation) affecting protein structure and function [204]. At the cellular level, homocysteine seems to particularly affect endothelial cell function. This specific sensitivity has been proposed to depend on the fact that human endothelial cells do not express an active form of cystathionine β-synthase and consequently cannot initiate homocysteine catabolism through the *trans*-sulfuration pathway [205]. In in vivo models of Parkinson's disease or Alzheimer's disease, where the neuronal loss is principally related to induction of apoptosis, homocysteine does not induce neurotoxicity itself but enhances the neuronal apoptosis caused by the neurotoxins administered. Homocysteine is also able to enhance excitotoxicity such as that determined by hyperstimulation of the NMDA receptor. In the nervous system, cytoplasmic calcium influx, a consequence of both excitotoxicity and oxidative stress, is associated with homocysteine exposure [206]. Calcium can both enter the mitochondria causing metabolic aberrations that induce cell death, and can enter the nucleus where it modulates gene transcription, which can also lead to neuronal cell apoptosis [207].

Probably the principal mechanisms by which homocysteine may trigger cell death by the mode of apoptosis is the occurrence of ER stress. This event has been demonstrated in cultured cells and in vivo [208, 209]. It was reported that elevated levels of intracellular homocysteine increased the expression of several ER stress-response genes, including GRP78, GRP94, and Herp [210, 211] and activation of unfolded protein response [209]. Homocysteine can also induce the expression of the pro-apoptotic GADD153 gene, which may be involved in linking ER stress to alterations in the expression of genes responsible for cell growth and proliferation [212]. The ER is the major site of intracellular calcium storage and ER stress induces loss of calcium from this compartment. Calcium is widely demonstrated to play an important role in apoptosis; indeed, increased calcium release leads to enhancement of apoptotic signal. Besides the induction of ER stress, homocysteine appears to induce calcium mobilization from the ER [209]. In conclusion, hyperhomocysteinemia appears to be associated with two independent cellular stress states: ER stress (via activation of stress-response and/or apoptotic genes) and oxidative stress.

10.6 CONCLUDING REMARKS AND RECENT PROGRESS

From the first evidence regarding the involvement of GSH in apoptosis up to date many improvements have been made, and results, which attempt to deeply dissect the mechanisms linking GSH to cell death phenomena, are added every day. In this chapter we have tried to summarize the evolution of knowledge regarding the implication of sulfur-containing molecules (amino acids, peptides, and proteins) in apoptosis by tracing the milestones of this field of research and showing how they fit together to outline a more general phenomenon. The scheme drawn clearly indicates that GSH is not the principal player, but a *weighty protagonist* of the huge network governing the decision between life and death. Such an intricate and highly complex scenario strongly depends on the redox state of the cell where GSH, sulfur amino acids, Trx, Grx, peroxiredoxins (together with the enzymes catalyzing their reduction) and the enzymatic antioxidant defense, as a whole, concur to modulate either ROS concentration, or the availability of cellular thiols, thus regulating the function of a large number of redox-sensitive proteins implicated in the induction and/or execution of apoptosis.

Many unsolved problems are now unraveling and, based on what has been emerging, the common idea is that, normally, a cascade of events is necessary in order to "channel" a definite alteration of the redox state into cell death by apoptosis. Only rarely, a single mechanism is able to completely account for the phenomenon observed; however, very recently a unique mechanism has been proposed to finally clarify the still unsolved relationship between Bcl-2 and GSH in the redox homeostasis of mitochondria and then in the induction of the intrinsic pathway of apoptosis [213]. Several hypotheses were made in the past years to explain the close association between GSH levels and Bcl-2 expression: from the alteration of mitochondrial volume induced by Bcl-2 itself [109], to a putative prooxidant action of Bcl-2, which was able to activate GSH neosynthesis [214]. Recently Zimmerman et al. demonstrated that GSH binds directly to the BH3 domain groove of Bcl-2, which is functional for the translocation of the tripeptide within the mitochondria [213]. The association of BH3-only pro-apoptotic members of the Bcl-2 family (e.g., Bid, Puma, and Noxa) with Bcl-2, by means of the same domain, could then represent a rationale for GSH decrease within the mitochondrial compartment during the induction phase of apoptosis and the correlation between GSH levels and Bcl-2 expression.

The remarkable progress accomplished in the last years allows one to assert that, even though the pathways implicated in the induction/execution of apoptosis have remained largely unaltered, many new "redox-dependent pieces" of the puzzle have been and are going to be added, thus rendering the redox signaling network upstream of cell death processes, of more general application and controlled at multiple levels.

ACKNOWLEDGMENTS

We apologize to researchers whose findings, which contribute daily to developments in the current state of knowledge in this progressing field, were not cited. This work was partially supported by grants from Ministero dell'Istruzione Università e Ricerca (MIUR), Ministero della Sanità and Fondo Investimento Ricerca di Base (FIRB).

REFERENCES

1. Brosnan, J.T., Brosnan, M.E. (2006). The sulfur-containing amino acids: An overview. *Journal of Nutrition*, *136*, 1636S–1640S.
2. Cooper, A.J.L. (1983). Biochemistry of sulfur-containing amino acids. *Annual Review of Biochemistry*, *58*, 187–222.
3. Stipanuk, M.H., Dominy, J.E., Lee, J., Coloso, R.M. (2006). Mammalian cysteine metabolism: New insights into regulation of cysteine metabolism. *Journal of Nutrition*, *136*, 1652S–1659S.

4. Kevresan, S., Kuhajada, K., Kandrac, J., Fawcett, J.P., Mikov, M. (2006). Biosynthesis of bile acids in mammalian liver. *European Journal of Drug Metabolism and Pharmacokinetics*, *31*, 145–156.

5. Hussy, N., Deleuze, C., Desarmenien, M.G., Moos, F.C. (2000). Osmotic regulation of neuronal activity: A new role for taurine and glial cells in a hypothalamic neuroendocrine structure. *Progress in Neurobiology*, *62*, 113–134.

6. Albrecht, J., Schousboe, A. (2005). Taurine interaction with neurotransmitter receptors in the CNS: An update. *Neurochemical Research*, *30*, 1615–1621.

7. Grimble, R.F. (2006). The effects of sulfur amino acid intake on immune function in humans. *Journal of Nutrition*, *136*, 1660S–1665S.

8. Finkel, T., Holbrook, N.J. (2000). Oxidants, oxidative stress and the biology of ageing. *Nature*, *408*, 239–247.

9. Filomeni, G., Rotilio, G., Ciriolo, M.R. (2002). Cell signaling and the glutathione redox system. *Biochemical Pharmacology*, *64*, 1057–1064.

10. Filomeni, G., Rotilio, G., Ciriolo, M.R. (2005). Disulfide relays and phosphorylative cascades: Partners in redox-mediated signaling pathways. *Cell Death & Differentiation*, *12*, 1555–1563.

11. Meister, A. (1995). Glutathione biosynthesis and its inhibition. *Methods in Enzymology*, *252*, 26–30.

12. Sies, H. (1999). Glutathione and its role in cellular functions. *Free Radicals in Biology and Medicine*, *27*, 916–921.

13. Cole, S.P., Deeley, R.G. (2006). Transport of glutathione conjugates by MRP1. *Trends in Pharmacological Sciences*, *27*, 438–446.

14. Cotgreave, I.A., Gerdes, R.G. (1998). Recent trends in glutathione biochemistry, glutathione-protein interactions: A molecular link between oxidative stress and cell proliferation? *Biochemical and Biophysical Research Communication*, *242*, 1–9.

15. Halestrap, A.P., Brennerb, C. (2003). The adenine nucleotide translocase: A central component of the mitochondrial permeability transition pore and key player in cell death. *Current Medicinal Chemistry*, *10*, 1507–1525.

16. Matsuzawa, A., Ichijo, H. (2005). Stress-responsive protein kinases in redox-regulated apoptosis signaling. *Antioxidants & Redox Signaling*, *7*, 472–481.

17. Griffith, O.W., Meister, A. (1985). Origin and turnover of mitochondrial glutathione. *Proceedings of the National Academic of Sciences USA*, *82*, 4668–4672.

18. Lash, L.H. (2006). Mitochondrial glutathione transport: Physiological, pathological and toxicological implications. *Chemico-Biological Interactions*, *163*, 54–67.

19. Meister, A., Anderson, M.E. (1983). Glutathione. *Annual Review of Biochemistry*, *52*, 711–760.

20. Soltaninassab, S.R., Sekhar, K.R., Meredith, M.J., Freeman, M.L. (2000). Multi-faceted regulation of γ-glutamylcysteine synthetase. *Journal of Cellular Physiology*, *182*, 163–170.

21. Seelig, G.F., Meister, A. (1985). Glutathione biosynthesis: γ-glutamylcysteine synthetase from rat kidney. *Methods in Enzymology*, *113*, 379–390.

22. Tu, Z., Anders, M.W. (1998). Identification of an important cysteine in human glutamate-cysteine ligase catalytic subunit by sited direct mutagenesis. *Biochemical Journal*, *336*, 675–680.

23. Krzywanski, D.M., Dickinson, D.A., Iles, K.E., Wigley, A.F., Franklin, C.C., Liu, R.M., Kavanagh, T.J., Forman, H.J. (2004). Variable regulation of glutamate cysteine ligase subunit proteins affects glutathione biosynthesis in response to oxidative stress. *Archives of Biochemistry and Biophysics, 423*, 116–125.

24. Chen, Y., Shertzer, H.G., Schneider, S.N., Nebert, D.W., Dalton, T.P. (2005). Glutamate cysteine ligase catalysis: Dependence on ATP and modifier subunit for regulation of tissue glutathione levels. *Journal of Biological Chemistry, 280*, 33766–33774.

25. Chang, L., Chang, C. (1994). Biochemical regulation of the activity of γ-glutamyl cysteine synthetase from rat liver and kidney by glutathione. *Biochemistry and Molecular Biology International, 32*, 697–703.

26. Sierra-Rivera, E., Summar, M.L., Dasouki, M., Krishnamani, M.R., Phillips, J.A., Freeman, M.L. (1995). Assignment of the gene (GLCLC) that encodes the heavy subunit of γ-glutamylcysteine synthetase to human chromosome 6. *Cytogenetics and Cell Genetics, 70*, 278–279.

27. Sierra-Rivera, E., Dasouki, M., Summar, M.L., Krishnamani, M.R., Meredith, M., Rao, P.N., Phillips, J.A., Freeman, M.L. (1996). Assignment of the human gene (GLCLR) that encodes the regulatory subunit of γ-glutamylcysteine synthetase to chromosome 1p21. *Cytogenetics and Cell Genetics, 72*, 252–254.

28. Dickinson, D.A., Levonen, A.L., Moellering, D.R., Arnold, E.K., Zhang, H., Darley-Usmar, V.M., Forman, H.J. (2004). Human glutamate cysteine ligase gene regulation through the electrophile response element. *Free Radicals in Biology and Medicine, 37*, 1152–1159.

29. Yang, H., Magilnick, N., Lee, C., Kalmaz, D., Ou, X., Chan, J.X., Lu, S.C. (2005). Nrf1 and Nrf2 regulate rat glutamate-cysteine ligase catalytic subunit transcription indirectly via NF-kappaB and AP-1. *Molecular and Cellular Biology, 25*, 5933–5946.

30. Griffith, O.W. (1999). Biologic and pharmacologic regulation of mammalian glutathione synthesis. *Free Radicals in Biology and Medicine, 27*, 922–935.

31. Lee, J.-I., Kang, J., Stipanuk, M.H. (2006), Differential regulation of glutamate-cysteine ligase subunit expression and increased holoenzyme formation in response to cysteine deprivation. *Biochemical Journal, 393*, 181–190.

32. Townsend, D.M., Tew, K.D., Tapiero, H. (2003). The importance of glutathione in human disease. *Biomedicine and Pharmacotherapy, 57*, 145–155.

33. D'Autreaux, B., Toledano, M.B. (2007). ROS as signaling molecules: Mechanisms that generate specificity in ROS homeostasis. *Nature Reviews in Molecular and Cellular Biology, 8*, 813–824.

34. Filomeni, G., Ciriolo, M.R. (2004). *Frontiers in Nurodegenerative Disorders and Aging: Fundamental Aspects, Clinical Perspective and New Insights.* Amsterdam: IOS Press, pp. 230–250.

35. Gallogly, M.M., Mieyal, J.J. (2007). Mechanisms of reversible protein glutathionylation in redox signaling and oxidative stress. *Current Opinion in Pharmacology, 7*, 381–391.

36. Schaffer, F.Q., Buettner, G.R. (2001). Redox environment of the cell as viewed through the redox state of the glutathione disulfide/glutathione couple. *Free Radicals in Biology and Medicine, 30*, 1191–1212.

37. Herrlich, P., Bohmer, F.D. (2000). Redox regulation of signal transduction in mammalian cells. *Biochemical Pharmacology, 59*, 35–41.

38. Pompella, A., Corti, A., Paolicchi, A., Giommarelli, C., Zumino, F. (2007). γ-glutamyltransferase, redox regulation and cancer drug resistance. *Current Opinion in Pharmacology*, *7*, 360–366.

39. Shimada, T. (2006). Xenobiotic-metabolizing enzymes involved in the activation and detoxification carcinogenic polycyclic aromatic hydrocarbons. *Drug Metabolism and Pharmacokinetics*, *21*, 257–276.

40. Zamek-Glisczynski, M.J., Hoffmster, K.A., Nezasa, K., Tallman, M.N., Brouwer, K.L. (2006). Integration of hepatic drug transporters and phase II metabolizing enzymes: Mechanisms of hepatic excretion of sulfate, glucuronide, and glutathione metabolites. *European Journal of Pharmaceutical Sciences*, *27*, 447–486.

41. Pastore, A., Federici, G., Bertini, E., Piemonte, F. (2003). Analysis of glutathione: Implication in redox and detoxification. *Clinica Chimica Acta*, *333*, 19–39.

42. Ketterer, B., Coles, B., Meyer, D.J. (1983). The role of glutathione in detoxification. *Environmental Health Perspectives*, *49*, 59–69.

43. Lo, H.W., Ali-osman, F. (2007). Genetic polymorphism and function of glutathione S-transferases in tumor drug resistance. *Current Opinion in Pharmacology*, *7*, 367–374.

44. Schmidt-Krey, I., Kanaoka, Y., Mills, D.J., Irikura, D., Haase, W., Lam, B.K., Austen, K.F., Luhlbrandt, W. (2004). Human leukotriene C4 synthase at 4.5 Å resolution in projection. *Structure*, *12*, 2009–2014.

45. Oakley, A.J. (2005). Glutathione trnsferases: New functions. *Current Opinion in Structural Biology*, *15*, 716–723.

46. Ladner, J.E., Parsons, J.F., Rife, C.L., Gilliland, G.L., Armstrong, R.N. (2004). Parallel evolutionary pathways for glutathione transferases: Structure and mechanism of the mitochondrial class kappa enzyme rGSTK1–1. *Biochemistry*, *43*, 352–361.

47. Thoren, S., Weinander, R., Saha, S., Jegerschold, C., Pettersson, P.L., Samuelsson, B., Hebert, H., Hamberg, M., Moegenstern, R., Jakobsson, P.J. (2003). Human microsomal prostaglandin E synthase-1. Purification, functional characterization, and projection structure determination. *Journal of Biological Chemistry*, *278*, 22199–22209.

48. Hebert, H., Jegerschold, C. (2007). The structure of membrane associated proteins in eicosanoid and glutathione metabolism as determined by electron crystallography. *Current Opinion in Structural Biology*, *17*, 396–404.

49. Landi, S. (2000). Mammalian class theta GST and differential susceptibility to carcinogens: A review. *Mutation Research*, *463*, 247–283.

50. Talalay, P. (2000). Chemoprotection against cancer by induction of phase 2 enzymes. *Biofactors*, *12*, 5–11.

51. Hayes, J.D., McLellen, L.I. (1999). Glutathione and glutathione-dependent enzymes reprent a co-ordinately regulated defense against oxidative stress. *Free Radicals Research*, *31*, 273–300.

52. Lei, X.G., Cheng, W.H., McClung, J.P. (2007). Metabolic regulation and function of glutathione peroxidase-1. *Annual Review of Nutrition*, *27*, 41–61.

53. Winterbourn, C.C. (2003). *Cellular Implications of Redox Signaling*. Singapore: ICP Press, pp. 175–190.

54. Kerwin, J.F., Lancaster, J.R, Feldman, P.L. (2005). Nitric oxide: A new paradigm for second messengers. *Journal Medicinal Chemistry*, *38*, 4343–4362.

55. Murphy, M.P. (1999). Nitric oxide and cell death. *Biochimica et Biophysica Acta, 1411*, 401–414.

56. Beckman, J.S., Koppenol, W.H. (1996). Nitric oxide, superoxide, and peroxynitrite: The good, the bad and the ugly. *American Journal of Physiology, 271*, C1424–C1437.

57. Wink, D.A, Ford, P.C. (1995). Nitric oxide reactions important to biological systems: A survey of some kinetics investigations. *Methods, 7*, 14–20.

58. Costa, N.J., Dahm, C.C., Hurrell, F., Taylor, E.R., Murphy, P.M. (2003). Interactions of mitochondrial thiols with nitric oxide. *Antioxidants & Redox Signaling, 5*, 291–305.

59. Moellering, D., McAndrew, J., Patel, R.P., Forman, H.J., Mulcahy, R.T., Jo, H., Darley-Usmar, V.M. (1999). The induction of GSH synthesis by nanomolar concentrations of NO in endothelial cells: A role for γ-glutamylcysteine synthetase and γ-glutamyl transpeptidase. *FEBS Letters, 448*, 292–296.

60. Moellering, D., McAndrew, J., Patel, R.P., Cornwell, T., Lincoln, T., Cao, X., Messina, J.L., Forman, H.J., Jo, H., Darley-Usmar, V.M. (1998). Nitric oxide-dependent induction of glutathione synthesis through increased expression of γ-glutamylcysteine synthetase. *Archives of Biochemistry and Biophysics, 358*, 74–82.

61. Dhakshinamoorthy, S., Porter, A.G. (2004). Nitric oxide-induced transcriptional up-regulation of protective genes by Nrf2 via the antioxidant response element counteracts apoptosis of neuroblastoma cells. *Journal of Biological Chemistry, 279*, 20096–20107.

62. Stamler, J.S., Jaraki, O., Osborne, J., Simon, D.I., Keaney, J., Vita, J., Singel, D., Valeri, C.R., Loscalzo, J. (1992). Nitric oxide circulates in mammalian plasma primarily as an *S*-nitroso adduct of serum albumin. *Proceedings of the National Academy of Sciences USA, 89*, 7674–7677.

63. Arnelle, D.R., Stamler, J.S. (1995). NO$^+$, NO, and NO$_2$ donation by *S*-nitrosothiols: Implications for regulation of physiological functions by *S*-nitrosylation and acceleration of disulfide formation. *Archives of Biochemistry and Biophysics, 318*, 279–285.

64. Gow, A.J., Chen, Q., Hess, D.T., Day, B.J., Ischiropoulos, H., Stamler, J.S. (2002). Basal and stimulated protein *S*-nitrosylation in multiple cell types and tissues. *Journal of Biological Chemistry, 277*, 9637–9640.

65. Jaffrey, S.R., Erdjument-Bromage, H., Ferris, C.D., Tempst, P., Snyder, S.H. (2001). Protein *S*-nitrosylation: A physiological signal for neuronal nitric oxide. *Nature Cell Biology, 3*, 193–197.

66. Nikitovic, D., Holmgren, A. (1996). *S*-Nitrosoglutathione is cleaved by the thioredoxin system with liberation of glutathione and redox regulating nitric oxide. *Journal of Biological Chemistry, 271*, 19180–19185.

67. Steffen, M., Sarkela, T.M., Gybina, A.A., Steele, T.W., Trasseth, N.J., Kuehl, D., Giulivi, C. (2001). Metabolism of *S*-nitrosoglutathione in intact mitochondria. *Biochemical Journal, 356*, 395–402.

68. Stamler, J.S., Hausladen, A. (1998). Oxidative modifications in nitrosative stress. *Nature Structural Biology, 5*, 247–249.

69. Stamler, J.S., Singel, D.J., Loscalzo, J. (1992). Biochemistry of nitric oxide and its redox activated forms. *Science, 258*, 1898–1902.

70. Wang, J., Boja, E.S., Tan, W., Tekle, E., Fales, H.M., English, S., Mieyal, J.J., Chock, P.B. (2001). Reversible glutathionylation regulates actin polymerization in A431 cells. *Journal of Biological Chemistry, 276*, 47763–47766.

71. Wang, J., Tekle, E., Oubrahim, H., Mieyal, J.J., Stadtman, E.R., Chock, P.B. (2003). Stable and controlled RNA interference: Investigating the physiological function of glutathionylated actin. *Proceedings of the National Academic of Sciences USA*, *100*, 5103–5106.

72. Adachi, T., Pimentel, D.R., Heibeck, T., Hou, X., Lee, Y.J., Jiang, B., Ido, Y., Cohen, R.A. (2004). S-glutathiolation of RAS mediates redox-sensitive signaling by angiotensin II in vascular smooth muscle cells. *Journal of Biological Chemistry*, *279*, 29857–29862.

73. Barret, W.C., DeGnore, J.P., Konig, S., Fales, H.M., Keng, Y.F., Zhang, Z.Y., Yim, M.B., Chock, P.B. (1999). Regulation of PTP1B via glutathionylation of the active site cysteine 215. *Biochemistry*, *38*, 6699–6705.

74. Klatt, P., Molina, E.P., De Lacoba, M.C., Padilla, C.A., Martinez-Galesteo, E., Barcena, J.A., Lamas, S. (1999). Redox regulation of c-Jun DNA binding by reversible S-glutathiolation. *FASEB Journal*, *13*, 1481–1490.

75. Akerboom, Y., Sies, H., Thomas, J.A. (1999). S-nitrosylation and S-glutathiolation of protein sulfhydryls by S-nitrosoglutathione. *Archives of Biochemistry and Biophysics*, *362*, 67–78.

76. Hill, B.G., Bhatnagar, A. (2007). Role of glutathiolation in preservation, restoration and regulation of protein function. *IUBMB Life*, *59*, 21–26.

77. Karoui, H., Hogg, N., Frejaville, C., Tordo, P., Kalyaraman, B. (1996). Characterization of sulfur-centered radical intermediates formed during the oxidation of thiols and sulfite by peroxynitrite. ESR-spin trapping and oxygen uptake studies. *Journal of Biological Chemistry*, *271*, 6000–6009.

78. Kwak, H.S., Yim, H.S., Chick, P.B., Yim, M.B. (1995). Endogenous intracellular glutathionyl radicals are generated in neuroblastoma cells under hydrogen peroxide oxidative stress. *Proceedings of the National Academic of Sciences USA*, *92*, 4582–4586.

79. Tew, K.D. (2007). Redox in redux: Emergent roles for glutathione S-transferase P (GSTP) in regulation of cell signaling and S-glutathionylation. *Biochemical Pharmacology*, *73*, 1257–1269.

80. Qanungo, S., Starke, D.W., Pal, H.V., Mieyal, J.J., Nieminen, A.L. (2007). Glutathione supplementation potentiates hypoxic apoptosis by S-glutathionylation of p65-NFkappaB. *Journal of Biological Chemistry*, *282*, 18427–18436.

81. Barret, W.C., DeGnore, J.P., Keng, Y.F., Zhang, Z.Y., Yim, M.B., Chock, P.B. (1999). Roles of superoxide radical anion in signal transduction mediated by reversible regulation of protein-tyrosine phosphatase 1B. *Journal of Biological Chemistry*, *274*, 34543–34546.

82. Adachi, T., Weisbrod, R.M., Pimentel, D.R., Ying, J., Sharov, V.S., Shoneich, C., Cohen, R.A. (2004). S-glutathiolation by peroxinitrite activates SERCA during arterial relaxation by nitric oxide. *Nature Medicine*, *10*, 1200–1207.

83. Reynaert, N.L., van der Vliet, A., Guala, A.S., McGovern, T., Hristova, M., Pantano, C., Heinz, N.H., Heim, J., Ho, Y.S., Matthews, D.E., Wouters, E.F., Janssen-Heininger, Y.M. (2006). Dynamic redox control of NF-kappaB through glutaredoxin-regulated S-glutathionylation of inhibitory kappaB kinase beta. *Proceedings of the National Academic of Sciences USA*, *103*, 13086–13091.

84. Beer, S.M., Taylor, E.R., Brown, S.E., Dahm, C.C., Costa, N.J., Runswich, M.J., Murphy, M.P. (2004). Glutaredoxin 2 catalyzes the reversible oxidation and glutathionylation of mitochondrial membrane thiol proteins: Implications for mitochondrial redox regulation and antioxidant defense. *Journal of Biological Chemistry*, *279*, 47939–47951.

85. Enoksson, M., Fernandes, A.P., Prast, S., Lillig, C.H., Holmgren, A., Orrenius, S. (2005). Overexpression of glutaredoxin 2 attenuates apoptosis by preventing cytochrome c release. *Biochemical and Biophysycal Research Communication, 327,* 774–779.

86. Fernando, M.R., Lechner, J.M., Löfgren, S., Gladyshev, V.N., Lou, M.F. (2006). Mitochondrial thioltransferase (glutaredoxin 2) has GSH-dependent and thioredoxin reductase-dependent peroxidase activities in vitro and in lens epithelial cells. *FASEB Journal, 20,* 2645–2647.

87. Lillig, C.H., Lönn, M.E., Enoksson, M., Fernandes, A.P., Holmgren, A. (2004). Short interfering RNA-mediated silencing of glutaredoxin 2 increases the sensitivity of HeLa cells toward doxorubicin and phenylarsine oxide. *Proceedings of the National Academic of Sciences USA, 101,* 13227–13232.

88. Garcerá, A., Barreto, L., Piedrafita, L., Tamarit, J., Herrero, E. (2006). Saccharomyces cerevisiae cells have three omega class glutathione S-transferases acting as 1-Cys thiol transferases. *Biochemical Journal, 398,* 187–196.

89. Raghavachari, N., Qiao, F., Lou, M.F. (1999). Does glutathione-S-transferase dethiolate lens protein-thiol mixed disulfides? A comparative study with thioltransferase. *Experimental Eye Research, 68,* 715–724.

90. Dal Monte, M., Cecconi, I., Buono, F., Vilardo, P.G., Del Corso, A., Mura, U. (1998). Thioltransferase activity of bovine lens glutathione S-transferase. *Biochemical Journal, 334,* 57–62.

91. Strasser, A., O'Connor, L., Dixit, V.M. (2000). Apoptosis signaling. *Annual Review of Biochemistry, 69,* 217–245.

92. Thornberry, N.A., Lazebnik, Y. (1998). Caspases: Enemies within. *Science, 281,* 1312–1316.

93. Chen, M., Wang, J. (2002). Initiator caspases in apoptosis signaling pathways. *Apoptosis, 7,* 313–319.

94. Cain, K., Bratton, S.B., Cohen, G.M. (2002). The Apaf-1 apoptosome: A large caspase-activating complex. *Biochimie, 84,* 203–214.

95. Adrain, C., Martin, S.J. (2001). The mitochondrial apoptosome: A killer unleashed by the cytochrome seas. *Trends in Biochemical Sciences, 26,* 390–397.

96. Mattson, M.P., Kroemer, G. (2003). Mitochondria in cell death: Novel targets for neuroprotection and cardioprotection. *Trends in Molecular Medicine, 9,* 196–205.

97. Martinou, J.C., Green, D.R. (2001). Breaking the mitochondrial barrier. *Nature Reviews in Molecular and Cellular Biology, 2,* 63–67.

98. Hockenbery, D.M., Oltvai, Z.N., Yin, X.M., Milliman, C.L., Korsmeyer, S.J. (1993). Bcl-2 functions in an antioxidant pathway to prevent apoptosis. *Cell, 75,* 241–251.

99. Van Gurp, M., Festjens, N., Van Loo, G., Saelens, X., Vandenabeele, P. (2003). Mitochondrial intermembrane proteins in cell death. *Biochemical and Biophysical Research Communication, 304,* 487–497.

100. Penninger, J.M., Kroemer, G. (2003). Mitochondria, AIF and caspases: Rivaling for cell death execution. *Nature Cell Biology, 5,* 97–99.

101. Ghibelli, L., Coppola, S., Rotilio, G., Lafavia, E., Maresca, V., Ciriolo, M.R. (1995). Non-oxidative loss of glutathione in apoptosis via GSH extrusion. *Biochemical and Biophysical Research Communication, 216,* 313–320.

102. Ghibelli, L., Fanelli, C., Rotilio, G., Lafavia, E., Coppola, S., Colussi, C., Civitareale, P., Ciriolo, M.R. (1998). Rescue of cells from apoptosis by inhibition of active GSH extrusion. *FASEB Journal, 12,* 479–486.

103. Ghibelli, L., Coppola, S., Fanelli, C., Rotilio, G., Civitareale, P., Scovassi, A.I., Ciriolo, M.R. (1999). Glutathione depletion causes cytochrome c release even in the absence of cell commitment to apoptosis. *FASEB Journal*, *13*, 2031–2036.

104. Filomeni, G., Aquilano, K., Rotilio, G., Ciriolo, M.R. (2005). Antiapoptotic response to induced GSH depletion: Involvement of heat shock proteins and NF-kappaB activation. *Antioxidants & Redox Signaling*, *7*, 446–455.

105. Hentze, H., Schmitz, I., Latta, M., Krueger, A., Krammer, P.H., Wendel, A. (2002). Glutathione dependence of caspase-8 activation at the death-inducing signaling complex. *Journal of Biological Chemistry*, *277*, 5588–5595.

106. Veis, D.J., Sorenson, C.M., Shutter, J.R., Korsmeyer, S.J. (1993). Bcl-2 deficient mice demonstrate fulminant lymphoid apoptosis, polycystic kidneys, and hypopigmented hair. *Cell*, *75*, 229–240.

107. Hochman, A., Sternin, H., Gorodin, S., Korsmeyer, S.J., Ziv, I., Melamed, E., Offen, D. (1998). Enhanced oxidative stress and altered antioxidants in brains of Bcl-2-deficient mice. *Journal of Neurochemistry*, *71*, 741–748.

108. Fabisiak, J.P., Kagan, V.E., Ritov, V.B., Johnson, D.E., Lazo, J.S. (1997). Bcl-2 inhibits selective oxidation and externalization of phosphatidylserine during paraquat-induced apoptosis. *American Journal of Physiology. Cell Physiology*, *272*, C675–C684.

109. Kowaltowski, A.J., Fiskum, G. (2005). Redox mechanisms of cytoprotection by Bcl-2. *Antioxidants and Redox Signaling*, *7*, 508–514.

110. Muchmore, S.W., Sattler, M., Liang, H., Meadows, R.P., Harlan, J.E., Yoon, H.S., Nettesheim, D., Chang, B.S., Thompson, C.B., Wong, S.L., Ng, S.L., Fesik, S.W. (1996). X-ray and NMR structure of the human Bcl-xL, an inhibitor of programmed cell death. *Nature*, *381*, 335–341.

111. Lee, M., Hyun, D.H., Marshall, K.A., Ellerby, L.M., Bredesen, D.E., Jenner, P., Halliwell, B. (2001). Effect of overexpression of BCL-2 on cellular oxidative damage, nitric oxide production, antioxidant defenses, and the proteasome. *Free Radicals in Biology and Medicine*, *31*, 1550–1559.

112. Schor, N.F., Rudin, C.M., Hartman, A.R., Thompson, C.B., Taurina, Y.Y., Kagan, V.E. (2000). Cell line dependence of Bcl-2-induced alteration of glutathione handling. *Oncogene*, *19*, 472–476.

113. Voehringer, D.W., McConkey, D.J., McDonnell, T.J., Brisbay, S., Meyn, R.E. (1998). Bcl-2 expression causes redistribution of glutathione to the nucleus. *Proceedings of the National Academic of Sciences USA*, *95*, 2956–2960.

114. Nencioni, L., Iuvara, A., Aquilano, K., Ciriolo, M.R., Cozzolino, F., Rotilio, G., Garaci, E., Palamara, A.T. (2003). Influenza A virus replication is dependent on an antioxidant pathway that involves GSH and Bcl-2. *FASEB Journal*, *17*, 758–760.

115. Meredith, M.J., Cusick, C.L., Soltaninassab, S., Sekhar, K.S., Lu, S., Freeman, M.L. (1998). Expression of Bcl-2 increases intracellular glutathione by inhibiting methionine-dependent GSH efflux. *Biochemical and Biophysical Research Communication*, *248*, 458–463.

116. Jang, J.H., Surh, Y.J. (2004). Bcl-2 attenuation of oxidative cell death is associated with up-regulation of γ-glutamylcysteine ligase via constitutive NF-κB activation. *Journal of Biological Chemistry*, *279*, 38779–38786.

117. Finkel, T. (2000). Redox-dependent signal transduction. *FEBS Letters*, *476*, 52–54.

118. Barford, D. (2004). The role of cysteine residues as redox-sensitive regulatory switches. *Current Opinion in Structural Biology*, *14*, 679–686.

119. Rhee, S.G., Kang, S.W., Jeong, W., Chang, T.S., Yang, K.S., Woo, H.A. (2005). Intracellular messenger function of hydrogen peroxide and its regulation by peroxiredoxins. *Current Opinion in Cellular Biology*, *17*, 183–189.

120. Helmann, J.D. (2002). OxyR: A molecular code for redox sensing? *Science STKE*, *5*, PE46.

121. Paget, M.S., Buttner, M.J. (2003). Thiol-based regulatory switches. *Annual Review of Genetics*, *37*, 91–121.

122. Georgiou, G. (2002). How to flip the (redox) switch. *Cell*, *111*, 607–610.

123. Zheng, M., Aslund, F., Storz, G. (1998). Activation of the OxyR transcription factor by reversible disulfide bond formation. *Science*, *279*, 1718–1721.

124. Kim, S.O., Merchant, K., Nudelman, R., Beyer, W.F., Jr., Keng, T., DeAngelo, J., Hausladen, A. Stamler, J.S. (2002). OxyR: A molecular code for redox-related signaling. *Cell*, *109*, 383–396.

125. Marshall, H.E., Merchant, K., Stamler, J.S. (2000). Nitrosation and oxidation in the regulation of gene expression. *FASEB Journal*, *14*, 1889–1900.

126. Pineda-Molina, E., Klatt, P., Vazquez, J., Marina, A., Garcia de Lacoba, M., Perez-Sala, D., Lamas, S. (2001). Glutathionylation of the p50 subunit of NF-kappaB: A mechanism for redox-induced inhibition of DNA binding. *Biochemistry*, *40*, 14134–14142.

127. Sun, X.Z., Vinci, C., Makmura, L., Han, S., Tran, D., Nguyen, J., Hamann, M., Grazziani, S., Sheppard, S., Gutova, M., Zhou, F., Thomas, J., Momand, J. (2003). Formation of disulfide bond in p53 correlates with inhibition of DNA binding and tetramerization. *Antioxidants & Redox Signaling*, *5*, 655–665.

128. Jacquier-Sarlin, M.R., Polla, B. (1996). Dual regulation of heat shock transcription factor (HSF) activation and DNA-binding activity by H_2O_2: Role of thioredoxin. *Biochemical Journal*, *318*, 187–193.

129. Itoh, K., Tong, K.I., Yamamoto, M. (2004). Molecular mechanism activating Nrf2-Keap1 pathway in regulation of adaptive response to electrophiles. *Free Radicals in Biology and Medicine*, *36*, 1208–1213.

130. Nguyen, T., Yang, C.S., Pickett, C.B. (2004). The pathways and molecular mechanisms regulating Nrf2 activation in response to chemical stress. *Free Radicals in Biology and Medicine*, *37*, 433–441.

131. Saitoh, M., Nishitoh, H., Fujii, M., Takeda, K., Tobiume, K., Sawada, Y., Kawabata, M., Miyazono, K., Ichijo, H. (1998). Mammalian thioredoxin is a direct inhibitor of apoptosis signal-regulating kinase (ASK) 1. *EMBO Journal*, *17*, 2596–2606.

132. Ichijo, H., Nishida, E., Irie, K., ten Dijke, P., Saitoh, M., Moriguchi, T., Takagi, M., Matsumoto, K., Miyazono, K., Gotoh, Y. (1997). Induction of apoptosis by ASK1, a mammalian MAPKKK that activates SAPK/JNK and p38 signaling pathways. *Science*, *5296*, 90–94.

133. Liu, Y., Min, W. (2002). Thioredoxin promotes ASK1 ubiquitination and degradation to inhibit ASK1-mediated apoptosis in a redox activity-independent manner. *Circulation Research*, *90*, 1259–1266.

134. Filomeni, G., Rotilio, G., Ciriolo, M.R. (2003). Glutathione disulfide induces apoptosis in U937 cells by a redox-mediated p38 MAP kinase pathway. *FASEB Journal*, *17*, 64–66.

135. Adler, V., Yin, Z., Fuchs, S.Y., Benezra, M., Rosario, L., Tew, K.D., Pincus, M.R., Sardana, M., Henderson, C.J., Wolf, C.R., Davis, R.J., Ronai, Z. (1999). Regulation of JNK signaling by GSTp. *EMBO Journal*, *18*, 1321–1334.

136. Adler, V., Yin, Z., Tew, K.D., Ronai, Z. (1999). Role of redox potential and reactive oxygen species in stress signaling. *Oncogene, 18*, 6104–6111.

137. Filomeni, G., Aquilano, K., Rotilio, G., Ciriolo, M.R. (2003). Reactive oxygen species-dependent c-Jun NH2-terminal kinase/c-Jun signaling cascade mediates neuroblastoma cell death induced by diallyl disulfide. *Cancer Research, 63*, 5940–5949.

138. Filomeni, G., Aquilano, K., Rotilio, G., Ciriolo, M.R. (2005). Glutathione-related systems and modulation of extracellular signal-regulated kinases are involved in the resistance of AGS adenocarcinoma gastric cells to diallyl disulfide-induced apoptosis. *Cancer Research, 65*, 11735–11742.

139. Levinthal, D.J., Defranco, D.B. (2005). Reversible oxidation of ERK-directed protein phosphatases drives oxidative toxicity in neurons. *Journal of Biological Chemistry, 280*, 5875–5883.

140. Dalle-Donne, I., Rossi, R., Giustarini, D., Colombo, R., Milzani, A. (2007). S-glutathionylation in protein redox regulation. *Free Radicals in Biology and Medicine, 43*, 883–898.

141. Dalle-Donne, I., Rossi, R., Milzani, A., Di Simplicio, P., Colombo, R. (2001). The actin cytoskeleton response to oxidants: From small heat shock protein phosphorylation to changes in the redox state of actin itself. *Free Radicals in Biology and Medicine, 31*, 1624–1632.

142. Dalle-Donne, I., Giustarini, D., Rossi, R., Colombo, R., Milzani, A. (2003). Reversible *S*-glutathionylation of Cys 374 regulates actin filament formation by inducing structural changes in the actin molecule. *Free Radicals in Biology and Medicine, 34*, 23–32.

143. Fiaschi, T., Cozzi, G., Raugei, G., Formigli, L., Ramponi, G., Chiarugi, P. (2006). Redox regulation of β-actin during integrin-mediated cell adhesion. *Journal of Biological Chemistry, 281*, 22983–22991.

144. Ponstingl, H., Krauhs, E., Little, M., Kempf, T. (1981). Complete amino acid sequence of alpha-tubulin from porcine brain. *Proceedings of the National Academy of Sciences USA, 78*, 2757–2761.

145. Krauhs, E., Little, M., Kempf, T., Hofer-Warbinek, R., Ade, W., Ponstingl, H. (1981). Complete amino acid sequence of beta-tubulin from porcine brain. *Proceedings of the National Academy of Sciences USA, 78*, 4156–4160.

146. Gupta, M.L., Jr., Bode, C.J., Dougherty, C.A., Marquez, R.T., Himes, R.H. (2001). Mutagenesis of beta-tubulin cysteine residues in Saccharomyces cerevisiae: Mutation of cysteine 354 results in cold-stable microtubules. *Cell Motility and the Cytoskeleton, 49*, 67–77.

147. Hosono, T., Fukao, T., Ogihara, J., Ito, Y., Shiba, H., Seki, T., Ariga, T. (2005). Diallyl trisulfide suppresses the proliferation and induces apoptosis of human colon cancer cells through oxidative modification of beta-tubulin. *Journal of Biological Chemistry, 280*, 41487–41493.

148. Osmanagic-Myers, S., Wiche, G. (2004). Plectin-RACK1 (receptor for activated C kinase 1) scaffolding: A novel mechanism to regulate protein kinase C activity. *Journal of Biological Chemistry, 279*, 18701–18710.

149. Wiche, G. (1998). Role of plectin in cytoskeleton organization and dynamics. *Journal of Cell Sciences, 111*, 2477–2486.

150. Spurny, R., Abdoulrahman, K., Janda, L., Rünzler, D., Köhler, G., Castañón, M.J., Wiche, G. (2007). Oxidation and nitrosylation of cysteines proximal to the intermediate filament

(IF)-binding site of plectin: Effects on structure and vimentin binding and involvement in IF collapse. *Journal of Biological Chemistry, 282*, 8175–8187.

151. Fulga, T.A., Elson-Schwab, I., Khurana, V., Steinhilb, M.L., Spires, T.L., Hyman, B.T., Feany, M.B. (2007). Abnormal bundling and accumulation of F-actin mediates tau-induced neuronal degeneration in vivo. *Nature Cell Biology, 9*, 139–148.

152. Zambrano, C.A., Egaña, J.T., Núñez, M.T., Maccioni, R.B., González-Billault, C. (2004). Oxidative stress promotes tau dephosphorylation in neuronal cells: The roles of cdk5 and PP1. *Free Radicals in Biology and Medicine, 36*, 1393–1402.

153. Hurd, T.R., Costa, N.J., Dahm, C.C., Beer, S.M., Brown, S.E., Filipovska, A., Murphy, M.P. (2005). Glutathionylation of mitochondrial proteins. *Antioxidants and Redox Signaling, 7*, 999–1010.

154. Fagian, M.M., Pereira-da Silva, L., Martins, I.S., Vercesi, A.E. (1990). Membrane protein thiol cross-linking associated with the permeabilization of the inner mitochondrial membrane by Ca^{2+} plus prooxidants. *Journal of Biological Chemistry, 265*, 19955–19960.

155. Costantini, P., Chernyak, B.V., Petronilli, V., Bernardi, P. (1996). Modulation of the mitochondrial permeability transition pore by pyridine nucleotides and dithiol oxidation at two separate sites. *Journal of Biological Chemistry, 271*, 6746–6751.

156. Taylor, E.R., Hurrell, F., Shannon, R.J., Lin, T.K., Hirst, J., Murphy, M.P. (2003). Reversible glutathionylation of complex I increases mitochondrial superoxide formation. *Journal of Biological Chemistry, 278*, 190603–190610.

157. Chen, C.L., Zhang, L., Yeh, A., Chen, C.A., Green-Church, K.B., Zweier, J.L., Chen, Y.R. (2007). Site-specific S-glutathiolation of mitochondrial NADH ubiquinone reductase. *Biochemistry, 46*, 5754–5765.

158. Fratelli, M., Demol, H., Puype, M., Casagrande, S., Villa, P., Eberini, I., Vandekerckhove, J., Gianazza, E., Grezzi, P. (2003). Identification of proteins undergoing glutathionylation in oxidatively stressed hepatocytes and hepatoma cells. *Proteomics, 3*, 1154–1161.

159. Di Monte, D.A., Chan, P., Sandy, M.S. (1992). Glutathione in Parkinson's disease: A link between oxidative stress and mitochondrial damage? *Annals of Neurology, 32*, S112–S111.

160. Chen, Y.R., Chen, C.L., Pfeiffer, D.R., Zweier, J.L. (2007). Mitochondrial complex II in the post-ischemic heart: Oxidative injury and the role of protein *S*-glutathionylation. *Journal of Biological Chemistry, 282*, 32640–32654.

161. Fratelli, M., Demol, H., Puype, M., Casagrande, S., Eberini, I., Salmona, M., Bonetto, V., Mengozzi, M., Duffieux, F., Miclet, E., Bachi, A., Vandekerckhove, J., Gianazza, E., Grezzi, P. (2002). Identification by redox proteomics of glutathionylated proteins in oxidatively stressed human T lymphocytes. *Proceedings of the National Academy of Sciences USA, 99*, 3505–3510.

162. Nulton-Persson, A.C., Starke, D.W., Mieyal, J.J., Szweda, L.I. (2003). Reversible inactivation of alpha-ketoglutarate dehydrogenase in response to alterations in the mitochondrial glutathione status. *Biochemistry, 42*, 4235–4242.

163. Odin, J.A., Huebert, R.C., Casciola-Rosen, L., LaRusso, N.F., Rosen, A. (2001). Bcl-2-dependent oxidation of pyruvate dehydrogenase-E2, a primary biliary cirrhosis autoantigen, during apoptosis. *Journal of Clinical Investigation, 108*, 187–188.

164. Eaton, P., Byers, H.L., Leeds, N., Ward, M.A., Shattock, M.J. (2002). Detection, quantitation, purification, and identification of cardiac proteins S-thiolated during ischemia and reperfusion. *Journal of Biological Chemistry, 277*, 9806–9811.

165. Halestrap, A.P., McStay, G.P., Clarke, S.J. (2001). The permeability transition pore complex: Another view. *Biochimie*, *84*, 153–166.

166. Zamzami, N., Kroemer, G. (2001). The mitochondrion in apoptosis: How Pandora's box opens. *Nature Reviews in Molecular and Cellular Biology*, *2*, 67–71.

167. Chernyak, B.V., Bernardi, P. (1996). The mitochondrial permeability transition pore is modulated by oxidative agents through both pyridine nucleotides and glutathione at two separate sites. *European Journal of Biochemistry*, *238*, 623–630.

168. McStay, G.P., Clarke, S.J., Halestrap, A.P. (2002). Role of critical thiol groups on the matrix surface of the adenine nucleotide translocase in the mechanism of the mitochondrial permeability transition pore. *Biochemical Journal*, *367*, 541–548.

169. Belzacq, A.S., Vieira, H.L., Kroemer, G., Brenner, C. (2002). The adenine nucleotide translocator in apoptosis. *Biochimie*, *84*, 167–176.

170. Perego, P., Paolicchi, A., Tongiani, R., Pompella, A., Tonarelli, P., Carenini, N., Romanelli, S., Zunino, F. (1997). The cell-specific anti-proliferative effect of reduced glutathione is mediated by γ-glutamyl transpeptidase-dependent extracellular pro-oxidant reactions. *International Journal of Cancer*, *71*, 246–250.

171. Sullivan, D.M., Wehr, N.B., Fergusson, M.M., Levine, R.L. Finkel, T. (2000). Identification of oxidant-sensitive proteins: TNF-alpha induces protein glutathiolation. *Biochemistry*, *39*, 11121–11128.

172. Nebreda, A.R., Porrai, A. (2000). p38 MAP kinases: Beyond the stress response. *Trends in Biochemical Sciences*, *25*, 257–260.

173. Choi, Y.B., Lipton, S.A. (2000). Redox modulation of the NMDA receptor. *Cellular and Molecular Life Science*, *57*, 1535–1541.

174. Lipton, S.A., Choi, Y.B., Pan, Z.H., Lei, S.Z., Chen, H.S., Sucher, N.J., Loscalzo, J., Singel, D.J., Stamler, J.S. (1993). A redox-based mechanism for the neuroprotective and neurodestructive effects of nitric oxide and related nitroso-compounds. *Nature*, *364*, 626–632.

175. Lipton, S.A., Choi, Y.B., Takahashi, H., Zhang, D., Li, W., Godzik, A., Bankston, L.A. (2002). Cysteine regulation of protein function: As exemplified by NMDA-receptor modulation. *Trends in Neuroscience*, *25*, 474–480.

176. Laragione, T., Bonetto, V., Casoni, F., Massignan, T., Bianchi, G., Gianazza, E., Ghezzi, P. (2003). Redox regulation of surface protein thiols: Identification of integrin alpha-4 as a molecular target by using redox proteomics. *Proceedings of the National Academy of Sciences USA*, *100*, 14737–14741.

177. Filomeni, G., Aquilano, K., Civitareale, P., Rotilio, G., Ciriolo, M.R. (2005). Activation of c-Jun-N-terminal kinase is required for apoptosis triggered by glutathione disulfide in neuroblastoma cells. *Free Radicals in Biology and Medicine*, *39*, 345–354.

178. Laragione, T., Gianazza, E., Tonelli, R., Bigini, P., Mennini, T., Casoni, F., Massignan, T., Bonetto, V., Ghezzi, P. (2006). Regulation of redox-sensitive exofacial protein thiols in CHO cells. *Biological Chemistry*, *387*, 1371–1376.

179. Reglinski, J., Hoey, S., Smith, W.E., Sturrock, R.D. (1988). Cellular response to oxidative stress at sulfhydryl group receptor sites on the erythrocyte membrane *Journal of Biological Chemistry*, *263*, 12360–12366.

180. Ciriolo, M.R., Paci, M., Sette, M., De Martino, A., Bozzi, A., Rotilio, G. (1993). Transduction of reducing power across the plasma membrane by reduced glutathione.

A 1H-NMR spin-echo study of intact human erythrocytes. *European Journal of Biochemistry*, *215*, 711–718.

181. Angelini, G., Gardella, S., Ardy, M., Ciriolo, M.R., Filomeni, G., Di Trapani, G., Clarke, F., Sitia, R., Rubartelli, A. (2002). Antigen-presenting dendritic cells provide the reducing extracellular microenvironment required for T lymphocyte activation. *Proceedings of the National Academy of Sciences USA*, *99*, 1491–1496.

182. Edinger, A.L., Thompson, C.B. (2002). Antigen-presenting cells control T cell proliferation by regulating amino acid availability. *Proceedings of the National Academy of Sciences USA*, *99*, 1107–1109.

183. Levine, R.L., Moskovitz, J., Stadtman, E.R. (2000). Oxidation of methionine in proteins: Roles in antioxidant defense and cellular regulation. *IUBMB Life*, *50*, 301–307.

184. Cabreiro, F., Picot, C.R., Friguet, B., Petropoulos, I. (2006). Methionine sulfoxide reductases: Relevance to aging and protection against oxidative stress. *Annals of the New York Academy of Sciences*, *1067*, 37–44.

185. Moskovitz, J. (2005). Methionine sulfoxide reductases: Ubiquitous enzymes involved in antioxidant defense, protein regulation, and prevention of aging-associated diseases. *Biochimica et Biophysica Acta*, *1703*, 213–219.

186. Yen, C.L., Mar, M.H., Craciunescu, C.N., Edwards, L.J., Zeisel, S.H. (2002). Deficiency in methionine, tryptophan, isoleucine, or choline induces apoptosis in cultured cells. *Journal of Nutrition*, *132*, 1840–1847.

187. Kokkinakis, D.M. (2006). Methionine-stress: A pleiotropic approach in enhancing the efficacy of chemotherapy. *Cancer Letters*, *233*, 195–207.

188. Hayes, K.C. (1985). Taurine requirement in primates. *Nutrition Review*, *43*, 65–70.

189. Foos, T.M., Wu, J.Y. (2002). The role of taurine in the central nervous system and the modulation of intracellular calcium homeostasis. *Neurochemical Research*, *27*, 21–26.

190. Rasmusson, R.L., Davis, D.G., Lieberman, M. (1993). Amino acid loss during volume regulatory decrease in cultured chick heart cells. *American Journal of Physiology. Cell Physiology*, *264*, C136–C145.

191. Schaffer, S., Takahashi, K., Azuma, J. (2000). Role of osmoregulation in the actions of taurine. *Amino Acids*, *19*, 527–546.

192. Wu, Q.D., Wang, J.H., Fennessy, F., Redmond, H.P., Bouchier-Haye, D. (1999). Taurine prevents high-glucose-induced human vascular endothelial cell apoptosis. *American Journal of Physiology*, *277*, C1229–C1238.

193. Maher, S.G., Condron, C.E., Bouchier-Hayes, D.J., Toomey, D.M. (2005). Taurine attenuates CD3/interleukin-2-induced T cell apoptosis in an in vitro model of activation-induced cell death (AICD). *Clinical & Experimental Immunology*, *139*, 279–86.

194. Tsujimoto, Y., Shimizu, S. (2002). The voltage-dependent anion channel: An essential player in apoptosis. *Biochimie*, *84*, 187–193.

195. Takatani, T., Takahashi, K., Uozumi, Y., Shikata, E., Yamamoto, Y., Ito, T., Matsuda, T., Schaffer, S.W., Fujio, Y., Azuma, J. (2004). Taurine inhibits apoptosis by preventing formation of the Apaf 1/caspase-9 apoptosome. *American Journal of Physiology. Cell Physiology*, *287*, C949–C953.

196. Taranukhin, A.G., Taranukhina, E.Y., Saransaari, P., Djatchkova, I.M., Pelto-Huikko, M., Oja, S.S. (2008). Taurine reduces caspase-8 and caspase-9 expression induced by ischemia in the mouse hypothalamic nuclei. *Amino Acids*, *1*, 169–174.

197. Warskulat, U., Heller-Stilb, B., Oermann, E., Zilles, K., Haas, H., Lang, F., Häussinger, D. (2007). Phenotype of the taurine transporter knockout mouse. *Methods in Enzymology*, *428*, 439–458.

198. Anderson, J.L., Muhlestein, J.B., Horne, B.D., Carlquist, J.F., Bair, T.L., Madsen, T.E., Pearson, R.R. (2000). Plasma homocysteine predicts mortality independently of traditional risk factors and C-reactive protein in patients with angiographically defined coronary artery disease. *Circulation*, *102*, 1227–1132.

199. Yoo, J.H., Lee, S.C. (2001). Elevated levels of plasma homocyst(e)ine and asymmetric dimethylarginine in elderly patients with stroke. *Atherosclerosis*, *158*, 425–430.

200. Mills, J.L., Scott, J.M., Kirke, P.N., McPartlin, J.M., Conley, M.R., Weir, D.G., Molloy, A.M, Lee, Y.J. (1996). Homocysteine and neural tube defects. *Journal of Nutrition*, *126*, 756S–760S.

201. Seshadri, S., Beiser, A., Selhub, J., Jacques, P.F., Rosenberg, I.H., D'Agostino, R.B., Wilson, P.W., Wolf, P.A. (2002). Plasma homocysteine as a risk factor for dementia and Alzheimer's disease. *New England Journal of Medicine*, *346*, 476–483.

202. Welch, G.N., Upchurch, G.R., Jr., Loscalzo, J. (1997). Homocysteine, oxidative stress, and vascular disease. *Hospital Practice*, *32*, 81–82.

203. Signorello, M.G., Pascale, R., Leoncini, G. (2002). Effect of homocysteine on arachidonic acid release in human platelets. *European Journal of Clinical Investigation*, *32*, 279–284.

204. Glushchenko, A.V., Jacobsen, D.W. (2007). Molecular targeting of proteins by L-homocysteine: Mechanistic implications for vascular disease. *Antioxidants and Redox Signaling*, *9*, 1883–1898.

205. Jacobsen, D.W. (1998). Homocysteine and vitamins in cardiovascular disease. *Clinical Chemistry*, *44*, 1833–1843.

206. Ziemińska, E., Stafiej, A., Łazarewicz, J.W. (2003). Role of group I metabotropic glutamate receptors and NMDA receptors in homocysteine-evoked acute neurodegeneration of cultured cerebellar granule neurones. *Neurochemistry International*, *43*, 481–492.

207. Ermak, G., Davies, K.J. (2002). Calcium and oxidative stress: From cell signaling to cell death. *Molecular Immunology*, *38*, 713–721.

208. Nogalska, A., Engel, W.K., McFerrin, J., Kokame, K., Komano, H., Askanas, V. (2006). Homocysteine-induced endoplasmic reticulum protein (Herp) is up-regulated in sporadic inclusion-body myositis and in endoplasmic reticulum stress-induced cultured human muscle fibers. *Journal of Neurochemistry*, *96*, 1491–1499.

209. Dickhout, J.G., Sood, S.K., Austin, R.C. (2007). Role of endoplasmic reticulum calcium disequilibria in the mechanism of homocysteine-induced ER stress. *Antioxidant & Redox Signaling*, *9*, 1863–1873.

210. Zhou, J., Werstuck, G.H., Lhoták, S., de Koning, A.B., Sood, S.K., Hossain, G.S., Møller, J., Ritskes-Hoitinga, M., Falk, E., Dayal, S., Lentz, S.R., Austin, R.C. (2004). Association of multiple cellular stress pathways with accelerated atherosclerosis in hyperhomocysteinemic apolipoprotein E-deficient mice. *Circulation*, *110*, 207–213.

211. Lenz, B., Bleich, S., Beutler, S., Schlierf, B., Schwager, K., Reulbach, U., Kornhuber, J., Bönsch, S. (2006). Homocysteine regulates expression of Herp by DNA methylation involving the AARE and CREB binding sites. *Experimental Cell Research*, *312*, 4049–4055.

212. Outinen, P.A., Sood, S.K., Pfeifer, S.I., Pamidi, S., Podor, T.J., Li, J., Weitz, J.I., Austin, R.C. (1999). Homocysteine-induced endoplasmic reticulum stress and growth arrest

leads to specific changes in gene expression in human vascular endothelial cells. *Blood*, *94*, 959–967.

213. Zimmermann, A.K., Loucks, F.A., Schroeder, E.K., Bouchard, R.J., Tyler, K.L., Linseman, D.A. (2007). Glutathione binding to the Bcl-2 homology-3 domain groove: A molecular basis for Bcl-2 antioxidant function at mitochondria. *Journal of Biological Chemistry*, *282*, 29296–29304.

214. Steinman, H.M. (1995). The Bcl-2 oncoprotein functions as a pro-oxidant. *Journal of Biological Chemistry*, *270*, 3487–3490.

CHAPTER 11

METHIONINE OXIDATION: IMPLICATION IN PROTEIN REGULATION, AGING, AND AGING-ASSOCIATED DISEASES

JACKOB MOSKOVITZ and DEREK B. OIEN

11.1 INTRODUCTION

The common hypothesis of aging is based on processes mediated by oxidative damage to cellular components, including nucleic acids, proteins, and lipids. These posttranslational modifications are caused by reactive oxygen species (ROS) and reactive nitrogen intermediates, for example, hydrogen peroxide, superoxide, oxygen, ozone, hypochlorous acid, chloramine T (sodium N-chloro-p-toluenesulfonchloramide), N-chlorosuccinimide, hydroxyl radicals, and peroxynitrite. Common ROS-mediated side-chain modifications can be in the form of a carbonyl or the oxidized sulfur atom of methionine (Met) or cysteine (Cys). Protein-carbonyls are nonenzymatic irreversible modifications. They are often catalyzed by metal ions and tend to form on the side chains of the amino acids proline, arginine, threonine, and lysine. In contrast, the sulfur-containing amino acids are readily oxidized and most modifications are reversible. Modifications of Cys residues have various consequences, including the alteration of protein structure, inactivation of proteins, and formation of disulfide bridges. Reversal of the posttranslational modifications to Cys residues can be achieved by several nonenzymatic reductants and reducing enzymes. However, the reduction of methionine sulfoxide (Met(o)) is exclusively performed by the methionine sulfoxide reductase (Msr) system.

Glutathione and Sulfur Amino Acids in Human Health and Disease. Edited by R. Masella and G. Mazza
Copyright © 2009 John Wiley & Sons, Inc.

11.2   THE METHIONINE SULFOXIDE REDUCTASE SYSTEM

The oxidation of Met residues results in either methionine sulfoxide (Met(o)) or methionine sulfone. Methionine sulfone is usually formed under extreme oxidant conditions following the formation of methionine sulfoxide. The modification of the Met side chain to a sulfone is considered irreversible. In contrast, Met(o) is readily formed, relative to other posttranslational modifications, and can be reduced by the Msr system. Oxidation of the Met sulfur atom can form either one of two possible enantiomers; denoted as *S* and *R*. With some specific exceptions, there is no general evidence to date predicting which enantiomer of Met(o) is more common in vivo. The *S* and *R* enantiomers can be readily reduced by the enzymes methionine sulfoxide reductase A and B (MsrA, MsrB), respectively. Methionine sulfoxide reductases reduce Met(o) using thioredoxin (Trx), thioredoxin reductase (TR), and NAD(P)H [1, 2]. In some forms of human MsrB, specifically hMsrB2 and hMsrB3, thioredoxin has been found less efficient for reduction. Additionally, a protein called thionein, especially for hMsrB3, and certain selenium compounds make better reducing enzymes to activate these reductases [3]. Under in vitro conditions, dithiothreitol is often used to reduce Msr, and lipoic acid also can act as a reductant [4].

The Cys at position 72 is vital for Msr activity and is highly conserved in most species [5]. When MsrA is inactivated, the Cys residue is oxidized and forms a disulfide bridge with another Cys near the C-terminal [6].

The Msr enzymes are ubiquitously expressed in many organisms. In a bacterial strain like *Escherichia coli*, there is one form of MsrA and one form of MsrB. However, in mammals there is one form of MsrA, and four forms of MsrB, denoted as MsrB1, MsrB2, MsrB3A, and MsrB3B. The MsrB1 form is a cytoplasmic selenoprotein [7, 8], MsrB2 and MsrB3B can be targeted to the mitochondria (like MsrA), and MsrB3A is targeted to the endoplasmic reticulum [2]. The *msr* genes are highly expressed in the liver and kidneys of mammals [9]. The Msr system is considered to be important for survival under oxidative stress conditions as manifested by *msrA* gene knockouts in various organisms [1].

The activity of the Msr system may prevent changes occurring to peptides, proteins, or compounds harboring Met(o) or methyl sulfoxide adducts [10]. Methionine is a hydrophobic amino acid, and the hydrophobicity decreases when the sulfur atom oxidized. However, the sulfoxide formation can alter the native folding and expose hydrophobic regions in a protein [11]. It was suggested, that protein-methionine can scavenge/detoxify ROS, and that the Msr system may facilitate this function by recycling Met(o) to Met. Thus, it is further speculated that surface-exposed methionines may play a protective role against ROS-mediated damage to proteins. Furthermore, lack of MsrA has been shown to increase protein-carbonyl accumulation in mice and yeast, either under hyperoxic/selenium deficient conditions or nonreplicative senescence, respectively [12–14], supporting the link between enhanced free radical damaging action and the aging process [15].

The role of protein-Met(o) in the pathogenesis of disease and general aging of cells is not yet completely revealed. Thus, the Msr system may prove to be a key component in preventing oxidative damage to proteins, in oxidative regulation of protein function, or a combination of both.

11.3 METHIONINE SULFOXIDE REDUCTASE AND SELENIUM

Selenium (Se) and MsrA are positive regulators of the expression level of MsrB1 (the selenoprotein form of MsrB) and TR [12, 16]. The first mouse generation (F1), fed with a selenium-deficient (SD) diet, exhibited higher protein-Met(o) and carbonyl levels detected at 6 months of age [16]. The protein-Met(o) and carbonyl levels observed in the 6-month-old mice fed with SD diet resembled the levels seen in mid-aged mice (13 months of age) fed with selenium-adequate (SA) diet [16]. Thus, it was concluded that Se deficiency shortens the time required to cause significant accumulation of faulty proteins due to age-related oxidative stress. Previously, it was shown that exposing mice to 100% oxygen (hyperoxia) caused higher elevation of protein-carbonyl [12]. However, exposing mice to a SD diet may better mimic the physiological conditions of oxidation, thereby facilitating monitoring the appearance of posttranslational modification (like protein-Met(o)), especially in the $MsrA^{-/-}$ mice. The effects of the SD at the F1 generation on both mouse strains were similar [16]. A recent study from our laboratory has shown that a prolonged SD diet had differential effects on these mouse strains [14]. The latter study examined the effects of SD diet through the second generation (F2) of $MsrA^{-/-}$ relative to wild-type (WT) mice with respect to their oxidized protein levels; activities and expression of seleno-enzymes and antioxidant enzymes (cellular-gluthathione peroxidase (GPx), TR, and selenoprotein P (SelP)), and the activities of the Msr system-related enzymes (MsrB, MsrA (in WT mice only), thioredoxin (Trx), TR, and glucose-6-phosphate dehydrogenase (G6PD); that is involved in NADPH production). Following the F1 generation of the SD diet, the mice are limited in their Se consumption only when they are weaned, as before then they acquire Se through their mother's milk. However, continuation of the SD diet through the F2 generation will cause the Se deficiency to start at birth, as the mother's milk will be already Se deficient. Moreover, following SD diet at the F1 generation, no significant observed phenotype has been noted in the $MsrA^{-/-}$ relative to WT mouse, except for an enhanced atypical walking pattern ("tip toe" walking) [16]. In contrast, continuing the SD diet through the F2 generation caused slower body weight gain in $MsrA^{-/-}$ mice up to 120 days of the diet (that started immediately after weanling) [14]. This phenotype may imply that a significant decrease in the levels of certain selenoproteins (including MsrB1 and TR) in conjunction with the absence of the MsrA protein may interfere with normal body growth at early stages of development. The observed phenotype may be related to the insufficient reduction of Met(o) residue(s) in key proteins participating in early stages of mouse growth. It will be of great interest to identify the specific proteins in which their methionine oxidation alters their ability to regulate directly or indirectly the function of growth-related enzymes.

The MsrA protein positively regulates TR expression (especially under oxidative stress conditions) [12] and MsrB1 (under nonstress conditions) [14, 16]. Following

SA diet, the most significant decrease in MsrB activity observed was mostly in liver and kidney tissues of $MsrA^{-/-}$ [14, 16]. However, only following SD diet through the F2 generation, the $MsrA^{-/-}$ mouse cerebellum showed a dramatic decline in MsrB activity compared to WT cerebellum [14]. Accordingly, it was suggested that a long-term SD diet exacerbates the negative effect on MsrB expression in the absence of MsrA only in the cerebellum. It is possible that in the cerebellum the expression levels of MsrA and Se tightly regulate the expression level of MsrB to avoid excess MsrB synthesis when the potential for full reduction of protein-S-Met(o) is limited. Thus, high level of S-Met(o) and low level of Se may be the secondary signals for reducing the synthesis of MsrB.

From these recent studies, it was concluded that enhanced protein oxidation that occurs in the $MsrA^{-/-}$ mouse tissues following a SD diet through the F2 generation, in comparison to the F1 generation, was even greater relative to WT mouse tissues, respectively. The MsrA protein is highly abundant in the brain cerebellum and lung alveolar macrophages [9]. Both cerebellum and alveolar macrophages require a high level of antioxidant defense to maintain their proper function. It is hypothesized that lower levels of Se reduce the basal transcriptional level of selenoproteins with antioxidant properties (including MsrB) and consequently lead to a compromised antioxidant defense, resulting in enhanced protein oxidation. Based on these observations, it appears that lack of MsrA exacerbates the effects caused by prolonged Se deficiency.

The mammalian TR is a selenoenzyme that plays an important role in antioxidant defense and is also a major component of the Msr system. Moreover, MsrA is positively upregulating TR expression under oxidative stress conditions [12]. As a result, WT and $MsrA^{-/-}$ mouse strains that were subjected to prolonged SD diet (through the F2 generation) demonstrated a dramatic decrease in their TR activity, mainly in the liver and kidneys [14]. The observed effects of the SD diet were again much stronger than the $MsrA$ knockout effects, except in the brain where the opposite is true (when both $MsrA^{-/-}$ mice and SD diet are applied through the F2 generation, the effect of MsrA absence is stronger) [14]. One possible explanation is that very low Se levels in brain contribute to the enhancement of oxidative stress that in turn is negatively affecting TR expression, especially in the absence of MsrA; similar to the effect of hyperoxia on TR levels in $MsrA^{-/-}$ mice [12]. Consequently, lowering TR activity by both dietary selenium and lack of MsrA may play a significant role in fostering oxidative damage to proteins.

The reduction of Trx by TR requires NADPH. The major supplier of NADPH is the pentose-phosphate pathway initiated by G6PD. Cells lacking G6PD are more sensitive to cell death that is mediated by oxidative stress [17, 18]. The hearts and lungs of $MsrA^{-/-}$ mice that were subjected to the SD diet through the F2 generation had significantly elevated expression and activity of G6PD, relative to control WT mice [14]. Both the lungs and heart are the first organs to be exposed to the high level of oxygen. Thus, it is essential to maintain sufficient reduction power (like NADPH) to prevent premature cell death in response to extensive oxidative stress conditions. It is possible that the elevation of G6PD in these tissues (subjected to SD diet) serves as a compensation mechanism for the lower antioxidant defense system in the $MsrA^{-/-}$ mice, under conditions of prolonged Se deficiency. It is important to note that neither a

SD diet nor a lack of MsrA alone showed the effect. The mechanism in which the upregulation of G6PD occurs in the $MsrA^{-/-}$ mice is yet to be identified. It may be that the signal mediators for this phenomenon are a combination of certain levels of cellular Se and Met(o) (as free or protein-bound) that initiate a signal transduction cascade leading to higher transcription level of *G6PD*.

One selenoprotein that is considered to be a good marker for Se deficiency is the secreted protein SelP [19]. Indeed, following SD diet through the F2 generation, the WT and $MsrA^{-/-}$ mice exhibited very low levels of plasma SelP that were below the assay's limits of detection [14]. However, contrary to expectations, the cellular levels of SelP were significantly higher in the $MsrA^{-/-}$ mice compared to control mice [14]. Normally, the SelP protein is secreted from cells to the plasma, and one of its possible roles is to deliver Se to tissues via its rich selenocysteine residue content [19, 20]. Another possible function of SelP is to act as an antioxidant by its potential reducing activity. SelP contains several redox centers in the form of Cys and seleno-cysteine residues. Saito et al. have shown that the human SelP can catalyze the oxidation of reduced gluthathione (GSH) by a phosphatidylcholine hydroperoxide [21]. Additionally, Trx was found to be a very good substitute for GSH as a reducing agent [22]. If indeed the elevation of SelP level in the $MsrA^{-/-}$ mice reflects a compensatory mechanism to accommodate higher cellular oxidative toxicity, it will suggest that SelP may have an important role as an antioxidant. Finally, supportive evidence for the possible role of SelP in protection against oxidative stress comes from the recent finding demonstrating that SelP may function as an antioxidant [23]. Taken together, the recent data about Se deficiency in $MsrA^{-/-}$ mice showed significant oxidative damage to proteins as a consequence of prolonged SD diet through the F2 generation. Additionally, the enhanced accumulation of posttranslational modifications in the $MsrA^{-/-}$ mice may be due to a compromised antioxidant defense. Not all tissues are equally affected by the Se restriction [14]. However, it is proposed that to compensate for the partial loss of selenoproteins, which function also as antioxidants, certain tissues may upregulate the activity/expression of specific proteins that are involved in reduction or peroxidation processes (like G6PD and SelP, respectively).

Unlike SelP and more like TR, the activity of the selenoprotein and antioxidant enzyme GPx sharply declined in brains and livers of $MsrA^{-/-}$ mice subjected to the SD diet through the F2 generation [14]. One possible explanation is that, similar to TR, GPx expression is also under the control of MsrA, especially under oxidative stress conditions mediated by prolonged Se deficiency. The levels of GPx were not dramatically altered following the F1 generation of the SD diet compared to the F2 generation (up to $\sim$50%, depending on the tissue [14]). However, following the SD diet at the F2 generation, a strong effect of the SD diet was observed and it is likely to occur due to Se deficiency during the weanling period.

Among all tested tissues, only cerebellum showed a major combined decrease in the specific activities of MsrB, TR, and GPx [14]. This observation may reflect a possible cerebellum malfunction associated with enhanced oxidative stress. It has been already noted that $MsrA^{-/-}$ mice exhibited an atypical "tip-toe" walking pattern that is exacerbated as a consequence of a SD diet [12, 16]. Since the cerebellum is also responsible for certain motor functions, it is possible that this form of ataxia is at least partially due to the significant loss of the above antioxidant activities. Further investigations are needed to determine the identity of the oxidized proteins resulting from the SD diet. Also, the data gathered will enable determining the signal transduction pathways and key regulatory proteins that are affected by oxidative stress, which is associated with Se deficiency.

11.4 METHIONINE SULFOXIDE REDUCTASE: A KNOCKOUT MOUSE AS A MODEL FOR NEURODEGENERATIVE DISEASES

Exposing mice to 100% oxygen causes a higher elevation of protein-carbonyl adducts in various tissues of $MsrA^{-/-}$ relative to control mice [12]. These results correlated with the loss of MsrA activity in brains with Alzheimer's disease (AD), while elevated levels of protein-carbonyl were observed in normal brains [24]. Methionine oxidation denatures proteins, and converts the hydrophobic properties of methionine into hydrophilic causing structural alterations [25]. Two major proteins, beta-amyloid (Aβ) and α-synuclein (αS), are involved in the toxicity associated with Alzheimer's and Parkinson's diseases, respectively. Both proteins have been shown to lose their fibrillation rate due to their methionine oxidation [26, 27]. In the case of Met(o)-αS, the oxidized protein was demonstrated to refibrillate in the presence of metal ions and ROS, in vitro [28]. Moreover, it appears that oxidation of Met35 in Aβ contributes significantly to its toxicity in vitro [29, 30]. It has also been demonstrated that Met(o)-Aβ adducts are present in postmortem senile plaques [31].

Our recent study showed that there is an elevated level of deposited Aβ in the hippocampal regions of mid-aged $MsrA^{-/-}$ mice [32]. The Aβ aggregates that were present in $MsrA^{-/-}$ mice at different sublayers of the CA1 pyramidal region were consistent with results that were reported earlier in the brains of transgenic mice models of AD. Also, the neuritic plaques that were preferentially localized in the areas of molecular layers of the dentate gyrus and stratum lacunosum may be due to the accumulative Aβ aggregates [32]. The interneurons of the CA1 hippocampal regions display a high spontaneous discharge rate and a pronounced action potential after hyperpolarization. These interneurons are vulnerable to extreme physiological conditions (like oxidative stress) that might lead to the release of an abnormal amount of Aβ and deposition at the sites of dying interneurons. Several Aβ aggregates were observed mainly in the $MsrA^{-/-}$ stratum lacunosum layer [32]. Previous reports have demonstrated that, in this layer, there were some interneurons that showed immunoreactivity with γ-aminobutyric acid (GABA) [33] and glutamic acid decarboxylase (GAD) [34, 35]. The latter result is in agreement with the selective deposition of Aβ in the amyloid precursor protein (APP) transgenic mouse to various regions of the hippocampus, including the stratum lacunosum and CA2 regions [36]. Since the stratum lacunosum is known to regulate declarative memory function, any cell death caused by either hyperexcitation or deposited Aβ aggregates can lead to a cognitive malfunction. Indeed, $MsrA^{-/-}$ mice exhibited a compromised complex task-learning capability when subjected to a behaviorally based reward system (unpublished results). It is expected that the observed Aβ deposition and the associated cognitive malfunction will be exacerbated with age, especially in the $MsrA^{-/-}$ mice. The region-specific Aβ deposition, accompanied by other pathological features, is associated clinically with progressive impairment of memory and intellectual function characteristic of the disease [37]. Consequently, we suggest that the results observed correlate with phenotypes associated with AD pathology in the $MsrA^{-/-}$ mice.

Tau protein microtubule-associated protein tau is abnormally hyperphosphorylated and aggregated into neurofibrillary tangles (NFTS) in the brains of individuals with AD and other tauopathies [38]. Additionally, developmentally and aging-induced alterations in brain oxidative status are a major factor in triggering enhanced predisposition to AD [39].

A significant immunostaining of tau-phosphorylation (p-tau) was observed mainly in the hippocampal CA3 region of the $MsrA^{-/-}$ brain, while it was not detected in the WT brain [32]. Among the many kinases that are involved in tau-phosphorylation is the active form of the extracellular signal-regulated kinase (p-ERK). In human and rhesus monkey brains, anti-ERK immunostaining showed that ERK levels are highest in the CA3 region, the mossy fiber zone, and the granule cell layer of the dentate gyrus [40, 41]. p-ERK is increased in neurons containing p-tau and NFTs, and in dystrophic neuritis of senile plaques in AD brains, and it is linked to oxidative stress. Additionally, zinc is present at high levels in the CA3 region of the hippocampus and can increase the levels of p-tau and p-ERK [42–46]. Taken together, it is suggested that the high p-tau level in the hippocampal CA3 region of the $MsrA^{-/-}$ brain has the similar characteristics of the elevated levels of zinc and p-ERK found in AD brains. To support this finding, it will be important to determine the levels of p-ERK and zinc in the $MsrA^{-/-}$ and WT brains. It is expected that the levels of zinc, p-ERK, and p-tau will be elevated with age relative to WT, especially in the CA3 region.

Synaptophysin is a calcium-binding glycoprotein that is present in the presynaptic vesicles of neurons and in the neurosecretory granules of neuroendocrine cells. Decreased levels of synaptophysin in AD correlate with the duration of the disease.

The strong immunoreactivity of the antibody against synaptophysin in the WT mice implies intact membrane structures in the presynaptic vesicles [32]. However, the overall weak and diminished synaptophysin immunostaining in the same regions of the $MsrA^{-/-}$ mice suggests severe axonal transport impairment and a gross failure in the synaptic transmission [32]. Consequently, it is concluded that the decreased synaptophysin level in the $MsrA^{-/-}$ mice reflects enhanced neuronal degeneration in the hippocampal areas that are similarly observed in mouse models of AD and human AD brains.

Glial fibrillary acidic protein (GFAP) is considered to be a highly specific marker for astroglial cells. A high number or enhanced apoptosis of the glial cells may reflect on the overall well-being of the neighboring neuronal cells. Generally, we expect the $MsrA$ ablation to accelerate pathologies associated with AD, which includes the induction of the GFAP level. Significantly greater GFAP levels were found in samples from individuals diagnosed with AD, mixed dementia, and vascular mediated dementia. Because elevated levels of GFAP reflect astroglial responses to even subtle forms of neural damage, GFAP may provide independent, supporting evidence for the damage underlying dementia, even in the absence of other evidence of neuropathology, such as the presence of neuritic plaques (NPs) and NFTs. In contrast, enhanced gliosis was observed throughout the course of the illness, and it was attributed to the cleavage of GFAP that may contribute to astrocyte injury and damage in the AD brain [47–49]. Indeed, our recent results demonstrated that the $MsrA^{-/-}$ hippocampal astrocytes are more damaged than astrocytes of the WT brain, suggesting the occurrence of a similar gliosis process described in AD [32]. Consequently, it is possible that the activated glia and astrocytes are trying to shift the Aβ deposits, but instead release H_2O_2 at them making the deposited Aβ bind to each other even tighter. Moreover, the H_2O_2 released may preferably damage the $MsrA^{-/-}$-astrocytes causing gliosis, as they are likely to be hypersensitive to H_2O_2. For example, primary-$MsrA^{-/-}$ hippocampal cells showed higher lethality rate following exposure to H_2O_2, compared to corresponding WT cells [32]. The latter result supports the proposed role of MsrA in protecting various brain cells against oxidative insult, including astrocytes. Moreover, the protecting effect of MsrA against oxidative stress has been shown to exist in other organisms/cells [1, 2]. Enhanced neurodegeneration in the $MsrA^{-/-}$ hippocampal and auditory regions were observed as well [32]. The hippocampal neurodegeneration is supported by the expression of the particular markers for AD as mentioned above, while the auditory nerve degeneration is a known phenomenon that is indicative of age-related neurodegeneration.

It is expected that all the observed differences between the $MsrA^{-/-}$ and WT mice, with regard to the expression and localization of the molecular markers associated with neurodegenerative diseases, will be exacerbated as a function of age. To better understand the possible role of MsrA in regulating the function of other brain proteins, it will be of great interest to compare the protein expression profiles of the two mouse strains. Identifying key proteins involved in regulating brain response to oxidative stress in the absence of MsrA will greatly contribute to our knowledge about the role of methionine oxidation in fostering neuronal damage. Ultimately, potential therapeutic interventions aimed at inducing MsrA or MsrB, or both, may facilitate preventing development and/or progression of neurodegenerative diseases.

11.5 REGULATION OF PROTEIN EXPRESSION/FUNCTION BY THE METHIONINE SULFOXIDE REDUCTASE SYSTEM

11.5.1 IκBα Function

The nuclear factor κB (NF-κB) is a transcription factor that regulates expression of genes that are essential for an adequate immune response during inflammation [50]. Under basal conditions, NF-κB is bound to proteins denoted as inhibitory κB (IκB), which inhibit its translocation to the cell nucleus [51]. During an inflammatory response one IκB form, IκBα, is phosphorylated, ubiquitinated, and degraded by the proteasome, allowing NF-κB to perform its transcriptional activity [52].

Recently, it has been shown that chloramines in the form of taurine chloramine and glycine chloramine have an inhibitory action on IκBα by the oxidation of its Met45 residue [53–55]. Moreover, it seems that the Met(o) formation on IκBα prevents its subsequent ubiquitin-mediated degradation when cells were activated with TNFα [55]. It is hypothesized that the structural change occurring due to Met45 oxidation prevents IκBα from being phosphorylated by the specific kinase [55]. Furthermore, it was demonstrated that reduced gluthathione (GSH) could not protect IκBα from oxidation by chloramines [55]. However, both MsrA and MsrB were able to reduce the oxidized Met45 in vitro [54, 55]. Thus, it is postulated that the inhibitory function of IκBα on NF-κB may be regulated by the redox state of its Met45, which can be oxidized by chloramines and reversibly reduced by the Msr system. In light of the above observations, the possibility of attenuating the functions of key proteins by methionine oxidation and reversal suggests a correlative signaling link between environmental conditions (e.g., oxidants) and cellular response (mediated by Met(o) reduction by the Msr system).

11.5.2 Cysteine Deoxygenase Expression

The enzyme cysteine deoxygenase (dioxygenase) (CDO) catalyzes the oxidation of Cys to cysteine sulfinic acid in the presence of Fe^{2+} that functions as a cofactor in mammals and yeast. The activity of CDO plays an important role in cysteine catabolism, taurine synthesis, and accumulation of pyruvate and sulfate [56–58]. The special significance of taurine synthesis, mediated by CDO, is mainly due to its involvement in bile salt synthesis, cardiac function, and protection of neuronal cells from ischemia-induced damage [59–61]. The cellular levels of the sulfur amino acids Cys and Met regulate the expression level of CDO [62]. Thus, in the absence of MsrA, it was predicted that enhanced oxidation of Cys and Met will cause changes in Cys metabolism and CDO expression (especially when both MsrA and CDO are highly expressed in liver). Indeed, under a SA diet the level of free thiol in the $MsrA^{-/-}$ was reduced to one-third of the level in WT mice [62]. Additionally, following a SD diet, the ratio between free thiol levels in the $MsrA^{-/-}$ and WT mice remained the same. However, absolute free thiol levels following the SD diet were reduced to about one-third of the corresponding levels following SA diet [62]. With respect to protein-thiol levels, no significant difference was observed between the WT and $MsrA^{-/-}$ mice under a SA diet [62]. In contrast, following SD diet the level of protein-thiol decreased by 18% and 50% in WT and $MsrA^{-/-}$ mice, respectively. One possible explanation is based on the $MsrA^{-/-}$ mice being hypersensitive to oxidative stress under the SA or SD diet [14]. Thus, enhanced oxidation of free and protein-bound thiols in $MsrA^{-/-}$ mice seems like a reasonable occurrence, which is exacerbated under SD diet [14]. The effect of thiol oxidation is more pronounced in the free thiol moiety because protein-bound thiols may not be as accessible to oxidation as free thiols (which are mostly present as L-cysteine). Lower L-cysteine can lead to decline in CDO expression [56]. Furthermore, studies performed on primary rat hepatocytes have demonstrated that when intracellular Cys levels were low, CDO became ubiquitinated and degraded by the 26S-proteasome. Reciprocally, when intracellular Cys levels were high, ubiquitination of CDO was altered causing a dramatic extension of its half-life [63]. Thereby, the levels of intracellular Cys attenuate the levels of CDO expression and degradation. Similarly, the relative lower levels of free thiols in $MsrA^{-/-}$ mice following either a SA or SD diet lead to a corresponding decline in CDO level [62]. These observations have a special importance when there is a cellular requirement to modulate the reduced versus oxidized levels of sulfur amino acids. For example, a compromised Msr system (i.e., lack of MsrA) leads to enhanced oxidation of sulfur amino acids. Consequently, there is an apparent need for lower enzymatic oxidation of Cys, which is accomplished by reduction of CDO expression. It is our hypothesis that like the indirect regulation of CDO by MsrA, there are other proteins that play a role in mechanisms involved in keeping adequate cellular redox balance and their expression is also mediated by thiol and/or Met levels. As no evidence for direct CDO-MsrA was detected, we have concluded that the expression of CDO is positively affected by the presence of MsrA. MsrA may either regulate CDO expression via the level of a secondary signal like reduced sulfur amino acids, or via a more direct influence on the activity of transcription factor(s) involved in CDO expression, or both. Cysteine levels need to be under very tight regulation to provide an adequate amount for GSH synthesis while avoiding high toxic levels of Cys. Thus, the down-regulation of CDO in the $MsrA^{-/-}$ mice may be an adaptive response to ensure sufficient level of GSH required for a compensatory antioxidant defense in the absence of MsrA. Identifying genes that are involved in the regulation of CDO in the $MsrA^{-/-}$ mice will enable better understanding of signal transduction events that are activated to protect cells from oxidative damage, which is mediated (at least in part) by lower levels of reduced sulfur amino acids.

11.6 CONCLUSIONS

The role of Met residue oxidation and reduction in various proteins is yet to be completely understood, but more evidence is emerging to support the importance of Met oxidation and reduction in cellular response mechanisms to oxidative stress. The most studied posttranslation modification to proteins that participates in signal transduction pathways is protein-phosphorylation. Similarly, Met oxidation and reduction may play a regulatory role under conditions of oxidative stress, as has been demonstrated for IκBα function and CDO expression. Failure of the Msr system in reducing pivotal methionine residues has also been shown to compromise antioxidant defense, resulting in premature cell death in several organisms. For example, lack of $MsrA$ in mice leads to enhanced neurodegeneration and shortened life span. Furthermore, abnormal behavioral traits exhibited by the $MsrA^{-/-}$ mice are currently under investigation to determine the link between an increase in Met(o) and atypical behavior phenotype. Overall, identification of major proteins that are affected by Met, in vivo, will strengthen the validity of the suggested roles of the Msr system.

REFERENCES

1. Moskovitz, J. (2005). Methionine sulfoxide reductases: Ubiquitous enzymes involved in antioxidant defense, protein regulation, and prevention of aging-associated diseases. *Biochimica et Biophysica Acta, 1703*, 213–219.

2. Moskovitz, J. (2005). Roles of methionine suldfoxide reductases in antioxidant defense, protein regulation and survival. *Current Pharmaceutical Design, 11*, 1451–1457.

3. Sagher, D., Brunell, D., Brot, N., Vallee, B.L., Weissbach, H. (2006). Selenocompounds can serve as oxidoreductants with the methionine sulfoxide reductase enzymes. *Journal of Biological Chemistry, 281*, 31184–31187.

4. Sagher, D., Brunell, D., Hejtmancik, J.F., Kantorow, M., Brot, N., Weissbach, H. (2006). Thionein can serve as a reducing agent for the methionine sulfoxide reductases. *Proceedings of the National Academy of Sciences USA, 103*, 8656–8661.

5. Moskovitz, J., Poston, J.M., Berlett, B.S., Nosworthy, N.J., Szczepanowski, R., Stadtman, E.R. (2000). Identification and characterization of a putative active site for peptide methionine sulfoxide reductase (MsrA) and its substrate stereospecificity. *Journal of Biological Chemistry, 275*, 14167–14172.

6. Brot, N., Weissbach, H. (2000). Peptide methionine sulfoxide reductase: Biochemistry and physiological role. *Biopolymers, 55*, 288–296.

7. Bar-Noy, S., Moskovitz, J. (2002). Mouse methionine sulfoxide reductase B: Effect of selenocysteine incorporation on its activity and expression of the seleno-containing enzyme in bacterial and mammalian cells. *Biochemical and Biophysical Research Communications, 297*, 956–961.

8. Moskovitz, J., Singh, V.K., Requena, J., Wilkinson, B.J., Jayaswal, R.K., Stadtman, E.R. (2002). Purification and characterization of methionine sulfoxide reductases from mouse and *Staphylococcus aureus* and their substrate stereospecificity. *Biochemical and Biophysical Research Communications, 290*, 62–65.

9. Moskovitz, J., Jenkins, N.A., Gilbert, D.J., Copeland, N.G., Jursky, F., Weissbach, H., Brot, N. (1996). Chromosomal localization of the mammalian peptide-methionine sulfoxide reductase gene and its differential expression in various tissues. *Proceedings of the National Academy of Sciences USA, 93*, 3205–3208.

10. Moskovitz, J., Weissbach, H., Brot, N. (1996). Cloning the expression of a mammalian gene involved in the reduction of methionine sulfoxide residues in proteins. *Proceedings of the National Academy of Sciences USA, 93*, 2095–2099.

11. Chao, C.C., Ma, Y.S., Stadtman, E.R. (1997). Modification of protein surface hydrophobicity and methionine oxidation by oxidative systems. *Proceedings of the National Academy of Sciences USA, 94*, 2969–2974.

12. Moskovitz, J., Bar-Noy, S., Williams, W.M., Requena, J., Berlett, B.S., Stadtman, E.R. (2001). Methionine sulfoxide reductase (MsrA) is a regulator of antioxidant defense and lifespan in mammals. *Proceedings of the National Academy of Sciences USA, 98*, 12920–12925.

13. Moskovitz, J. (2007). Prolonged selenium-deficient diet in MsrA knockout mice causes enhanced oxidative modification to proteins and affects the levels of antioxidant enzymes in a tissue-specific manner. *Free Radical Research, 41*, 162–171.

14. Oien, D., Moskovitz, J. (2007). Protein-carbonyl accumulation in the non-replicative senescence of the methionine sulfoxide reductase A (msrA) knockout yeast strain. *Amino Acids, 32*, 603–606.

15. Stadtman, E.R., Moskovitz, J., Berlett, B.S., Levine, R.L. (2002). Cyclic oxidation and reduction of protein methionine residues is an important antioxidant mechanism. *Molecular and Cellular Biochemistry, 234–235*, 3–9.

16. Moskovitz, J., Stadtman, E.R. (2003). Selenium-deficient diet enhances protein oxidation and affects methionine sulfoxide reductase (MsrB) protein level in certain mouse tissues. *Proceedings of the National Academy of Sciences USA, 100*, 7486–7490.

17. Filosa, S., Fico, A., Paglialunga, F., Balestrieri, M., Crooke, A., Verde, P., Abrescia, P., Bautista, J.M., Martini, G. (2003). Failure to increase glucose consumption through the pentose-phosphate pathway results in the death of glucose-6-phosphate dehydrogenase gene-deleted mouse embryonic stem cells subjected to oxidative stress. *Biochemical Journal, 370*, 935–943.

18. Juhnke, H., Krems, B., Kotter, P., Entian, K.D. (1996). Mutants that show increased sensitivity to hydrogen peroxide reveal an important role for the pentose phosphate pathway in protection of yeast against oxidative-stress. *Molecular and General Genetics, 252*, 56–64.

19. Burk, R.F., Hill, K.E. (2005). Selenoprotein P: An extracellular protein with unique physical characteristics and a role in selenium homeostasis. *Annual Review of Nutrition, 25*, 215–235.

20. Schomburg, L., Schweizer, U., Holtmann, B., Flohe, L., Sendtner, M., Kohrle, J. (2003). Gene disruption discloses role of selenoprotein P in selenium delivery to target tissues. *Biochemical Journal, 370*, 397–402.

21. Saito, Y., Hayashi, T., Tanaka, A., Watanabe, Y., Suzuki, M., Saito, E., Takahashi, K. (1999). Selenoprotein P in human plasma as an extracellular phospholipid hydroperoxide glutathione peroxidase. Isolation and enzymatic characterization of human selenoprotein P. *Journal of Biological Chemistry, 274*, 2866–2871.

22. Takebe, G., Yarimizu, J., Saito, Y., Hayashi, T., Nakamura, H., Yodoi, J., Nagasawa, S., Takahashi, K. (2002). A comparative study on the hydroperoxide and thiol specificity of the glutathione peroxidase family and selenoprotein P. *Journal of Biological Chemistry, 277*, 41254–41258.

23. Steinbrenner, H., Alili, L., Bilgic, E., Sies, H., Nakamura, H., Brenneisen, P. (2006). Involvement of selenoprotein P in protection of human astrocytes from oxidative damage. *Free Radical Biology and Medicine, 40*, 1513–1523.

24. Gabbita, S.P., Aksenov, M.Y., Lovell, M.A., Markesbery, W.R. (1999). Decrease in peptide methionine sulfoxide reductase in Alzheimer's disease brain. *Journal of Neurochemistry, 73*, 1660–1666.

25. Stadtman, E.R., Moskovitz, J., Levine, R.L. (2003). Oxidation of methionine residues of proteins: Biological consequences. *Antioxidants and Redox Signaling, 5*, 577–582.

26. Palmblad, M., Westlind-Danielsson, A., Bergquist, J. (2002). Oxidation of methionine 35 attenuates formation of amyloid beta-peptide 1–40 oligomers. *Journal of Biological Chemistry, 277*, 19506–19510.

27. Uversky, V.N., Yamin, G., Souillac, P.O., Goers, J., Glaser, C.B., Fink, A.L. (2002). Methionine oxidation inhibits fibrillation of human alpha-synuclein in vitro. *FEBS Letters, 517*, 239–244.

28. Yamin, G., Glaser, C.B., Uversky, V.N., Fink, A.L. (2003). Certain metals trigger fibrillation of methionine-oxidized alpha-synuclein. *Journal of Biological Chemistry*, *278*, 27630–27635.

29. Butterfield, D.A., Boyd-Kimball, D. (2005). The critical role of methionine 35 in Alzheimer's amyloid beta-peptide (1-42)-induced oxidative-stress and neurotoxicity. *Biochimica et Biophysica Acta*, *1703*, 149–156.

30. Schoneich, C. (2005). Methionine oxidation by reactive oxygen species: Reaction mechanisms and relevance to Alzheimer's disease. *Biochimica et Biophysica Acta*, *1703*, 111–119.

31. Dong, J., Atwood, C.S., Anderson, V.E., Siedlak, S.L., Smith, M.A., Perry, G., Carey, P.R. (2003). Metal binding and oxidation of amyloid-beta within isolated senile plaque cores: Raman microscopic evidence. *Biochemistry*, *42*, 2768–2773.

32. Pal, R., Oien, D.B., Ersen, F.Y., Moskovitz, J. (2007). Elevated levels of brain-pathologies associated with neurodegenerative diseases in the methionine sulfoxide reductase A knockout mouse. *Experimental Brain Research*, *180*, 765–774.

33. Gamrani, H., Onteniente, B., Seguela, P., Geffard, M., Calas, A. (1986). γ-aminobutyric acid-immunoreactivity in the rat hippocampus. A light and electron microscopic study with anti-GABA antibodies. *Brain Research*, *364*, 30–38.

34. Ribak, C.E., Vaughn, J.E., Saito, K. (1978). Immunocytochemical localization of glutamic acid decarboxylase in neuronal somata following colchicine inhibition of axonal transport. *Brain Research*, *140*, 315–332.

35. Kunkel, D.D., Hendrickson, A.E., Wu, J.Y., Schwartzkroin, P.A. (1986). Glutamic acid decarboxylase (GAD) immunocytochemistry of developing rabbit hippocampus. *Journal of Neurosciences*, *6*, 541–552.

36. Su, Y., Ni, B. (1998). Selective deposition of amyloid-beta protein in the entorhinal-dentate projection of a transgenic mouse model of Alzheimer's disease. *Journal of Neuroscience Research*, *53*, 177–186.

37. Morris, J.C., Storandt, M., McKeel, D.W., Jr., Rubin, E.H., Price, J.L., Grant, E.A., Berg, L. (1996). Cerebral amyloid deposition and diffuse plaques in "normal" aging: evidence for presymptomatic and very mild Alzheimer's disease. *Neurology*, *46*, 707–719.

38. Blennow, K., Vanmechelen, E., Hampel, H. (2001). CSF total tau, Abeta42 and phosphorylated tau protein as biomarkers for Alzheimer's disease. *Molecular Neurobiology*, *24*, 87–97.

39. Apelt, J., Bigl, M., Wunderlich, P., Schliebs, R. (2004). Aging-related increase in oxidative-stress correlates with developmental pattern of beta-secretase activity and beta-amyloid plaque formation in transgenic Tg2576 mice with Alzheimer-like pathology. *International Journal of Developmental Neuroscience*, *22*, 475–484.

40. Hyman, B.T., Elvhage, T.E., Reiter, J. (1994). Extracellular signal regulated kinases. Localization of protein and mRNA in the human hippocampal formation in Alzheimer's disease. *American Journal of Pathology*, *144*, 565–572.

41. Hyman, B.T., Reiter, J., Moss, M., Rosene, D., Pandya, D. (1994). Extracellular signal-regulated kinase (MAP kinase) immunoreactivity in the rhesus monkey brain. *Neuroscience Letters*, *166*, 113–116.

42. Trojanowski, J.Q., Mawal-Dewan, M., Schmidt, M.L., Martin, J., Lee, V.M. (1993). Localization of the mitogen activated protein kinase ERK2 in Alzheimer's disease neurofibrillary tangles and senile plaque neurites. *Brain Research*, *618*, 333–337.

43. Perry, G., Roder, H., Nunomura, A., Takeda, A., Friedlich, A.L, Zhu, X., Raina, A.K., Holbrook, N., Siedlak, S.L., Harris, P.L., Smith, M.A. (1999). Activation of neuronal extracellular receptor kinase (ERK) in Alzheimer disease links oxidative stress to abnormal phosphorylation. *Neuroreport, 10*, 2411–2415.

44. Pei, J.J., Braak, H., An, W.L., Winblad, B., Cowburn, R.F., Iqbal, K., Grundke-Iqbal, I. (2002). Up-regulation of mitogen-activated protein kinases ERK1/2 and MEK1/2 is associated with the progression of neurofibrillary degeneration in Alzheimer's disease. *Brain Research. Molecular Brain Research, 109*, 45–55.

45. Ferrer, I., Blanco, R., Carmona, M., Ribera, R., Goutan, E., Puig, B., Rey, M.J., Cardozo, A., Vinals, F., Ribalta, T. (2001). Phosphorylated map kinase (ERK1, ERK2) expression is associated with early tau deposition in neurones and glial cells, but not with increased nuclear DNA vulnerability and cell death, in Alzheimer disease, Pick's disease, progressive supranuclear palsy and corticobasal degeneration. *Brain Pathology, 11*, 144–158.

46. Harris, F.M., Brecht, W.J., Xu, Q., Mahley, R.W., Huang, Y. (2004). Increased tau phosphorylation in apolipoprotein E4 transgenic mice is associated with activation of extracellular signal-regulated kinase: Modulation by zinc. *Journal of Biological Chemistry, 279*, 44795–44801.

47. Hol, E.M., Roelofs, R.F., Moraal, E., Sonnemans, M.A., Sluijs, J.A., Proper, E.A., De Graan, P.N., Fischer, D.F., Van Leeuwen, F.W. (2003). Neuronal expression of GFAP in patients with Alzheimer pathology and identification of novel GFAP splice forms. *Molecular Psychiatry, 8*, 786–796.

48. Ingelsson, M., Fukumoto, H., Newell, K.L., Growdon, J.H., Hedley-Whyte, E.T., Frosch, M.P., Albert, M.S., Hyman, B.T., Irizarry, M.C. (2004). Early Abeta accumulation and progressive synaptic loss, gliosis, and tangle formation in AD brain. *Neurology, 62*, 925–931.

49. Mouser, P.E., Head, E., Ha, K.H., Rohn, T.T. (2006). Caspase-mediated cleavage of glial fibrillary acidic protein within degenerating astrocytes of the Alzheimer's disease brain. *American Journal of Pathology, 168*, 936–946.

50. Baeuerle, P.A., Henkel, T. (1994). Function and activation of NF-κB in the immune system. *Annual Review of Immunology, 12*, 141–179.

51. Baeuerle, P.A., Baltimore, D. (1988). IκBα: A specific inhibitor of the NF-κB transcription factor. *Science, 242*, 540–546.

52. Henkel, T., Machleidt, T., Alkalay, I., Kronke, M., Ben-Neriah, Y., Baeuerle, P.A. (1993). Rapid proteolysis of IκBα is necessary for activation of transcription factor NF-κB. *Nature, 365*, 182–185.

53. Kanayama, A., Inoue, J., Sugita-Konishi, Y., Shimizu, M., Miyamoto, Y. (2002). Oxidation of Ikappa B alpha at methionine 45 is one cause of taurine chloramine-induced inhibition of NF-kappa B activation. *Journal of Biological Chemistry, 277*, 24049–24056.

54. Mohri, M., Reinach, P.S., Kanayama, A., Shimizu, M., Moskovitz, J., Hisatsune, T., Miyamoto, Y. (2002). Suppression of the TNFα-induced increase in IL-1α expression by hypochlorite in human corneal epithelial cells. *Investigative Ophthalmology & Visual Science, 43*, 3190–3195.

55. Midwinter, R.G., Cheah, F.C., Moskovitz, J., Vissers, M.C., Winterbourn, C.C. (2006). IkappaB is a sensitive target for oxidation by cell-permeable chloramines: Inhibition of NF-kappaB activity by glycine chloramine through methionine oxidation. *Biochemical Journal, 396*, 71–78.

56. Stipanuk, M.H., Dominy, J.E., Jr., Lee, J.I., Coloso, R.M. (2006). Mammalian cysteine metabolism: New insights into regulation of cysteinemetabolism. *Journal of Nutrition*, *136*, 1652S–1659S.

57. Simmons, C.R., Liu, Q., Huang, Q., Hao, Q., Begley, T.P., Karplus, P.A., Stipanuk, M.H. (2006). Crystal structure of mammalian cysteine dioxygenase. A novel mononuclear iron center for cysteine thiol oxidation. *Journal of Biological Chemistry*, *281*, 18723–18733.

58. Chai, S.C., Jerkins, A.A., Banik, J.J., Shalev, I., Pinkham, J.L., Uden, P.C., Maroney, M.J. (2005). Heterologous expression, purification, and characterization of recombinant rat cysteine dioxygenase. *Journal of Biological Chemistry*, *280*, 9865–9869.

59. Huxtable, R.J. (2000). Expanding the circle 1975–1999: Sulfur biochemistry and insights on the biological functions of taurine. *Advances in Experimental Medicine and Biology*, *483*, 1–25.

60. Satoh, H. (1996). Electrophysiological and electro pharmacological actions of taurine on cardiac cells. *Advances in Experimental Medicine and Biology*, *403*, 285–296.

61. Saransarri, P., Oja, S.S. (1996). Taurine and neural cell damage: Transport of taurine in adult and developing mice. *Advances in Experimental Medicine and Biology*, *403*, 481–490.

62. Oien, D.B., Moskovitz, J. (2007). Ablation of the mammalian methionine sulfoxide reductase A affects the expression level of cysteine deoxygenase. *Biochemical and Biophysical Research Communications*, *352*, 556–559.

63. Dominy, J.E., Jr., Hirschberger, L.L., Coloso, R.M., Stipanuk, M.H. (2006). Regulation of cysteine dioxygenase degradation is mediated by intracellular cysteine levels and the ubiquitin-26 S proteasome system in the living rat. *Biochemical Journal*, *394*, 267–273.

CHAPTER 12

SULFUR AMINO ACIDS, GLUTATHIONE, AND IMMUNE FUNCTION

ROBERT GRIMBLE

12.1 THE BIOCHEMISTRY OF SULFUR AMINO ACIDS

12.1.1 Sulfur Amino Acid Metabolism

The sulfur amino acids are methionine and cysteine. Their metabolism is closely interlinked. As a result of this relationship the sulfur moiety is incorporated into a number of end products, three of which, glutathione, taurine, and proteins, have important roles in immune function.

Methionine is nutritionally essential due to the inability of mammals to synthesize its carbon skeleton. Cysteine is considered to be semiessential because it is synthesized from methionine, provided that the dietary supply of the latter is sufficient (Fig. 12.1). The methyl group of methionine can be removed from, and reattached to, the carbon skeleton of the amino acid by a cyclical process referred to as the transmethylation pathway (Fig. 12.1). The formation of homocysteine, part of the way along the transmethylation pathway, is an important branch point in metabolism of methionine. Homocysteine can be remethylated to form methionine, or can be metabolized by the transsulfuration pathway to form cysteine (Fig. 12.1). Both the remethylation of homocysteine and the formation of cysteine utilize serine. This latter amino acid forms the carbon skeleton of cysteine and acts as a methyl group donor to tetrahydrofolic acid, once the methyl version of the latter compound has donated its methyl group to homocysteine during the formation of methionine. Thus, a holistic consideration of the effects of sulfur amino acids on biological processes should involve some awareness of serine metabolism (Fig. 12.1). Furthermore, glycine should be considered in this holistic approach as it is a precursor of serine and one three amino acids comprising the sulfur-containing antioxidant glutathione (GSH).

In addition to incorporation into proteins, cysteine can be incorporated into GSH, or converted to taurine and inorganic sulfate (Fig. 12.1). The possession of an SH group

Glutathione and Sulfur Amino Acids in Human Health and Disease. Edited by R. Masella and G. Mazza
Copyright © 2009 John Wiley & Sons, Inc.

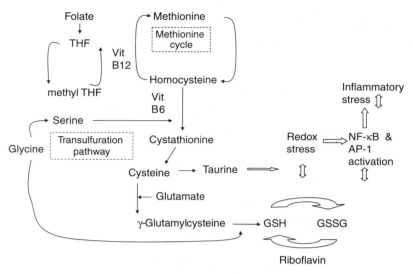

Figure 12.1   Outline of sulfur amino acid metabolism and its relationship to inflammatory stress. Abbreviations: AP-1, activator protein 1; GSH, reduced glutathione; GSSG, oxidized glutathione; NF-κB, nuclear factor kappa B; THF, tetrahydrofolic acid; Vit B6, vitamin B6; Vit B12, vitamin B12.

by cysteine and GSH allows the formation of an S-S bridge between two molecules of cysteine or of GSH to form cystine and oxidized glutathione (GSSG), respectively. Taurine has many roles, including formation of the bile salt taurocholic acid and is an antioxidant and cell membrane stabilizer. Taurine is the predominant nitrogenous compound in immune cells.

The synthesis of glutathione from its three constituent amino acids is mainly limited to the liver. The rate limiting enzyme in the pathway is γ-glutamylcysteine synthetase. Under normal physiological conditions there is feedback on the activity of this enzyme by GSH. Thus, conversion of cysteine to GSH is strongly influenced by the rate of utilization/transport of GSH within, and between, the cells of the body. In other words, synthesis is a "demand led" process, provided that cysteine is available.

From the organs of its synthesis glutathione is transferred to the blood and transported around the body in both plasma and cells mainly in its reduced form (GSH).

12.1.2   Control of Sulfur Amino Acid Metabolism

The biochemical characteristics of the enzymes regulating sulfur amino acid metabolism have an innate capacity for determining which of the products of sulfur amino acid metabolism are most affected when the cellular availability of sulfur amino acids is influenced by diet and disease. For example, the Km values for the homocysteine transferase enzymes (which lead to the recycling of methionine) are two orders of magnitude lower than those for cystathionine synthase (Fig. 12.1) (which processes methionine towards catabolism via the transulfuration pathway). Thus, at low intracellular concentrations of methionine, remethylation will be favored over transulfuration and methionine will be conserved. When these two pathways were examined in vivo, in rats fed diets containing 3, 15, and 30 g L-methionine/kg of diet, the percentage of methionine metabolized by the two competing pathways changed [1, 2]. With increasing dietary methionine intake, substrate flux through the transmethylation pathway fell and flux through the transulfuration pathway increased.

Examination of the Km values for rate-limiting enzymes processing the major cysteine metabolites provides a further insight into how sulfur amino acid metabolism is influenced by alteration in the supply of cysteine. The Km for L-cysteinyl-tRNA synthetase (essential for incorporation of cysteine into protein) is less than one-tenth of that for γ-glutamylcysteine synthetase (the rate-limiting enzyme for GSH synthesis) or cysteine dioxygenase (forming cysteine sulfinate, the precursor for sulfate and taurine). Thus, under conditions of low cysteine availability protein synthesis will be maintained and synthesis of sulfate, taurine, and GSH curtailed.

From the kinetics of the key enzymes in sulfur amino acid metabolism, reported above, it can be seen that when the diet is low in sulfur amino acids cellular methionine is highly conserved. Flux down the transulfuration pathway, which ultimately leads to methionine catabolism, increases only as dietary methionine intake increases. It can also be seen that at low flux rates of substrate down the transulfuration pathway conversion of cysteine into its main metabolites will be affected so that protein synthesis will be relatively maintained while sulfate and GSH synthesis rates will fall. Synthesis of GSH and sulfate will increase in concert as increasing levels of substrate flow through the pathway. In a study in rats, 7 molecules of cysteine were incorporated into GSH for every 10 incorporated into protein in liver at adequate sulfur amino acid intake [3]. At inadequate sulfur amino acid intake the ratio fell to less than 3 : 10. This response to a low intake of sulfur amino acids will not necessarily be advantageous since GSH is an important component of antioxidant defense. Thus, at low sulfur amino acid intakes antioxidant defenses will become weakened. The immune response makes large demands on these defenses and sulfur amino acid metabolism in particular.

12.2 SULFUR AMINO ACID AND GLUTATHIONE METABOLISM FOLLOWING INFECTION AND INJURY

The immune system has great capacity for immobilizing invading microbes, creating a hostile environment for them and bringing about their destruction. It can also become activated, in a similar way to the response to microbial invasion, by a wide range of stimuli and conditions. These include burns, penetrating and blunt injury, the presence of tumor cells, environmental pollutants, radiation, exposure to allergens, and the presence of chronic inflammatory diseases. The strength of the response to this disparate range of stimuli will vary, but it will contain many of the hallmarks of the response to invading pathogens. The immune response has a high metabolic cost, and inappropriate prolongation of the response will exert a deleterious effect on the nutritional status of the host.

The pro-inflammatory cytokines interleukin (IL)-1, IL-6, and tumor necrosis factor alpha (TNFα), have widespread metabolic effects on the body and stimulate the process of inflammation. Many of the signs and symptoms experienced after infection and injury, such as fever, loss of appetite, weight loss, negative nitrogen, sulfur, and mineral balance, and lethargy are caused directly or indirectly by pro-inflammatory cytokines. The indirect effects of cytokines are mediated by actions on the adrenal glands and endocrine pancreas resulting in increased secretion of the catabolic hormones adrenalin, noradrenalin, glucocorticoids, and glucagon. Insulin insensitivity occurs in addition to this "catabolic state." The biochemistry of an infected individual is thus fundamentally changed in a way which will ensure that the immune system receives nutrients from within the body. Muscle protein is catabolized to provide amino acids for synthesizing new cells, GSH, and proteins for the immune response. Furthermore, amino acids are converted to glucose (a preferred fuel, together with glutamine, for the immune system). An increase in urinary nitrogen and sulfur excretion occurs as a result of this catabolic process. The extent of this process is highlighted by the significant increase in urinary nitrogen excretion from 9 g/d in mild infection to 20–30 g/d following major burn or severe traumatic injury [4]. The loss of nitrogen from the body of an adult during a bacterial infection may be equivalent to 60 g of tissue protein and in a period of persistent malarial infection, equivalent to over 500 g of protein. However, during the response to infection and injury the urinary excretion of sulfur increases to a lesser extent than that of nitrogen [5], suggesting that sulfur amino acids are preferentially retained and so "spared" from catabolism. Infection with human immunodeficiency virus (HIV), however, has been shown to cause substantial excretion of sulfate in the urine during the asymptomatic phase of the disease [6]. The losses reported were equivalent to 10 g of cysteine per day, in contrast to losses of approximately 3 g/d for healthy individuals on a "Westernized diet". As cysteine is the precursor for both sulfate and GSH this finding may be linked with the decline in tissue glutathione pools that has been observed in HIV infection [7]. Clearly such a depletion of antioxidant defenses will not be sustainable over a long period.

Large decreases in plasma glycine, serine, and taurine concentrations occur following infection and injury. These changes may be due to enhanced utilization of a closely related group of amino acids, namely glycine, serine, methionine, and cysteine. Many substances produced in enhanced amounts in response to pro-inflammatory cytokines are particularly rich in these amino acids. These substances include GSH (comprised of glycine, glutamic acid, and cysteine), metallothionein (the major zinc transport protein), in which glycine, serine, cysteine, and methionine make up 56% of the total amino acids, and a range of acute phase proteins which contain up to 25% of these amino acids in their structure. If an increased demand for sulfur and related amino acids is created by the inflammatory response then provision of additional supplies of these amino acids may assist the response.

Many of the components of antioxidant defense interact to maintain antioxidant status. Glutathione and the enzymes that maintain it in its reduced form are central to effective antioxidant status. For example, when oxidants interact with cell membranes, the oxidized form of vitamin E that results is restored to its reduced form by ascorbic acid. Dehydroascorbic acid formed in this process is reconverted to ascorbic

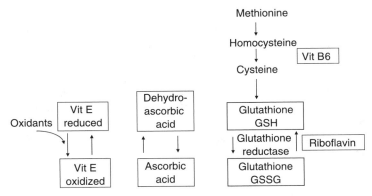

Figure 12.2 Interrelationships between antioxidant vitamins and amino acids. GSH, reduced glutathione; GSSG, oxidized glutathione; Vit B6, vitamin B6; Vit E, vitamin E.

acid by interaction with the reduced form of glutathione. Subsequently, oxidized glutathione formed in the reaction is reconverted to the reduced form of glutathione by glutathione reductase (Fig. 12.2). Vitamins E and C and glutathione are thus intimately linked in antioxidant defense. The interdependence of the various nutritional components of antioxidant defense is illustrated in a study in which healthy subjects were given 500 mg ascorbic acid per day for six weeks [8]. A 47% increase in glutathione content of red blood cells occurred. Vitamin B6 and riboflavin, which have no antioxidant properties per se, also contribute to antioxidant defenses indirectly. Vitamin B6 is the cofactor in the metabolic pathway for the biosynthesis of cysteine (Fig. 12.1). Cellular cysteine concentration is rate limiting for glutathione synthesis. Riboflavin is a cofactor for glutathione reductase, which maintains the major part of cellular glutathione in the reduced form (Fig. 12.1).

12.2.1 Changes in Antioxidant Defenses Following Injury and Infection

Although proinflammatory cytokines are essential for the normal operating of the immune system, they play a major damaging role in many inflammatory diseases such as rheumatoid arthritis, inflammatory bowel disease, asthma, psoriasis, multiple sclerosis, and cancer [9, 10]. They are also thought to be important in the development of atheromatous plaques in cardiovascular disease [11]. In conditions such as cerebral malaria, meningitis, and sepsis, they are produced in excessive amounts and are an important factor in increased mortality [9].

In malaria, tuberculosis, sepsis, cancer, HIV infection, and rheumatoid arthritis, inflammatory cytokines bring about a loss of lean tissue, which is associated with depleted tissue GSH content, and an increased output of nitrogenous and sulfur-containing excretion products in the urine (see above).

Although the body strives to maintain the integrity of antioxidant defenses, observations in experimental animals and patients indicate that, paradoxically, antioxidant defenses become depleted during infection and after injury. For example, in mice infected with influenza virus, there were 27%, 42%, and 45% decreases in the vitamin C, vitamin E, and glutathione contents of blood, respectively [12]. In asymptomatic HIV infection substantial decreases in glutathione concentrations in blood and lung epithelial lining fluid have been noted [13]. In patients undergoing elective abdominal operations the glutathione content of blood and skeletal muscle fell by over 10% and 42%, respectively, within 24 hours of the operation [14]. While values in blood slowly returned to preoperative values, concentrations in muscle were still depressed 48 h postoperative.

Furthermore, a reduced tissue glutathione concentration has been noted in hepatitis C, ulcerative colitis, and cirrhosis. In patients with malignant melanoma, metastatic hypernephroma, and metastatic colon cancer, plasma ascorbic acid concentrations fell from normal to almost undetectable levels within 5 days of commencement of treatment with IL-2 [15]. In patients with inflammatory bowel disease, substantial reductions in ascorbic acid concentrations occurred in inflamed gut mucosa [16].

As a general consequence of the weakening of antioxidant defenses during disease that is illustrated in the examples referred to earlier, oxidative damage is apparent in a wide range of clinical conditions in which cytokines are produced. Lipid peroxides and increased thiobarbituric acid reactive substances are present in blood of patients with septic shock, asymptomatic HIV infection, chronic hepatitis C, breast cancer, cystic fibrosis, diabetes mellitus, and alcoholic liver disease. When glutathione status was reduced in rats by injection of diethyl maleate, which binds irreversibly to GSH rendering it inactive, a sublethal dose of TNF became lethal [17], thus illustrating the importance of GSH in protection from the adverse effects of pro-inflammatory cytokines. The onset of sepsis in patients leads to a transient decrease in the total antioxidant capacity of blood plasma (a functional measure of the total antioxidant content) [18]. The capacity returns to normal values over the following 5 days. However, this was not the case for patients who subsequently died, in whom values remained well below the normal range.

As well as increasing the risk of direct oxidant damage, a reduction in the strength of antioxidant defenses also indirectly increases the risk of damage to the host via transcription factor activation leading to upregulation of pro-inflammatory cytokine production (see below).

12.3 GLUTATHIONE AND THE IMMUNE SYSTEM

12.3.1 Direct Effects of Glutathione

One of the first indications that glutathione influences lymphocyte function came from a study in which the GSH content of lymphocytes was measured in a group of healthy volunteers [19]. The numbers of helper (CD4$^+$) and cytotoxic (CD8$^+$) T cells increased in parallel with intracellular glutathione concentrations up to 30 nmol/mg protein. However, the relationship between cellular glutathione concentrations and cell numbers was complex, with numbers of both subsets declining at intracellular glutathione concentrations between 30 and 50 nmol/mg protein. The study also revealed that cell numbers were responsive to long-term changes in GSH content.

When the subjects engaged in a program of intensive physical exercise daily for 4 weeks (an activity that increases superoxide radical production), a fall in glutathione concentrations occurred. Individuals with glutathione concentrations in the optimal range before exercise, who experienced a fall in concentration after exercise, showed a 30% fall in $CD4^+$ T cell numbers. The decline in T cell number was prevented by administration of N-acetyl cysteine (NAC is metabolized to cysteine, see later). This study suggests that immune cell function may be sensitive to a range of intracellular sulfydryl compounds, including glutathione and cysteine. In HIV + individuals and patients with AIDS a reduction in cellular and plasma glutathione has been noted [13]. It is unclear at present whether the depletion in lymphocyte population that occurs in these subjects is related to this phenomenon. However, in a large randomized, double blind, placebo controlled trial, administration of 600 mg/d of NAC for 7 months resulted in both anti-inflammatory and immunoenhancing effects [6]. A decrease in plasma IL-6 concentration occurred, together with an increase in lymphocyte count and in the stimulation index of T lymphocytes in response to tetanus toxin. The precise mechanism underlying the complex effects of changes in cellular glutathione content are not clear, and whether they are related to GSH function as an antioxidant or to some other property is not apparent. However, a recent study suggests that glutathione promotes IL-12 production by antigen presenting cells so driving T helper cells along the Th1 pathway of differentiation [20].

12.3.2 Indirect Effects from Nutrients which Might Impact on Glutathione Status

12.3.2.1 Vitamin B6 Vitamin B6, although having no antioxidant properties, plays an important part in antioxidant defenses because of its action in the metabolic pathway for the formation of cysteine, which, as indicated earlier, is the rate-limiting precursor in glutathione synthesis. Vitamin B6 status has widespread effects on immune function [21]. Vitamin B6 deficiency causes thymic atrophy and lymphocyte depletion in lymph nodes and spleen. Antigen processing is unaffected. However, the ability to make antibodies to sheep red blood cells is depressed. In human studies the ability to make antibodies to tetanus and typhoid antigens is not seriously affected. Various aspects of cell-mediated immunity are also influenced by vitamin B6 deficiency. Skin grafts in rats and mice survive longer during deficiency, and guinea-pigs exhibit decreased delayed hypersensitivity reactions to bacilli Calmette-Guerin (BCG) administration. Deficiency of vitamin B6 is rare in humans but can be precipitated with the anti-tuberculosis drug isoniazid. However, experimental deficiency in elderly subjects has been shown to reduce total blood lymphocyte numbers and decrease the proliferative response of lymphocytes to mitogens [22]. Likewise IL-2 production is reduced by deficiency of the vitamin. Restoration of vitamin B6 intake to normal by dietary supplements restores immune function. However, intakes that are higher than currently recommended values are required to normalize all immune functions. It is unclear, at present, whether a similar situation occurs in younger subjects. One mechanism for the effect of vitamin B6 on immune function may be due to the importance of the vitamin in cysteine synthesis, as outlined earlier. Deficiency of the vitamin may limit the availability of cysteine for glutathione synthesis. In rats, vitamin B6 deficiency resulted in decreases of 12% and 21% in glutathione concentrations in plasma and spleen, respectively [23]. In healthy young women large doses of vitamin B6 (27 mg/d for 2 weeks) resulted in a 50% increase in plasma cysteine content [24], presumably by increased flux through the transulfuration pathway. As cysteine is a rate-limiting substrate for glutathione synthesis, these findings may have implications for the response to pathogens because of the importance of glutathione in lymphocyte proliferation and antioxidant defense. However, while vitamin B6 has cellular effects on the immune system, evidence is lacking of any effect on the inflammatory response.

12.3.2.2 Ascorbic Acid   High concentrations of vitamin C are found in phagocytic cells. Although the role of vitamin C as a key component of antioxidant defense is well established (Fig. 12.2), most studies have shown only minor effects on a range of immune functions, except in cases where the vitamin may be acting by interacting with GSH metabolism. Unlike deficiencies in vitamins B6, E and riboflavin, deficiency of vitamin C does not cause atrophy of lymphoid tissue. In a study of ultra marathon runners, dietary supplementation with 600 mg/d of ascorbic acid reduced the incidence of upper respiratory tract infections after a race by 50% [25]. It is interesting to note that strenuous exercise has been shown to deplete tissue glutathione content. The interrelationship between glutathione and ascorbic acid may therefore play a role in the effect of exercise on immune function.

When immunological parameters and antioxidant status were measured in adult males fed 250 mg/d of vitamin C for 4 days followed by 5 mg/d for 32 days, plasma ascorbic acid and glutathione decreased and impairment of antioxidant status became evident from a doubling in semen 8-hydroxydeoxyguanosine concentration (a measure of oxidative damage to nucleic acids) during the second dietary period [26]. A fall in vitamin content in peripheral blood mononuclear cells was noted and the delayed type hypersensitivity reaction to seven recall antigens was significantly reduced in intensity.

12.4 MECHANISM OF THE EFFECT OF OXIDANTS AND ANTIOXIDANTS ON INFLAMMATION AND IMMUNE FUNCTION

There is a growing body of evidence that antioxidants suppress inflammatory components of the response to infection and trauma and enhance components related to cell-mediated immunity. The reverse situation applies when antioxidant defenses become depleted.

The oxidant molecules produced by the immune system to kill invading organisms may activate at least two important families of proteins that are sensitive to changes in cellular redox state. The families are nuclear transcription factor kappa B (NF-κB) and activator protein 1 (AP-1). These transcription factors act as "control switches" for biological processes, not all of which are of advantage to the individual. NF-κB is present in the cytosol in an inactive form, by being linked to IκB. Phosphorylation and dissociation of IκB renders the remaining NF-κB dimer active. Activation of NF-κB can be brought about by a wide range of stimuli, including pro-inflammatory cytokines, hydrogen peroxide, mitogens, bacteria and viruses and their related products, and UV and ionizing radiations. The dissociated IκB is degraded and the active NF-κB is translocated to the nucleus where it binds to response elements in the enhancer and promoter regions of genes. A similar translocation of AP-1, a transcription factor composed of the protooncogenes c-fos and c-jun, from cytosol to nucleus, also occurs in the presence of oxidant stress. Binding of the transcription factors is implicated in activation of a wide range of genes associated with inflammation and the immune response, including those encoding cytokines, cytokine receptors, cell adhesion molecules, acute phase proteins, and growth factors [27].

Unfortunately NF-κB also activates transcription of the genes of some viruses, such as HIV. This sequence of events in the case of HIV accounts for the ability of minor infections to speed the progression of individuals who are infected with HIV towards AIDS since, if antioxidant defenses are poor, each encounter with general infections results in cytokine and oxidant production, NF-κB activation, and an increase in viral replication. It is thus unfortunate that reduced cellular concentrations of GSH are a common feature of asymptomatic HIV infection [13].

Oxidant damage to cells will indirectly create a pro-inflammatory effect by the production of lipid peroxides. This situation may lead to upregulation of NF-κB activity, since the transcription factor has been shown to be activated in endothelial cells cultured with linoleic acid, the main dietary n-6 polyunsaturated fatty acid, an effect inhibited by vitamin E and NAC [28]. The interaction between oxidant stress and an impaired ability to synthesize glutathione that results in enhanced inflammation is clearly seen in cirrhosis, a disease that results in high levels of oxidative stress and an impaired ability to synthesize GSH [29]. In this study, an inverse relationship between glutathione concentration and the ability of monocytes to produce IL-1, IL-8, and TNFα was observed. Furthermore, treatment of the patients with the GSH pro-drug, oxothiazalidine-4-carboxylate (procysteine) (Fig. 12.3) increased monocyte GSH content and reduced IL-1, IL-8, and TNFα production. Thus, antioxidants might act to prevent NF-κB activation by quenching oxidants. However, not all transcription factors respond to changes in cell redox state in the same way. When rats were subjected to depletion of effective tissue GSH pools by administration of diethyl

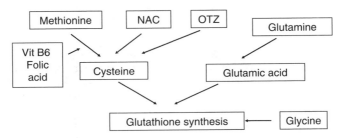

Figure 12.3 Nutrients and drugs that are important for enhancing glutathione synthesis. Abbreviations: NAC, *N*-acetyl cysteine; OTZ, L-2-oxothiazolidine-4-carboxylate.

maleate there was a significant reduction in lymphocyte proliferation in spleen and mesenteric lymph nodes [30]. In an in vitro study using HeLa cells and cells from human embryonic kidney, both TNF and hydrogen peroxide resulted in activation of NF-κB and AP-1 [31]. Addition of the antioxidant sorbitol to the medium suppressed NF-κB activation (as expected) but (unexpectedly) activation of AP-1 occurred. Thus, the antioxidant environment of the cell might exert opposite effects on transcription factors closely associated with inflammation (e.g., NF-κB) and cellular proliferation (e.g., AP-1). Evidence for this biphasic effect was seen when glutathione was incubated with immune cells from young adults [32]. A rise in cellular glutathione content was accompanied by an increase in IL-2 production and lymphocyte proliferation, and a decrease in production of the inflammatory mediators, PGE_2 and LTB_4. Modification of the glutathione content of liver, lung, spleen, and thymus in young rats, by feeding diets containing a range of casein (a protein with a low sulfur amino acid content) concentrations, changed immune cell numbers in lung [33]. It was found that in unstressed animals the number of lung neutrophils decreased as dietary protein intake and tissue glutathione content fell. However, in animals given an inflammatory challenge (endotoxin) liver and lung GSH concentrations increased directly in relation to dietary protein intake. Lung neutrophils, however, became related inversely with tissue glutathione content. Addition of methionine to the protein-deficient diets normalized tissue glutathione content and restored lung neutrophil numbers to those seen in unstressed animals fed a diet of adequate protein content.

Thus, it can be hypothesized that antioxidants exert an immuno-enhancing effect by activating transcription factors that are strongly associated with cell proliferation (e.g., AP-1) and an anti-inflammatory effect by preventing activation of NF-κB by oxidants produced during the inflammatory response.

12.5 STRATEGIES FOR MODULATING TISSUE GLUTATHIONE CONTENT AND INFLUENCING IMMUNE FUNCTION

A number of strategies have evolved to raise levels of glutathione in depleted individuals. There are at least three potential ways of enhancing cellular GSH content: administration of the three amino acids (cysteine, glutamic acid, and glycine) which comprise the tripeptide, either singly or in various combinations; administration of cofactors for the metabolic pathways leading to GSH production, that is, vitamin B6, riboflavin, and folic acid; and administration of synthetic compounds which become converted to precursors of GSH.

While cysteine supplies are the primary determinant of the ability to synthesize GSH, in some circumstances an insufficiency in the other two amino acids from which it is made might limit synthesis. Glutamine (a precursor of glutamate), for example, has been shown to maintain hepatic GSH in animals poisoned with acetaminophen, to enhance gut GSH synthesis in rats when given by gavage and to enhance hepatic GSH synthesis when given intravenously to rats [34]. In human studies a similar effect on gut GSH concentrations was noted [35]. Glycine supplements have been shown to raise hepatic GSH in rats exposed to hemorrhagic shock [36]. In this condition, however, the metabolic demand for glycine is increased since glycine is the sole nitrogen donor for haem synthesis and would therefore become rate limiting for GSH synthesis. There are many studies that illustrate the ability of sulfur amino acid availability to influence tissue GSH concentrations, for example, see Reference 37.

Studies using animal models of inflammation have shown that a low protein diet will suppress glutathione synthesis, a situation that is reversed by provision of cysteine or methionine [33, 38]. Beneficial effects on immune function, morbidity, and mortality were observed in burned children when additional protein in the form of whey protein (the milk protein richest in sulfur amino acids) was fed [39]. In HIV positive patients a whey protein formulation was clearly demonstrated to increase plasma GSH concentrations [40].

Because cysteine is unstable in its reduced form, is toxic in high doses, and is mostly degraded in the extracellular compartment, several compounds have been used to deliver cysteine directly to cells. These are L-2-oxothiazalidine-4-carboxylate (OTC) and NAC. OTC is an analog of 5-oxoproline in which the 4-methylene moiety has been replaced with sulfur. It provides an excellent substrate for 5-oxoprolinase (an intracellular enzyme). The enzyme converts OTC to S-carboxy-L-cysteine which is rapidly hydrolyzed to L-cysteine. NAC rapidly enters the cell and is speedily deacylated to yield L-cysteine. Recent animal and clinical trials with NAC and OTC have demonstrated the ability of the compounds to enhance GSH status [7, 41, 42]. In studies on patients with sepsis NAC infusion was shown to increase blood GSH, decrease plasma concentrations of IL-8 and soluble TNF receptors (an index of TNF production), improve respiratory function, and shorten the number of days needed in intensive care [42, 43]. While not affecting mortality rates, NAC shortened hospital length of stay by >60%. OTZ increased whole blood GSH in peritoneal dialysis patients, normalized tissue GSH in rats fed a sulfur amino acid deficient diet, and decreased the extent of inflammation in a rat peritonitis model [42]. In a randomized double blind controlled study on asymptomatic HIV-infected patients, oral OTC treatment increased GSH concentrations in whole blood [6]. Other randomized studies on asymptomatic HIV positive patients in the presence and absence of antiretroviral therapy (ART) have shown that NAC can raise blood GSH, increase natural killer cell activity, and enhance stimulation indices of T cells incubated with mitogen or tetanus toxin [6, 44]. Interestingly the rise in T cell function was accompanied by a fall in plasma IL-6 in subjects receiving ART as well as the drug. Furthermore studies have shown that survival time was improved in HIV+ patients who maintained high concentrations of GSH in CD4+ T lymphocytes [45]. It could therefore be surmised that improved T cell function and reduced inflammation are modulated by improvement in antioxidant status in these patients.

Alpha-lipoic acid provides a further means of enhancing tissue GSH content [41]. The compound is reduced to dihydrolipoic acid, which converts cystine to cysteine. This change has functional significance for glutathione status in lymphocytes, since the xc-transport system which is needed to take up cystine into the cells is weakly expressed and is inhibited by glutamate, while the neutral amino acid transport system which takes up cysteine is functional. Cysteine, on gaining entry to the immune cells, is rapidly converted to GSH. Flow cytometric analysis of freshly prepared human peripheral blood lymphocytes shows that lipoic acid is able to normalize a subpopulation of cells with severely compromised thiol status rather than increasing the level in all cells above normal values [46]. Hence lipoic acid may also prove to be a useful clinical agent for restoring cellular GSH concentration in immunocompromised subjects.

12.6   TAURINE AND IMMUNE FUNCTION

Taurine, together with sulfate, can be regarded as a biochemical end product of cysteine metabolism. However, it is apparent that taurine also plays a role in immune function. It is the most abundant free nitrogenous compound (often incorrectly classified as an amino acid) in cells. It is a membrane stabilizer and regulates calcium flux thereby controlling cell stability. It has been shown to possess antioxidant properties and to regulate the release of pro-inflammatory cytokines in hamsters, rats, and humans [47–49].

The possibility that taurine might have immunomodulatory properties was indicated in studies in obligate carnivores, such as cats, in which taurine is an essential nutrient due to an inability to synthesize the compound. Premature infants have similar metabolic difficulties. In cats deprived of taurine substantial impairment of immune function occurs [48]. A large decline in lymphocytes, an increase in mononuclear cells, and a decrease in the ability of these cells to produce a "respiratory burst" and to phagocytose bacteria, occurs. There was a rise in γ-globulin concentrations in deficient animals. Spleen and lymph nodes showed regression of follicular centers and depletion of mature and immature B lymphocyte numbers. The changes were reversed by inclusion of taurine in the diets. Studies in other species have also reported effects of supplementation on immune system and function. In mice administration of taurine prevented the decline in T cell number that occurs with aging and enhanced the proliferative responses of T cells in both young and old mice [15]. The effect was more marked in cells from old than young animals. Taurine has been shown to ameliorate inflammation in trinitrobenzene sulfonic acid-induced colitis.

Taurine interacts with hypochlorous acid, produced during the "oxidant burst" of stimulated macrophages, to produce taurine chloramine (TauCl). This compound may have important immunomodulatory properties and may be responsible for properties that have been ascribed earlier to taurine. TauCl has been shown to inhibit NO, PGE_2, $TNF\alpha$, and IL-6 production from stimulated macrophages in culture and to inhibit the ability of antigen presenting cells to process and present ovalbumin [15]. In in vitro studies with murine dendritic cells the compound altered the balance of Th1 to Th2 cytokines, suggesting that it might play a role in maintaining the balance between the inflammatory response and the acquired immune response.

12.7   CONCLUSIONS

Oxidant stress is both an integral part of the body's response to invasion by pathogens and a modulator of immune function. The modulation may take the form of an upregulation of inflammatory components of the response and downregulation of cell-mediated immunity. This apparent paradoxical response is due in part to the action of oxidant stress on the activity of transcription factors such as NF-κB and AP-1. The former has an impact on inflammation and the latter on cell-mediated immunity. In addition to these molecular factors the age of the host may influence the balance between inflammation and cell-mediated immunity. As aging proceeds inflammation increases in intensity, even in the absence of pathogenic invasion of the body. Cell-mediated immunity may also weaken. Studies on PPARα in mice indicate that the normal restraining influence of this group of transcription factors on inflammation may weaken, thereby contributing to an inflammatory phenotype in the aged. Paradoxically the inflammatory response may deplete antioxidant defenses, an action that may lead to upregulation of inflammation and impairment of cell-mediated immunity.

Many studies in humans and animals have shown that nutrients that contribute to antioxidant defenses within the body in general have an anti-inflammatory, immuno-stimulatory influence. For some nutrients such as ascorbic acid, glutathione, and its precursors, the modulatory effect is via actions on NF-κB; for other nutrients, such as α-tocopherol, actions may be via an influence on AP-1 activity or by unknown mechanisms.

REFERENCES

1. Finkelstein, J.D., Martin, J.J. (1984). Methionine metabolism in mammals: Distribution of homocysteine between competing pathways. *Journal of Biological Chemistry, 259,* 9508–9513.

2. Finkelstein, J.D., Martin, J.J. (1986). Methionine metabolism in mammals: Adaptation to methionine excess. *Journal of Biological Chemistry, 261,* 1582–1587.

3. Grimble, R.F., Grimble, G.K. (1998). Immunonutrition: Role of sulfur amino acids, related amino acids, and polyamines. *Nutrition, 14,* 605–610.

4. Wilmore, D.W. (1983). Alterations in protein, carbohydrate, and fat metabolism in injured and septic patients. *Journal of the American College of Nutrition, 2,* 3–13.

5. Cuthbertson, D.P. (1931). The distribution of nitrogen and sulphur in the urine during conditions of increased catabolism. *Biochemical Journal, 25,* 236–240.

6. Breitkreutz, R., Pittack, N., Nebe, C.T., Schuster, D., Brust, J., Beichert, M., Hack, V., Daniel, V., Edler, L., Droge, W. (2000). Improvement of immune functions in HIV infection by sulfur supplementation: Two randomized trials. *Journal of Molecular Medicine, 78,* 55–62.

7. De Rosa, S.C., Zaretsky, M.D., Dubs, J.G., Roederer, M., Anderson, M., Green, A., Mitra, D., Watanabe, N., Nakamura, H., Tjioe, I., Deresinski, S.C., Moore, W.A., Ela, S.W., Parks, D., Herzenberg, L.A., Herzenberg, L.A. (2000). N-acetylcysteine replenishes glutathione in HIV infection. *European Journal of Clinical Investigation, 30,* 915–929.

8. Johnston, C.S., Meyer, C.G., Srilakshmi, J.C. (1993). Vitamin C elevates red blood cell glutathione in healthy adults. *American Journal of Clinical Nutrition, 58,* 103–105.

9. Tracey, K.J., Cerami, A. (1993). Tumor necrosis factor, other cytokines and disease. *Annual Review of Cell Biology, 9,* 317–343.

10. Grimble, R.F. (1996). Interaction between nutrients, pro-inflammatory cytokines and inflammation. *Clinical Science*, *91*, 121–130.

11. Ross, R. (1993). The pathogenesis of atherosclerosis: A perspective for the 1990s. *Nature*, *362*, 801–809.

12. Hennett, T., Peterhans, E., Stocker, R. (1992). Alterations in antioxidant defences in lung and liver of mice infected with influenza A virus. *Journal of General Virology*, *73*, 39–46.

13. Staal, F.J.T., Ela, S.W., Roederer, M. (1992). Glutathione deficiency in human immunodeficiency virus infection. *Lancet*, *339*(8798), 909–912.

14. Luo, J.L., Hammarqvist, F., Andersson, K., Wernerman, J. (1996). Skeletal muscle glutathione after surgical trauma. *Annals of Surgery*, *223*, 420–427.

15. Grimble, R.F. (1996). Theory and efficacy of antioxidant therapy. *Current Opinion in Critical Care*, *2*, 260–266.

16. Buffinton, G.D., Doe, W.F. (1995). Altered ascorbic acid status in the mucosa from inflammatory bowel patients. *Free Radical Research*, *22*, 131–143.

17. Zimmerman, R.J., Marafino, B.J., Chan, A. (1989). The role of oxidant injury in tumor cell sensitivity to recombinant tumor necrosis factor in vivo. *Journal of Immunology*, *142*, 1405–1409.

18. Cowley, H.C., Bacon, P.J., Goode, H.F., Webster, N.R., Jones, J.G., Menon, D.K. (1996). Plasma antioxidant potential in severe sepsis: A comparison of survivors and nonsurvivors. *Critical Care Medicine*, *24*, 1179–1183.

19. Kinscherf, R., Fischbach, T., Mihm, S., Roth, S., Hohen-Sievert, E., Weiss, C., Edler, L., Bartsch, P., Droge, W. (1994). Effect of glutathione depletion and oral N-acetyl-cysteine treatment on $CD4^+$ and $CD8^+$ cells. *FASEB Journal*, *8*, 448–451.

20. Peterson, J.D., Herzenberg, L.A., Vasquez, K., Waltenbaugh, C. (1998). Glutathione levels in antigen-presenting cells modulate Th1 versus Th2 response patterns. *Proceedings of the National Academy of Sciences USA*, *95*, 3071–3076.

21. Rall, L.C., Meydani, S.N. (1993). Vitamin B6 and immune competence. *Nutrition Reviews*, *8*, 217–225.

22. Meydani, S.N., Ribaya-Mercado, J.D., Russell, R.M., Sahyoun, N., Morrow, R.D., Gershoff, S.N. (1991). Vitamin B_6 deficiency impaires IL-2 production and lymphocyte proliferation in elderly adults. *American Journal of Clinical Nutrition*, *53*, 1275–1280.

23. Takeuchi, F., Izuta, S., Tsubouchi, R., Shibata, Y. (1991). Glutathione levels and related enzyme activities in vitamin B-6 deficient rats fed a high methionine and low cysteine diet. *Journal of Nutrition*, *121*, 1366–1373.

24. Kang-Yoon, S.A., Kirksey, A. (1992). Relation of short-term pyridoxine hydrochloride supplements to plasma vitamin B_6 vitamers and amino acid concentration in young women. *American Journal of Clinical Nutrition*, *55*, 865–872.

25. Peters, E.M., Goetzsche, G.M., Grobelaar, B., Noakes, T.D. (1993). Vitamin C supplementation reduces the incidence of post-race symptoms of upper-respiratory tract infection in ultramarathon runners. *American Journal of Clinical Nutrition*, *57*, 170–174.

26. Jacob, R.A., Kelley, D.S., Pianalto, F.S., Swendseid, M.E., Henning, S.M., Zhang, J.Z., Ames, B.N., Fraga, C.G., Peters, J.H. (1991). Immunocompetence and oxidant defence during ascorbate depletion of healthy men. *American Journal of Clinical Nutrition*, *54*, 1302S–1309S.

27. Schreck, R., Rieber, P., Baeurerle, P.A. (1991). Reactive oxygen intermediates as apparently widely used messengers in the activation of nuclear transcription factor-kB and HIV-1. *EMBO Journal, 10*, 2247–2256.

28. Hennig, B., Taborek, M., Joshi-Barve, S., Barger, S.W., Barve, S., Mattson, M.P., McClain, C.J. (1996). Linoleic acid activates NFkB and induces NFkB dependent transcription in cultured endothelial cells. *American Journal of Clinical Nutrition, 63*, 322–328.

29. Pena, L.R., Hill, D.B., McClain, C.J. (1999). Treatment with glutathione precursor decreases cytokine activity. *Journal of Parenteral and Enteral Nutrition, 23*, 1–6.

30. Robinson, M.K., Rodrick, M.L., Jacobs, D.O., Rounds, J.D., Collins, K.H., Saporoschetz, I.B., Mannick, J.A., Wilmore, D.W. (1993). Glutathione depletion in rats impairs T-cell and macrophage immune function. *Archives of Surgery, 128*, 29–34.

31. Wesselborg, S., Bauer, M.K.A., Vogt, M., Schmitz, M.L., Schulze-Osthoff, K. (1997). Activation of transcription factor NF-kappa B and p38 mitogen-activated protein kinase is mediated by distinct and separate stress effector pathways. *Journal of Biological Chemistry, 272*, 12422–12429.

32. Wu, D., Meydani, S.N., Sastre, J., Hayek, M., Meydani, M. (1994). In vitro glutathione supplementation enhances interleukin-2 production and mitogenic response of peripheral blood mononuclear cells from young and old subjects. *Journal of Nutrition, 124*, 655–663.

33. Hunter, E.A.L., Grimble, R.F. (1994). Cysteine and methionine supplementation modulate the effect of tumor necrosis factor α on protein synthesis, glutathione and zinc content of tissues in rats fed a low-protein diet. *Journal of Nutrition, 124*, 2319–2328.

34. Cao, Y., Feng, Z., Hoos, A., Klimberg, V.S. (1998). Glutamine enhances gut glutathione production. *Journal of Parenteral and Enteral Nutrition, 22*, 224–227.

35. O'Riordain, M.G., De Beaux, A., Fearon, K.C. (1996). Effect of glutamine on immune function in the surgical patient. *Nutrition, 12*(Suppl), S82–S84.

36. Spittler, A., Reissner, C.M., Oehler, R., Gornikiewicz, A., Gruenberger, T., Manhart, N., Brodowicz, T., Mittlboeck, M., Boltz-Nitulescu, G., Roth, E. (1999). Immunomodulatory effects of glycine on LPS-treated monocytes: Reduced TNF-alpha production and accelerated IL-10 expression. *FASEB Journal, 13*, 563–571.

37. Stipanuk, M.H., Coloso, R.M., Garcia, R.A.G. (1992). Cysteine concentration regulates cysteine metabolism to glutathione, sulfate and taurine in rat hepatocytes. *Journal of Nutrition, 122*, 420–427.

38. Hunter, E.A.L., Grimble, R.F. (1997). Dietary sulphur amino acid adequacy influences glutathione synthesis and glutathione-dependent enzymes during the inflammatory response to endotoxin and tumour necrosis factor-α in rats. *Clinical Science, 92*, 297–305.

39. Alexander, J.W., MacMillan, B.G., Stinnett, J.D., Ogle, C.K., Bozian, R.C., Fischer, J.E., Oakes, J.B., Morris, M.J., Krummel, R. (1980). Beneficial effects of aggressive protein feeding in severely burned children. *Annals of Surgery, 192*, 505–517.

40. Micke, P., Beeh, K.M., Schlook, J.F., Buhl, R. (2001). Oral supplementation with whey proteins increases plasma glutathione levels in HIV-infected patients. *European Journal of Clinical Investigation, 31*, 171–178.

41. Deneke, S.M. (2000). Thiol-based antioxidants. *Current Topics in Cellular Regulation, 36*, 151–180.

42. Bernard, G.R., Wheeler, A.P., Arons, M.M., Morris, P.E., La Paz, H., Russell, J.A., Wright, P.E., the Antioxidant in ARDS Study Group. (1997). A trial of antioxidants N-acetylcysteine and procysteine in ARDS. *Chest, 112*, 164–172.

43. Spapen, H., Zhang, H., Demanet, C., Velminckx, W., Vincent, J.L., Huyghens, L. (1998). Does N-acetyl cysteine influence the cytokine response during early human septic shock? *Chest, 113*, 1616–1624.

44. Simon, G., Moog, C., Obert, G. (1994). Effects of glutathione precursors on human immunodeficiency virus replication. *Chemico-Biological Interactions, 91*, 217–224.

45. Herzenberg, L.A., De Rosa, S.C., Dubs, J.G., Roederer, M., Anderson, M.T., Ela, S.W., Deresinski, S.C., Herzenberg, L.A. (1997). Glutathione deficiency is associated with impaired survival in HIV disease. *Proceedings of the National Academy of Sciences USA, 94*, 1967–1972.

46. Sen, C.K., Roy, S., Han, D., Packer, L. (1997). Regulation of cellular thiols in human lymphocytes by alpha-lipoic acid: A flow cytometric analysis. *Free Radical Biology and Medicine, 22*, 1241–1257.

47. Kontny, E., Szczepanska, K., Kowalczewski, J., Kurowska, M., Janicka, I., Marcinkiewicz, J., Maslinski, W. (2000). The mechanism of taurine chloramine inhibition of cytokine (interleukin-6, interleukin-8) production by rheumatoid arthritis fibroblast-like synoviocytes. *Arthritis and Rheumatism, 43*, 169–177.

48. Grimble, R.F. (1994). Sulphur amino acids and the metabolic response to cytokines. *Advances in Experimental Medicine and Biology, 359*, 41–49.

49. Huxtable, R.J. (1996). Taurine past, present, and future. *Advances in Experimental Medicine and Biology, 403*, 641–650.

PART V

GSH AND SULFUR AMINO ACIDS IN PATHOLOGICAL PROCESSES

CHAPTER 13

SULFUR AMINO ACID DEFICIENCY AND TOXICITY: RESEARCH WITH ANIMAL MODELS

DAVID H. BAKER and RYAN N. DILGER

13.1 INTRODUCTION

Quantitative studies of methionine (Met) utilization, requirement, and toxicity are difficult and complicated, because a plethora of factors, both nutritional and metabolic, can impact these studies. Accurate assessment of dietary concentrations of Met and cyst(e)ine (cysteine and/or cystine) is problematic, digestibility of protein-bound Met and cyst(e)ine must be considered, transsulfuration of Met to cysteine (Cys) must be factored in, and interacting (or confounding) factors such as Met : Cys ratio, level of choline (or betaine), taurine, glutathione (GSH), S-methylmethionine, lanthionine, and inorganic sulfate in the experimental diet used cannot be ignored. The review that follows will cover sulfur amino acid (SAA), that is, Met + cyst(e)ine studies done with animal models, and the focus will be on requirement and toxicity assessment.

13.2 SULFUR AMINO ACID DEFICIENCY

When considering SAA deficiency, it is necessary to consider not only Met and cyst(e)ine, but also GSH, taurine, inorganic sulfate, 3-phosphoadenosine-5′-phosphosulfate (PAPS), choline, betaine, S-methylmethionine, creatine, and lanthionine. Assessment of Met and cyst(e)ine in foods is complicated by the fact that acid hydrolysis results in some degree of destruction of Met and, particularly, cyst(e)ine. Thus, performic acid preoxidation of food samples prior to the HCl hydrolysis is necessary for accurate quantification of both Met and cyst(e)ine in food proteins [1–4]. Because body protein synthesis requires both Met and Cys, levels of both of these SAA in experimental diets must be known prior to carrying out research on SAA deficiency,

Glutathione and Sulfur Amino Acids in Human Health and Disease. Edited by R. Masella and G. Mazza
Copyright © 2009 John Wiley & Sons, Inc.

adequacy, or excess. Moreover, digestibility of these SAA must also be known. Studies with animals have shown rather conclusively that among the 20 amino acids in food proteins, Met is among the most efficiently digested, whereas cyst(e)ine is among the most poorly digested [5–7]. Clearly, any determination of a requirement for Met, cyst(e)ine, or SAA must consider not only the concentration of digestible Met and cyst(e)ine in the basal diet, but also the so-called cyst(e)ine-sparing effect on the Met requirement.

Deficiency of SAA in the food supply of humans is not well characterized. Nonetheless, Met (or cyst(e)ine) is likely deficient in the food supply of several population groups. Lysine, however, which is in low concentration in all cereal crops [8], is virtually always more deficient than SAA in the food supply of population groups in the poorer countries of the world. These populations usually have to contend with multiple nutrient deficiencies of not only amino acids but also vitamins and minerals [9].

Accurate food composition tables are necessary when assessing SAA deficiency and adequacy for various population groups. Bos et al. [10] have reviewed the SAA content of dietary proteins. Other food components can also impact responses to supplemental SAA. Thus, choline or betaine [11], S-methylmethionine [12], GSH [13], lanthionine [14, 15], and taurine [16] are compounds in foods that are closely related to SAA and therefore should not be ignored.

13.2.1 Cyst(e)ine Sparing of Methionine

Transsulfuration involves transfer of the sulfur from Met to serine (Ser), resulting in Cys biosynthesis [17–21]. On a molar basis, Met is 100% efficient as a precursor of Cys [22, 23]. The reaction between Cys and cystine is freely reversible such that both compounds are equal in furnishing Cys bioactivity for support of protein synthesis. In young, rapidly growing animals, cyst(e)ine can furnish 50% of the requirement (wt : wt) for SAA [21–29]. For older animals (i.e., adult maintenance), cyst(e)ine can furnish >50% of the SAA requirement [30–33].

Fukagawa et al. [34] and Young [35] questioned whether Cys can spare Met in adult humans. Data from Di Buono et al. [36, 37], however, showed that the Met requirement of adult men was less than half as high when determined in the presence of excess dietary Cys as when determined with Met alone (i.e., no dietary Cys). More recently, Humayun et al. [38] reported similar results with school-age children. These studies suggested that excess dietary Cys lowers the dietary Met requirement by increasing the remethylation of homocysteine (Hcy) to Met and decreasing the flux of Hcy transsulfuration to Cys [39]. Dietary SAA requirements of humans are expressed as $mg \cdot kg^{-1} \cdot d^{-1}$. Therefore, the molecular weight difference between Met (149.2 mg/mmol) and Cys (121.2 mg/mmol) comes into play. Thus, even though transsulfuration conversion of Met sulfur to Cys sulfur is 100% efficient [22, 23, 27, 29, 39], 149.2 mg of Met (1 mmol) yields only 121.2 mg (1 mmol) of Cys. This, then, should result in a lower total SAA requirement when a proper ratio of Met and Cys is consumed than when Met alone is used to meet the SAA requirement.

TABLE 13.1 Illustration of Three Separate Bioassays Required to Evaluate Met Sparing by Cyst(e)ine[*]

Requirement Bioassay	Dietary Condition	Result
1. Met	No dietary Cys	700
2. Met[a]	Excess dietary Cys	314
3. Cys[b]	Dietary Met at 314	314

[*]Illustration from SAA requirement studies in young chicks [22, 40]. All requirement values expressed as $mg \cdot kg^{-1} \cdot d^{-1}$.
[a]The difference between 700 (assay I) and 314 (assay 2) is 386 $mg \cdot kg^{-1} \cdot d^{-1}$, which is an incorrect estimate of the Cys requirement.
[b]The total SAA requirement is $314 + 314 = 628$ $mg \cdot kg^{-1} \cdot d^{-1}$, lower than the 700 $mg \cdot kg^{-1} \cdot d^{-1}$ estimated for all Met in assay 1. The correct estimate of the Cys requirement is 314 $mg \cdot kg^{-1} \cdot d^{-1}$, which is 81% of the 386 $mg \cdot kg^{-1} \cdot d^{-1}$ (fallacious) estimate arrived at in assays 1 and 2. Note that 81% is the same percentage arrived at by dividing the molecular weight of Cys (121.2) by the molecular weight of Met (149.2).

As illustrated by the work of Graber and Baker [22] and Baker [40], three separate bioassays (requirement studies) are necessary to clarify the issue of Met sparing by Cys, and purified amino acid diets are required for all three bioassays (Table 13.1). Requirements were based on quantities of SAA needed to achieve maximal body weight gain and food utilization. In several instances where SAA requirement studies have been done, only assays 1 and 2 have been completed, and these two assays lead to an erroneous estimate of Cys sparing. Hence, the results of assays 2 and 3 make it clear that Cys can furnish 50% (wt : wt) of the dietary requirement for SAA, whereas assays 1 and 2 suggest that Cys can furnish 55% (700 − 314 ÷ 700) of the total requirement for SAA.

Inorganic sulfate is also a factor that can influence the Cys-sparing effect. Work with chicks [23, 41] and rats [42] has shown that 200 mg/kg sulfate addition to a Met-adequate diet that is deficient in Cys and devoid of sulfate can produce a marked growth response. Presumably, sulfate under these conditions is being used for PAPS biosynthesis and thereby (indirectly) sparing Cys so that more of the Cys can be used for synthesis of protein, GSH, and (or) taurine. This sulfate-sparing effect has also been observed in humans [43]. However, virtually all animal and human diets contain surfeit sulfate (from SAA metabolism, sulfate salts, and food sources) such that sulfate sparing of Cys is primarily of academic interest.

A fourth bioassay may help if questions persist about the efficiency with which Met furnishes Cys via transsulfuration. This (slope-ratio) bioassay uses the Met requirement (314 $mg \cdot kg^{-1} \cdot d^{-1}$) established in assay 2 (Table 13.1) wherein the assay diet contained excess Cys. The basal diet for this assay would therefore provide no Cys but enough Met to furnish a Met intake of 314 $mg \cdot kg^{-1} \cdot d^{-1}$. Then, dietary levels of Met or Cys would be supplemented to provide 0, 125, or 250 $mg \cdot kg^{-1} \cdot d^{-1}$ of L-Met or L-Cys (i.e., three levels of each SAA below the requirement). If done carefully, slope (weight gain in grams vs. intake in milligrams) of the Met response curve should be about 81% that of the Cys response curve in a common-intercept multiple linear regression model [22, 23, 40]. If an assay such as this is done using indirect (e.g., phenylalanine) oxidation methodology in either animals or humans, one would expect the slope of the Cys response curve to be more steeply negative than that of the Met response curve.

13.2.2 Methionine and Cyst(e)ine Growth Responses

There are numerous instances where it is desirable to construct assay diets that are specifically deficient in Met or cyst(e)ine per se. Thus, Met-deficient diets are needed to quantify the bioefficacy of Met precursors, isomers, and analogs such as D-Met, DL-Met, DL-OH-Met, Keto-Met, N-acetyl-L-Met, L-Met sulfoxide, L-Met sulfone, S-methyl-L-Met, L-Hcy, and D-Hcy. Likewise, diets specifically deficient in cyst(e)ine are needed for Cys bioefficacy studies on D-cystine, Keto-Cys, cysteic acid, DL-lanthionine, GSH, N-acetyl-L-Cys, S-methyl-L-Cys, L-Met, L-Hcy, D-Hcy, taurine, and L-2-oxothiazolidine-4-carboxylic acid (OTC). We have made good use of an SAA-deficient purified diet containing 198.6 g/kg of an SAA-free amino acid mixture, 40 g/kg soy protein isolate, and 25 g/kg casein [44]. This diet for young chicks was analyzed to contain 0.5 g/kg cyst(e)ine and 1.2 g/kg Met, with the requirement for young chicks fed this diet being close to 3 g/kg Met and 3 g/kg Cys. For studies of N-acetyl-L-Cys bioefficacy (relative to L-Cys), the diet was fortified with 2 g/kg L-Met; for studies on L-Met precursor bioactivity, the diet was fortified with cyst(e)ine levels of 1.5 to 3.5 g/kg.

Often overlooked in Met dosing studies is the profound effect dietary cyst(e)ine concentration can have on the magnitude of growth responses to Met (Fig. 13.1). In situations where Met is singly deficient in the Met dosing response range (i.e., excess dietary Cys), every incremental dose of Met produces a marked growth response that is attributable not only to Met but also to Met allowing a portion (equal to the Met dose) of the excess dietary Cys to be used. In dietary scenarios where Met and Cys are equally deficient, however, each dose of Met must be partitioned 50 : 50 to furnish both Met and, via transsulfuration, Cys. Thus, the magnitude of the growth response to Met when Cys is also deficient is less than half as great as that occurring when Met is singly deficient throughout the Met dosing range. Hence, in the illustration shown in Fig. 13.1, it took 1.11 g/kg supplemental L-Met in diets with deficient Met and deficient Cys to produce the same growth response as that obtained from 0.5 g/kg L-Met in the diet containing excess Cys. With excess Cys, 0.5 g/kg supplemental Met also allowed 0.5 g/kg Cys to be used, but with deficient Cys, 1.11 g/kg supplemental Met was partitioned to 0.5 g/kg Met plus 0.5 g/kg ÷ 0.81 (wt : wt efficiency of Met conversion to Cys) or 0.61 g/kg Met for Cys biosynthesis. On several occasions in our laboratory, we have observed responses to Met very similar to those shown in Fig. 13.1.

With Cys dose-response studies, similar pitfalls exist. Thus, as long as Cys is always singly deficient throughout its dosing range, each dose of Cys will allow an equal increment of Met to be used. In this case, however, it is important for dietary Met to be set at its minimal requirement (i.e., no excess) established in diets with excess Cys (see assay 2 of Table 13.1). Clearly, if Met and Cys are equally deficient, Cys supplementation will not elicit a growth response. More common in practice,

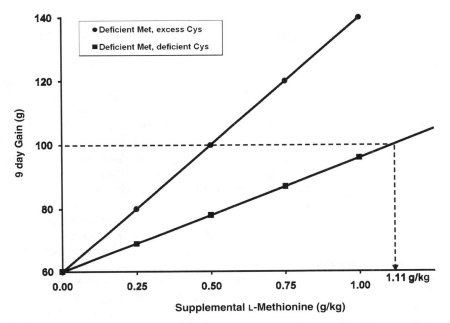

Figure 13.1 Growth response to L-Met. Illustration of growth responses of young chicks to L-Met in Met-deficient diets containing either excess or deficient Cys. The basal diet contained 1.2 g/kg Met and either 3.0 (excess) or 1.2 (deficient) g/kg Cys. Adapted from Dilger and Baker [76].

however, are situations where Cys is more deficient than Met, but Met is also deficient. In these cases, responses to Cys will be curvilinear rather than linear.

13.2.3 Requirement Studies

Numerous SAA requirement studies have been done with growing chicks, rats, mice, pigs, cats, dogs, and fish. SAA requirements have been studied for maintenance, gestation, and lactation in pigs and for egg production in laying hens [6, 45]. For growing animals, maximal growth rate, maximal nitrogen retention, or minimal plasma urea nitrogen (for mammals) has generally been used to establish dietary requirements. Also, it is now popular to express animal amino acid requirements (percent of diet, percent of calories, or grams per day) as ratios or percentages of the dietary lysine requirement. In general, SAA requirements of growing animals range from 60% to 70% of the requirement for lysine. But for adult animals, as illustrated with pigs, the SAA maintenance requirement is well over 100% of the lysine requirement [30, 32, 45].

Early work on the SAA requirement of adult humans was based on attainment of zero nitrogen balance [33], but more recent studies have based requirements on attainment of a breakpoint in oxidation (i.e., $^{13}CO_2$ expiration) of the limiting amino acid (34), that is, direct oxidation, or of a target excess amino acid, generally phenylalanine [36, 46], that is, indirect oxidation. Using this methodology, human studies have suggested that the SAA requirement of adult humans is less than 50% of the requirement for lysine [36, 46, 47]. An illustration of how oxidation methodology is used to estimate a requirement for Met (Fig. 13.2) involves graded doses of Met, with at least three doses below and two or three doses above the expected requirement. With direct oxidation, $^{13}CO_2$ production remains low and relatively constant until the requirement is reached, after which it increases rapidly. The inflection point (or breakpoint) represents the estimated requirement. With indirect oxidation, often called indicator amino acid oxidation, $^{13}CO_2$ production from 1 ^{13}C-phenylalanine (an excess amino acid) declines rapidly (and linearly) with increasing doses of Met, until the Met requirement is reached, after which it tends to plateau.

Because oxidation methodology predicts an SAA requirement of adult humans that is less than 50% of the lysine requirement [47], whereas nitrogen balance methodology in both humans [48] and pigs [30, 32, 49] predicts an SAA requirement that exceeds the lysine requirement, some have questioned whether the oxidation methodology may underestimate the requirement for SAA [39, 50]. Thus, SAA [especially cyst(e)ine] unlike other amino acids, are rich in certain tissues (keratoid) and compounds (mucin) that are sloughed from the body. It seems unreasonable that adult humans can have SAA needs relative to lysine that are less than 50%, but that adult pigs have SAA requirements that are over 100% of the maintenance lysine requirement. The use of Cys for synthesis of GSH, taurine, coenzyme A, and specialized high-Cys proteins such as metallothionein, keratoid proteins (hair, skin, toenails, etc.), and mucin may also be a complicating factor in SAA requirement assessment using

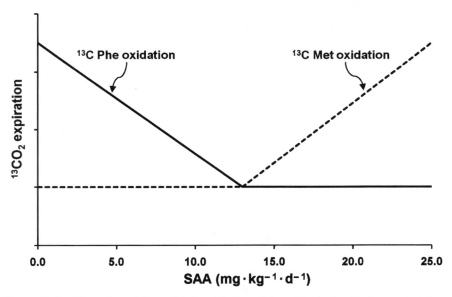

Figure 13.2 Illustration of direct (Met) and indirect (phenylalanine) oxidation methodology for determining a Met requirement. See text for details. SAA, sulfur amino acids.

the oxidation methodology. Interestingly, the indirect oxidation methodology has predicted a minimal SAA requirement of about $13 \, \text{mg} \cdot \text{kg}^{-1} \cdot \text{d}^{-1}$ for both adult humans and school-age children [36, 38], and about 60% of this need can be furnished by Cys.

13.2.4 Sulfur Amino Acid Precursors

The SAA bioefficacy of several precursors, isomers, or analogs of Met or Cys has been extensively reviewed previously [24, 51]. Glutathione, however, deserves special mention here. It can serve as a fully effective endogenous reservoir of Cys, and the GSH found in food products [13] is 100% efficacious on a molar basis in furnishing bioavailable Cys [24, 51–54]. Because of the important body compounds, including GSH, derived from Cys, one could question how Cys is partitioned for its various functions during times of Cys deficiency. Our work with chickens fed diets singly deficient in cyst(e)ine suggested that protein synthesis is prioritized over GSH synthesis during periods of Cys deficiency. Thus, Cys deficiency resulted in reduced liver GSH, and it remained low during graded Cys dosing until the Cys requirement (for maximal growth rate) was reached, after which hepatic GSH increased rapidly [52, 55]. How Cys is partitioned for taurine, coenzyme A, and PAPS synthesis during periods of Cys deficiency is not known [56].

Cyst(e)ine and Met responses have also been studied in animals fed a protein-free diet. Several investigators have observed that Met supplementation of a protein-free diet reduces body weight loss and improves nitrogen retention in rats [57], chickens [58], pigs [59], and dogs [60]. Our work with young chicks [61] has confirmed an earlier suggestion [62] that the Met response does not result from Met per se but instead from Met furnishing sulfur for Cys biosynthesis via transsulfuration. Thus, Cys supplementation of a protein-free diet elicits a response equal to or greater than Met. During protein turnover (degradation and synthesis), a portion of the amino acids released from body protein is oxidized and therefore not available for resynthesis of new protein. The Cys response observed when a protein-free diet is fed implies that this amino acid is substantially depleted from body pools, making it the first-limiting amino acid for endogenous protein synthesis.

13.2.4.1 *N-Acetyl-L-Cysteine* Transsulfuration may provide inadequate Cys in preterm infants and certain members of the geriatric population. Some have also suggested that Cys should be considered a conditionally indispensable amino acid, contingent on Met status of the animal or human [63]. Sulfur amino acid supplementation of human diets, however, presents problems. Thus, Met is unpalatable, Cys is unstable, and cystine is insoluble. In both its reduced (Cys) and oxidized (cystine) forms, cyst(e)ine is considered a poor choice for both enteral and parenteral nutrition formulas. *N*-acetyl-L-cysteine (NAC) serves as an effective precursor for Cys because most tissues in the body possess the ability to remove the acetyl group and therefore furnish Cys [44, 63, 64]. Because the α-amino group of Cys is acetylated, NAC is protected against Maillard destruction [65], and NAC is also soluble. Clinical interest in NAC (and lipoic acid, which causes increased intracellular cysteine and

GSH [66]) stems from its antioxidant activity and its role in treating acetaminophen hepatotoxicity, chronic bronchitis, diabetes, cancer, sepsis, HIV infection, heart disease, and acute myocardial infarction [67–73].

13.2.4.2 Other Sulfur Amino Acid Precursors

Several compounds, both food components and synthetic compounds, can contribute to, or affect, SAA responses and requirements. Glutathione, inorganic sulfate, and NAC have already been discussed. Regarding isomers of Met and cyst(e)ine, neither D-Cys [74] nor the keto analog of Cys [75] have L-Cys bioactivity. Both D-Met and keto-Met, however, are well utilized as Met precursors by most animals [51, 76, 77], although D-Met is utilized poorly by apes and humans [43, 78, 79]. The DL-α-hydroxy analog of Met is a synthetic compound that is widely used as a Met precursor in animal nutrition [51]. It has been used in low nitrogen formulations for renal patients [80, 81]. Its efficacy as a source of Met is good, although not 100% on a molar basis [51, 82, 83]. Another synthetic compound, L-2-oxothiazolidine-4-carboxylic acid (OTC), has been shown to have excellent L-Cys (and GSH) bioactivity [55, 84].

Several other SAA compounds can exist in variable quantities in foods and feeds. Taurine in animal products has no Met or Cys precursor bioactivity for either chicks [23] or rats [85], although taurine per se has been suggested as being a possible limiting nutrient for neonates [86]. Plant-based food products contain both *S*-methylmethionine and dimethylsulfonio-propionate [12, 87], and *S*-methylmethionine can spare the dietary need for Met when diets are low in either choline or betaine; it also can replace *S*-adenosylmethionine as a methyl donor in choline biosynthesis from phosphatidylaminoethanol [12]. Lanthionine is a cross-linked SAA that is formed in food products exposed to heat and alkaline conditions [14, 88, 89]. It can be prominent in high cyst(e)ine products such as feather meal and poultry by-product meal used in animal feeds. The lanthionine absorbed from the gut can be cleaved by cystathionase [90], yielding both L- and D-Cys. Synthetic DL-lanthionine was found to possess 35% L-Cys activity when administered orally to chickens [15].

Milk-based foods may contain small quantities of SAA oxidation products (Met sulfoxide, Met sulfone, cysteic acid), because hydrogen peroxide is often used in milk sterilization processes [1–4]. Among these compounds, only Met sulfoxide has Met-sparing bioactivity, about 70% relative to L-Met [51]. Small amounts of Hcy also are present in some foods. Work with chicks using synthetic L-Hcy indicated that when serving as a source of Met, L-Hcy had 65% of the growth promoting efficacy of L-Met. As a source of Cys, however, in a Met adequate but Cys deficient diet, L-Hcy had a Cys replacement value of near 100% [91–93].

Choline is not a sulfur containing compound, but among its three primary functions (precursor for acetyl choline, phospholipid, and betaine formation), its role in biological methylation (via betaine and its contribution of methyl groups to the folate pool) seems to result in a Met-sparing effect. This effect is well known in animal nutrition where excess dietary Met is known to be capable of sparing (or eliminating) the dietary need for preformed choline in mammals, and excess dietary choline can reduce the dietary requirement for Met [6, 45, 94–96]. Unfortunately, the choline-Met interrelationship has not been clearly defined in humans.

13.3 SULFUR AMINO ACID TOXICITY

Characterization of the toxicity profiles for Met and Cys is important for human health and nutrition. In this regard, toxicity refers to the adverse effects of ingesting SAA compounds in excess [97]. Because of poor organoleptic properties, humans would not typically consume diets containing excess concentrations of Met or Cys [10, 51], but ingestion of pharmacologic doses as dietary supplements could lead to health issues [97]. Dietary SAA supplements are gaining popularity in the clinical setting due to their relation to Hcy and GSH. Moreover, nonprescription dietary SAA supplements are available to the general public where they are marketed purporting such claims as enhanced protein synthesis, restoration of hair growth, and protection against toxins. Animal research is critical for defining upper tolerance limits for SAA, and the best approach to elucidate potential risks to humans is through comparative species investigations. For a complete literature review on the adverse effects of ingesting SAA by animals and humans, the reader is encouraged to read the 1992 document prepared by the Life Sciences Research Office of the Federation of American Societies for Experimental Biology [97].

13.3.1 Methionine Toxicity

Methionine was first discovered as part of a dipeptide with phenylalanine by Mueller in 1922 [98, 99], and later characterized after being isolated from a casein hydrolysate [100]. Among the classic 10 "essential" amino acids for animal growth originally defined by Rose and coworkers [101–103], Met in excess of its requirement is considered the most growth depressing and noxious [51, 97, 104–110]. Because of this and also because inborn errors of SAA metabolism, particularly homocystinuria and homocysteinemia, are well-studied problems, the literature is extensive on manifestations of excess Met ingestion [51, 111–116]. However, a review of literature in this area reveals the complexities of the integrative metabolic pathways involving SAA. For instance, the Met cycle, irreversible transsulfuration of Met into Cys, and alternate pathways allow for a diverse array of metabolites and end products resulting from Met. Moreover, influences of diet composition cannot be ignored, and previous research highlights the importance of both level and source of dietary protein on the toxic effects of Met [51, 105, 110, 117].

Most rat studies have used young, growing rats fed low-protein, purified diets containing casein [97, 106, 110, 117]. While informative, the application of these studies toward defining upper tolerances for humans is limited. The toxic effects of supplementing individual amino acids in excess of physiological requirements are lessened as dietary protein content increases [110, 117]. Thus, interpretation of data from studies using low-protein diets may lead to erroneous conclusions, because Met toxic effects are amplified under these dietary circumstances. When growing rats [104], chicks [108], and pigs [107, 109] were fed diets adequate in protein for each respective species, Met was found to be the most noxious amino acid in terms of reduced growth and food intake. These studies may be more beneficial in defining upper tolerance limits for humans. However, caution must be exercised when extrapolating data from animal models to humans. True effects of excess Met can only come from direct administration of Met to humans, or by studying individuals displaying congenital errors in SAA metabolism. To this end, human subjects receiving 30 g of Met intravenously experienced untoward effects including nausea, vomiting, increased sweating, chill followed by fever, moderate hypotension, tachycardia, and intermittent disorientation [118]. Thus, strong evidence suggests that ingestion of Met in excess of its physiological requirement results in adverse effects.

The biochemical basis by which Met exerts its noxious effects has long been debated. Methionine is interesting because of the many unique metabolic intermediates produced during its degradation. Homocysteine is produced through transmethylation, Cys through transsulfuration, and 2-keto-4-(methylthio)butyric acid, 3-methylthiopropionate, methanethiol, and hydrogen sulfide through the transaminative pathway [119, 120]. Under conditions of Met deficiency, the Met cycle (i.e., transmethylation to Hcy and remethylation of Hcy back to Met) predominates to conserve Met [121]. When dietary levels of Met approach adequacy, more Met is converted to Cys via transsulfuration, making Cys a conditionally essential amino acid. The balance between remethylation and transsulfuration (with Hcy poised at the metabolic branch-point) is responsible for Met flux [21, 121–124], and this balance is known to depend on Hcy concentration [122]. Plasma Hcy has been shown to increase after ingestion of excess Met by some researchers [111, 112, 125], but not by others [126, 127]. Confusion in this area may be related to vitamin deficiency of the experimental animals under conditions of excess Met [105, 110]; notably, the vitamin B6 requirement of chicks was shown to be increased 44% when chicks were fed 3% excess Met in a soy-based diet containing 20% protein [128]. While the effect of excess Met on plasma Hcy concentrations seems to be variable, this point is critical in light of the fact that elevated plasma Hcy has been implicated as an independent risk factor for cardiovascular disease [129, 130]. Whether ingestion of equimolar excess quantities of Hcy and Met results in similar physiological outcomes remains a debatable point [127, 131–133].

When chicks were fed a purified diet (containing the equivalent of 14.8% crude protein) supplemented with either 1.5% Met or 1.36% Hcy (equimolar to 1.5% Met), rate and efficiency of weight gain were reduced [127]. However, chicks fed excess Hcy did not display the tissue damage characteristic of Met toxicity. Pathologies associated with ingestion of excess Met by rats, guinea pigs, and chicks include hypoglycemia, opisthotonus, fatty liver, reduced hepatic ATP concentration, renal hypertrophy due to tubule dilatation, and extensive pancreatic acinar damage [134–137]. Evidence from three neonates with congenital hypermethioninemia confirms such tissue damage also occurs in humans [138]; these infants each exhibited progressive drowsiness and opisthotonus, and died by 12 weeks of age. Most strikingly, 2-keto-4-(methylthio)butyric acid, the keto-analog of Met and first intermediate in the transamination (i.e., alternative) pathway of Met, was found at high concentrations in the urine of these infants. In animal models, excess Hcy leads to some of these symptoms, but it does not produce the hallmark signs of Met toxicity: hemolytic anemia, darkened spleens due to iron deposition, and splenic hemosiderosis [127, 136, 139, 140]. Evidence suggests that while the transmethylation and transsulfuration pathways aid in adaptation to high Met intake [141], the alternative pathway becomes increasingly more important as Met ingestion exceeds the physiological requirement, thus serving as an "overflow" mechanism [119, 133].

It was originally believed that the labile methyl group of Met was at least partly responsible for the toxicity of Met [110, 132, 133]. Thus, addition of glycine or serine to low-protein diets containing excess Met has been shown to partially ameliorate Met toxicity by enhancing Met oxidation [110, 127, 132, 139, 142, 143]. However, it is still unclear whether the ameliorative effect of glycine is due to its role in eliminating excess methyl groups (e.g., synthesis of sarcosine by glycine N-methyltransferase) or as a precursor for serine, which condenses with Hcy to form cystathionine. While glycine and serine partly alleviate toxicity of both Met and Hcy, differences in tissue damage between Met and Hcy would suggest that Hcy cannot be solely responsible for Met toxicity [110]. Moreover, when choline, betaine, or sarcosine are used to supply methyl equivalents similar to levels supplied by Met, no signs of Met toxicity are observed [105]. This is important because recent reviews [144, 145] have emphasized the need for supplemental betaine, in combination with B vitamins, to prevent homocystinuria. Thus, while evidence suggests the methyl group of Met may be partly involved in Met toxicity, it cannot fully explain the adverse effects observed in experimental animal models.

Interestingly, incorporation of some methyl-containing compounds, including dimethylthetin [110], S-methyl-L-cysteine [146], and 3-methylthiopropionate [120, 127], to low-protein diets reduces weight gain and feed intake, and causes gross tissue damage strikingly similar to the effects of Met per se. This suggests that metabolism of the methylthiol moiety, not the methyl group, is at the heart of Met toxicity [120]. Transamination of Met produces 2-keto-4-(methylthio)butyric acid, which is oxidatively decarboxylated to 3-methylthiopropionate, an intermediate in the Met transamination pathway [147]. It was Steele and Benevenga [120] who first suggested that methanethiol and hydrogen sulfide, two very toxic products, could be produced from 3-methylthiopropionate. Reports of elevated blood concentrations of 2-keto-4-(methylthio)butyric acid, 3-methylthiopropionate, and methanethiol in humans confirm that aberrations in Met metabolism can result in noxious metabolites [148–151].

It is still unclear whether the transaminative pathway is more or less important when subjects receive excess dietary Met, or if they display elevated tissue Met concentrations due to inborn metabolic errors. Recent evidence suggests the gut possesses significant capacity for transmethylation and transsulfuration [152]. Additionally, the gut may play a critical role in SAA detoxification by demethylation of methanethiol to hydrogen sulfide, and subsequent oxidation of hydrogen sulfide primarily to thiosulfate, an innocuous compound [153, 154]. In contrast to dietary effects of excess Met, human patients displaying hypermethioninemia have been known to survive childhood with few medical complications [148]. Thus, more research is required to elucidate the effects of excess dietary Met, but it seems that exogenous excesses of Met may have the potential to cause more acute adverse effects than inborn metabolic errors.

13.3.2 Cyst(e)ine Toxicity

Cystine (oxidized) or cysteine (reduced, i.e., Cys) was the second amino acid discovered after asparagine. It was isolated from urinary stones by Wollaston in 1810 [155]; he termed the compound "cystic oxide." This SAA was later properly renamed "cystine" by Berzelius [156] and further characterized chemically by Thaulow in 1838 [157]. Therefore, it comes as no surprise that a great deal of research has been amassed on cyst(e)ine. The toxic nature of cystine has been known for some time [158, 159], and many studies have referenced deleterious effects due to this amino acid [110]. However, few studies have investigated differences in toxicity profiles between the reduced (Cys) and oxidized (cystine) forms of this SAA. The dearth of information regarding cyst(e)ine toxicity is likely because Cys is considered a conditionally essential amino acid, based on Met status of the animal [17–21]. Additionally, inborn metabolic errors resulting in high urinary excretion of cystine (i.e., cystinuria) were documented long ago [160], but such aberrations have been associated with minimal risk if renal calculi are minimized. Only recently has emphasis been placed on elucidating whether toxicity is due to Cys per se or perhaps one of its metabolites.

Similar to Met, the noxious effects of cyst(e)ine have often been tested in low-protein diets [106, 117, 158], which may amplify the toxic effects. However, there are reports available where excess cyst(e)ine was included in diets containing adequate concentrations of SAA and protein [52, 104, 158, 161]. These data will be useful in defining upper tolerance limits for humans, who often supplement their diets with bolus tablets of amino acids. There has been a lack of emphasis on separating the differential noxious effects of cyst(e)ine redox forms. While both forms are known to support growth equally well [22], evidence suggests Cys and cystine cause very different outcomes when supplied at pharmacological levels [161, 162]. Also striking is the fact that excess cyst(e)ine has been consistently shown to cause mortality in rats and chicks [106, 117, 158, 161], yet little attention has been paid to this deleterious outcome. Few would argue that the tissue damage, anorexia, and reduced growth resulting from excess Met ingestion is more pernicious than death resulting from excess cyst(e)ine ingestion.

Ingestion of excess cyst(e)ine causes depressed weight gain and food intake in rats, chicks, and pigs [104, 106, 117, 161, 163], though not nearly to the extent of Met. There is also evidence that a small excess of Cys, relative to Met, supplied in an SAA-deficient diet causes a nutritional imbalance [22, 76, 164, 165]. Tissue damage in rats having ingested large excesses of supplemental cyst(e)ine (i.e., 1% to 20% of diet) has been characterized by renal tubule necrosis [158, 163], hemorrhagic hepatic necrosis [166], and pulmonary congestion and pleural effusion [161]. Evidence from injection studies with infant rodents also suggests severe neurodegenerative changes in the retina and hypothalamus [167–171], which has led some researchers to suggest that Cys is an endogenous excitotoxin [172, 173]. This theory is based on evidence suggesting Cys selectively activates N-methyl-D-aspartate receptors, much like glutamate, to cause brain damage [174]. However, caution must be exercised when interpreting these results because only through subcutaneous administration of a large L-Cys dose (10 mmol/kg body weight) to immature rodents were neurotoxic effects observed. Due to the extensive oxidation of dietary Cys by splanchnic tissues, it is unlikely that excess oral Cys would elevate blood, much less brain, concentrations to levels capable of causing neurotoxic damage in normal subjects. It is clear, though, that the biochemical lesions caused by excess Cys ingestion are quite different from those caused by excess Met.

Strong evidence suggests that tissue concentrations of Cys are maintained at low levels under myriad physiological conditions, mainly through synthesis of cysteine-sulfinate by Cys dioxygenase [122, 175]. Cysteinesulfinate-independent catabolism of Cys occurs through a host of desulfhydration systems which remove the sulfur moiety of Cys before it is oxidized to pyruvate. Hydrogen sulfide is a physiologically relevant product of each desulfhydration pathway [175, 176], and while these pathways are thought to be only minimally responsive to excess Cys, the likelihood is great that this toxic metabolite is produced with elevated levels of tissue Cys [177]. Endogenously produced hydrogen sulfide is a smooth muscle relaxant [178] and likely serves as a neuromodulator [179, 180]. Hydrogen sulfide chemistry has been studied for several hundred years, and it is well established that this lipid-soluble gas is toxic due to its inhibition of cytochrome c oxidase [181, 182]. Thus, hydrogen sulfide serves as a cellular asphyxiant by disrupting oxidative phosphorylation, and it is far more potent than even cyanide. Moreover, hydrogen sulfide was recently shown to be a direct genotoxic agent [183]. Abe and Kimura [179] showed that hydrogen sulfide enhanced N-methyl-D-aspartate currents in rat hippocampal slices by increasing neuronal intracellular cAMP levels; a role concurrent with initial findings that Cys was an excitotoxic mimetic. Interestingly, hydrogen sulfide is a common intermediate in the catabolic pathways of both Met and Cys, providing a link between these SAA that may have important physiological consequences in times of dietary excess. As it stands, the splanchnic tissues appear to provide a critical buffer between excess dietary SAA intake and lethal production of toxic metabolites.

13.3.3 *N*-Acetyl-L-Cysteine Toxicity

Inclusion of cyst(e)ine in enteral or parenteral formulas is problematic because (1) free L-Cys is highly susceptible to oxidation, and is therefore unstable, and (2) L-cystine is the least soluble crystalline amino acid. N-acetyl-L-cysteine has been studied for many years, both as a therapeutic agent and dietary precursor of Cys. Oral administration of NAC remains a primary treatment for acetaminophen overdose in humans [71], and it has also been shown to positively affect overall antioxidant status [72]. In this regard, NAC serves as a direct antioxidant per se, but more importantly, as a precursor for Cys, the availability of which is rate limiting for hepatic GSH synthesis. Recent evidence from our laboratory suggests NAC is much less toxic than L-Cys [44]. Ingestion of 2% excess Cys as NAC was innocuous to chick growth, and 4% excess Cys supplied as NAC (i.e., nine times the dietary Cys requirement) reduced growth just 34% [44]. *N*-acetyl-L-cysteine is advantageous because it is highly soluble and is more heat stable than Cys due to its α-amino nitrogen being protected from Maillard destruction.

Due to the increased demand for nutritional supplements and the ease with which they can be obtained by consumers, it seems prudent to eliminate L-Cys as a nutritional supplement and replace it with NAC.

13.3.4   Glutathione and Other Sulfur Amino Acid Precursors

There are no reports of adverse effects of ingesting excess concentrations of GSH. Unpublished work from our laboratory showed that when GSH supplied 2% excess Cys, no deleterious effects on chick growth or well-being were observed. What is important in understanding the lack of toxicity of GSH is that this compound is simply a tripeptide of glutamate, Cys, and glycine. Thus, while GSH may be absorbed by peptide transporters in the proximal intestine, GSH is more likely degraded to its constituent amino acids in the gut. Moreover, any GSH entering the portal circulation would definitely be degraded by hepatic γ-glutamyltransferase. While there have been reports suggesting oral GSH can increase tissue GSH levels [184–187], one must scrutinize the experimental conditions in which these studies were conducted. Rat diets used in some of these studies were likely deficient in Cys, considering they were based on AIN-76A formulations [188]. Because these diets were Cys-deficient, there was definite potential to reduce GSH synthesis and ultimately shift the physiological redox status towards an oxidized state. Thus, it cannot be excluded that oral GSH supplied to these SAA-deficient rats simply served as a source of dietary Cys, while the GSH synthesis rate was elevated to counteract the oxidized environment in vivo. Without a doubt, GSH is 100% efficacious as a source of dietary Cys in chicks and rats [51], and GSH synthesis is known to be a "demand-led" process [189], increasing under conditions in which endogenous GSH is depleted. Regardless of whether dietary GSH supplements affect tissue GSH levels, the public's general perception is most definitely positive towards exogenous antioxidants, and there exists no evidence that consuming large quantities of GSH is harmful to humans.

Another point that requires further investigation is whether excess dietary Cys affects tissue GSH levels. It is well established that Cys availability is limiting for GSH synthesis, and provision of increasing Cys from deficient to adequate levels results in concomitant increases in tissue GSH levels [52]. Additionally, work with chicks and rats [55] suggests that increases in hepatic GSH levels are possible when Cys is supplied in excess of the dietary requirement for growth. While not entirely clear, this phenomenon lends credence to the prioritization of dietary nutrients for physiological functions, with growth almost always the primary function for amino acids. In this respect, the use of dietary Cys for synthesis of GSH should not theoretically occur until after the physiological requirement of Cys for growth has been met [190]. Prioritization of nutrients for various physiological purposes is an area of research that requires more focus, especially for amino acids such as Cys that have many roles beyond protein synthesis.

Neither cysteic acid nor taurine are efficacious as sources of Cys for growth of rats and chicks [51]. However, ingestion of excess cysteic acid by rats causes histopathological lesions similar to those described for cystine [191, 192]. In contrast, taurine consumed at concentrations up to 10% of the diet produces no adverse effects whatsoever in rats [191]. The lack of toxicity is not entirely surprising considering taurine is the most abundant free SAA in the body. Moreover, supplemental taurine is unlikely to have high metabolic value because it is rapidly excreted in the urine without being metabolized [193]. Finally, L-2-oxothiazolidine-4-carboxylate, a Cys precursor, has been shown to be safe when administered to mice and rats at high concentrations [194]. Thus, current evidence suggests only certain Cys catabolites have the potential to cause adverse effects.

REFERENCES

1. Fox, P.F., Kosikowski, F.V. (1967). Some effects of hydrogen peroxide on casein and its implications in cheese making. *Journal of Dairy Science, 50,* 1183–1188.

2. Yang, S.F. (1970). Sulfoxide formation from methionine or its sulfide analogs during aerobic oxidation of sulfite. *Biochemistry, 9,* 5008–5014.

3. Anderson, G.H., Li, G.S., Jones, J.D., Bender, F. (1975). Effect of hydrogen peroxide treatment on the nutritional quality of rapeseed flour fed to weanling rats. *Journal of Nutrition, 105,* 317–325.

4. Anderson, G.H., Ashley, D.V., Jones, J.D. (1976). Utilization of L-methionine sulfoxide, L-methionine sulfone and cysteic acid by the weanling rat. *Journal of Nutrition, 106,* 1108–1114.

5. Parsons, C.M., Hashimoto, K., Wedekind, K.J., Han, Y., Baker, D.H. (1992). Effects of overprocessing on availability of amino acids and energy in soybean meal. *Poultry Science, 71,* 133–140.

6. National Research Council. (1994). *Nutrient Requirements of Poultry.* Washington, D.C.: National Academies Press.

7. Miller, E.L., Huang, Y.X., Kasinathan, S., Rayner, B., Luzzana, U., Moretti, V.M., Valfr, F., Torrissen, K.R., Jensen, H.B., Opstvedt, J. (2001). Heat-damaged protein has reduced ileal true digestibility of cystine and aspartic acid in chicks. *Journal of Animal Science, 79*(Suppl 1), 65.

8. Howe, E.E., Jansen, G.R., Gilfillan, E.W. (1965). Amino acid supplementation of cereal grains as related to the world food supply. *American Journal of Clinical Nutrition, 16,* 315–320.

9. Baker, D.H., Edwards, H.M. III, Strunk, C.S., Emmert, J.L., Peter, C.M., Mavromichalis, I., Parr, T.M. (1999). Single versus multiple deficiencies of methionine, zinc, riboflavin, vitamin B-6 and choline elicit surprising growth responses in young chicks. *Journal of Nutrition, 129,* 2239–2245.

10. Bos, C., Huneau, J.F., Gaudichon, C. (2009). Sulfur amino acid contents of dietary proteins: Daily intake and requirements. In Masella, R. and Mazza, G., eds., *Glutathione and Sulfur Amino Acids in Human Health and Disease.* New York: Wiley.

11. Zeisel, S.H., Mar, M.H., Howe, J.C., Holden, J.M. (2003). Concentrations of choline-containing compounds and betaine in common foods. *Journal of Nutrition, 133,* 1302–1307.

12. Augspurger, N.R., Scherer, C.S., Garrow, T.A., Baker, D.H. (2005). Dietary S-methyl-methionine, a component of foods, has choline-sparing activity in chickens. *Journal of Nutrition, 135,* 1712–1717.

13. Wiezlicker, G.T., Hagen, T.M., Tones, D.P. (1989). Glutathione in food. *Journal of Food Composition Analogy*, 2, 327–337.

14. Jones, D.B., Caldwell, A., Horn, M.J. (1948). The availability of DL-lanthionine for the promotion of growth in young rats when added to a cystine- and methionine-deficient diet. *Journal of Biological Chemistry*, 176, 65–69.

15. Robbins, K.R., Baker, D.H., Finley, J.W. (1980). Studies on the utilization of lysino-alanine and lanthionine. *Journal of Nutrition*, 110, 907–915.

16. Laidlaw, S.A., Grosvenor, M., Kopple, J.D. (1990). The taurine content of common food-stuffs. *Journal of Parenteral and Enteral Nutrition*, 14, 183–188.

17. Womack, M., Rose, W.C. (1942). The partial replacement of dietary methionine by cystine for purposes of growth. *Journal of Biological Chemistry*, 141, 375–379.

18. du Vigneaud, V., Kilmer, G.W., Rachele, J.R., Cohn, M. (1944). On the mechanism of the conversion *in vivo* of methionine to cystine. *Journal of Biological Chemistry*, 155, 645–651.

19. du Vigneaud, V. (1952). *Trail of Research in Sulfur Chemistry and Metabolism and Related Fields*. Ithaca, NY: Cornell University Press.

20. Finkelstein, J.D., Mudd, S.H. (1967). Trans-sulfuration in mammals. The methionine-sparing effect of cystine. *Journal of Biological Chemistry*, 242, 873–880.

21. Finkelstein, J.D., Martin, J.J., Harris, B.J. (1988). Methionine metabolism in mammals. The methionine-sparing effect of cystine. *Journal of Biological Chemistry*, 263, 11750–11754.

22. Graber, G., Baker, D.H. (1971). Sulfur amino acid nutrition of the growing chick: Quantitative aspects concerning the efficacy of dietary methionine, cysteine and cystine. *Journal of Animal Science*, 33, 1005–1011.

23. Sasse, C.E., Baker, D.H. (1974). Sulfur utilization by the chick with emphasis on the effect of inorganic sulfate on the cystine-methionine interrelationship. *Journal of Nutrition*, 104, 244–251.

24. Baker, D.H., Utilization of precursors for L-amino acids. (1994). In D'Mello, J.P.F., ed., *Amino Acids in Farm Animal Nutrition*, pp. 37–64. Wallingford, Oxon, UK: CAB International.

25. Sowers, J.E., Stockland, W.L., Meade, R.J. (1972). L-methionine and L-cystine require-ments of the growing rat. *Journal of Animal Science*, 35, 782–788.

26. Teeter, R.G., Baker, D.H., Corbin, J.E. (1978). Methionine and cystine requirements of the cat. *Journal of Nutrition*, 108, 291–295.

27. Halpin, K.M., Baker, D.H. (1984). Selenium deficiency and transsulfuration in the chick. *Journal of Nutrition*, 114, 606–612.

28. Hirakawa, D.A., Baker, D.H. (1985). Sulfur amino acid nutrition of the growing puppy: Determination of dietary requirements for methionine and cystine. *Nutrition Research*, 5, 631–642.

29. Chung, T.K., Baker, D.H. (1992). Maximal portion of the young pig's sulfur amino acid requirement that can be furnished by cystine. *Journal of Animal Science*, 70, 1182–1187.

30. Baker, D.H., Becker, D.E., Norton, H.W., Jensen, A.H., Harmon, B.G. (1966). Quantitat-ive evaluation of the tryptophan, methionine and lysine needs of adult swine for mainten-ance. *Journal of Nutrition*, 89, 441–447.

31. Said, A.K., Hegsted, D.M. (1970). Response of adult rats to low dietary levels of essential amino acids. *Journal of Nutrition, 100*, 1363–1375.

32. Fuller, M.F., McWilliam, R., Wang, T.C., Giles, L.R. (1989). The optimum dietary amino acid pattern for growing pigs. II. Requirements for maintenance and for tissue protein accretion. *British Journal of Nutrition, 62*, 255–267.

33. Rose, W.C., Wixom, R.L. (1955). The amino acid requirements of man. XIII. The sparing effect of cystine on the methionine requirement. *Journal of Biological Chemistry, 216*, 753–773.

34. Fukagawa, N.K., Yu, Y.M., Young, V.R. (1998). Methionine and cysteine kinetics at different intakes of methionine and cysteine in elderly men and women. *American Journal of Clinical Nutrition, 68*, 380–388.

35. Young, V.R. (2001). Got some amino acids to spare? *American Journal of Clinical Nutrition, 74*, 709–711.

36. Di Buono, M., Wykes, L.J., Ball, R.O., Pencharz, P.B. (2001). Dietary cysteine reduces the methionine requirement in men. *American Journal of Clinical Nutrition, 74*, 761–766.

37. Di Buono, M., Wykes, L.J., Cole, D.E., Ball, R.O., Pencharz, P.B. (2003). Regulation of sulfur amino acid metabolism in men in response to changes in sulfur amino acid intakes. *Journal of Nutrition, 133*, 733–739.

38. Humayun, M.A., Turner, J.M., Elango, R., Rafii, M., Langos, V., Ball, R.O., Pencharz, P.B. (2006). Minimum methionine requirement and cysteine sparing of methionine in healthy school-age children. *American Journal of Clinical Nutrition, 84*, 1080–1085.

39. Ball, R.O., Courtney-Martin, G., Pencharz, P.B. (2006). The in vivo sparing of methionine by cysteine in sulfur amino acid requirements in animal models and adult humans. *Journal of Nutrition, 136*, 1682S–1693S.

40. Baker, D.H. (1986). Problems and pitfalls in animal experiments designed to establish dietary requirements for essential nutrients. *Journal of Nutrition, 116*, 2339–2349.

41. Sasse, C.E., Baker, D.H. (1974). Factors affecting sulfate-sulfur utilization by the young chick. *Poultry Science, 53*, 652–662.

42. Smith, J.T. (1973). An optimal level of inorganic sulfate for the diet of a rat. *Journal of Nutrition, 103*, 1008–1011.

43. Zezulka, A.Y., Calloway, D.H. (1976). Nitrogen retention in men fed isolated soybean protein supplemented with L-methionine, D-methionine, N-acetyl-L-methionine, or inorganic sulfate. *Journal of Nutrition, 106*, 1286–1291.

44. Dilger, R.N., Baker, D.H. (2007). Oral N-acetyl-L-cysteine is a safe and effective precursor of cysteine. *Journal of Animal Science, 85*, 1712–1718.

45. National Research Council. (1998). *Nutrient Requirements of Swine*. Washington, D.C.: National Academies Press.

46. Di Buono, M., Wykes, L.J., Ball, R.O., Pencharz, P.B. (2001). Total sulfur amino acid requirement in young men as determined by indicator amino acid oxidation with L-[1–13C]phenylalanine. *American Journal of Clinical Nutrition, 74*, 756–760.

47. Food and Nutrition Board, Institute of Medicine. (2002). *Dietary Reference Intakes for Energy, Carbohydrate, Fiber, Fat, Fatty Acids, Cholesterol, Protein, and Amino Acids (Macronutrients): Preliminary Report*. Washington, D.C.: National Academy Press.

48. Rose, W.C., Wixom, R.L., Lockhart, H.B., Lambert, G.F. (1955). The amino acid requirements of man. XV. The valine requirement; summary and final observations. *Journal of Biological Chemistry, 217,* 987–995.

49. Heger, J., Van Phung, T., Krizova, L. (2002). Efficiency of amino acid utilization in the growing pig at suboptimal levels of intake: Lysine, threonine, sulphur amino acids, and tryptophan. *Journal of Animal Physiology and Animal Nutrition, 86,* 153–165.

50. Baker, D.H. (2005). Tolerance for branched-chain amino acids in experimental animals and humans. *Journal of Nutrition, 135,* 1585S–1590S.

51. Baker, D.H. (2006). Comparative species utilization and toxicity of sulfur amino acids. *Journal of Nutrition, 136,* 1670S–1675S.

52. Boebel, K.P., Baker, D.H. (1983). Blood and liver concentrations of glutathione, and plasma concentrations of sulfur-containing amino acids in chicks fed deficient, adequate, or excess levels of dietary cysteine. *Proceedings of the Society for Experimental Biology and Medicine, 172,* 498–501.

53. Dyer, H.M., du Vigneaud, V. (1936). The utilization of glutathione in connection with a cystine-deficient diet. *Journal of Biological Chemistry, 115,* 543–549.

54. Harter, J.M., Baker, D.H. (1977). Sulfur amino acid activity of glutathione, DL-α-hydroxy-methionine, and α-keto-methionine in chicks. *Proceedings of the Society for Experimental Biology and Medicine, 156,* 201–204.

55. Chung, T.K., Funk, M.A., Baker, D.H. (1990). L-2-oxothiazolidine-4-carboxylate as a cysteine precursor: Efficacy for growth and hepatic glutathione synthesis in chicks and rats. *Journal of Nutrition, 120,* 158–165.

56. Baker, D.H. (2005). Comparative nutrition and metabolism: Explication of open questions with emphasis on protein and amino acids. *Proceedings of the National Academy of Sciences USA, 102,* 17897–17902.

57. Yoshida, A., Moritoki, K. (1974). Nitrogen sparing action of methionine and threonine in rats receiving a protein free diet. *Nutrition Reports International, 9,* 159–168.

58. Okumura, J., Muramatsu, T. (1978). Effect of dietary methionine and arginine on the excretion of nitrogen in cocks fed a protein-free diet. *Japanese Poultry Science, 15,* 69–73.

59. Lubaszewska, S., Pastuszewska, B., Kielanowski, J. (1973). Effect of methionine supplementation of a protein-free diet on the nitrogen excretion in rats and pigs. *Zeitschrift fur Tierphysiologie, Tierernahrung, und Futtermittelkunde, 31,* 120–128.

60. Allison, J.B., Anderson, J.A., Seeley, R.D. (1947). Some effects of methionine on the utilization of nitrogen in the adult dog. *Journal of Nutrition, 33,* 361–370.

61. Webel, D.M., Baker, D.H. (1999). Cystine is the first-limiting amino acid for the utilization of endogenous amino acids in chicks fed a protein-free diet. *Nutrition Research, 19,* 569–577.

62. Muramatsu, T., Okumura, J. (1980). The nitrogen-sparing effect of methionine in chicks receiving a protein-free diet supplemented with arginine: Effect of various methionine substituents. *British Poultry Science, 21,* 273–280.

63. Shoveller, A.K., Brunton, J.A., Brand, O., Pencharz, P.B., Ball, R.O. (2006). N-acetylcysteine is a highly available precursor for cysteine in the neonatal piglet receiving parenteral nutrition. *Journal of Parenteral and Enteral Nutrition, 30,* 133–142.

64. Baker, D.H., Han, Y. (1993). Bioavailable level and source of cysteine determine protein quality of a commercial enteral product: Adequacy of tryptophan but deficiency of

cysteine for rats fed an enteral product prepared fresh or stored beyond shelf life. *Journal of Nutrition*, *123*, 541–546.

65. Baker, D.H., Bafundo, K.W., Boebel, K.P., Czarnecki, G.L., Halpin, K.M. (1984). Methionine peptides as potential food supplements: Efficacy and susceptibility to Maillard browning. *Journal of Nutrition*, *114*, 292–297.

66. Han, D., Handelman, G., Marcocci, L., Sen, C.K., Roy, S., Kobuchi, H., Tritschler, H.J., Flohe, L., Packer, L. (1997). Lipoic acid increases de novo synthesis of cellular glutathione by improving cystine utilization. *Biofactors*, *6*, 321–338.

67. Atmaca, G. (2004). Antioxidant effects of sulfur-containing amino acids. *Yonsei Medical Journal*, *45*, 776–788.

68. Santangelo, F. (2003). Intracellular thiol concentration modulating inflammatory response: Influence on the regulation of cell functions through cysteine prodrug approach. *Current Medicinal Chemistry*, *10*, 2599–2610.

69. Quadrilatero, J., Hoffman-Goetz, L. (2005). N-acetyl-l-cysteine protects intestinal lymphocytes from apoptotic death after acute exercise in adrenalectomized mice. *American Journal of Physiology. Regulatory, Integrative, and Comparative Physiology*, *288*, R1664–R1672.

70. Hsu, C.C., Yen, H.F., Yin, M.C., Tsai, C.M., Hsieh, C.H. (2004). Five cysteine-containing compounds delay diabetic deterioration in Balb/cA mice. *Journal of Nutrition*, *134*, 3245–3249.

71. Vale, J.A., Proudfoot, A.T. (1995). Paracetamol (acetaminophen) poisoning. *Lancet*, *346*, 547–552.

72. Ahola, T., Fellman, V., Laaksonen, R., Laitila, J., Lapatto, R., Neuvonen, P.J., Raivio, K.O. (1999). Pharmacokinetics of intravenous N-acetylcysteine in pre-term new-born infants. *European Journal of Clinical Pharmacology*, *55*, 645–650.

73. Baker, D.H., Wood, R.J. (1992). Cellular antioxidant status and human immunodeficiency virus replication. *Nutrition Reviews*, *50*, 15–18.

74. Baker, D.H., Harter, J.M. (1978). D-cystine utilization by the chick. *Poultry Science*, *57*, 562–563.

75. Meister, A., Fraser, P.E., Tice, S.V. (1954). Enzymatic desulfuration of beta-mercaptopyruvate to pyruvate. *Journal of Biological Chemistry*, *206*, 561–575.

76. Dilger, R.N., Baker, D.H. (2007). DL-Methionine is as efficacious as L-methionine, but modest L-cystine excesses are anorexigenic in sulfur amino acid-deficient purified and practical-type diets fed to chicks. *Poultry Science*, *86*, 2367–2374.

77. Dilger, R.N., Kobler, C., Weckbecker, C., Hoehler, D., Baker, D.H. (2007). 2-keto-4-(methylthio)butyric acid (keto analog of methionine) is a safe and efficacious precursor of L-methionine in chicks. *Journal of Nutrition*, *137*, 1868–1873.

78. Kies, C., Fox, H., Aprahamian, S. (1975). Comparative value of L-, and D-methionine supplementation of an oat-based diet for humans. *Journal of Nutrition*, *105*, 809–814.

79. Stegink, L.D., Moss, J., Printen, K.J., Cho, E.S. (1980). D-Methionine utilization in adult monkeys fed diets containing DL-methionine. *Journal of Nutrition*, *110*, 1240–1246.

80. Anonymous. (1976). Dietary substitution of essential amino acids by their alpha-keto and alpha-hydroxy analogues. *Nutrition Reviews*, *34*, 22–23.

81. Baker, D.H. (1976). Letter: Utilization of methionine analogues. *Journal of Nutrition*, *106*, 1376–1377.

82. Boebel, K.P., Baker, D.H. (1982). Efficacy of calcium salt and free acid forms of methionine hydroxy analog for chicks. *Poultry Science, 61*, 1167–1175.

83. Baker, D.H., Boebel, K.P. (1980). Utilization of the D- and L-isomers of methionine and methionine hydroxy analogue as determined by chick bioassay. *Journal of Nutrition, 110*, 959–964.

84. Williamson, J.M., Meister, A. (1981). Stimulation of hepatic glutathione formation by administration of L-2-oxothiazolidine-4-carboxylate, a 5-oxo-L-prolinase substrate. *Proceedings of the National Academy of Sciences USA, 78*, 936–939.

85. Martir, W.G., Truex, C.R., Tarka, S.M., Hill, L.J., Gorby, W.G. (1974). The synthesis of taurine from sulfate. VIII. A constitutive enzyme in mammals. *Proceedings of the Society for Experimental Biology and Medicine, 147*, 563–565.

86. Rigo, J., Senterre, J. (1977). Is taurine essential for the neonates? *Biology of the Neonate, 32*, 73–76.

87. Hanson, A.D., Rivoal, J., Paquet, L., Gage, D.A. (1994). Biosynthesis of 3-dimethyl-sulfoniopropionate in *Wollastonia biflora* (L.) DC. Evidence that S-methylmethionine is an intermediate. *Plant Physiology, 105*, 103–110.

88. Jones, D.B., Divine, J.P., Horn, M.J. (1942). A study of the availability of mesolanthionine for the promotion of growth when added to a cystine-deficient diet. *Journal of Biological Chemistry, 146*, 571–575.

89. Snow, J.T., Finley, J.W., Friedman, M. (1976). Relative reactivities of sulfhydryl groups with N-acetyl dehydroalanine and N-acetyl dehydroalanine methyl ester. *International Journal of Peptide and Protein Research, 8*, 57–64.

90. Cavallini, D., De Marco, C., Mondovi, B., Mori, B.G. (1960). The cleavage of cystine by cystathionase and the transsulfuration of hypotaurine. *Enzymologia, 22*, 161–173.

91. Dyer, H.M., du Vigneaud, V. (1935). A study of the availability of D- and L-homocysteine for growth purposes. *Journal of Biological Chemistry, 109*, 477–480.

92. Harter, J.M., Baker, D.H. (1978). Sulfur amino acid activity of D- and L-homocysteine for chicks. *Proceedings of the Society for Experimental Biology and Medicine, 157*, 139–143.

93. Baker, D.H., Czarnecki, G.L. (1985). Transmethylation of homocysteine to methionine: Efficiency in the rat and chick. *Journal of Nutrition, 115*, 1291–1299.

94. Anderson, P.A., Baker, D.H., Sherry, P.A., Corbin, J.E. (1979). Choline-methionine interrelationship in feline nutrition. *Journal of Animal Science, 49*, 522–527.

95. Baker, D.H., Halpin, K.M., Czarnecki, G.L., Parsons, C.M. (1983). The choline-methionine interrelationship for growth of the chick. *Poultry Science, 62*, 133–137.

96. Czarnecki, G.L., Halpin, K.M., Baker, D.H. (1983). Precursor (amino acid): Product (vitamin) interrelationship for growing chicks as illustrated by tryptophan-niacin and methionine-choline. *Poultry Science, 62*, 371–374.

97. Anderson, S.A., Raiten, D.J. (1992). *Safety of Amino Acids Used as Dietary Supplements.* Bethesda, MD: Life Sciences Research Office, Federation of American Societies for Experimental Biology.

98. Mueller, J.H. (1922). Studies on cultural requirements of bacteria. II. *Journal of Bacteriology, 7*, 325–338.

99. Mueller, J.H. (1922). A new sulphur-containing amino acid isolated from casein. *Proceedings of the Society for Experimental Biology and Medicine, 19*, 161–163.

100. Mueller, J.H. (1923). A new sulfur-containing amino-acid isolated from the hydrolytic products of protein. *Journal of Biological Chemistry*, *56*, 157–169.

101. Rose, W.C. (1938). The nutritive significance of the amino acids. *Physiological Reviews*, *18*, 109–136.

102. McCoy, R.H., Meyer, C.E., Rose, W.C. (1935). Feeding experiments with mixtures of highly purified amino acids. VIII. Isolation and identification of a new essential amino acid. *Journal of Biological Chemistry*, *112*, 283–302.

103. Rose, W.C., McCoy, R.H., Meyer, C.E., Carter, H.E., Womack, M., Mertz, E.T. (1935). Isolation of the "unknown" essential present in proteins. *Journal of Biological Chemistry*, *109*, 77–78.

104. Daniel, R.G., Waisman, H.A. (1968). The effects of excess amino acids on the growth of the young rat. *Growth*, *32*, 255–265.

105. Benevenga, N.J., Steele, R.D. (1984). Adverse effects of excessive consumption of amino acids. *Annual Review of Nutrition*, *4*, 157–181.

106. Muramatsu, K., Odagiri, H., Morishita, S., Takeuchi, H. (1971). Effect of excess levels of individual amino acids on growth of rats fed casein diets. *Journal of Nutrition*, *101*, 1117–1125.

107. Edmonds, M.S., Baker, D.H. (1987). Amino acid excesses for young pigs: Effects of excess methionine, tryptophan, threonine, or leucine. *Journal of Animal Science*, *64*, 1664–1671.

108. Edmonds, M.S., Baker, D.H. (1987). Comparative effects of individual amino acid excesses when added to a corn-soybean meal diet: Effects on growth and dietary choice in the chick. *Journal of Animal Science*, *65*, 699–705.

109. Edmonds, M.S., Gonyou, H.W., Baker, D.H. (1987). Effect of excess levels of methionine, tryptophan, arginine, lysine, or threonine on growth and dietary choice in the pig. *Journal of Animal Science*, *65*, 179–185.

110. Harper, A.E., Benevenga, N.J., Wohlhueter, R.M. (1970). Effects of ingestion of disproportionate amounts of amino acids. *Physiological Reviews*, *50*, 428–558.

111. Toue, S., Kodama, R., Amao, M., Kawamata, Y., Kimura, T., Sakai, R. (2006). Screening of toxicity biomarkers for methionine excess in rats. *Journal of Nutrition*, *136*, 1716S–1721S.

112. Garlick, P.J. (2006). Toxicity of methionine in humans. *Journal of Nutrition*, *136*, 1722S–1725S.

113. Selhub, J. (2006). The many facets of hyperhomocysteinemia: Studies from the Framingham cohorts. *Journal of Nutrition*, *136*, 1726S–1730S.

114. Refsum, H., Nurk, E., Smith, A.D., Ueland, P.M., Gjesdal, C.G., Bjelland, I., Tverdal, A., Tell, G.S., Nygard, O., Vollset, S.E. (2006). The Hordaland Homocysteine Study: A community-based study of homocysteine, its determinants, and associations with disease. *Journal of Nutrition*, *136*, 1731S–1740S.

115. Jakubowski, H. (2006). Pathophysiological consequences of homocysteine excess. *Journal of Nutrition*, *136*, 1741S–1749S.

116. Finkelstein, J.D. (2006). Inborn errors of sulfur-containing amino acid metabolism. *Journal of Nutrition*, *136*, 1750S–1754S.

117. Sauberlich, H.E. (1961). Studies on the toxicity and antagonism of amino acids for weanling rats. *Journal of Nutrition*, *75*, 61–72.

118. Floyd, J.C., Jr., Fajans, S.S., Conn, J.W., Knopf, R.F., Rull, J. (1966). Stimulation of insulin secretion by amino acids. *Journal of Clinical Investigation, 45*, 1487–1502.

119. Meister, A. (1965). Intermediary metabolism of the amino acids. In Meister, A., ed., *Biochemistry of the Amino Acids*, p. 785. New York: Academic Press.

120. Steele, R.D., Benevenga, N.J. (1979). The metabolism of 3-methylthiopropionate in rat liver homogenates. *Journal of Biological Chemistry, 254*, 8885–8890.

121. Finkelstein, J.D., Martin, J.J. (1984). Methionine metabolism in mammals. Distribution of homocysteine between competing pathways. *Journal of Biological Chemistry, 259*, 9508–9513.

122. Stipanuk, M.H. (2004). Sulfur amino acid metabolism: Pathways for production and removal of homocysteine and cysteine. *Annual Review of Nutrition, 24*, 539–577.

123. Storch, K.J., Wagner, D.A., Burke, J.F., Young, V.R. (1990). [1-^{13}C;methyl-^{2}H$_3$]-methionine kinetics in humans: Methionine conservation and cystine sparing. *American Journal of Physiology, 258*, E790–E798.

124. Finkelstein, J.D. (1978). Regulation of methionine metabolism in mammals. In Usdin, E., Borchardt, R.T., and Creveling, C.R., eds., *Transmethylation*, pp. 49–58. New York: Elsevier/North-Holland.

125. Fau, D., Peret, J., Hadjiisky, P. (1988). Effects of ingestion of high protein or excess methionine diets by rats for two years. *Journal of Nutrition, 118*, 128–133.

126. Daniel, R.G., Waisman, H.A. (1969). The influence of excess methionine on the free amino acids of brain and liver of the weanling rat. *Journal of Neurochemistry, 16*, 787–795.

127. Harter, J.M., Baker, D.H. (1978). Factors affecting methionine toxicity and its alleviation in the chick. *Journal of Nutrition, 108*, 1061–1070.

128. Scherer, C.S., Baker, D.H. (2000). Excess dietary methionine markedly increases in the vitamin B-6 requirement of young chicks. *Journal of Nutrition, 130*, 3055–3058.

129. Ueland, P.M., Refsum, H. (1989). Plasma homocysteine, a risk factor for vascular disease: Plasma levels in health, disease, and drug therapy. *Journal of Laboratory and Clinical Medicine, 114*, 473–501.

130. McCully, K.S. (1969). Vascular pathology of homocysteinemia: Implications for the pathogenesis of arteriosclerosis. *American Journal of Pathology, 56*, 111–128.

131. Katz, R.S., Baker, D.H. (1975). Toxicity of various organic sulfur compounds for chicks fed crystalline amino acid diets containing threonine and glycine at their minimal dietary requirements for maximal growth. *Journal of Animal Science, 41*, 1355–1361.

132. Benevenga, N.J., Harper, A.E. (1967). Alleviation of methionine and homocystine toxicity in the rat. *Journal of Nutrition, 93*, 44–52.

133. Benevenga, N.J. (1974). Toxicities of methionine and other amino acids. *Journal of Agricultural and Food Chemistry, 22*, 2–9.

134. Kaufman, N., Klavins, J.V., Kinney, T.D. (1960). Pancreatic damage induced by excess methionine. *Archives of Pathology, 70*, 331–337.

135. Hardwick, D.F., Applegarth, D.A., Cockcroft, D.M., Ross, P.M., Cder, R.J. (1970). Pathogenesis of methionine-induced toxicity. *Metabolism, 19*, 381–391.

136. Klavins, J.V., Johansen, P.V. (1965). Pathology of amino acid excess. IV. Effects and interactions of excessive amounts of dietary methionine, homocystine, and serine. *Archives of Pathology, 79*, 600–614.

137. Klavins, J.V., Kinney, T.D., Kaufman, N. (1963). Histopathologic changes in methionine excess. *Archives of Pathology*, *75*, 661–673.

138. Perry, T.L., Hardwick, D.F., Dixon, G.H., Dolman, C.L., Hansen, S. (1965). Hypermethioninemia: A metabolic disorder associated with cirrhosis, islet cell hyperplasia, and renal tubular degeneration. *Pediatrics*, *36*, 236–250.

139. Cohen, H.P., Choitz, H.C., Berg, C.P. (1958). Response of rats to diets high in methionine and related compounds. *Journal of Nutrition*, *64*, 555–569.

140. Roth, J.S., Allison, J.B. (1949). The effect of feeding excess glycine, L-arginine and DL-methionine to rats on a casein diet. *Proceedings of the Society for Experimental Biology and Medicine*, *70*, 327–330.

141. Finkelstein, J.D., Martin, J.J. (1986). Methionine metabolism in mammals. Adaptation to methionine excess. *Journal of Biological Chemistry*, *261*, 1582–1587.

142. Benevenga, N.J., Harper, A.E. (1970). Effect of glycine and serine on methionine metabolism in rats fed diets high in methionine. *Journal of Nutrition*, *100*, 1205–1214.

143. Klain, G.J., Vaughan, D.A., Vaughan, L.N. (1963). Some metabolic effects of methionine toxicity in the rat. *Journal of Nutrition*, *80*, 337–341.

144. Benevenga, N.J. (2007). Consideration of betaine and one-carbon sources of N^5-methyltetrahydrofolate for use in homocystinuria and neural tube defects. *American Journal of Clinical Nutrition*, *85*, 946–949.

145. Anonymous. (1984). Betaine therapy for homocystinuria. *Nutrition Reviews*, 42, 180–182.

146. Case, G.L., Benevenga, N.J. (1972). S-Methylcysteine as a methionine analogue in methionine toxicity studies. *Federation Proceedings*, *31*, 715 (Abstr).

147. Benevenga, N.J. (1984). Evidence for alternative pathways of methionine catabolism. *Advances in Nutritional Research*, *6*, 1–18.

148. Mudd, S.H., Levy, H.L., Tangerman, A., Boujet, C., Buist, N., Davidson-Mundt, A., Hudgins, L., Oyanagi, K., Nagao, M., Wilson, W.G. (1995). Isolated persistent hypermethioninemia. *American Journal of Human Genetics*, *57*, 882–892.

149. Blom, H.J., Boers, G.H., van den Elzen, J.P., Gahl, W.A., Tangerman, A. (1989). Transamination of methionine in humans. *Clinical Science (London)*, *76*, 43–49.

150. Gahl, W.A., Bernardini, I., Finkelstein, J.D., Tangerman, A., Martin, J.J., Blom, H.J., Mullen, K.D., Mudd, S.H. (1988). Transsulfuration in an adult with hepatic methionine adenosyltransferase deficiency. *Journal of Clinical Investigation*, *81*, 390–397.

151. Tangerman, A., Wilcken, B., Levy, H.L., Boers, G.H., Mudd, S.H. (2000). Methionine transamination in patients with homocystinuria due to cystathionine beta-synthase deficiency. *Metabolism*, *49*, 1071–1077.

152. Burrin, D.G., Stoll, B. (2007). Emerging aspects of gut sulfur amino acid metabolism. *Current Opinion in Clinical Nutrition and Metabolic Care*, *10*, 63–68.

153. Furne, J., Springfield, J., Koenig, T., DeMaster, E., Levitt, M.D. (2001). Oxidation of hydrogen sulfide and methanethiol to thiosulfate by rat tissues: A specialized function of the colonic mucosa. *Biochemical Pharmacology*, *62*, 255–259.

154. Levitt, M.D., Furne, J., Springfield, J., Suarez, F., DeMaster, E. (1999). Detoxification of hydrogen sulfide and methanethiol in the cecal mucosa. *Journal of Clinical Investigation*, *104*, 1107–1114.

155. Wollaston, W.H. (1810). On cystic oxide, a new species of urinary calculus. *Philosophical Transactions of the Royal Society of London*, *100*, 223–230.

156. Berzelius, J.J. (1833). Calculus urinaries. In Fréres, F.D., ed., *Traité de chimie*, Vol. 7, p. 424. Paris.

157. Thaulow, M.C.J. (1838). Sur la composition de la cystine. *Journal de Pharmacie*, *24*, 629–632.

158. Curtis, A.C., Newburgh, L.H., Thomas, F.H. (1927). The toxic action of cystine on the kidney. *Archives of Internal Medicine*, *39*, 817–827.

159. Blum, L. (1904). Über das schicksal des cystins im tierkörper. *Beiträge zur Chemischen Physiologie und Pathologie*, *5*, 1–14.

160. Knox, W.E. (1960). Cystinuria. In Stanbury, J.B., Wyngaarden, J.B., and Dredrickson, D.S., eds., *The Metabolic Basis of Inherited Disease*, pp. 1302–1337. New York: McGraw-Hill.

161. Dilger, R.N., Toue, S., Kimura, T., Sakai, R., Baker, D.H. (2007). Excess dietary L-cysteine, but not L-cystine, is lethal for chicks but not for rats or pigs. *Journal of Nutrition*, *137*, 331–338.

162. Baker, D.H., Czarnecki-Maulden, G.L. (1987). Pharmacologic role of cysteine in ameliorating or exacerbating mineral toxicities. *Journal of Nutrition*, *117*, 1003–1010.

163. Klavins, J.V. (1963). Pathology of Amino Acid Excess. II. effects of administration of excessive amounts of sulphur containing amino acids: L-cystine. *British Journal of Experimental Pathology*, *44*, 516–519.

164. Sell, D.R., Featherston, W.R., Rogler, J.C. (1980). Methionine-cystine interrelationships in chicks and rats fed diets containing suboptimal levels of methionine. *Poultry Science*, *59*, 1878–1884.

165. Lerner, J., Taylor, M.W. (1967). A common step in the intestinal absorption mechanisms of D- and L-methionine. *Biochimica et Biophysica Acta*, *135*, 990–999.

166. Curtis, A.C., Newburgh, L.H. (1927). The toxic action of cystine on the liver of the albino rat. *Archives of Internal Medicine*, *39*, 828–832.

167. Pedersen, O.O., Karlsen, R.L. (1980). The toxic effect of L-cysteine on the rat retina. A morphological and biochemical study. *Investigative Ophthalmology & Visual Science*, *19*, 886–892.

168. Olney, J.W., Ho, O.L. (1970). Brain damage in infant mice following oral intake of glutamate, aspartate or cysteine. *Nature*, *227*, 609–611.

169. Olney, J.W., Ho, O.L., Rhee, V. (1971). Cytotoxic effects of acidic and sulphur containing amino acids on the infant mouse central nervous system. *Experimental Brain Research*, *14*, 61–76.

170. Olney, J.W., Ho, O.L., Rhee, V., Schainker, B. (1972). Cysteine-induced brain damage in infant and fetal rodents. *Brain Research*, *45*, 309–313.

171. Sharpe, L.G., Olney, J.W., Ohlendorf, C., Lyss, A., Zimmerman, M., Gale, B. (1975). Brain damage and associated behavioral deficits following the administration of L-cysteine to infant rats. *Pharmacology, Biochemistry, and Behavior*, *3*, 291–298.

172. Olney, J.W., Zorumski, C., Price, M.T., Labruyere, J. (1990). L-cysteine, a bicarbonate-sensitive endogenous excitotoxin. *Science*, *248*, 596–599.

173. Puka-Sundvall, M., Eriksson, P., Nilsson, M., Sandberg, M., Lehmann, A. (1995). Neurotoxicity of cysteine: Interaction with glutamate. *Brain Research*, *705*, 65–70.

174. Janaky, R., Varga, V., Hermann, A., Saransaari, P., Oja, S.S. (2000). Mechanisms of L-cysteine neurotoxicity. *Neurochemical Research, 25*, 1397–1405.

175. Stipanuk, M.H., Dominy, J.E., Jr., Lee, J.I., Coloso, R.M. (2006). Mammalian cysteine metabolism: New insights into regulation of cysteine metabolism. *Journal of Nutrition, 136*, 1652S–1659S.

176. Kamoun, P. (2004). Endogenous production of hydrogen sulfide in mammals. *Amino Acids, 26*, 243–254.

177. Dominy, J.E., Stipanuk, M.H. (2004). New roles for cysteine and transsulfuration enzymes: Production of H2S, a neuromodulator and smooth muscle relaxant. *Nutrition Reviews, 62*, 348–353.

178. Hosoki, R., Matsuki, N., Kimura, H. (1997). The possible role of hydrogen sulfide as an endogenous smooth muscle relaxant in synergy with nitric oxide. *Biochemical and Biophysical Research Communications, 237*, 527–531.

179. Abe, K., Kimura, H. (1996). The possible role of hydrogen sulfide as an endogenous neuromodulator. *Journal of Neuroscience, 16*, 1066–1071.

180. Kimura, H. (2002). Hydrogen sulfide as a neuromodulator. *Molecular Neurobiology, 26*, 13–19.

181. Beck, J.F., Donini, J.C., Maneckjee, A. (1983). The influence of sulfide and cyanide on axonal function. *Toxicology, 26*, 37–45.

182. Truong, D.H., Eghbal, M.A., Hindmarsh, W., Roth, S.H., O'Brien, P.J. (2006). Molecular mechanisms of hydrogen sulfide toxicity. *Drug Metabolism Reviews, 38*, 733–744.

183. Attene-Ramos, M.S., Wagner, E.D., Plewa, M.J., Gaskins, H.R. (2006). Evidence that hydrogen sulfide is a genotoxic agent. *Molecular Cancer Research, 4*, 9–14.

184. Hagen, T.M., Wierzbicka, G.T., Bowman, B.B., Aw, T.Y., Jones, D.P. (1990). Fate of dietary glutathione: Disposition in the gastrointestinal tract. *American Journal of Physiology, 259*, G530–G535.

185. Jones, D.P., Hagen, T.M., Weber, R., Wierzbicka, G.T., Bonkovsky, H.L. (1989). Oral administration of glutathione (GSH) increases plasma GSH concentration humans. *FASEB Journal, 3*, A1250 (Abstr).

186. Aw, T.Y., Wierzbicka, G., Jones, D.P. (1991). Oral glutathione increases tissue glutathione in vivo. *Chemico-Biological Interactions, 80*, 89–97.

187. Hagen, T.M., Wierzbicka, G.T., Sillau, A.H., Bowman, B.B., Jones, D.P. (1990). Bioavailability of dietary glutathione: Effect on plasma concentration. *American Journal of Physiology, 259*, G524–G529.

188. Reeves, P.G. (1997). Components of the AIN-93 diets as improvements in the AIN-76A diet. *Journal of Nutrition, 127*, 838S–841S.

189. Grimble, R.F. (2006). The effects of sulfur amino acid intake on immune function in humans. *Journal of Nutrition, 136*, 1660S–1665S.

190. Baker, D.H. (1991). Partitioning of nutrients for growth and other metabolic functions: Efficiency and priority considerations. *Poultry Science, 70*, 1797–1805.

191. Earle, D.P., Jr., Smull, K., Victor, J. (1942). Effects of excess dietary cysteic acid, DL-methionine, and taurine on the rat liver. *Journal of Experimental Medicine, 76*, 317–323.

192. Earle, D.P., Jr., Kendall, F.E. (1942). Liver damage and urinary excretion of sulfate in rats fed L-cystine, DL-methionine, and cysteic acid. *Journal of Experimental Medicine, 75*, 191–195.

193. Sturman, J.A., Hepner, G.W., Hofmann, A.F., Thomas, P.J. (1975). Metabolism of [^{35}S]taurine in man. *Journal of Nutrition*, *105*, 1206–1214.

194. Anderson, M.E., Meister, A. (1989). Marked increase of cysteine levels in many regions of the brain after administration of 2-oxothiazolidine-4-carboxylate. *FASEB Journal*, *3*, 1632–1636.

CHAPTER 14

HUMAN PATHOLOGIES AND ABERRANT SULFUR METABOLISM

DANYELLE M. TOWNSEND, HAIM TAPIERO, and KENNETH D. TEW

14.1 INTRODUCTION

Sulfur is found in relatively small quantities in biological molecules. It has numerous properties that make it valuable in facilitating protein structure–function relationships that are critical to life processes. Sulfur has the essential chemical properties to exist in a biologically reduced sulfhydryl state where the pKa of the thiol group is ~9.65, accounting for its nucleophilicity. Sulfur and thiol homeostasis are maintained in cells by a complex series of balanced pathways. Methionine, cysteine, and glutathione (GSH) sequester the majority of cellular sulfur. Within pathways that regulate these molecules there exist defects that translate into human disease states. In this chapter (and others within this volume) we will discuss some of the phenotypes that can result in aberrant physiologies in human populations.

14.2 BIOSYNTHESIS AND METABOLISM OF METHIONINE AND CYSTEINE

Methionine is required for protein synthesis, while its activated form, S-adenosyl-methionine (SAM), serves as a methyl donor in numerous biological reactions. ATP is attached to the sulfur atom of methionine to form SAM, a reaction catalyzed by methionine adenosyl transferase (MAT) and SAM condenses with glycine, releasing a methyl group and sarcosine, to form S-adenosylhomocysteine (SAH). This reaction is catalyzed by the cytosolic enzyme glycine N-methyltransferase (GNMT) [1], a regulator of the SAM : SAH ratio. Where the methyl group supply is limiting, GNMT activity is reduced in order to provide a greater supply for other SAM-dependent methyltransferases. Conversion of SAH to homocysteine is

Glutathione and Sulfur Amino Acids in Human Health and Disease. Edited by R. Masella and G. Mazza
Copyright © 2009 John Wiley & Sons, Inc.

the intersect between the transulfuration pathway and the folic acid cycle. Indeed, GNMT is a folate binding protein, but can also act as a sensor to maintain cellular thiol balance.

14.2.1 Folic Acid Metabolism

A functional link between sulfur amino acid metabolism and the metabolism of methyl groups is provided by the conversion of homocysteine to methionine, resulting in the formation of tetrahydrofolate (THF), the active form of the water-soluble vitamin folic acid. Folic acid is synthesized by two sequential reductions both requiring NADPH and catalyzed by dihydrofolate reductase (DHFR). 5,10-Methenyl-THF while also involved in the metabolism of glycine and serine can be thought of as a central compound with respect to the various folate derivatives. It can be generated from THF either through conversion of serine to glycine or through the decarboxlyation of glycine. Its reduction to 5-methyl-THF is essentially irreversible and with the possible exception of some central nervous system functions, 5-methyl-THF is of limited direct biological consequence.

This compound is the predominant extracellular form of folic acid and once transported into cells it must be demethylated to THF. Because of the irreversibility of the reaction catalyzed by DHFR it cannot be oxidized to 5,10-methylene-THF. Demethylation may be achieved where homocysteine accesses the methyl acceptor and is converted back to methionine. This is a reaction in which both folic acid and vitamin B12 participate. While this reaction is of central significance to folic acid homeostasis, it is relatively minor in terms of regeneration of methionine, one characteristic that makes methionine an essential amino acid.

Inhibition of GNMT is achieved by SAM-induced allosteric inhibition of 5,10-methylene tetrahydrofolate reductase (MTHFR) with concomitant decreased levels of 5-methyl-THF [2]. GNMT is a folate-binding protein and is subject to inhibition by 5-methyl-THF [3]. Thus, under conditions of low availability of methyl groups, low SAM levels prevail and this leads to an increase in 5-methyl-THF with subsequent inhibition of GNMT [4]. Conversely, with excess methyl groups, SAM levels increase, with subsequent decrease in MTHFR and 5-methyl-THF and enhancement of GNMT activity.

14.2.2 Transulfuration Pathway

Homocysteine is a sulfur-containing amino acid that plays a significant role in one-carbon metabolism and methylation reactions. In humans, the sole source of homocysteine is through dietary methionine intake and subsequent metabolism. The inability of certain individuals to metabolize homocysteine via methylation and/or transulfuration can result in its systemic build up in the circulation. In the initial step of the transulfuration pathway, serine is combined with homocysteine in a reaction catalyzed by the B6-dependent enzyme cystathionine β-synthase (CBS) to form cystathionine, which is converted to cysteine via c-cystathionine. Subsequent metabolism of cysteine may eventually lead to taurine, a nonstandard amino acid that is critical in fetal and childhood development and is usually added as a supplement in many infant formulas. While high plasma concentrations of cysteine can prove to be toxic, the amino acid can be limiting in the synthesis and maintenance of cellular glutathione pools. Glutathione is a primary source of cellular nucleophiles and critical to the maintenance of a reduced environment by maintaining a balanced cellular redox potential. Of equal biological importance, sulfur amino acids contribute to critical regulatory pathways that involve one carbon metabolism.

14.2.3 One-Carbon Metabolism

One-carbon metabolism is the transfer of one-carbon groups from one compound to another in a complex array of interrelated biochemical reactions that in its most simple view serves two critical functions: methylation of nucleic acids and synthesis of nucleotides and thymidylate [5, 6]. THF can function as a coenzyme in the transfer of one-carbon units, critical in a number of important cellular synthetic reactions, perhaps the most important of which is the synthesis of thymidylate. The conversion of 5-methyl-THF to THF provides the one-carbon group that is used in the remethylation of homocysteine to produce methionine, a reaction catalyzed by the B12-dependent enzyme methionine synthase. It is also worth noting that an oxidized metabolite of choline, betaine (trimethylglycine), can also serve as a methyl donor. Its participation in the remethylation of homocysteine to methionine produces dimethylglycine, which is not a methyl donor. However, when the methyl groups are removed as formaldehyde, oxidation to formate can lead to the formation of 10-formyl-THF. Although the major significance of this pathway probably relates to the biosynthesis of phospholipids, a conversion of choline to glycine can be thought of as a salvage pathway for one-carbon units. One-carbon metabolism has been attributed to >80 reactions and frequently has folate and the B vitamins as coenzymes. Modest dietary deficiencies of these coenzymes are associated with important diseases, including neural tube defects (NTD), cardiovascular disease, and cancer. Although cysteine is not directly involved in one-carbon metabolism, it can be synthesized from serine and methionine and these two amino acids are directly involved. Thus, overall, serine and methionine together with glycine, homocysteine and various THF moieties are major contributors to one-carbon metabolism.

14.3 DEFECTS IN THE TRANSULFURATION PATHWAY

14.3.1 Homocysteinuria

Previous studies have suggested that homocysteine is a specific risk factor and/or a marker for human pathologies such as cardiovascular disease [7–9]. Whether homocysteine is a cause or effect of the increased incidence of vascular disease is not clear; however, there is a meaningful correlation between elevated plasma homocysteine and mortality from all causes [10].

Both methionine and homocysteine accumulate within cells and bodily fluids of individuals with homocysteinuria, with the result that cysteine biosynthesis is impaired, reducing the availability of this amino acid. The build up of homocysteine has numerous pathological effects, including the alteration of normal collagen cross-linking [11]. Interference with normal collagen formation may contribute to ocular, skeletal, and vascular complications in patients. In the eye, changes in the ligaments of the optic lens can affect lens stability. In bones, the matrix may be compromised, leading to progressive osteoporosis. Interference with vascular wall formation and maintenance may contribute towards arterial and venous thrombotic disease. Increased homocysteine accumulation may also contribute towards enhanced platelet adhesiveness, thereby providing the baseline for thrombotic occlusive disease.

In addition to homocysteinuria, an elevated plasma concentration of homocysteine is common among patients with cardiovascular disease. While treatments to solve the underlying metabolic malfunction would be optimal, there is evidence that lowering homocysteine levels pharmacologically may provide some therapeutic benefit. Several studies have shown an inverse relationship between homocysteine levels and folic acid and/or the B vitamins [11]. Hence, dietary supplementation with the corresponding vitamin deficiency is beneficial. Numerous studies have shown that folic acid supplementation (dietary or supplements) can reduce plasma homocysteine levels [12, 13].

14.3.2 Homocystinuria

Homocystinuria is a metabolic disorder discovered in the 1960s independently in the United States and Ireland by observations of elevated homocystine (the disulfide of homocysteine) levels in the urine of mentally retarded individuals [14, 15]. While the worldwide incidence is 1 in 344,000, Celtic regions have a significantly higher incidence of 1 in 65,000. Homocystinuria affects the eyes, central nervous system, skeletal and vascular systems. The disorder is characterized by seven biochemically distinct alterations, resulting in increased concentrations of homocystine and methionine in body fluids. The most prevalent form of the disease is characterized by decreased activity of CBS, while other forms have resulted from impaired conversions of homocysteine to methionine [16]. Decreased CBS activity has been classified in three categories: (1) no residual activity, (2) decreased activity with normal affinity for the cofactor pyridoxal phosphate, and (3) decreased activity with low affinity for the cofactor [17]. CBS is a 63 kDa heme containing enzyme that forms a homotetramer and catalyzes the condensation of homocysteine with serine to form cystathionine. CBS requires SAM that can stimulate both pyridoxal phosphate and heme and its activity. The locus for the enzyme is the q21 region of chromosome 21 [18, 19]. The gene contains 23 exons and has an unusually high number of Alu repeats that may predispose it to deleterious rearrangement [20]. Nearly 92 disease-associated mutations in the CBS gene have been identified in laboratories around the world [21]. The most common mutation in the Celtic region is the G307S mutation [22]. Individuals homozygous for this allele have been shown not to respond to pyridoxine supplementation [21], whereas individuals with an I278T mutation respond favorably to dietary supplementation [21]. Moreover, >80% of homozygous individuals for complete synthase deficiency have optical defects. Mental retardation can occur in approximately 50% of the patients and this is sometimes accompanied by behavioral symptoms. It is interesting to note the wide range of cognitive abilities in individuals with homocystinuria. Nearly one-third of individuals with this disorder have normal intelligence [23]. Of the individuals that show altered capabilities, two categories have been defined; those that respond to B6 supplementation (mean IQ of 79) and B6 nonresponsive (mean IQ of 57) [16]. Approximately one-quarter of the patients die from vascular occlusive disease before the age of 30. Heterozygote patients may also be at increased risk of premature peripheral and cerebral occlusive vascular disease. Heterozygocity shows a dominant negative effect as enzyme levels are $\sim$25% to 30% of normal, rather than 50%. This may be attributed to the formation of the homodimer. Effective treatment is enhanced by early diagnosis. Newborn screening for decreased CBS activity began in Ireland in 1971. Infants diagnosed have been successfully treated with methionine-restricted cystine-supplemented diets. In addition, oral supplementation with pyridoxine can provide a reduction in urinary methionine and homocystine. This benefit reflects the capacity of residual enzyme activity to be enhanced by the presence of the cofactor.

14.3.3 Cystathioninuria

Cystathioninuria is an autosomal recessive disorder attributed to a defect in the cystathionase γ-lyase (CTH) gene that involves the cleavage of cystathione to cysteine. Because of the elevated plasma concentrations, there is an increase in urinary excretion of cystathione. Mutations in the CTH gene result in a decreased capacity for the enzyme to bind its cofactor, pyridoxal phosphate [24]. Cystathioninuria is considered to be a benign biochemical anomaly that has a low occurrence of 1 per 14,000 live births [25]. Cystathioninuria is not clinically associated with consistent or striking pathologic features; however, some individuals may have developmental defects, convulsions, thrombocytopenia, and mental retardation.

14.4 INHERITED DEFECTS IN MEMBRANE TRANSPORT

14.4.1 Methionine Malabsorption

At least 10 disorders of amino acid transport have been described. Both cysteine and methionine are represented in these disease states of methionine malabsorption, folate malabsorption, and cystinuria. Frequently, these conditions affect transport in the kidney and the gastrointestinal tract, or both. Only rarely is there an impact on other tissues. For example, the autosomal recessive methionine malabsorption trait has direct effects on jejunal mucosa, with clinical manifestations that include mental retardation, convulsions, hyperpneic attacks, white hair, and α-hydroxybutyricaciduria [26]. The disorder is diagnosable primarily as a consequence of urinary excretion of α-hydroxybutyric acid, a by-product of the breakdown of unabsorbed methionine by intestinal flora and adds an odor reminiscent of malt to the urine. Treatment of such individuals with a methionine-restricted diet can produce improvement in the symptoms.

14.4.2 Folate Malabsorption

Folate malabsorption is a hereditary defect in transport of folic acid in the intestine as well as the blood–brain barrier [27]. Individuals with this disorder experience megaloblastic anemia, mental retardation, convulsions, and movement disorders. Some studies show that treatment of such individuals with folic acid reduces seizures while others show the condition to be aggravated [28, 29].

14.4.3 Cystinuria

Cystinuria, one of the most common inborn errors of amino acid transport, is inherited as an autosomal recessive trait resulting from mutations in membrane transport proteins for structurally related amino acids. In the early 1800s, Wollaston [30] identified yellow stones in the urine of some patients that he proposed were composed of sulfur-containing amino acids, and termed the substance cystic oxide, and referred to the syndrome as cystinuria. The disease is characterized by excessive urinary excretion of lysine, arginine, ornithine, and cystine and is a consequence of restricted tubular reabsorption of these amino acids. Although a similarly impaired absorption also occurs in the intestinal tract, clinical symptoms of cystinuria manifest as a build up of cystine stones in renal, ureteral, and bladder calculi. These calculi occur primarily because cystine is one of the least water-soluble amino acids and is more likely to precipitate in target organs. Characteristic of the disease is the fact that at physiological pH, the solubility of cysteine is approximately 300 mg per liter. Individuals who suffer from the disease frequently excrete 600 to 1800 mg of cysteine per day, producing an environment conducive to the formation of stones. While these stones are characteristically found in the second or third decade of life, in some individuals they can occur in the first year.

Type I, II, and III cystinuria have been described. These designations are based on the excretion of cystine and dibasic amino acids in the urine of heterozygous individuals. Specifically, type I refers to heterozygotes who excrete normal amounts of cystine and dibasic amino acids; in type II, heterozygotes excrete 9 to 15 times more; in type III, heterozygotes excrete twice the normal range. Type III patients respond to cystine supplementation whereas type I and type II do not. The underlying mechanism leading to this disorder has been attributed to mutations in at least two amino acid transporters. Type I cystinuria has been attributed to the SLC3A1 amino acid transport gene localized to chromosome 2 [31, 32]. Mutations in a second amino acid transporter that contains a heavy and light chain and is encoded by two genes (SLC7A9 and SLC7A3) were identified in type II and type III patients [32]. Mutations in SCL7A9 are characteristic of mild (A182T allele) to severe (G105R, V170M, and R33W alleles) cystinuria [33]. Medical treatment of the disease includes a high fluid ingestion, usually in excess of 4:1 per day. Ideal urinary cysteine excretion should be less than 250 to 300 mg per liter. These high levels of water intake can serve either to prevent crystal formation, or to dissolve existing crystals. While alkalinization of urine can also positively impact on stone formation, such a treatment modality must be balanced with the possibility of inducing calcium-based stones and other nephrology complications. A further treatment modality involves the use of penicillamine, which can redox exchange with cysteine to form mixed disulfides of penicillamine and cysteine. This disulfide is significantly more soluble than cystine and can therefore help to reduce the physiological concentrations of amino acids.

14.5 PATHOLOGIES ASSOCIATED WITH FOLIC ACID METABOLIZING ENZYMES

14.5.1 Methionine Synthase Reductase Deficiency

Methylation of homocysteine via methionine synthase results in the formation of methionine. Methionine synthase requires the cofactor cob(I)alamin, which becomes oxidized to cob(II)alamin, resulting in the inactivation of the enzyme. Hence, a second enzyme, methionine synthase reductase (MTRR) is required to maintain methionine synthase in a functional state [34]. MTRR is a 77.7 kDa protein containing 698 amino acids [34]. RT-PCR analyses have identified a variety of mutations in the MTRR gene that are associated with homocystinuria–megaloblastic anemia and spina bifida [34–37].

14.5.2 Methylenetetrahydrofolate Reductase Deficiency

5,10-Methylenetetrahydrofolate reductase (MTHFR) is the enzyme that catalyzes the conversion of 5,10-methylene-THF to 5-methyl-THF, the cosubstrate for remethylation of homocysteine to methionine. A 7.2 kb transcript of MTHFR was identified in all tissues; however, a 9 kb transcript was identified in brain, muscle, placenta, and stomach [38]. The tissue-specific transcript has been shown to be a product of an alternate transcriptional start site and polyadenylation signal.

A number of polymorphisms exist within the MTHFR gene and some are associated with a decrease in enzyme activity that leads to MTHFR deficiency, a process that alters folate metabolism and is associated with a variety of disorders, including homocystinuria, homocysteinemia, NTD, and coronary heart disease. While 24 point mutations have so far been identified that alter enzyme activity [39], a high degree of MTHFR deficiency has been causally associated with nine of these [40]. The C559T mutation which gives rise to a termination codon was identified in Native Americans who lack MTHFR activity and have severe homocystinuria [41]. A second mutation (G482A) also decreased enzyme capacity [41] and this allele was associated with a milder disorder.

Perhaps one of the most widely studied allelic variants of MTHFR is the thermolabile C667T allele that has decreased enzyme activity [41]. This allele has been identified in all populations studied and ranges in frequency of 0.1 to 0.38 [42–44] Chromatographic studies showed that the distribution of red blood cell (RBC) folates is altered in individuals carrying the C667T allele [45]. High pressure liquid chromatography and mass spectrum analysis of DNA from the RBC of individuals homozygous for the C667T allele showed a positive correlation of DNA methylation and an inverse correlation with plasma homocysteine levels [46]. Folate can stabilize the thermolabile enzyme [42]. Subsequent studies have shown that increasing serum folate levels >15.4 nM appear to neutralize the clinical manifestations due to the thermolabile allele [47].

Homozygous individuals carrying the C667T allele have a threefold increased risk of developing premature cardiovascular disease [48]. The risk factor of the thermolabile allele with coronary disease was confirmed in a meta-analysis of dozens of independent studies [49]. The risk was particularly enhanced when serum folate levels were decreased.

14.5.3 Neural Tube Defects (NTD) and MTHFR Deficiency

NTD are developmental abnormalities of the spinal cord that are recessively inherited. NTD include a wide variety of disorders, such as spina bifida occulta, diastematomyelia, and intradural or extradural lipoma. The C667T allele of MTHFR was characterized as the first genetic risk factor for NTD at the molecular level [50]. Ou et al. [51] showed that C667T homozygosity was associated with a 7.2-fold increased risk for neural tube disorders. Conflicting results with the thermolabile allele and NTD exist [51–53]. These studies provide evidence that a number of factors contribute to the development of NTD.

Folic acid can serve to lower homocysteine levels by providing the factors necessary for the remethylation of homocysteine to cysteine. Evidence from the Centers for Disease Control suggest that administration of folic acid prior to conception and during the first 4 weeks of pregnancy can prevent ~50% of NTD [54]. In 1998, the United States mandated that grain products were to be fortified with folic acid (140 μg/100 g) to prevent NTD in pregnant women. It is important to note that NTD do not arise from a nutritional deficiency of folate but from metabolic defects that can be corrected by large doses of folic acid at developmentally critical times.

14.5.4 Polymorphisms in MTHFR and MTRR as Risk Factors for Spina Bifida

Spina bifida is one of the disorders associated with NTD and is prevalent in the general population (0.14%). Polymorphisms of the MTHFR (C677T), MTRR (A66G), and methionine synthase (A2756G) genes have been studied in families who have members with spina bifida and compared to individuals from unaffected families [34, 55]. Determining the significance of these enzymes to the disease is complicated by consideration of other maternal and embryonic risk factors. Pietrzyk et al. [55] concluded that maternal homozygosity for polymorphisms in MTHFR and methionine synthase genes confers a high risk. In prior studies, [56] this same causal relationship was shown and it was suggested that the risk of having a child with spina bifida increased with the number of maternal alleles. From these and other studies, enzymes involved in the homocysteine-folate metabolic axis should be considered as independent risk factors for spina bifida.

14.5.5 Down Syndrome

Down syndrome, trisomy 21, is one of the most common human disorders associated with chromosomal imbalance. Clearly the location of the CBS gene on chromosome 21 has a significant impact on affected individuals who have an additional chromosome. The CBS protein is overexpressed in individuals with Down syndrome and alters homocysteine metabolism, resulting in a metabolic imbalance such that folate-dependent resynthesis of methionine is compromised [57].

In a manner similar to potential risk factors for spina bifida, polymorphisms in the MTHFR (C667T) and MTRR (A66G) genes were examined and have been linked to the etiology of Down syndrome [58]. Wisniewski et al. [59] reported the presence of senile plaques and neurofibrillary tangles in the brains of patients with Down syndrome. These findings are neuropathologic hallmarks of Alzheimer's disease; however, the presence of plaques appears at an earlier age. Polymorphisms in the MTHFR gene, as well as increased plasma homocysteine levels, have been associated with Alzheimer's disease in some populations [60]. In general, MTHFR polymorphisms have been linked to a wide variety of disorders that are associated with impaired mental dysfunction, including Alzheimer's disease [60], Down syndrome [59], and spina bifida [55, 56]. Studies are ongoing to clarify the impact of allelic variation for folate metabolizing enzymes in individuals who have Down syndrome.

14.5.6 Cancer

Some cancer cell primary cultures and cell lines express an unusual dependence on methionine for growth [61]. Conversely, most nontransformed cells are methionine independent [62]. Initially, a defect in the enzyme methionine synthase was considered a viable explanation for the methionine dependence. Indeed, decreased activity of this enzyme has been demonstrated in some tumor cell lines [63], but not all [64]. Furthermore, some methionine-dependent cells have defects in cobalamin metabolism [65], while others are associated with defective expression of methylthioadenosine phosphorylase [66]. Thus, methionine dependence is multifactorial. Matsuo et al. [67] examined polymorphisms of methionine synthase reductase (MTRR), methionine synthase, and MTHFR in rectal cancer patients and compared the incidence to noncancer patients. Individuals homozygous for the A66G polymorphism in MTRR had a significantly higher risk of colorectal cancer than other genotypes in Japanese populations [68]. These same three genes were analyzed in Caucasians with non-Hodgkin's lymphoma, multiple myeloma, and noncancer patients. The methionine synthaseA2756G polymorphism was shown to confer a 2.4-fold lower risk in lymphoma patients. Alterations in one-carbon metabolism have also been associated with the pathology of cancer. Indeed, aberrant DNA methylation is a common phenotype in human neoplasias. Decreased SAM levels could contribute to altered DNA methylation in tumor cells. The underlying cause could be a consequence of nutritional imbalance or allelic variation in genes governing SAM metabolism. Paz et al. [68] analyzed a wide range of cancer types for the methylation status of three genes involved in methyl group metabolism. A positive correlation was found among the C677T allele of MTHFR and the 2756G allele of methionine synthase [68]. Efforts continue to unravel what role, if any, these enzymes may have in tumor progression. Whether therapeutic targeting of these pathways could be used to achieve anticancer effects remains to be established. 5,10-Methylene-THF and its 5,10 precursors play critical roles in purine and pyrimidine biosynthesis. The pool of 5,10-methylene-THF increases with diminished activity of MTHFR. Skibola et al. [69] hypothesized that the enhanced 5,10-methylene-THF pools could result in decreased misincorporation of uracil into DNA, thereby resulting in fewer double strand breaks. Hence, folate status would be critical in the development of rapidly proliferating cancers (colorectal and leukemias) that have high DNA synthesis rates. The 667TT genotype was shown to confer a 4.3-fold decreased risk among patients with acute lymphocytic leukemia (ALL) [69]. Further studies in pediatric leukemia patients showed a significant association with the C667T genotype when compared to healthy newborns [70]. 5-Formyl-THF (leucovorin) is used pharmaceutically as a rescue agent in combination with cancer drugs of the antimetabolite class. The role that folate-metabolizing enzymes play in the etiology of cancer is not clearly understood. However, a better understanding of the intricate relationship between cancer risk and thiol status may unravel new initiatives that could incorporate folate supplementation as a means of chemoprevention in high-risk individuals.

14.6 HETEROGENEITY OF GSH METABOLIZING ENZYMES AND ASSOCIATED HUMAN PATHOLOGIES

Alterations in GSH levels are associated with a wide variety of pathologies, including cancer, HIV, lung disease, and Parkinson's disease. Hence, polymorphisms in the genes governing GSH levels are considered contributory to the etiology of these disorders. Polymorphisms within the γ-GCS gene have been identified within the heavy subunit [71]. The gene, located on chromosome 1, encompasses 22 kb and contains seven exons and six introns. Three alleles of the γ-GCS-HS subunit have been identified that differ by the number of GAG trinucleotide repeats in the 5 coding and noncoding region. The contribution of these alleles toward GSH homeostasis pathologies remains unclear. There are examples of altered γ-GCS activity associated with a variety of diseases. The essential role of γ-GCS in GSH synthesis has been demonstrated in knockout mice that were incompetent to form the heavy chain of γ-GCS [72]. The mutation was shown to be embryonic lethal; however, cell lines were derived from the mutants when supplemented with either GSH or N-acetyl cysteine (NAC). In humans, γ-GCS activity is diminished in patients with hemolytic anemia [73]. These patients were shown to carry an A → T mutation at nucleotide 1109 that results in a histidine to leucine transition at amino acid 370. Two additional alterations were identified in an intron (+206) and a CGC repeat in the 3-untranslated region [73]. Some patients with malignant mesothelioma have a deletion on chromosome 1 in the region that encompasses the γ-GCS gene [74]. This deletion can lead to γ-GCS deficiency and it was proposed that this could contribute to the malignant phenotype of this disease.

14.6.1 Diseases Associated with Altered Glutathione Metabolism

14.6.1.1 Defects in Enzymes of the γ-Glutamyl Cycle

To date, hereditary defects have been described in four of the major enzymes that mediate glutathione metabolism through the γ-glutamyl cycle [75]. Polymorphic variants of γ-GCS have been linked to syndromes that include hemolytic anemia, either with or without hepatosplenomegaly. Hereditary defects in glutathione synthetase are autosomal recessive and can lead to mental retardation and neuropsychiatric dysfunction in approximately 50% of patients, while this deficiency is routinely accompanied by metabolic acidosis and hemolytic anemia. The cycle intermediate 5-oxoproline is found in excess in the bloodstream of these patients, presumably because of the lack of feedback inhibition by GSH on γ-GCS. Where glutathione synthetase deficiency is restricted to erythrocytes, the hemolytic anemia is not accompanied by a generalized oxoprolinuria [76]. Glutathionemia (excess GSH in the blood) occurs with aberrant expression of γ-glutamyl-transpeptidase. This can lead to an imbalance in glutamic acid homeostasis, classifying the disease as an inherited disorder of dicarboxylic acid catabolism. Symptoms can include mental retardation, but it is not clear whether there is a straightforward inheritance pattern for this genetic abnormality.

14.6.1.2 Parkinson's Disease

While GSH is found in millimolar concentrations in the brain [77] this organ is more susceptible to oxidative damage than other tissues [78]. Hence an alteration in GSH homeostasis that may lead to oxidative stress has been associated with neurodegenerative diseases, such as Parkinson's disease (PD). Parkinson's disease, affecting nearly 1% of individuals over the age of 65, is a progressive neurodegenerative disorder that results in impaired motor and cognitive functions [79]. The underlying cause of the disease stems from the destruction of dopaminergic neurons in the substantia nigra pars compacta (SNpc) region of the midbrain [80]. These cells are involved in the metabolism of dopamine and PD is characterized by a dopamine deficiency. During normal endogenous dopamine metabolism, ROS are generated and their removal by GSH serves to protect the SNpc. The progression of PD is associated with a depletion of GSH levels and an increase in ROS within the SNpc [81, 82]. Using a murine model, it was shown that BSO treatment depleted GSH and resulted in selective damage to the neurons within the SNpc [83]. In a clinical study, improvements in patients with PD were observed following administration of reduced GSH [83]. Whether prolonged, systemic treatments with reductive agents that cross the blood–brain barrier would prove to be an effective preventive treatment for patients at high risk remains to be established.

14.6.1.3 HIV

Nearly 21.8 million deaths associated with HIV/AIDS were reported worldwide between 1981 and 2000. Prior to clinical manifestations of the disease, the immune system is compromised. GSH levels have an impact on many immune functions, including activation of lymphocytes. Consequently, it was postulated that GSH deficiency could lead to the progression of immune dysfunction, a hallmark of AIDS. Glutathione levels are depleted in plasma, epithelial lining fluid (ELF), peripheral blood mononuclear cells, and monocytes in asymptomatic

HIV-infected individuals and in AIDS patients [84]. Systemic glutathione deficiency has also been reported in symptom-free HIV seropositive individuals. [84]. Clinical studies have shown that GSH deficiency is correlated with morbidity [85]. It seems reasonable to conclude that a generally impaired antioxidant system is an obvious contributory factor that may contribute to these clinical findings. However, the precise importance of GSH deficiency is a more complex scenario. Decreased GSH levels have been shown to activate NF-κB, leading to a series of downstream signal transduction events that allow HIV expression [86]. The long terminal repeat of HIV (HIV LTR) contains an NF-κB site. In vitro studies have shown that NF-κB binds to and activates genes controlled by the HIV LTR [87]. *N*-acetyl-cysteine (NAC) supplementation blocked HIV LTR gene expression, thereby confirming the importance of thiol status in HIV-positive cells [86]. Depletion of the CD4+ T cell lymphocytes accompanies the etiology of HIV progression. Decreased GSH levels are known to be one contributory factor in the induction of apoptosis in CD4+ T lymphocytes [88]. Oxidative stress indices were measured in blood samples from HIV/AIDS patients and compared to healthy individuals [89]. These studies showed that reduced GSH levels were accompanied by an increase of DNA fragmentation in lymphocytes, indicative of apoptosis [89].

These factors suggest that maintenance or restoration of GSH levels is a potential therapeutic approach in HIV patients. Several studies have shown that NAC restores GSH levels, prevents the activation of NF-κB and replication of HIV [90]. Treatment with NAC has provided beneficial effects for HIV-infected individuals, even though GSH levels in lymphocytes are not altered [90]. Plasma GSH levels in HIV-infected individuals were increased to 89% of the uninfected controls following an 8-week treatment with oral NAC [91]. Supplementation with cysteine-rich whey proteins achieves short-term increases in plasma GSH levels [92]. In concordance with other dietary protocols, GSH precursor amino acid supplements seem, at least on the surface, to be a beneficial additive.

14.6.1.4 *Liver Disease*

High intracellular content of GSH in liver are congruous with the detoxification functions of this organ. Inherited disorders in glutathione synthesis and metabolism can significantly disrupt liver function and in some instances can be conditionally lethal. In humans, regular dietary intake of precursor sulfur containing amino acids will maintain hepatic intracellular GSH levels in the 5 to 10 mM range. Alterations in liver GSH are either the cause or effect of a number of pathologies. For example, in alcoholics, pools of mitochondrial GSH are depleted, with the concomitant result that ROS damage can be exacerbated producing cell death and contributing to cirrhosis. The defect that leads to reduced levels of mitochondrial GSH involves a partial inactivation of a specific mitochondrial membrane transport protein [93]. Thus, while a build up of cytosolic GSH occurs, inability to transport this into mitochondria is caused by physicochemical alterations to the inner mitochondrial membrane caused by long-term alcohol exposure. The selective depletion of GSH in this organelle can sensitize hepatocytes to the oxidative effects of cytokines such as tumor necrosis factor (TNF) [94]. In patients with chronic hepatitis C infections, GSH levels are severely depleted in hepatic and plasma fractions and also in peripheral blood mononuclear cells. These conditions were more pronounced in patients who had a concomitant HIV infection [95].

14.6.1.5 Cystic Fibrosis

Cystic fibrosis (CF) is a genetic disorder afflicting nearly 250,000 children worldwide per year. The lung dysfunction that characterizes the disease is due to an alteration in an ion transport protein, cystic fibrosis transmembrane conductance regulator (CFTR). The recessive mutation renders the channel dysfunctional or absent. CFTR is an organic anion efflux channel with functional properties that are redundant to MRP, a related class of ATP binding cassette transporters. CFTR maintains a cellular homeostatic balance of ions, including sodium, chloride, and GSH. Normal levels of GSH in the ELF of the lung are 150 times higher than other tissues [96] where it serves as an essential antioxidant that protects the tissue from inhaled toxins. However, the presence of GSH in the ELF also provides a sensor system for maintaining surfactant production, as well as a trigger for inflammation. CF is characterized by systemic GSH deficiency that progresses over time [97]. Cellular GSH deficiency has been associated with an increase in transcription of NF-κB, which participates in the regulation of the inflammatory cytokines [96]. Low levels of GSH lead to inflammation, a hallmark of CF, and oxidative stress that can lead to damage to cell membranes, cellular proteins, and DNA. In support of the causative influence of ROS in CF, these patients frequently have higher levels of lipid peroxidation by-products [98, 99]. Adding to the complexity of disease progression is the expression pattern of GSTM in CF patients. GSTM1 plays a role in the detoxification of hydroperoxides. Additionally, GSTM1 is a negative regulator of ASK1, a kinase involved in the regulation of apoptotic pathways [100]. CF patients with the null phenotype for GSTM1 (GSTM*0) have a poorer prognosis than individuals with other GSTM1 alleles [101]. At this time, the impact of allelic variation on the regulation of kinase signaling is unknown. We do know, however, that CF patients have a diminished immune response that is attributed to decreased GSH levels leading to premature apoptosis in macrophages and neutrophils recruited to the lung [96].

Some therapeutic strategies for CF are aimed at restoring GSH levels, particularly in the ELF. Cysteine supplementation has been undertaken in other disorders associated with GSH depletion, including PD. Because GSH deficiency is due to an aberration in efflux rather than synthesis, augmentation with GSH is desirable. Three clinical strategies to supplement GSH have included intravenous, oral, or inhalation of GSH or N-acetyl cysteine [102]. Due to stability and uptake, inhalation methods appear more promising. Recent studies in seven CF patients treated with 600 mg of a GSH aerosol administered twice daily for 3 days showed an increase in ELF GSH levels and should provide a platform for future clinical trials [103].

14.6.1.6 Aging

Much has been written concerning the plausible inverse correlation between the generation of free radicals and subsequent ROS and the longevity of an organism. Intuitively, one might assume that natural selection would provide an adaptive force to secure cellular protective mechanisms that permit more efficient protection against such stresses. However, a number of issues cloud this principle and influence the selective advantage of efficient ROS detoxification systems. Specifically, protection of organisms early in life to permit the attainment of reproduction will serve to propagate the species and provide selective advantage. Thus, when diseases of prepuberty result in production of ROS through, for example, a protective inflammatory response, the consequence would be survival to reach a reproductive age. To achieve this, unavoidable cumulative collateral damage may adversely influence the organism in the later stages of life. This outcome would have little consequence to the success of the individual in terms of selective advantage. In other words, the biological advantage of protecting somatic cells in old age will not have a major impact on survival of the species, whereas energy expended at younger ages will be a strong selective advantage. Therefore, there is significant advantage to counteracting childhood infections with macrophage-mediated ROS defenses. Notwithstanding the age-related relevance of the cellular defense mechanisms, the pleiotropic and redundant array of protective enzyme systems that counteract ROS include many that utilize GSH directly. The type and complement of these protective systems can vary significantly, both between tissues and between organisms. In the blood and tissues of numerous organisms any or all of the following can contribute to protection against ROS: water soluble radical scavengers, including GSH, ascorbate, or urate; lipid soluble scavengers, α-tocopherol, γ-tocopherol, flavonoids, carotenoids, ubiquinol; enzymatic scavengers such as superoxide dismutase (SOD), catalase and glutathione peroxidase and some glutathione S-transferases; small molecule thiol-rich antioxidants such as thioredoxin and metallothionein; the enzymes that maintain small molecule antioxidants in a reduced state, thioredoxin reductase, glutathione reductase, dehydroascorbate reductase, the glyoxalase sytem; the complement of enzymes that maintain a reduced cellular environment, including glucose-6-phosphate dehydrogenase, in part responsible for maintaining levels of NADPH. The functional redundancy and cooperative interactions between these defense pathways illustrates just how critical protection against ROS is to survival.

Numerous reports have correlated age-related induction of oxidized or glycated proteins with a decreased ratio of GSH to GSSG in both invertebrates and vertebrates. A number of important metabolic enzymes, including aconitase III, can be inactivated by oxidation [104]. This enzyme participates in the citric acid cycle and possesses an active site iron-sulfur cluster which is sensitive to inactivation by superoxide ($O_2^{\cdot-}$) [105]. Carbonic anhydrase III has two reactive sulfhydryls that are subject to conversion to cysteine sulfinic acid or cysteic acid in the presence of H_2O_2, peroxy radicals, or hypochlorous acid (HOCl). These reactions are competitively inhibited by GSH, perhaps as a consequence of S-glutathionylation of the affected cysteine residues [106]. These authors reported that in menadione-treated rats, the extent of cysteine sulfinic acid damage to aconitase III was higher in older animals compared to young ones. In light of the potential widespread occurrence of protein S-glutathionylation, it seems reasonable to propose that this mechanism may prove to be functionally protective for a number of critical cellular proteins.

Some credence has been given to the relevance of ROS-induced cell membrane damage as a causative event in cell aging and senescence. In this context, oxygen toxicity can be promoted by metals (such as iron and copper) that catalyze the cleavage of ROOH groups. This Fenton reaction generates hydroxyl radicals (OH$^{\bullet}$) which can abstract protons to initiate lipid peroxidation reactions. In healthy individuals, the potential catalytic activity of these metals is negatively regulated through binding to proteins such as ferritin and transferrin [78]. In aging humans the total body content of iron increases with age (in women after menopause). It was proposed that this increase would promote the occurrence of oxidative damage during the aging process [107] and that perhaps lipid peroxide-induced membrane damage could be crucial to the onset of geriatric disease. A further indication that lipid peroxidation may be linked to aging is provided by studies in *Drosophila* [108]. By disrupting a microsomal glutathione-*S*-transferase (mGST)-like gene these authors showed that the mutant flies had a significantly reduced lifespan compared to controls. One of the characteristic properties of mGSTs is their efficacy in detoxifying products of lipid peroxidation, particularly in the membrane compartments of cells.

A recent small scale study in healthy humans aged 19 to 85 measured the ratios of cysteine to cystine and GSH to GSSG in plasma [109]. For the former, a linear oxidation rate was observed throughout life. For GSH : GSSG ratios, there was no alteration in the redox balance until age 45, after which there was an enhanced oxidation at a nearly linear rate. While the correlation between low GSH levels or low GSH : GSSG ratios and aging seems clear, the precise reasons for the age-related change in the content of GSH is less well characterized. One recent report has shown that a downregulation of the regulatory subunit of γ-GCS occurs in the rat brain during aging [110]. As the combination of catalytic and regulatory subunits of GCS contributes to the de novo synthesis of GSH, this age-related alteration in expression of this enzyme subunit may be a contributory factor in leading to the lower GSH levels.

Support for the free radical theory of aging is also provided from clinical studies in accelerated aging diseases such as Down syndrome, progeria—both adult (Werner syndrome) and childhood (Hutchison–Gilford). In each case a significantly shortened lifespan is accompanied by evidence of increased oxidative stress and disturbance in the redox balance of host cells [111].

The immune response with respect to balance of Th1 and Th2 production can also be influenced by redox conditions. For example, thioredoxin transgenic mice had a longer life expectancy than their wild-type counterparts. In these mice, peritoneal resident macrophages showed a higher ratio of GSH to GSSG compared to age-matched wild-type animals [112]. These so-called reductive macrophages predominated and were associated with sustained maintenance of Th1 prevalence during aging until 2 years in the transgenic mice, while wild-type littermates showed a rapid polarization to Th2 at 8 months. Cytokine production was different in these animals, suggesting that altered redox balance, particularly as a consequence of GSH changes, could influence immune response.

Dietary supplements frequently claim to be enriched in antioxidants and free radical scavengers. Are such claims of value to prevention of aging and the diseases associated with age? In the absence of carefully controlled (and possibly long-term) clinical studies, this is a difficult question to answer. Inclusion of GSH in over-the-counter supplements is of limited value, since the reduced state will not be maintained when exposed to normal atmospheric conditions and room temperature. Perhaps the oxidized product (GSSG) will provide a supply of the constituent amino acids, where, in particular, cysteine may be useful in stimulating gastrointestinal synthesis of GSH. There is sufficient evidence that thiol-containing compounds can rescue patients from acute exposure to oxidative or electrophilic stress (for example, *N*-acetyl cysteine in acetaminophen overdose). It is also a general principle that cells prefer (and thrive in) a mildly reduced environment and that mild oxidative stress can stimulate growth in a manner not conducive to benign cellular homeostasis. As such, there would seem to be no harm in supplementing a diet with reducing equivalents. However, whether this will prove to be the elixir of longevity remains to be seen.

14.6.2   Diseases Associated with Glutathione *S*-Transferase Polymorphisms

Glutathione *S*-transferases (GSTs) are a family of phase II detoxification enzymes that have co-evolved with GSH and are abundant throughout most phyla. GSTs catalyze the conjugation of GSH to a wide variety of endogenous and exogenous electrophilic compounds. Human GSTs are divided into the membrane-bound microsomal and cytosolic family members. Microsomal GSTs play a key role in the endogenous metabolism of leukotrienes and prostaglandins [113]. Cytosolic GSTs are divided into 6 classes: α, μ, ω, π, θ, and ζ. GSTs can be induced by structurally unrelated compounds known to result in chemical stress and carcinogenesis, including phenobarbital, planar aromatic compounds, ethoxyquin, butylated hydroxyanisole (BHA), and trans-stilbene oxide [114]. Some of the compounds known to induce GSTs are themselves substrates of the enzyme, suggesting that induction is an adaptive response. Many clinically useful drugs are also potential substrates for GST and development of drug resistance can frequently be a key element in cancer treatment failure. GSTs have been linked with the development of resistance toward chemotherapy agents, insecticides, herbicides, and microbial antibiotics [115].

In addition to their catalytic function, GSTs have been shown to form protein-protein interactions with members of the Mitogen Activated Protein (MAP) kinase pathway, thereby serving a regulatory role in the balance between cell survival and apoptosis. By interacting directly with MAP kinases, including c-Jun N-terminal kinase 1 (JNK1) and ASK1 (apoptosis signal-regulating kinase), GSTs function to sequester the ligand in a complex, preventing interactions with their downstream targets [100]. Many anticancer agents induce apoptosis via activation of MAP kinase pathways, in particular those involving JNK and p38 [116]. This novel, non-enzymatic role for GSTs has direct relevance to the GST overexpressing phenotypes of many drug-resistant tumors. As an endogenous switch for the control of signaling cascade pathways, elevated expression of GST alters the balance of regulation of kinase pathways during drug treatment, thereby conferring a potential selective advantage. This process can also provide a plausible explanation for the numerous examples of drug resistance linking GST overexpression with agents that are not substrates for these enzymes.

While polymorphisms have been identified within each class of GSTs, only a limited number have been shown to contribute to human pathologies or clinical drug response. The μ and τ class of GST have a null phenotype (GSTM*0 and GSTT*0) where individuals do not express catalytically active protein. The presumed inability to detoxify carcinogens is associated with an increased risk toward a variety of cancers. The GSTM1*0 allele is observed in $\sim$50% of the Caucasian population [117] and is associated with an increased risk of lung, colon, and bladder cancer and is a risk factor for pulmonary asbestosis [118, 119]. The GSTT*0 phenotype varies between ethnic groups and is found to be highest in Chinese (65%) and lowest in Mexican American (9%) populations [120]. The GSTT*0 phenotype is associated with an increased risk of tumors of the head and neck, oral cavity, pharynx, and larynx [121, 122].

The μ class of GSTs has five genes (GSTM1-5) [123] that are found in a gene cluster on chromosome 1 [124]. The GSTM1 gene contains four alleles and has been the most widely studied. GSTM1*A has been associated with a decreased risk of bladder cancer and has an allele frequency of 20% [117]. Neurodegenerative diseases such as Parkinson's disease and schizophrenia are characterized by the degeneration of dopaminergic neurons. GSTM2-2 has been shown to catalyze the conjugation of GSH to aminochrome, a reactive oxygen species generated in the redox cycling of orthoquinones within dopaminergic neurons [125]. Hence, GSTM2-2 has been proposed to play a protective role against neurodegenerative diseases.

A single gene spanning $\sim$3 kb located on chromosome 11 encodes for proteins designated in the π class of GSTs [126]. Polymorphisms at the GSTP1 locus result in four alleles, GSTP1*A-D, that differ structurally and functionally [127]. The promoter region contains a TATA box, two SP1 sites, an insulin response element, and an antioxidant response element within an AP-1 site [127]. GSTP1*A plays a role in the acquisition of resistance to cisplatin by enhancing the capacity of the cell to form platinum-glutathione conjugates [128]. GSTP1*B is an allele in which a single nucleotide (A $\rightarrow$ G) substitution at position 313 substantially diminishes catalytic activity [129]. Homozygocity for GSTP1*B is favorable in the treatment of cancer patients because they have a diminished capacity to detoxify platinum-based anticancer agents [130]. GSTP1*C or an allelic variant that is more predominant in malignant glioma cells differs from other GSTP1 variants by two transitions resulting in Ile104Val and Ala113Val [127c]. No major functional property has yet been assigned to this polymorphism.

REFERENCES

1. Wagner, C., Decha-Umphai, W., Corbin, J. (1989). Phosphorylation modulates the activity of glycine N-methyltransferase, a folate binding protein. In vitro phosphorylation is inhibited by the natural folate ligand. *Journal of Biological Chemistry*, *264*(16), 9638–9642.

2. Jencks, D.A., Mathews, R.G. (1987). Allosteric inhibition of methylenetetrahydrofolate reductase by adenosylmethionine. Effects of adenosylmethionine and NADPH on the equilibrium between active and inactive forms of the enzyme and on the kinetics of approach to equilibrium. *Journal of Biological Chemistry*, *262*(6), 2485–2493.

3. Wagner, C., Briggs, W.T., Cook, R.J. (1985). Inhibition of glycine N-methyltransferase activity by folate derivatives: Implications for regulation of methyl group metabolism. *Biochemical and Biophysical Research Communications, 127*(3), 746–752.

4. Kutzbach, C., Stokstad, E.L. (1967). Feedback inhibition of methylene-tetrahydrofolate reductase in rat liver by S-adenosylmethionine. *Biochimica et Biophysica Acta, 139*(1), 217–220.

5. Choi, S.W., Mason, J.B. (2000). Folate and carcinogenesis: An integrated scheme. *Journal of Nutrition, 130*(2), 129–132.

6. Mason, J.B. (2003). Biomarkers of nutrient exposure and status in one-carbon (methyl) metabolism. *Journal of Nutrition, 133* (Suppl 3), 941S–947S.

7. McCully, K.S. (1969). Vascular pathology of homocysteinemia: Implications for the pathogenesis of arteriosclerosis. *American Journal of Pathology, 56*(1), 111–128.

8. Clarke, R., Daly, L., Robinson, K., Naughten, E., Cahalane, S., Fowler, B., Graham, I. (1991). Hyperhomocysteinemia: An independent risk factor for vascular disease. *New England Journal of Medicine, 324*(17), 1149–1155.

9. Kang, S.S., Wong, P.W., Malinow, M.R. (1992). Hyperhomocyst(e)inemia as a risk factor for occlusive vascular disease. *Annual Review of Nutrition, 12*, 279–298.

10. Vollset, S.E., Refsum, H., Tverdal, A., Nygard, O., Nordrehaug, J.E., Tell, G.S., Ueland, P.M. (2001). Plasma total homocysteine and cardiovascular and noncardiovascular mortality: The Hordaland Homocysteine Study. *American Journal of Clinical Nutrition, 74*(1), 130–136.

11. Ubbink, J.B., Vermaak, W.J., van der Merwe, A., Becker, P.J. (1993). Vitamin B-12, vitamin B-6, and folate nutritional status in men with hyperhomocysteinemia. *American Journal of Clinical Nutrition, 57*(1), 47–53.

12. Jacques, P.F., Selhub, J., Bostom, A.G., Wilson, P.W., Rosenberg, I.H. (1999). The effect of folic acid fortification on plasma folate and total homocysteine concentrations. *New England Journal of Medicine, 340*(19), 1449–1454.

13. Riddell, L.J., Chisholm, A., Williams, S., Mann, J.I. (2000). Dietary strategies for lowering homocysteine concentrations. *American Journal of Clinical Nutrition, 71*(6), 1448–1454.

14. Carson, N.A., Neill, D.W. (1962). Metabolic abnormalities detected in a survey of mentally backward individuals in Northern Ireland. *Archives of Disease in Childhood, 37*, 505–513.

15. Gerritsen, T., Vaughn, J.G., Waisman, H.A. (1962). The identification of homocystine in the urine. *Biochemical and Biophysical Research Communications, 9*, 493–496.

16. Mudd, S.H., Skovby, F., Levy, H.L., Pettigrew, K.D., Wilcken, B., Pyeritz, R.E., Andria, G., Boers, G.H., Bromberg, I.L., Cerone, R. (1985). The natural history of homocystinuria due to cystathionine beta-synthase deficiency. *American Journal of Human Genetics, 37*(1), 1–31.

17. Fowler, B., Kraus, J., Packman, S., Rosenberg, L.E. (1978). Homocystinuria: Evidence for three distinct classes of cystathionine beta-synthase mutants in cultured fibroblasts. *Journal of Clinical Investigation, 61*(3), 645–653.

18. Skovby, F., Krassikoff, N., Francke, U. (1984). Assignment of the gene for cystathionine beta-synthase to human chromosome 21 in somatic cell hybrids. *Human Genetics, 65*(3), 291–294.

19. Munke, M., Kraus, J.P., Ohura, T., Francke, U. (1988). The gene for cystathionine beta-synthase (CBS) maps to the subtelomeric region on human chromosome 21q and to proximal mouse chromosome 17. *American Journal of Human Genetics*, *42*(4), 550–559.

20. Kraus, J.P., Oliveriusova, J., Sokolova, J., Kraus, E., Vlcek, C., de Franchis, R., Maclean, K.N., Bao, L., Bukovsk, L., Patterson, D., Paces, V., Ansorge, W., Kozich, V. (1998). The human cystathionine beta-synthase (CBS) gene: Complete sequence, alternative splicing, and polymorphisms. *Genomics*, *52*(3), 312–324.

21. Kraus, J.P., Janosik, M., Kozich, V., Mandell, R., Shih, V., Sperandeo, M.P., Sebastio, G., de Franchis, R., Andria, G., Kluijtmans, L.A., Blom, H., Boers, G.H., Gordon, R.B., Kamoun, P., Tsai, M.Y., Kruger, W.D., Koch, H.G., Ohura, T, Gaustadnes, M. (1999). Cystathionine beta-synthase mutations in homocystinuria. *Human Mutation*, *13*(5), 362–375.

22. Kraus, J.P. (1994). Komrower Lecture. Molecular basis of phenotype expression in homocystinuria. *Journal of Inherited Metabolic Disease*, *17*(4), 383–390.

23. Abbott, M.H., Folstein, S.E., Abbey, H., Pyeritz, R.E. (1987). Psychiatric manifestations of homocystinuria due to cystathionine beta-synthase deficiency: Prevalence, natural history, and relationship to neurologic impairment and vitamin B6-responsiveness. *American Journal of Medical Genetics*, *26*(4), 959–969.

24. Frimpter, G.W. (1965). Cystathioninuria: Nature of the defect. *Science*, *149*(688), 1095–1096.

25. Wong, L.T., Hardwick, D.F., Applegarth, D.A., Davidson, A.G. (1979). Review of Metabolic Screening Program of Children's Hospital, Vancouver, British Columbia. 1971–1977. *Clinical Biochemistry*, *12*(5), 167–172.

26. Smith, A.J., Strang, L.B. (1958). An inborn error of metabolism with the urinary excretion of alpha-hydroxy-butyric acid and phenylpyruvic acid. *Archives of Disease in Childhood*, *33*(168), 109–113.

27. Tapiero, H., Tew, K.D., Gate, L., Machover, D. (2001). Prevention of pathologies associated with oxidative stress and dietary intake deficiencies: Folate deficiency and requirements. *Biomedicine & Pharmacotherapy*, *55*(7), 381–390.

28. Luhby, A.L., Cooperman, J.M., Pesci-Bourel, A. (1965). A new inborn error of metabolism: Folic acid responsive megaloblastic anemia, ataxia, mental retardation, and convulsions. *Journal of Pediatrics*, *67*, 1052.

29. Lanzkowsky, P., Erlandson, M.E., Bezan, A.I. (1969). Isolated defect of folic acid absorption associated with mental retardation and cerebral calcification. *Blood*, *34*(4), 452–465.

30. Wollaston, W.H. (1810). On cystic oxide, a new species of urinary calculus. *Philosophical Transactions of the Royal Society of London. Series B, Biological Sciences*, *100*, 223–230.

31. Calonge, M.J., Gasparini, P., Chillaron, J., Chillon, M., Gallucci, M., Rousaud, F., Zelante, L., Testar, X., Dallapiccola, B., Di Silverio, F., Barceló, P., Estivill, X., Zorzano, A., Nunes, V., Palacín, M. (1994). Cystinuria caused by mutations in rBAT, a gene involved in the transport of cystine. *Nature Genetics*, *6*(4), 420–425.

32. Lee, W.S., Wells, R.G., Sabbag, R.V., Mohandas, T.K., Hediger, M.A. (1993). Cloning and chromosomal localization of a human kidney cDNA involved in cystine, dibasic, and neutral amino acid transport. *Journal of Clinical Investigation*, *91*(5), 1959–1963.

33. Feliubadalo, L., Font, M., Purroy, J., Rousaud, F., Estivill, X., Nunes, V., Golomb, E., Centola, M., Aksentijevich, I., Kreiss, Y., Goldman, B., Pras, M., Kastner, D. L., Pras, E., Gasparini, P., Bisceglia, L., Beccia, E., Gallucci, M., de Sanctis, L., Ponzone, A., Rizzoni, G.F., Zelante, L., Bassi, M.T., George, A.L., Jr., Manzoni, M., De Grandi, A., Riboni, M., Endsley, J.K., Ballabio, A., Borsani, G., Reig, N., Fernandez, E., Estevez, R., Pineda, M., Torrents, D., Camps, M., Lloberas, J., Zorzano, A., Palacin, M. (1999). Non-type I cystinuria caused by mutations in SLC7A9, encoding a subunit (bo,+AT) of rBAT. *Nature Genetics*, *23*(1), 52–57.

34. Leclerc, D., Wilson, A., Dumas, R., Gafuik, C., Song, D., Watkins, D., Heng, H.H., Rommens, J.M., Scherer, S.W., Rosenblatt, D.S., Gravel, R.A. (1998). Cloning and mapping of a cDNA for methionine synthase reductase, a flavoprotein defective in patients with homocystinuria. *Proceedings of the National Academy of Sciences USA*, *95*, 3059–3064.

35. Wilson, A., Leclerc, D., Rosenblatt, D.S., Gravel, R.A. (1999). Molecular basis for methionine synthase reductase deficiency in patients belonging to the cblE complementation group of disorders in folate/cobalamin metabolism. *Human Molecular Genetics*, *8*(11), 2009–2016.

36. Wilson, A., Platt, R., Wu, Q., Leclerc, D., Christensen, B., Yang, H., Gravel, R.A., Rozen, R. (1999). A common variant in methionine synthase reductase combined with low cobalamin (vitamin B12) increases risk for spina bifida. *Molecular Genetics and Metabolism*, *67*(4), 317–323.

37. Hobbs, C.A., Sherman, S.L., Yi, P., Hopkins, S.E., Torfs, C.P., Hine, R.J., Pogribna, M., Rozen, R., James, S.J. (2000). Polymorphisms in genes involved in folate metabolism as maternal risk factors for Down syndrome. *American Journal of Human Genetics*, *67*(3), 623–630.

38. Gaughan, D.J., Barbaux, S., Kluijtmans, L.A., Whitehead, A.S. (2000). The human and mouse methylenetetrahydrofolate reductase (MTHFR) genes: Genomic organization, mRNA structure and linkage to the CLCN6 gene. *Gene*, *257*(2), 279–289.

39. Sibani, S., Christensen, B., O'Ferrall, E., Saadi, I., Hiou-Tim, F., Rosenblatt, D.S., Rozen, R. (2000). Characterization of six novel mutations in the methylenetetrahydrofolate reductase (MTHFR) gene in patients with homocystinuria. *Human Mutation*, *15*(3), 280–287.

40. Rozen, R. (1996). Molecular genetics of methylenetetrahydrofolate reductase deficiency. *Journal of Inherited Metabolic Disease*, *19*(5), 589–594.

41. Goyette, P., Sumner, J.S., Milos, R., Duncan, A.M., Rosenblatt, D.S., Matthews, R.G., Rozen, R. (1994). Human methylenetetrahydrofolate reductase: Isolation of cDNA, mapping and mutation identification. *Nature Genetics*, *7*(2), 195–200.

42. Frosst, P., Blom, H.J., Milos, R., Goyette, P., Sheppard, C.A., Matthews, R.G., Boers, G.J., den Heijer, M., Kluijtmans, L.A., van den Heuvel, L.P., Rozen, R. (1995). A candidate genetic risk factor for vascular disease: A common mutation in methylenetetrahydrofolate reductase. *Nature Genetics*, *10*(1), 111–113.

43. Schneider, J.A., Rees, D.C., Liu, Y.T., Clegg, J.B. (1998). Worldwide distribution of a common methylenetetrahydrofolate reductase mutation. *American Journal of Human Genetics*, *62*(5), 1258–1260.

44. McAndrew, P.E., Brandt, J.T., Pearl, D.K., Prior, T.W. (1996). The incidence of the gene for thermolabile methylene tetrahydrofolate reductase in African Americans. *Thrombosis Research*, *83*(2), 195–198.

45. Bagley, P.J., Selhub, J. (1998). A common mutation in the methylenetetrahydrofolate reductase gene is associated with an accumulation of formylated tetrahydrofolates in red blood cells. *Proceedings of the National Academy of Sciences USA, 95*(22), 13217–13220.

46. Friso, S., Choi, S.W., Girelli, D., Mason, J.B., Dolnikowski, G.G., Bagley, P.J., Olivieri, O., Jacques, P.F., Rosenberg, I.H., Corrocher, R., Selhub, J. (2002). A common mutation in the 5,10-methylenetetrahydrofolate reductase gene affects genomic DNA methylation through an interaction with folate status. *Proceedings of the National Academy of Sciences USA, 99*(8), 5606–5611.

47. Jacques, P.F., Bostom, A.G., Williams, R.R., Ellison, R.C., Eckfeldt, J.H., Rosenberg, I.H., Selhub, J., Rozen, R. (1996). Relation between folate status, a common mutation in methylenetetrahydrofolate reductase, and plasma homocysteine concentrations. *Circulation, 93*(1), 7–9.

48. Kluijtmans, L.A., van den Heuvel, L.P., Boers, G.H., Frosst, P., Stevens, E.M., van Oost, B.A., den Heijer, M., Trijbels, F.J., Rozen, R., Blom, H.J. (1996). Molecular genetic analysis in mild hyperhomocysteinemia: A common mutation in the methylenetetrahydrofolate reductase gene is a genetic risk factor for cardiovascular disease. *American Journal of Human Genetics, 58*(1), 35–41.

49. Klerk, M., Verhoef, P., Clarke, R., Blom, H.J., Kok, F.J., Schouten, E.G. (2002). MTHFR 677C → T polymorphism and risk of coronary heart disease: A meta-analysis. *JAMA, 288*(16), 2023–2031.

50. Christensen, B., Arbour, L., Tran, P., Leclerc, D., Sabbaghian, N., Platt, R., Gilfix, B.M., Rosenblatt, D.S., Gravel, R.A., Forbes, P., Rozen, R. (1999). Genetic polymorphisms in methylenetetrahydrofolate reductase and methionine synthase, folate levels in red blood cells, and risk of neural tube defects. *American Journal of Medical Genetics, 84*(2), 151–157.

51. Ou, C.Y., Stevenson, R.E., Brown, V.K., Schwartz, C.E., Allen, W.P., Khoury, M.J., Rozen, R., Oakley, G.P., Jr., Adams, M.J., Jr. (1996). 5,10-Methylenetetrahydrofolate reductase genetic polymorphism as a risk factor for neural tube defects. *American Journal of Medical Genetics, 63*(4), 610–614.

52. Mornet, E., Muller, F., Lenvoisé-Furet, A., Delezoide, A.L., Col, J.Y., Simon-Bouy, B., Serre, J.L. (1997). Screening of the C677T mutation on the methylenetetrahydrofolate reductase gene in French patients with neural tube defects. *Human Genetics, 100*(5–6), 512–514.

53. Speer, M.C., Worley, G., Mackey, J.F., Melvin, E., Oakes, W.J., George, T.M. (1997). The thermolabile variant of methylenetetrahydrofolate reductase (MTHFR) is not a major risk factor for neural tube defect in American Caucasians. The NTD Collaborative Group. *Neurogenetics, 1*(2), 149–150.

54. Motulsky, A.G. (1996). Nutritional ecogenetics: Homocysteine-related arteriosclerotic vascular disease, neural tube defects, and folic acid. *American Journal of Human Genetics, 58*(1), 17–20.

55. Pietrzyk, J.J., Bik-Multanowski, M., Sanak, M., Twardowska, M. (2003). Polymorphisms of the 5,10-methylenetetrahydrofolate and the methionine synthase reductase genes as independent risk factors for spina bifida. *Journal of Applied Genetics, 44*(1), 111–113.

56. Doolin, M.T., Barbaux, S., McDonnell, M., Hoess, K., Whitehead, A.S., Mitchell, L.E. (2002). Maternal genetic effects, exerted by genes involved in homocysteine

remethylation, influence the risk of spina bifida. *American Journal of Human Genetics,* *71*(5), 1222–1226.

57. Pogribna, M., Melnyk, S., Pogribny, I., Chango, A., Yi, P., James, S.J. (2001). Homocysteine metabolism in children with Down syndrome: In vitro modulation. *American Journal of Human Genetics, 69*(1), 88–95.

58. O'Leary, V.B., Parle-McDermott, A., Molloy, A.M., Kirke, P.N., Johnson, Z., Conley, M., Scott, J.M., Mills, J.L. (2002). MTRR and MTHFR polymorphism: Link to Down syndrome? *American Journal of Medical Genetics, 107*(2), 151–155.

59. Wisniewski, K.E., Wisniewski, H.M., Wen, G.Y. (1985). Occurrence of neuropathological changes and dementia of Alzheimer's disease in Down's syndrome. *Annals of Neurology, 17*(3), 278–282.

60. Religa, D., Styczynska, M., Peplonska, B., Gabryelewicz, T., Pfeffer, A., Chodakowska, M., Luczywek, E., Wasiak, B., Stepien, K., Golebiowski, M., Winblad, B., Barcikowska, M. (2003). Homocysteine, apolipoproteine E and methylenetetrahydrofolate reductase in Alzheimer's disease and mild cognitive impairment. *Dementia and Geriatric Cognitive Disorders, 16*(2), 64–70.

61. Hoffman, R.M. (1982). Methionine dependence in cancer cells: A review. *In Vitro, 18*(5), 421–428.

62. Hoffman, R.M. (1985). Altered methionine metabolism and transmethylation in cancer. *Anticancer Research, 5*(1), 1–30.

63. Liteplo, R.G., Hipwell, S.E., Rosenblatt, D.S., Sillaots, S., Lue-Shing, H. (1991). Changes in cobalamin metabolism are associated with the altered methionine auxotrophy of highly growth autonomous human melanoma cells. *Journal of Cellular Physiology, 149*(2), 332–338.

64. Tautt, J.W., Anuszewska, E.L., Koziorowska, J.H. (1982). Methionine regulation of N-5-methyltetrahydrofolate: Homocysteine methyltransferase and its influence on the growth and protein synthesis in normal, neoplastic, and transformed cells in culture. *Journal of the National Cancer Institute, 69*(1), 9–14.

65. Fiskerstrand, T., Christensen, B., Tysnes, O.B., Ueland, P.M., Refsum, H. (1994). Development and reversion of methionine dependence in a human glioma cell line: Relation to homocysteine remethylation and cobalamin status. *Cancer Research, 54*(18), 4899–4906.

66. Tang, B., Li, Y.N., Kruger, W.D. (2000). Defects in methylthioadenosine phosphorylase are associated with but not responsible for methionine-dependent tumor cell growth. *Cancer Research, 60*(19), 5543–5547.

67. Matsuo, K., Hamajima, N., Hirai, T., Kato, T., Inoue, M., Takezaki, T., Tajima, K. (2002). Methionine synthase reductase gene A66G polymorphism is associated with risk of colorectal cancer. *Sian Pacific Journal of Cancer Prevention, 3*(4), 353–359.

68. Paz, M.F., Avila, S., Fraga, M.F., Pollan, M., Capella, G., Peinado, M.A., Sanchez-Cespedes, M., Herman, J.G., Esteller, M. (2002). Germ-line variants in methyl-group metabolism genes and susceptibility to DNA methylation in normal tissues and human primary tumors. *Cancer Research, 62*(15), 4519–4524.

69. Skibola, C.F., Smith, M.T., Kane, E., Roman, E., Rollinson, S., Cartwright, R.A., Morgan, G. (1999). Polymorphisms in the methylenetetrahydrofolate reductase gene are associated with susceptibility to acute leukemia in adults. *Proceedings of the National Academy of Sciences USA, 96*(22), 12810–12815.

70. Wiemels, J.L., Smith, R.N., Taylor, G.M., Eden, O.B., Alexander, F.E., Greaves, M.F. (2001). Methylenetetrahydrofolate reductase (MTHFR) polymorphisms and risk of molecularly defined subtypes of childhood acute leukemia. *Proceedings of the National Academy of Sciences USA*, *98*(7), 4004–4009.

71. Walsh, A.C., Li, W., Rosen, D.R., Lawrence, D.A. (1996). Genetic mapping of GLCLC, the human gene encoding the catalytic subunit of γ-glutamylcysteine synthetase, to chromosome band 6p12 and characterization of a polymorphic trinucleotide repeat within its 5′ untranslated region. *Cytogenetics and Cell Genetics*, *75*(1), 14–16.

72. Shi, Z.Z., Osei-Frimpong, J., Kala, G., Kala, S.V., Barrios, R.J., Habib, G.M., Lukin, D.J., Danney, C.M., Matzuk, M.M., Lieberman, M.W. (2000). Glutathione synthesis is essential for mouse development but not for cell growth in culture. *Proceedings of the National Academy of Sciences USA*, *97*(10), 5101–5106.

73. Beutler, E., Gelbart, T., Kondo, T., Matsunaga, A.T. (1999). The molecular basis of a case of γ-glutamylcysteine synthetase deficiency. *Blood*, *94*(8), 2890–2894.

74. Rozet, J.M., Gerber, S., Perrault, I., Calvas, P., Souied, E., Châtelin, S., Viegas-Péquignot, Molina-Gomez, D., Munnich, A., Kaplan, J. (1998). Structure and refinement of the physical mapping of the γ-glutamylcysteine ligase regulatory subunit (GLCLR) gene to chromosome 1p22.1 within the critically deleted region of human malignant mesothelioma. *Cytogenetics and Cell Genetics*, *82*(1–2), 91–94.

75. Ristoff, E., Larsson, A. (1998). Patients with genetic defects in the γ-glutamyl cycle. *Chemico-Biological Interactions*, *111–112*, 113–121.

76. Shi, Z.Z., Habib, G.M., Rhead, W.J., Gahl, W.A., He, X., Sazer, S., Lieberman, M.W. (1996). Mutations in the glutathione synthetase gene cause 5-oxoprolinuria. *Nature Genetics*, *14*(3), 361–365.

77. Dringen, R., Gutterer, J.M., Hirrlinger, J. (2000). Glutathione metabolism in brain metabolic interaction between astrocytes and neurons in the defense against reactive oxygen species. *European Journal of Biochemistry*, *267*(16), 4912–4916.

78. Halliwell, B., Gutteridge, J.M. (1986). Oxygen free radicals and iron in relation to biology and medicine: Some problems and concepts. *Archives of Biochemistry and Biophysics*, *246*(2), 501–514.

79. Youdim, M.B., Riederer, P. (1997). Understanding Parkinson's disease. *Scientific American*, *276*(1), 52–59.

80. Forno, L.S. (1996). Neuropathology of Parkinson's disease. *Journal of Neuropathology and Experimental Neurology*, *55*(3), 259–272.

81. Sofic, E., Lange, K.W., Jellinger, K., Riederer, P. (1992). Reduced and oxidized glutathione in the substantia nigra of patients with Parkinson's disease. *Neuroscience Letters*, *142*(2), 128–130.

82. Adams, J.D., Jr., Chang, M.L., Klaidman, L. (2001). Parkinson's disease: Redox mechanisms. *Current Medicinal Chemistry*, *8*(7), 809–814.

83. Sechi, G., Deledda, M.G., Bua, G., Satta, W.M., Deiana, G.A., Pes, G.M., Rosati, G. (1996). Reduced intravenous glutathione in the treatment of early Parkinson's disease. *Progress in Neuro-Psychopharmacology & Biological Psychiatry*, *20*(7), 1159–1170.

84. Buhl, R., Jaffe, H.A., Holroyd, K.J., Wells, F.B., Mastrangeli, A., Saltini, C., Cantin, A.M., Crystal, R.G. (1989). Systemic glutathione deficiency in symptom-free HIV-seropositive individuals. *Lancet*, *2*(8675), 1294–1298.

85. Herzenberg, L.A., De Rosa, S.C., Dubs, J.G., Roederer, M., Anderson, M.T., Ela, S.W., Deresinski, S.C., Herzenberg, L.A. (1997). Glutathione deficiency is associated with impaired survival in HIV disease. *Proceedings of the National Academy of Sciences USA*, *94*(5), 1967–1672.

86. Staal, F.J., Roederer, M., Herzenberg, L.A., Herzenberg, L.A. (1990). Intracellular thiols regulate activation of nuclear factor kappa B and transcription of human immunodeficiency virus. *Proceedings of the National Academy of Sciences USA*, *87*(24), 9943–9947.

87. Duh, E.J., Maury, W.J., Folks, T.M., Fauci, A.S., Rabson, A.B. (1989). Tumor necrosis factor alpha activates human immunodeficiency virus type 1 through induction of nuclear factor binding to the NF-kappa B sites in the long terminal repeat. *Proceedings of the National Academy of Sciences USA*, *86*(15), 5974–5978.

88. Suthanthiran, M., Anderson, M.E., Sharma, V.K., Meister, A. (1990). Glutathione regulates activation-dependent DNA synthesis in highly purified normal human T lymphocytes stimulated via the CD2 and CD3 antigens. *Proceedings of the National Academy of Sciences USA*, *87*(9), 3343–3347.

89. Gil, L., Martínez, G., González, I., Tarinas, A., Alvarez, A., Giuliani, A., Molina, R., Tápanes, R., Pérez, J., León, O.S. (2003). Contribution to characterization of oxidative stress in HIV/AIDS patients. *Pharmacological Research*, *47*(3), 217–224.

90. Nakamura, H., Masutani, H., Yodoi, J. (2002). Redox imbalance and its control in HIV infection. *Antioxidant Redox Signaling*, *4*(3), 455–464.

91. DeRosa, S.C., Zaretsky, M.D., Dubs, J.G., Roederer, M., Anderson, M., Green, A., Mitra, D., Watanabe, N., Nakamura, H., Tjioe, I., Deresinski, S.C., Moore, W.A., Ela, S.W., Parks, D., Herzenberg, L.A., Herzenberg, L.A. (2000). N-acetylcysteine replenishes glutathione in HIV infection. *European Journal of Clinical Investigation*, *30*(10), 915–929.

92. Micke, P., Beeh, K.M., Schlaak, J.F., Buhl, R. (2001). Oral supplementation with whey proteins increases plasma glutathione levels of HIV-infected patients. *European Journal of Clinical Investigation*, *31*(2), 171–178.

93. Fernandez-Checa, J.C., Colell, A., Garcia-Ruiz, C. (2002). S-Adenosyl-L-methionine and mitochondrial reduced glutathione depletion in alcoholic liver disease. *Alcohol*, *27*(3), 179–183.

94. Fernandez-Checa, J.C., Kaplowitz, N., García-Ruiz, C., Colell, A. (1998). Mitochondrial glutathione: Importance and transport. *Seminars in Liver Disease*, *18*(4), 389–401.

95. Barbaro, G., Di Lorenzo, G., Soldini, M., Parrotto, S., Bellomo, G., Belloni, G., Grisorio, B., Barbarini, G. (1996). Hepatic glutathione deficiency in chronic hepatitis C: Quantitative evaluation in patients who are HIV positive and HIV negative and correlations with plasmatic and lymphocytic concentrations and with the activity of the liver disease. *American Journal of Gastroenterology*, *91*(12), 2569–2573.

96. Hudson, V.M. (2001). Rethinking cystic fibrosis pathology: The critical role of abnormal reduced glutathione (GSH) transport caused by CFTR mutation. *Free Radical Biology & Medicine*, *30*(12), 1440–1461.

97. Roum, J.H., Buhl, R., McElvaney, N.G., Borok, Z., Crystal, R.G. (1993). Systemic deficiency of glutathione in cystic fibrosis. *Journal of Applied Physiology*, *75*(6), 2419–2424.

98. Brown, R.K., McBurney, A., Lunec, J., Kelly, F.J. (1995). Oxidative damage to DNA in patients with cystic fibrosis. *Free Radical Biology & Medicine*, *234*, 137–146.

99. Brown, R.K., Wyatt, H., Price, J.F., Kelly, F.J. (1996). Pulmonary dysfunction in cystic fibrosis is associated with oxidative stress. *European Respiratory Journal*, *9*(2), 334–339.

100. Cho, S.G., Lee, Y.H., Park, H.S., Ryoo, K., Kang, K.W., Park, J., Eom, S.J., Kim, M.J., Chang, T.S., Choi, S.Y., Shim, J., Kim, Y., Dong, M.S., Lee, M.J., Kim, S.G., Ichijo, H., Choi, E.J. (2001). Glutathione S-transferase mu modulates the stress-activated signals by suppressing apoptosis signal-regulating kinase 1. *Journal of Biological Chemistry*, *276*, 12749–12755.

101. Hull, J., Thomson, A.H. (1998). Contribution of genetic factors other than CFTR to disease severity in cystic fibrosis. *Thorax*, *53*(12), 1018–1021.

102. Buhl, R., Vogelmeier, C., Critenden, M., Hubbard, R.C., Hoyt, R.F., Jr., Wilson, E.M., Cantin, A.M., Crystal, R.G. (1990). Augmentation of glutathione in the fluid lining the epithelium of the lower respiratory tract by directly administering glutathione aerosol. *Proceedings of the National Academy of Sciences USA*, *87*(11), 4063–4067.

103. Roum, J.H., Borok, Z., McElvaney, N.G., Grimes, G.J., Bokser, A.D., Buhl, R., Crystal, R.G. (1999). Glutathione aerosol suppresses lung epithelial surface inflammatory cell-derived oxidants in cystic fibrosis. *Journal of Applied Physiology*, *87*(1), 438–443.

104. Flint, D.H., Tuminello, J.F., Emptage, M.H. (1993). The inactivation of Fe-S cluster containing hydro-lyases by superoxide. *Journal of Biological Chemistry*, *268*(30), 22369–22376.

105. Gardner, P.R., Fridovich, I. (1991). Superoxide sensitivity of the *Escherichia coli* aconitase. *Journal of Biological Chemistry*, *266*(29), 19328–19333.

106. Mallis, R.J., Hamann, M.J., Zhao, W., Zhang, T., Hendrich, S., Thomas, J.A. (2002). Irreversible thiol oxidation in carbonic anhydrase III, protection by S-glutathiolation and detection in aging rats. *Biological Chemistry*, *383*(3–4), 649–662.

107. Koster, J.F., Sluiter, W. (1995). Is increased tissue ferritin a risk factor for atherosclerosis and ischaemic heart disease? *British Heart Journal*, *73*(3), 208.

108. Toba, G., Aigaki, T. (2000). Disruption of the microsomal glutathione S-transferase-like gene reduces life span of *Drosophila melanogaster*. *Gene*, *253*(2), 179–187.

109. Jones, D.P., Mody, V.C., Jr., Carlson, J.L., Lynn, M.J., Sternberg, P., Jr. (2002). Redox analysis of human plasma allows separation of pro-oxidant events of aging from decline in antioxidant defenses. *Free Radical Biology & Medicine*, *33*(9), 1290–1300.

110. Liu, R.M. (2002). Down-regulation of γ-glutamylcysteine synthetase regulatory subunit gene expression in rat brain tissue during aging. *Journal of Neuroscience Research*, *68*(3), 344–351.

111. Knight, J.A. (2000). The biochemistry of aging. *Advances in Clinical Chemistry*, *35*, 1–62.

112. Murata, Y., Amao, M., Yoneda, J., Hamuro, J. (2002). Intracellular thiol redox status of macrophages directs the Th1 skewing in thioredoxin transgenic mice during aging. *Molecular Immunology*, *38*(10), 747–757.

113. Jakobsson, P.J., Thorén, S., Morgenstern, R., Samuelsson, B. (1999). Identification of human prostaglandin E synthase: A microsomal, glutathione-dependent, inducible enzyme, constituting a potential novel drug target. *Proceedings of the National Academy of Sciences USA*, *96*(13), 7220–7225.

114. Mannervik, B. (1985). The isoenzymes of glutathione transferase. *Advances in Enzymology and Related Areas of Molecular Biology*, *57*, 357–417.

115. Tew, K.D. (1994). Glutathione-associated enzymes in anticancer drug resistance. *Cancer Research*, *54*(16), 4313–4320.

116. Davis, R.J. (2000). Signal transduction by the JNK group of MAP kinases. *Cell*, *103*(2), 239–252.

117. Smith, G., Stanley, L.A., Sim, E., Strange, R.C., Wolf, C.R. (1995). Metabolic polymorphisms and cancer susceptibility. *Cancer Surveys*, *25*, 27–65.

118. Strange, R.C., Jones, P.W., Fryer, A.A. (2000). Glutathione S-transferase: Genetics and role in toxicology. *Toxicology letters*, *112–113*, 357–363.

119. Smith, C.M., Kelsey, K.T., Wiencke, J.K., Leyden, K., Levin, S., Christiani, D.C. (1994). Inherited glutathione-S-transferase deficiency is a risk factor for pulmonary asbestosis. *Cancer Epidemiology, Biomarkers & Prevention*, *3*(6), 471–477.

120. Nelson, H.H., Wiencke, J.K., Christiani, D.C., Cheng, T.J., Zuo, Z.F., Schwartz, B.S., Lee, B.K., Spitz, M.R., Wang, M., Xu, X., Kelsey, K.T. (1995). Ethnic differences in the prevalence of the homozygous deleted genotype of glutathione S-transferase theta. *Carcinogenesis*, *16*(5), 1243–1245.

121. Strange, R.C., Fryer, A.A. (1999). The glutathione S-transferases: Influence of polymorphism on cancer susceptibility. *IARC Scientific Publications*, *148*, 231–249.

122. Chenevix-Trench, G., Young, J., Coggan, M., Board, P. (1995). Glutathione S-transferase M1 and T1 polymorphisms: Susceptibility to colon cancer and age of onset. *Carcinogenesis*, *16*(7), 1655–1657.

123. Pearson, W.R., Vorachek, W.R., Xu, S.J., Berger, R., Hart, I., Vannais, D., Patterson, D. (1993). Identification of class-mu glutathione transferase genes GSTM1-GSTM5 on human chromosome 1p13. *American Journal of Human Genetics*, *53*(1), 220–233.

124. DeJong, J.L., Mohandas, T., Tu, C.P. (1991). The human Hb (mu) class glutathione S-transferases are encoded by a dispersed gene family. *Biochemical and Biophysical Research Communications*, *180*(1), 15–22.

125. Baez, S., Segura-Aguilar, J., Widersten, M., Johansson, A.S., Mannervik, B. (1997). Glutathione transferases catalyse the detoxication of oxidized metabolites (o-quinones) of catecholamines and may serve as an antioxidant system preventing degenerative cellular processes. *Biochemical Journal*, *324* (Pt 1), 25–28.

126. Cowell, I.G., Dixon, K.H., Pemble, S.E., Ketterer, B., Taylor, J.B. (1988). The structure of the human glutathione S-transferase pi gene. *Biochemical Journal*, *255*(1), 79–83.

127. Lo, H.W., Ali-Osman, F. (1998). Structure of the human allelic glutathione S-transferase-pi gene variant, hGSTP1 C, cloned from a glioblastoma multiforme cell line. *Chemico-Biological Interactions*, *111–112*, 91–102.

128. Goto, S., Iida, T., Cho, S., Oka, M., Kohno, S., Kondo, T. (1999). Overexpression of glutathione S-transferase pi enhances the adduct formation of cisplatin with glutathione in human cancer cells. *Free Radical Research*, *31*(6), 549–558.

129. Watson, M.A., Stewart, R.K., Smith, G.B., Massey, T.E., Bell, D.A. (1998). Human glutathione S-transferase P1 polymorphisms: Relationship to lung tissue enzyme activity and population frequency distribution. *Carcinogenesis*, *19*(2), 275–280.

130. Stoehlmacher, J., Park, D.J., Zhang, W., Groshen, S., Tsao-Wei, D.D., Yu, M.C., Lenz, H.J. (2002). Association between glutathione S-transferase P1, T1, and M1 genetic polymorphism and survival of patients with metastatic colorectal cancer. *Journal of the National Cancer Institute*, *94*(12), 936–942.

CHAPTER 15

INBORN ERRORS OF GSH METABOLISM

ELLINOR RISTOFF

15.1 INTRODUCTION

Glutathione is metabolized by six enzymes in the γ-glutamyl cycle (Fig. 15.1). In this chapter, known inborn errors of the γ-glutamyl cycle in humans will be discussed, with special emphasis on clinical presentation, diagnostic evaluation, molecular genetics, and treatment. Other disorders of GSH metabolism, such as GSH peroxidase deficiency, GSH reductase deficiency, and glucose-6-phosphate dehydrogenase deficiency, will not be addressed.

Glutathione is a tripeptide composed of glutamate, cysteine, and glycine (L-γ-glutamyl-L-cysteinylglycine). It is present in most living cells at substantial concentrations (0.1 to 10 mM) and plays a critical role in protecting organisms against toxicity and disease. The unusual γ-peptide bond prevents the hydrolysis of GSH by all but one peptidase, and a thiol moiety is key to its physiological and biochemical functions.

Glutathione is involved in detoxification of xenobiotics and carcinogens, amino acid transport, synthesis of proteins and DNA, and drug metabolism. By affecting the cellular redox status, GSH may also modulate gene expression and other cellular mechanisms [1]. Glutathione depletion is linked to a number of disease states, including liver cirrhosis [2], various pulmonary diseases [3–6], myocardial ischemia and reperfusion injury [7], sepsis [8], aging [9], Parkinson's disease [10], and Alzheimer's disease [11]. Low intracellular levels of GSH may contribute to the immunodeficiency observed in later stages of HIV infection [12], as adequate concentrations of GSH are needed for proper lymphocyte function.

Reduced concentrations of GSH in combination with advanced age are associated with an increased risk of chronic diseases such as chronic renal failure, malignancies, diabetes, alcoholism, Parkinson's disease, and cataract development [10]. In these pathological conditions, it is uncertain whether the synthesis or the metabolism of

Glutathione and Sulfur Amino Acids in Human Health and Disease. Edited by R. Masella and G. Mazza
Copyright © 2009 John Wiley & Sons, Inc.

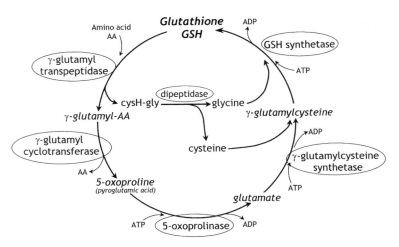

Figure 15.1   The γ-glutamyl cycle.

GSH is affected. Julius et al. [9] measured GSH concentrations in the blood of 33 people aged 60 to 79 years and related the data to health, number of illnesses, and other risk factors for chronic disease. A direct relationship was found between higher GSH concentrations and increasing age with good health. People with chronic diseases had lower mean GSH concentrations than healthy people.

Oxidative stress is thought to contribute significantly to atherogenesis [13]. Rosenblat et al. showed that GSH may retard the development of atherosclerosis by reducing cellular oxidative stress in apolipoprotein E-deficient (apo e $-/-$) mice [14]. These authors also found in animal studies that vitamin E and GSH could act together in scavenging free radicals, leading to a synergistic effect. The brain is especially prone to oxidative stress due to a high content of polyunsaturated fatty acids and very high oxygen consumption. The cells of the brain utilize 20% of the oxygen consumed by the body but constitute only 2% of the body weight. Oxidative stress has been connected with neuron loss during the progression of neuro-logical diseases. The mammalian brain contains 1 to 3 mM GSH in all regions [15], and GSH plays a key role in the defense of brain cells against oxidative stress [16–18].

Very little GSH appears to be transported across the blood–brain barrier in rats [19]. Every enzyme in the γ-glutamyl cycle is present in the brain, as well as other enzymes needed for free radical scavenging, such as GSSG reductase, GSH peroxi-dase, thiol transferases, GSH-S-transferases, SOD, and catalase. Astrocytes contain substantially higher levels of GSH than neurons, and astrocytes may protect the brain against reactive oxygen species and provide cysteine to restore GSH pools in neurons [20, 21]. Apart from GSH, ascorbate is an important antioxidant in the brain, and GSH and ascorbate may act synergistically. Astrocytes and the spinal cord contain high-affinity binding sites for GSH, and it has been postulated that GSH may be an endogenous agonist of N-methyl-D-aspartate (NMDA) glutamate receptors with neuromodulator and neurotransmitter functions in the central nervous system (CNS) [22].

Another equally important role of GSH is to store cysteine [23]. Cysteine is a potentially toxic amino acid that has been reported to damage the CNS [24, 25]. Intracellular concentrations of cysteine are usually much lower than those of GSH. In rat brain, the level of GSH is ~2 mM, or 35 times that of free cysteine, which is ~55 μM [16].

Premature infants have reduced defenses against oxidative stress compared with term infants, and they are at risk of exposure to high concentrations of oxygen in inhaled air and of increased oxidative stress resulting from infections and inflammation [26]. Prematurely born newborns exhibit GSH deficiency (on average, 30% of the normal mean GSH level) that increases with the degree of prematurity [27]. Oxidative stress seems to play an important role in the pathogenesis of several conditions in newborn infants, such as bronchopulmonary dysplasia, retinopathy of prematurity, necrotizing enterocolitis, and periventricular leukomalacia [26]. These conditions are far more common than inborn errors in the metabolism of GSH.

By studying patients with inborn errors in GSH metabolism, the biological functions of GSH and the pathophysiological mechanisms of GSH deficiency may be clarified. This knowledge is essential for greater understanding of diseases resulting from defects in GSH metabolism, for genetic counseling of affected families, and for developing improved treatments to prevent damage to the CNS and elsewhere.

15.2 DEFINITIONS

In man, hereditary deficiencies have been found in five of the six enzymes of the γ-glutamyl cycle (Fig. 15.1). Glutathione synthetase deficiency is the most commonly recognized disorder that in its severe form is associated with hemolytic anemia, metabolic acidosis, 5-oxoprolinuria, CNS damage, and recurrent bacterial infections. γ-Glutamylcysteine synthetase deficiency is also associated with hemolytic anemia, and some patients with this disorder exhibit neurological symptoms and generalized aminoaciduria. γ-Glutamyl transpeptidase deficiency has been found in patients with CNS involvement and glutathionuria. 5-Oxoprolinase deficiency is a heterogeneous disease associated with 5-oxoprolinuria. Dipeptidase deficiency has been described in only one patient. Diagnosis is made by measuring enzyme activity and the concentrations of different metabolites in the γ-glutamyl cycle. In GSH synthetase and γ-glutamylcysteine synthetase deficiencies, diagnosis is also made by mutation analysis. Prenatal diagnosis has been performed in GSH synthetase deficiency. All of these disorders are very rare, and because few patients are known, the prognosis is difficult to predict. However, the prognosis appears to vary significantly among different patients. The aims of the treatment of defects in GSH synthesis are to avoid hemolytic crises and to increase the defense against reactive oxygen species. No treatment has been recommended for γ-glutamyl transpeptidase, 5-oxoprolinase, or dipeptidase deficiency.

15.3 THE γ-GLUTAMYL CYCLE

Six enzymes comprise the γ-glutamyl cycle, which catalyzes the synthesis and degradation of GSH (Fig. 15.1). The γ-glutamyl cycle was identified by Orlowski and

Meister in 1970 [28]. Since then, a large body of experimental evidence supports its function in vivo. For diagnostic purposes, it is important to note that erythrocytes, which are anucleate, lack γ-glutamyl transpeptidase and 5-oxoprolinase. Both of these enzymes must be analyzed in nucleated cells, such as leukocytes or cultured fibroblasts.

Glutathione is synthesized intracellularly by the consecutive actions of γ-glutamyl-cysteine synthetase and GSH synthetase. Both enzymes are cytosolic and use ATP, which is hydrolyzed to ADP and P_i. GSH is exported from most cells. Different tissues have distinct rates of GSH turnover.

Glutathione acts as a feedback inhibitor of γ-glutamylcysteine synthetase. The initial degradative step is catalyzed by γ-glutamyl transpeptidase, which transfers the γ-glutamyl group to an acceptor (i.e., an amino acid) to form γ-glutamyl amino acids. These dipeptides are substrates of γ-glutamyl cyclotransferase, which catalyzes the release of the γ-glutamyl residue as 5-oxoproline (pyroglutamic acid), which is then converted to glutamate by 5-oxoprolinase. In most tissues, including the brain, 5-oxoprolinase is the enzyme of the γ-glutamyl cycle with the lowest catalytic capacity. In man, hereditary deficiencies have been found in five of the six enzymes of the γ-glutamyl cycle: γ-glutamylcysteine synthetase, GSH synthetase, γ-glutamyl transpeptidase, 5-oxoprolinase, and dipeptidase [29, 30]. Mutants in γ-glutamyl cyclotransferase have not yet been identified. Most of the mutations are "leaky," meaning that the patients have considerable residual enzyme activity. Cultured cells from patients with inborn errors in the metabolism of GSH provide unique experimental model systems. Animal models are also used to study the biological roles of GSH.

The γ-glutamyl cycle may be involved in the active transport of amino acids [28]. According to this view, interaction of the membrane-bound γ-glutamyl transpeptidase with intracellular GSH and extracellular amino acids leads to the formation of γ-glutamyl amino acids, which are transported into the cell. γ-Glutamyl transpeptidase is found on the outer surface of the cell membrane, especially in the epithelia of tissues widely involved in transport (e.g., the kidney).

15.4 INBORN ERRORS IN THE METABOLISM OF GSH

Because GSH plays a role in many fundamental cellular functions, it might be expected that humans with severe GSH deficiency would not survive. Nevertheless, patients with mutations in the γ-glutamyl cycle exist, although they are rare. All five verified defects are inherited as autosomal recessive traits.

15.4.1 γ-Glutamylcysteine Synthetase Deficiency

15.4.1.1 Clinical Presentation γ-Glutamylcysteine synthetase deficiency (OMIM 230450) has been described worldwide in nine patients from seven families (the United States, Germany, Japan, The Netherlands, Poland, and Spain). All of these patients had well-compensated hemolytic anemia [31–38]. Two patients who were siblings (brother and sister) also had generalized aminoaciduria and developed in their 30s spinocerebellar degeneration and a neuromuscular disorder with peripheral neuropathy and myopathy [34, 38]. The sister became psychotic after being treated with sulfonamide for a urinary tract infection. Another patient, reported to have a learning disability with dyslexia, was regarded as mentally retarded [35]. However, she had no abnormalities on physical examination, including a neurological evaluation. Yet another patient had delayed psychomotor development and progressive sensory neuropathy of the lower extremities, ataxia, hyperreflexia, dysarthria, and probably a spinocerebellar degeneration with peculiar gait [33]. Other symptoms found in patients with γ-glutamylcysteine synthetase deficiency are transient jaundice, reticulocytosis, and hepatosplenomegaly.

15.4.1.2 *Molecular Genetic Data*

Human γ-glutamylcysteine synthetase is a heterodimer consisting of a heavy (catalytic) and a light (regulatory) subunit. The gene for the heavy subunit is located on chromosome 6p12 [39], and the gene for the light subunit is on chromosome 1p21 [40]. The heavy subunit (molecular weight 73 kDa) has the catalytic activity of the native enzyme; it is also feedback-inhibited by GSH. The light subunit (molecular weight 28 kDa) is catalytically inactive but plays an important regulatory role by lowering the K_m of γ-glutamylcysteine synthetase for glutamate and by raising the K_i for GSH [41]. Many compounds, including those forming GSH-conjugates and those generating reactive oxygen species (ROS), have been shown to induce GSH biosynthesis by increasing transcription of γ-glutamylcysteine synthetase [42]. Four different mutations in the heavy subunit have been identified in four families affected by γ-glutamylcysteine synthetase deficiency [31–33, 35].

15.4.1.3 *Diagnostic Test*

The diagnosis of γ-glutamylcysteine synthetase deficiency is established by the finding of low activity of γ-glutamylcysteine synthetase in red blood cells, leukocytes, and/or cultured skin fibroblasts, in combination with low levels (1% to 20% of the normal mean) of γ-glutamylcysteine and GSH in red blood cells and/or cultured skin fibroblasts. Mutation analysis can also be performed. The patients whose results have been published have had homozygous mutations in the gene encoding the heavy subunit of the enzyme. In red blood cells, heterozygous carriers have an enzyme activity of ~50% of the normal mean and normal levels of glutathione [32].

Glutathione and sulfhydryl compounds in erythrocytes can be measured using 5,5'-dithiobis (2-nitrobenzoic acid), whereas GSH in fibroblasts can be measured with the 5,5'-dithiobis (2-nitrobenzoic acid) GSH recycling assay [43] or by using high performance liquid chromatography (HPLC) [44]. γ-Glutamylcysteine synthetase in erythrocytes and/or cultured fibroblasts can be measured as described elsewhere [32].

Sequence analysis can be performed by polymerase chain reaction (PCR) and sequencing of the γ-glutamylcysteine synthetase genes (*GLCLC*, *GLCLR*) [32].

15.4.1.4 *Treatment*

Patients with γ-glutamylcysteine synthetase deficiency should avoid drugs known to precipitate hemolytic crises in patients with glucose-6-phosphate dehydrogenase deficiency, for example, phenobarbital, acetylsalicylic acid, and sulfonamides. It is possible that patients would benefit from treatment with antioxidants, but as yet no studies have been conducted. The prognosis and the relationship between symptoms reported in various patients and the primary enzyme deficiency remain to be established.

15.4.2 Glutathione Synthetase Deficiency

15.4.2.1 Clinical Presentation
Glutathione synthetase deficiency (OMIM 266130) has been confirmed in more than 70 patients from more than 50 families worldwide. Glutathione synthetase catalyzes the final step in the synthesis of glutathione, and a deficiency results in low levels of GSH. Approximately 25% of all patients with this condition have died in childhood, often in the neonatal period, of electrolyte imbalance and infections.

According to the clinical symptoms, GSH synthetase deficiency can be classified as mild, moderate, or severe [45]. Patients with mild GSH synthetase deficiency show mild hemolytic anemia as their only clinical symptom. In very rare cases, these patients may excrete excessive amounts of 5-oxoproline in their urine (reference range <0.1 mol/mol creatinine), but they usually maintain sufficient cellular levels of GSH to prevent accumulation of 5-oxoproline in body fluids. Those with moderate GSH synthetase deficiency usually present in the neonatal period with severe and chronic metabolic acidosis, 5-oxoprolinuria, and mild or moderate hemolytic anemia.

Patients with severe GSH synthetase deficiency have the symptoms observed in moderate glutathione synthetase deficiency. In addition, they develop progressive neurological symptoms, such as psychomotor retardation, mental retardation, seizures, spasticity, ataxia, and intention tremor. Some patients with severe glutathione synthetase deficiency also develop recurrent bacterial infections, probably due to defective granulocyte function. Retinal dystrophy with decreased visual acuity has also been observed in some patients. Two adult sisters with severe GSH synthetase deficiency were investigated and found to have signs of progressive retinal dystrophy affecting both the macular and midperiphery and both the inner and outer retinal layers, with attenuated or nearly abolished electroretinograms [46]. They had no obvious signs of abnormalities in the optic nerve or central visual pathways. It was proposed that the ocular findings were related to low levels of GSH and that decreased ROS scavenging capacity and/or increased oxidative stress may cause the retinal dystrophy [46]. Treatment with antioxidants, such as vitamins E and C, seems to prevent the progression of CNS damage, and it has been suggested that these antioxidants might also prevent retinal dystrophy in patients with GSH synthetase deficiency.

The mechanism behind metabolic acidosis and 5-oxoprolinuria in this condition involves decreased levels of cellular GSH, which leads to decreased feedback inhibition of γ-glutamylcysteine synthetase. This results in excessive formation of the dipeptide γ-glutamylcysteine, which is converted by γ-glutamyl cyclotransferase into 5-oxoproline. The overproduction of 5-oxoproline exceeds the capacity of 5-oxoprolinase. Therefore, 5-oxoproline accumulates in body fluids and is excreted in the urine. Patients having moderate or severe GSH synthetase deficiency usually excrete gram quantities (up to 30 g/d) of 5-oxoproline in the urine, but those with mild GSH synthetase deficiency maintain cellular levels of GSH, which are usually sufficient to prevent the accumulation of 5-oxoproline.

Patients with GSH synthetase deficiency accumulate the dipeptide γ-glutamylcysteine and the amino acid cysteine in fibroblasts [47]. Because γ-glutamylcysteine contains both reactive groups of GSH (i.e., the sulfhydryl and γ-glutamyl groups), it may to some extent compensate for GSH in the cellular defense against oxidative stress. Thus, γ-glutamylcysteine may alleviate, but only partly prevent, the serious consequences of insufficient GSH levels in affected patients. Because the sum of the levels of GSH and γ-glutamylcysteine in GSH synthetase-deficient cells is similar to the level of GSH alone in control cells, it was proposed that cultured fibroblasts may have a mechanism to coordinately regulate the levels of GSH and γ-glutamylcysteine, for example, both compounds acting as feedback inhibitors of γ-glutamylcysteine synthetase.

Further evidence that γ-glutamylcysteine can compensate for GSH is provided by the finding that GSH-deficient cells are no more prone to DNA damage than control cells [48]. Oxidative DNA damage, including background levels of oxidative damage and sensitivity to an oxidative agent (ionizing radiation), was studied in cultured fibroblasts from 11 patients with GSH synthetase deficiency. No significant differences in oxidative DNA damage were observed between the patients and controls ($n = 5$). The patient and control cells were equally sensitive to the induction of single-stranded DNA breaks by γ-irradiation. Therefore, factors other than GSH also protect DNA from oxidative damage.

Glutathione participates in the synthesis of leukotriene C4 (LTC4), the primary cysteinyl leukotriene. Synthesis of cysteinyl leukotrienes is impaired in patients with GSH synthetase deficiency [49].

Several patients with GSH synthetase deficiency have died, but few have been autopsied. The first patient described with GSH synthetase deficiency died at 28 years of age. The autopsy of the CNS showed selective atrophy of the granule cell layer of the cerebellum, focal lesions in the frontoparietal cortex, and bilateral lesions in the visual cortex and thalamus [50]. The lesions in the brain resemble those seen after intoxication with mercury (i.e., Minamata disease), and it has been suggested that treatment of GSH synthetase deficiency with antioxidants may be beneficial [50]. The autopsy findings in another patient with GSH synthetase deficiency, who died at 10 days of age, resemble those of the above case, with distinct loss of the granular cell layer and almost complete loss of Purkinje cells. The pathological findings in patients with GSH synthetase deficiency confined especially to the granule cell layer of the cerebellum support the view that GSH is an important scavenger of ROS. The brain damage may also be due to excessive apoptosis arising from GSH deficiency. Low levels of GSH are thought to trigger apoptosis by changing the intracellular redox potential [51]. A localized decline in GSH, and thus in the capacity to withstand oxidative stress, may increase the levels of excitotoxic molecules. These events may initiate apoptotic cell death in certain neural subsets [52].

Another hypothesis to explain why some patients with GSH synthetase deficiency develop neurological symptoms is based on data suggesting that GSH is a neuromodulator and neurotransmitter in the CNS. Specific high-affinity binding sites for

GSH exist in the astrocytes and spinal cord [22]. Moreover, human brain tissue can synthesize leukotrienes, which in addition to being mediators of inflammation and host defense may have neuromodulatory functions in the brain [53]. More studies are needed to elucidate the pathogenetic mechanism of GSH synthetase deficiency, how low levels of GSH affect apoptosis, and the defense against ROS in these patients.

Several studies have been done on cultures of fibroblasts from patients with GSH synthetase deficiency. Such cells are more sensitive to radiation and excess oxygen in terms of DNA strand breaks [54]. Isolated lymphocytes from GSH-deficient patients are also more sensitive to certain drugs, for example, acetaminophen and nitrofurantoin [55]. However, patient fibroblasts have a normal content of the enzymatic scavengers SOD, catalase, and GSH peroxidase [56] and normal activities of thioredoxin and thioredoxin reductase [57]. In other words, there seems to be no compensatory increase in alternative cellular scavenger systems in GSH-deficient cells in vitro.

15.4.2.2 *Molecular Genetic Data*

Human GSH synthetase is a homodimer with a subunit size of 52 kDa. The three-dimensional structure of the GSH synthetase enzyme has been established [58]. The GSH synthetase gene (*GSS*) gene was localized to chromosome 20q11.2, and its structure was determined [59, 60]. Because the human genome contains only one GSH synthetase gene, the various clinical forms of GSH synthetase deficiency reflect different mutations or epigenetic modifications of the GSH synthetase gene. Less is known about the regulation of GSH synthetase than that of γ-glutamylcysteine synthetase. The 5′-untranslated region of GSH synthetase has not been cloned, and is not well represented in the expressed sequence tag databases. Possible regulatory elements for this gene remain unknown.

In 41 patients with GSH synthetase deficiency from 33 families, nearly 30 different mutations in the *GSS* gene have been identified (missense, splicing, deletion, insertion, and nonsense mutations) [61]. Twenty-three patients were homozygous for the respective mutation, and 18 were compound heterozygous. The moderate and severe clinical phenotypes could not be distinguished based on enzyme activity, GSH, or γ-glutamylcysteine levels in cultured fibroblasts. However, in fibroblasts the residual GSH synthetase activity correlates with the GSH level. All mutations causing frameshifts, premature stop codons, or aberrant splicing were associated with moderate or severe clinical phenotypes, including hemolytic anemia, 5-oxoprolinuria, and neurological symptoms (in several forms). To some extent, the type of mutation involved can predict a mild versus a more severe phenotype [61].

Known missense mutations in the *GSS* gene have been expressed in vitro in *Escherichia coli* expression systems [62, 63]. Most of the known mutations in GSH synthetase deficiency affect the K_m and/or the V_{max} value for glycine, causing decreased substrate affinity and/or maximal velocity. One mutation has been shown to decrease the stability of the enzyme [62]. Further insight into the molecular basis of GSH synthetase deficiency can be achieved by deducing how various mutations affect the three-dimensional GSH synthetase structure. This has already been done for some mutations in patients with GSH synthetase deficiency [58, 63]. Many of these mutations are thought to affect ligand binding or catalysis, whereas others likely affect enzyme dimerization or folding.

15.4.2.3 Diagnostic Tests
The diagnosis of GSH synthetase deficiency is established by urinary 5-oxoproline (up to 1 g/kg/day), a low activity of GSH synthetase (1% to 30% of the normal mean), and low levels of GSH (5% to 20% of the normal mean) in erythrocytes and/or nucleated cells. The diagnosis can be confirmed by mutation analysis. Heterozygous carriers have normal levels of GSH and an enzyme activity of ~50% of the normal mean [61].

Urinary 5-oxoproline can be determined by gas chromatography-mass spectrometry [64]. Glutathione and sulfhydryls in erythrocytes can be measured using 5,5′-dithiobis (2-nitrobenzoic acid). GSH in fibroblasts can be measured by using the 5,5′-dithiobis (2-nitrobenzoic acid) GSH recycling assay [43] or HPLC [44]. Glutathione synthetase in erythrocytes and/or cultured fibroblasts can be measured as described elsewhere [32]. Mutation analysis of *GSS* can be performed as described by Njålsson et al. [65] and Shi et al. [66].

Prenatal diagnosis of GSH synthetase deficiency can be made by mutation analysis of chorionic villi (the method of choice if the mutation in the family is known), mesurement of 5-oxoproline in amniotic fluid [67, 68], or analysis of GSH synthetase activity in cultured amniocytes or chorionic villi [67].

15.4.2.4 Treatment
A long-term follow-up study of 28 patients with GSH synthetase deficiency showed that the factors most predictive of survival and long-term outcome are early diagnosis, correction of acidosis, and early supplementation with the antioxidants vitamin C and vitamin E [45]. The acidosis can be corrected with bicarbonate, citrate, or tris-hydroxymethyl aminomethane (THAM). The recommended dose of the antioxidant vitamin C (ascorbic acid) is 100 mg/kg/day and of vitamin E (α-tocopherol) is 10 mg/kg/day. Short-term treatment of GSH synthetase-deficient patients with vitamin C has been reported to increase lymphocyte GSH levels [69]. Vitamin E has been reported to correct the defective granulocyte function [70]. Vitamin C and GSH can spare each other in a rodent model [71].

Patients with GSH synthetase deficiency should avoid the drugs known to precipitate hemolytic crises in patients with glucose-6-phosphate dehydrogenase deficiency. Because *N*-acetylcysteine (NAC) protects cells from oxidative stress in vitro, it has been suggested that NAC supplements (15 mg/kg/d) should be given to GSH-deficient patients. However, patients with GSH synthetase deficiency accumulate γ-glutamylcysteine and cysteine, at least in cultured fibroblasts [47]. Because cysteine is known to be neurotoxic in excessive amounts [72], it has been suggested that treatment with NAC should not be recommended for patients with GSH synthetase deficiency as this may further increase intracellular cysteine levels.

Treatment with GSH esters has been attempted in animal models of GSH deficiency and in two patients with GSH synthetase deficiency [73]. The GSH esters are more lipid soluble than GSH and are readily transported into cells and converted into GSH. The esters increased GSH levels in several tissues, but their use is limited due to associated toxic effects, that is, when they are hydrolyzed to release GSH, alcohols are produced as by-products.

15.4.3   γ-Glutamyltranspeptidase Deficiency

15.4.3.1   Clinical Presentation   γ-Glutamyl transpeptidase deficiency (OMIM 231950) has been reported in seven patients from five families worldwide [74–79]. Five of these patients had involvement of the CNS with psychomotor retardation, mental retardation, and absence epilepsy. It is uncertain whether these symptoms are directly related to the enzyme deficiency. All patients had glutathionuria (up to 1 g/day; controls < 10 mg/day). In addition, patients had increased urinary levels of γ-glutamylcysteine and cysteine. Three patients with γ-glutamyl transpeptidase deficiency have been studied and were found to have a complete deficiency of leukotriene D4 biosynthesis [80].

15.4.3.2   Molecular Genetic Data   The γ-glutamyl transpeptidase gene family in humans contains at least seven different gene loci, several of which are located on the long arm of chromosome 22 [29]. γ-Glutamyltranspeptidase is a heterodimer with subunits of 21 kDa and 38 kDa that result from the processing of a single precursor polypeptide. The enzyme is membrane bound, with its active site facing the external side of the cell. No mutations have yet been identified in patients with γ-glutamyl transpeptidase deficiency.

15.4.3.3   Diagnostic Tests   The diagnosis of γ-glutamyl transpeptidase deficiency is based on glutathionuria (up to 1 g/day in urine; controls < 10 mg), elevated levels of GSH in plasma, and decreased activity of γ-glutamyl transpeptidase in nucleated cells such as leukocytes or cultured skin fibroblasts (< 10% of the normal mean). Erythrocytes lack γ-glutamyl transpeptidase under normal conditions. Cellular levels of GSH in these patients are normal. The patients also have increased urinary levels of γ-glutamylcysteine and cysteine.

Glutathione in plasma and urine can be determined by various chromatographic or calorimetric techniques. γ-Glutamyl transpeptidase in nucleated cells can be determined with the method described by Wright et al. [77].

15.4.3.4   Treatment and Prognosis   No specific treatment has been proposed or attempted in patients with γ-glutamyl transpeptidase deficiency. However, administration of N-acetylcysteine to γ-glutamyl transpeptidase-deficient mutant mice for 2 weeks restored their fertility [81].

15.4.4   5-Oxoprolinase Deficiency

15.4.4.1   Clinical Presentation   5-Oxoprolinase deficiency (OMIM 260005) has been reported in eight patients from six families [82–87]. 5-Oxoprolinase deficiency is a very heterogeneous condition. A variety of clinical symptoms have been reported, for example, mental retardation, microcephaly, neonatal hypoglycemia, microcytic anemia, formation of renal stones, and enterocolitis [76, 83–87]. All patients had 5-oxoprolinuria (4 to 10 g/day, reference range <0.1 mol/mol creatinine) [29]. The 5-oxoprolinuria is due to decreased activity of 5-oxoprolinase in nucleated cells, which reduces the conversion of 5-oxoproline to glutamate and increases 5-oxoproline in body fluids and urine. The amounts of 5-oxoproline are less than those found in patients with GSH synthetase deficiency, and metabolic acidosis is usually not present.

15.4.4.2 Molecular Genetic Data The mammalian 5-oxoprolinase enzyme has not been studied extensively, but it appears to be composed of two identical subunits of 140 kDa.

15.4.4.3 Diagnostic Tests The diagnosis of 5-oxoprolinase deficiency is based on low activity of 5-oxoprolinase in nucleated cells, elevated levels of 5-oxoproline in body fluids, and 5-oxoprolinuria. The level of 5-oxoproline in urine can be determined by gas chromatography-mass spectrometry [64]. The activity of 5-oxoprolinase in leukocytes and/or cultured fibroblasts can be measured according to the method described by Larsson et al. [82].

15.4.4.4 Treatment No specific treatment has been proposed or attempted in patients with 5-oxoprolinase deficiency.

15.4.5 Dipeptidase Deficiency

15.4.5.1 Clinical Presentation Dipeptidase deficiency has been suggested in only a single patient worldwide [30].

The diagnosis has not been confirmed by enzyme analysis in this patient. Dipeptidase deficiency is characterized by increased urinary excretion of cysteinylglycine and a pathological excretion pattern of leukotrienes.

The 15-year-old boy presented with mental retardation, mild motor impairment, and partial deafness. Biochemical investigations showed a normal level of cysteinylglycine in plasma, an abnormal urinary profile with increased excretion of cysteinylglycine (4972 mmol/mol of creatinine), and abnormal leukotriene excretion. Leukotriene E4, the major urinary metabolite in humans, was completely absent, whereas the concentration of leukotriene D4, which is usually not detectable, was highly increased. These data suggest membrane-bound dipeptidase deficiency [30].

15.4.5.2 Molecular Genetic Data Membrane-bound dipeptidase (E.C. 3.4.13.19) is 42 kDa when unglycosylated and 63 kDa when glycosylated. The crystal structure of human membrane-bound dipeptidase has been solved [88]. The renal dipeptidase gene has been mapped to human chromosome 16q24 [89]. Membrane-bound dipeptidase hydrolyzes dipeptides, including cysteinylglycine compounds such as the oxidized γ-glutamyltranspeptidase product cystinyl-bis-glycine, and catalyzes the conversion of leukotriene D4 to E4 [90]. Dipeptidase also hydrolyzes certain β-lactam antibiotics.

15.4.5.3 Diagnostic Tests The diagnosis of dipeptidase deficiency is based on increased urinary excretion of cysteinylglycine, a normal concentration of cysteinyl-glycine in plasma, and a low activity of dipeptidase in cultured skin fibroblasts and/or red blood cells.

The levels of cysteinylglycine in urine can be determined by quantitative amino acid analysis of urine. The activity of dipeptidase in cultured skin fibroblasts and/or red blood cells can be assayed with an HPLC method using glycyl-D-phenylalanine, according to the procedure described by Littlewood et al. [91]. To date, dipeptidase enzyme activity has not been assayed in the patient with suspected dipeptidase deficiency.

15.4.5.4 Treatment No specific treatment has been proposed or attempted in the patient with suspected dipeptidase deficiency.

15.4.6 Other Causes of 5-Oxoprolinuria

Other causes of 5-oxoprolinuria, apart from GSH synthetase deficiency and 5-oxoprolinase deficiency, should be considered in diagnostic work [29, 92]. For example, 5-oxoprolinuria is observed in the following patients:

1. Patients on certain diets. Some infant formulas and tomato juices contain proteins modified by preparation, resulting in increased 5-oxoproline content [93].

2. Patients with severe burns or Stevens–Johnson syndrome, who may have increased metabolism of collagen, fibrinogen, or other proteins that contain substantial amounts of 5-oxoproline [94].

3. Some patients with inborn errors of metabolism outside the γ-glutamyl cycle (e.g., X-linked ornithine transcarbamylase deficiency, urea cycle defects, tyrosinemia) lack ATP in vital organs (e.g., liver, kidney). Because ATP is needed for 5-oxoproline conversion to glutamate, its deficiency may result in 5-oxoprolinuria [29, 92].

4. Patients with homocystinuria may have excessive formation of 5-oxoproline because homocysteine can replace cysteine as a substrate for γ-glutamyl-cysteine synthetase, resulting in γ-glutamylhomocysteine. This dipeptide is efficiently split by γ-glutamylcyclotransferase to 5-oxoproline and homocysteine [95].

5. Patients on various medications, for example, paracetamol, vigabatrin, and antibiotics (flucloxacillin, netimicin), which likely interact with the γ-glutamyl cycle [96–99].

6. Very preterm infants who may have transient 5-oxoprolinuria of unknown etiology [92, 100].

7. Malnourished patients and pregnant women, likely due to limited availability of glycine [101].

8. Patients with nephropathic cystinosis may have 5-oxoprolinuria, likely due to decreased availability of free cysteine, resulting in a secondary impairment of the γ-glutamyl cycle. Cysteamine therapy normalizes the 5-oxoprolinuria [102].

15.5 ANIMAL MODELS

Numerous experimental methods to induce enzyme deficiency have been used to study the roles of individual enzymes in the γ-glutamyl cycle, including the use of cultured cells, tissue slices, and knockout mice [29].

A selective inhibitor of γ-glutamylcysteine synthetase, L-buthionine-S,R-sulfoximine (BSO), is transported into many tissues but not across the blood–brain barrier. After a few doses of BSO, the levels of GSH decline in rodent tissues such as liver, pancreas, kidney, and plasma to about 10% to 20% of control levels [103]. γ-Glutamylcysteine synthetase knockout mice have been developed for both the heavy and the light subunits [104–106]. In the knockout mice of the heavy subunit, homozygous embryos fail to gastrulate and die before day 8.5 of gestation [104]. This mouse model has a complete GSH deficiency, and the authors conclude that lethality is caused by apoptosis rather than by reduced cell proliferation. However, cell lines from homozygous mutant blastocysts grow indefinitely in GSH-free medium supplemented with N-acetylcysteine as a replacement for GSH. The authors concluded that GSH is needed for mammalian development but is dispensable in cell culture, and the functions of GSH (not GSH itself) are essential for cell growth. The knockout mice of the light subunit are viable and fertile and have no overt phenotype [106].

No selective inhibitor of mammalian GSH synthetase has been found, and so far no knockout mouse is available.

Several inhibitors of γ-glutamyl transpeptidase exist. The administration of these inhibitors to mice causes glutathionuria and glutathionemia. After acivicin treatment, urinary thiols (i.e., GSH, γ-glutamylcysteine, and cysteine) increase. A knockout mouse for γ-glutamyl transpeptidase has been developed, and these mice suffer from glutathionuria, glutathionemia, postnatal growth failure, cataracts, lethargy, reduced life span, and infertility [107]. A study of the reproductive phenotype of γ-glutamyl transpeptidase-deficient mice showed that they are hypogonadal and infertile [81]. Administration of N-acetylcysteine to γ-glutamyl transpeptidase-deficient mutant mice for 2 weeks restored their fertility [81].

In mice, the administration of competitive inhibitors of 5-oxoprolinase, such as L-2-imidazolidone-4-carboxylate or D,L-3-methyl-5-oxoproline, significantly reduces the metabolism of 5-oxoproline and increases its concentration in urine [108].

ACKNOWLEDGMENTS

These studies were supported by grants from the Swedish Research Council (4792), the Free Masons in Stockholm for Children's Welfare, the Memory Foundation of Golje, the HRH Crown Princess Lovisa Foundation, the Åke Wiberg Foundation, the Ronald McDonald Foundation, the Linnéa and Josef Carlsson Foundation, the Lennanders Foundation, the Swedish Society of Medicine, and the Samariten Foundation, which are gratefully acknowledged.

REFERENCES

1. Taylor, C.G., Nagy, L.E., Bray, T.M. (1996). Nutritional and hormonal regulation of glutathione homeostasis. *Current Topics in Cellular Regulation*, *34*, 189–208.
2. Chawla, R.K., Lewis, F.W., Kutner, M.H., Bate, D.M., Roy, R.G., Rudman, D. (1984). Plasma cysteine, cystine, and glutathione in cirrhosis. *Gastroenterology*, *87*, 770–776.
3. Bridgeman, M.M., Marsden, M., Selby, C., Morrison, D., MacNee, W. (1994). Effect of N-acetyl cysteine on the concentrations of thiols in plasma, bronchoalveolar lavage fluid, and lung tissue. *Thorax*, *49*, 670–675.
4. Pacht, E.R., Timerman, A.P., Lykens, M.G., Merola, A.J. (1991). Deficiency of alveolar fluid glutathione in patients with sepsis and the adult respiratory distress syndrome. *Chest*, *100*, 1397–1403.
5. Grigg, J., Barber, A., Silverman, M. (1993). Bronchoalveolar lavage fluid glutathione in intubated premature infants. *Archives of Disease in Childhood*, *69*, 49–51.
6. Smith, L.J., Houston, M., Anderson, J. (1993). Increased levels of glutathione in bronchoalveolar lavage fluid from patients with asthma. *American Review of Respiratory Diseases*, *147*, 1461–1464.
7. Singh, A., Lee, K.J., Lee, C.Y., Goldfarb, R.D., Tsan, M.F. (1989). Relation between myocardial glutathione content and extent of ischemia-reperfusion injury. *Circulation*, *80*, 1795–1804.
8. Henderson, A., Hayes, P. (1994). Acetylcysteine as a cytoprotective antioxidant in patients with severe sepsis: Potential new use for an old drug. *Annals of Pharmacotherapy*, *28*, 1086–1088.
9. Julius, M., Lang, C.A., Gleiberman, L., Harburg, E., DiFranceisco, W., Schork, A. (1994). Glutathione and morbidity in a community-based sample of elderly. *Journal of Clinical Epidemiology*, *47*, 1021–1026.
10. Lomaestro, B.M., Malone, M. (1995). Glutathione in health and disease: Pharmacotherapeutic issues. *Annals of Pharmacotherapy*, *29*, 1263–1273.
11. Ginsberg, S.D., Hemby, S.E., Lee, V.M., Eberwine, J.H., Trojanowski, J.Q. (2000). Expression profile of transcripts in Alzheimer's disease tangle-bearing CA1 neurons. *Annals of Neurology*, *48*, 77–87.
12. Staal, F.J., Roederer, M., Israelski, D.M., Bubp, J., Mole, L.A., McShane, D., Deresinski, S.C., Ross, W., Sussman, H., Raju, P.A. (1992). Intracellular glutathione levels in T cell subsets decrease in HIV- infected individuals. *AIDS Research and Human Retroviruses*, *8*, 305–311.
13. Griendling, K.K., Alexander, R.W. (1997). Oxidative stress and cardiovascular disease. *Circulation*, *96*, 3264–3265.
14. Rosenblat, M., Coleman, R., Aviram, M. (2002). Increased macrophage glutathione content reduces cell-mediated oxidation of LDL and atherosclerosis in apolipoprotein E-deficient mice. *Atherosclerosis*, *163*, 17–28.

15. Shaw, C. (Ed.). (1998). *Glutathione in the Nervous System*. Bristol: Taylor & Francis.

16. Cooper, A. (Ed.). (1997). *Glutathione in the Brain: Disorders of Glutathione Metabolism*, 2nd edition. Boston: Butterworth-Heinemann.

17. Cooper, A.J., Kristal, B.S. (1997). Multiple roles of glutathione in the central nervous system. *Biological Chemistry, 378*, 793–802.

18. Dringen, R., Gutterer, J.M., Hirrlinger, J. (2000). Glutathione metabolism in brain metabolic interaction between astrocytes and neurons in the defense against reactive oxygen species. *European Journal of Biochemistry, 267*, 4912–4916.

19. Jain, A., Martensson, J., Stole, E., Auld, P.A., Meister, A. (1991). Glutathione deficiency leads to mitochondrial damage in brain. *Proceedings of the National Academy of Sciences USA, 88*, 1913–1917.

20. Sen, C.K. (2000). Cellular thiols and redox-regulated signal transduction. *Current Topics in Cell Regulation, 36*, 1–30.

21. Dringen, R. (2000). Metabolism and functions of glutathione in brain. *Progress in Neurobiology, 62*, 649–671.

22. Janaky, R., Ogita, K., Pasqualotto, B.A., Bains, J.S., Oja, S.S., Yoneda, Y., Shaw, C.A. (1999). Glutathione and signal transduction in the mammalian CNS. *Journal of Neurochemistry, 73*, 889–902.

23. Tateishi, N., Higashi, T., Naruse, A., Nakashima, K., Shiozaki, H. (1977). Rat liver glutathione: Possible role as a reservoir of cysteine. *Journal of Nutrition, 107*, 51–60.

24. Olney, J.W., Ho, O.L., Rhee, V. (1971). Cytotoxic effects of acidic and sulphur containing amino acids on the infant mouse central nervous system. *Experimental Brain Research, 14*, 61–76.

25. Karlsen, R.L., Grofova, I., Malthe-Sorenssen, D., Fonnum, F. (1981). Morphological changes in rat brain induced by L-cysteine injection in newborn animals. *Brain Research, 208*, 167–180.

26. Saugstad, O.D. (2001). Update on oxygen radical disease in neonatology. *Current Opinion in Obstetrics and Gynecology, 13*, 147–153.

27. Jain, A., Mehta, T., Auld, P.A., Rodrigues, J., Ward, R.F., Schwartz, M.K., Martensson, J. (1995). Glutathione metabolism in newborns: Evidence for glutathione deficiency in plasma, bronchoalveolar lavage fluid, and lymphocytes in prematures. *Pediatric Pulmonology, 20*, 160–166.

28. Orlowski, M., Meister, A. (1970). The γ-glutamyl cycle: A possible transport system for amino acids. *Proceedings of the National Academy of Sciences USA, 67*, 1248–1255.

29. Larsson, A., Ristoff, E., Anderson, M., (2005). Glutathione synthetase deficiency and other disorders of the γ-glutamyl cycle. In Scriver, C., Beaudet, A., Sly, W., Valle, D., Vogelstein, B., Childs, B., and Kinzler, K., eds., *The Metabolic and Molecular Bases of Inherited Disease*. New York: McGraw-Hill. Online. http://genetics.accessmedicine. com.

30. Mayatepek, E., Badiou, S., Bellet, H., Lehmann, W.D. (2005). A patient with neurological symptoms and abnormal leukotriene metabolism: A new defect in leukotriene biosynthesis. *Annals of Neurology, 58*, 968–970.

31. Hamilton, D., Wu, J.H., Alaoui-Jamali, M., Batist, G. (2003). A novel missense mutation in the γ-glutamylcysteine synthetase catalytic subunit gene causes both decreased enzymatic activity and glutathione production. *Blood, 102*, 725–730.

32. Ristoff, E., Augustson, C., Geissler, J., de Rijk, T., Carlsson, K., Luo, J.L., Andersson, K., Weening, R.S., van Zwieten, R., Larsson, A., Roos, D. (2000). A missense mutation in the heavy subunit of γ-glutamylcysteine synthetase gene causes hemolytic anemia. *Blood, 95,* 2193–2196.

33. Mañú Pereira, M., Gelbart, T., Ristoff, E., Crain, K.C., Bergua, J.M., López Lafuente, A., Kalko, S.G., García Mateos, E., Beutler, E., Vives Corrons, J.L. (2007). Chronic non-spherocytic haemolytic anaemia associated with severe neurological disease due to γ-glutamylcysteine synthetase deficiency in a patient of Moroccan origin. *Haematologica, 92*(11), e102–e105.

34. Richards, F.D., Cooper, M.R., Pearce, L.A., Cowan, R.J., Spurr, C.L. (1974). Familial spinocerebellar degeneration, hemolytic anemia, and glutathione deficiency. *Archives of Internal Medicine, 134,* 534–537.

35. Beutler, E., Gelbart, T., Kondo, T., Matsunaga, A.T. (1999). The molecular basis of a case of γ-glutamylcysteine synthetase deficiency. *Blood, 94,* 2890–2894.

36. Hirono, A., Iyori, H., Sekine, I., Ueyama, J., Chiba, H., Kanno, H., Fujii, H., Miwa, S. (1996). Three cases of hereditary nonspherocytic hemolytic anemia associated with red blood cell glutathione deficiency. *Blood, 87,* 2071–2074.

37. Beutler, E., Moroose, R., Kramer, L., Gelbart, T., Forman, L. (1990). γ-glutamylcysteine synthetase deficiency and hemolytic anemia. *Blood, 75,* 271–273.

38. Konrad, P.N., Richards, F.D., Valentine, W.N., Paglia, D.E. (1972). γ-glutamylcysteine synthetase deficiency. A cause of hereditary hemolytic anemia. *New England Journal of Medicine, 286,* 557–561.

39. Sierra-Rivera, E., Summar, M.L., Dasouki, M., Krishnamani, M.R., Phillips, J.A., Freeman, M.L. (1995). Assignment of the gene (GLCLC) that encodes the heavy subunit of γ-glutamylcysteine synthetase to human chromosome 6. *Cytogenetics and Cell Genetics, 70,* 278–279.

40. Sierra-Rivera, E., Dasouki, M., Summar, M.L., Krishnamani, M.R., Meredith, M., Rao, P.N., Phillips, J.A. Freeman, M.L. III (1996). Assignment of the human gene (GLCLR) that encodes the regulatory subunit of γ-glutamylcysteine synthetase to chromosome 1p21. *Cytogenetics and Cell Genetics, 72,* 252–254.

41. Huang, C.S., Chang, L.S., Anderson, M.E. and Meister, A. (1993). Catalytic and regulatory properties of the heavy subunit of rat kidney γ-glutamylcysteine synthetase. *Journal of Biological Chemistry, 268,* 19675–19680.

42. Wild, A.C., Mulcahy, R.T. (2000). Regulation of γ-glutamylcysteine synthetase subunit gene expression: Insights into transcriptional control of antioxidant defenses. *Free Radical Research, 32,* 281–301.

43. Anderson, M.E. (1985). Determination of glutathione and glutathione disulfide in biological samples. *Methods in Enzymology, 113,* 548–555.

44. Luo, J.L., Hammarqvist, F., Andersson, K., Wernerman, J. (1998). Surgical trauma decreases glutathione synthetic capacity in human skeletal muscle tissue. *American Journal of Physiology, 275,* E359–E365.

45. Ristoff, E., Mayatepek, E., Larsson, A. (2001). Long-term clinical outcome in patients with glutathione synthetase deficiency. *Journal of Pediatrics, 139,* 79–84.

46. Ristoff, E., Burstedt, M., Larsson, A., Wachtmeister, L. (2007). Progressive retinal dystrophy in two sisters with glutathione synthetase (GS) deficiency. *Journal of Inherited Metabolic Diseases, 30,* 102.

47. Ristoff, E., Hebert, C., Njalsson, R., Norgren, S., Rooyackers, O., Larsson, A. (2002). Glutathione synthetase deficiency: Is γ-glutamylcysteine accumulation a way to cope with oxidative stress in cells with insufficient levels of glutathione? *Journal of Inherited Metabolic Diseases, 25*, 577–584.

48. Nygren, J., Ristoff, E., Carlsson, K., Moller, L., Larsson, A. (2005). Oxidative DNA damage in cultured fibroblasts from patients with hereditary glutathione synthetase deficiency. *Free Radical Research, 39*, 595–601.

49. Mayatepek, E., Hoffmann, G.F., Carlsson, B., Larsson, A., Becker, K. (1994). Impaired synthesis of lipoxygenase products in glutathione synthetase deficiency. *Pediatric Research, 35*, 307–310.

50. Skullerud, K., Marstein, S., Schrader, H., Brundelet, P.J., Jellum, E. (1980). The cerebral lesions in a patient with generalized glutathione deficiency and pyroglutamic aciduria (5-oxoprolinuria). *Acta Neuropathologica, 52*, 235–238.

51. Hall, A.G. (1999). Review: The role of glutathione in the regulation of apoptosis. *European Journal of Clinical Investigations, 29*, 238–245.

52. Bains, J.S., Shaw, C.A. (1997). Neurodegenerative disorders in humans: The role of glutathione in oxidative stress-mediated neuronal death. *Brain Research Reviews, 25*, 335–358.

53. Mayatepek, E. (2000). Leukotriene C4 synthesis deficiency: A member of a probably underdiagnosed new group of neurometabolic diseases. *European Journal of Pediatrics, 159*, 811–818.

54. Edgren, M., Revesz, L., Larsson, A. (1981). Induction and repair of single-strand DNA breaks after X-irradiation of human fibroblasts deficient in glutathione. *International Journal of Radiation Biology and Related Studies in Physics, Chemistry, and Medicine, 40*, 355–363.

55. Spielberg, S.P. (1984). In vitro assessment of pharmacogenetic susceptibility to toxic drug metabolites in humans. *Federation Proceedings, 43*, 2308–2313.

56. Marklund, S.L., Midander, J., Westman, G. (1984). CuZn superoxide dismutase, Mn superoxide dismutase, catalase, and glutathione peroxidase in glutathione-deficient human fibroblasts. *Biochimica et Biophysica Acta, 798*, 302–305.

57. Larsson, A., Holmgren, A., Bratt, I. (1978). Thioredoxin and glutathione in cultured fibroblasts from human cases with 5-oxoprolinuria and cystinosis. *FEBS Letters, 87*, 61–64.

58. Polekhina, G., Board, P.G., Gali, R.R., Rossjohn, J., Parker, M.W. (1999). Molecular basis of glutathione synthetase deficiency and a rare gene permutation event. *EMBO Journal, 18*, 3204–3213.

59. Gali, R.R., Board, P.G. (1995). Sequencing and expression of a cDNA for human glutathione synthetase. *Biochemistry Journal, 310*, 353–358.

60. Whitbread, L., Gali, R.R., Board, P.G. (1998). The structure of the human glutathione synthetase gene. *Chemico-Biological Interactions, 111–112*, 35–40.

61. Njalsson, R., Ristoff, E., Carlsson, K., Winkler, A., Larsson, A., Norgren, S. (2005). Genotype, enzyme activity, glutathione level, and clinical phenotype in patients with glutathione synthetase deficiency. *Human Genetics, 116*, 384–389.

62. Njalsson, R., Carlsson, K., Olin, B., Carlsson, B., Whitbread, L., Polekhina, G., Parker, M.W., Norgren, S., Mannervik, B., Board, P.G., Larsson, A. (2000). Kinetic properties of missense mutations in patients with glutathione synthetase deficiency. *Biochemical Journal, 349*, 275–279.

63. Njalsson, R., Carlsson, K., Bhansali, V., Luo, J.L., Nilsson, L., Ladenstein, R., Anderson, M., Larsson, A., Norgren, S. (2004). Human hereditary glutathione synthetase deficiency: Kinetic properties of mutant enzymes. *Biochemical Journal*, *381*, 489–494.

64. Hoffmann, G., Aramaki, S., Blum-Hoffmann, E., Nyhan, W.L., Sweetman, L. (1989). Quantitative analysis for organic acids in biological samples: Batch isolation followed by gas chromatographic-mass spectrometric analysis. *Clinical Chemistry*, *35*, 587–595.

65. Njålsson, R., Carlsson, K., Winkler, A., Larsson, A., Norgren, S. (2003). Diagnostics in patients with glutathione synthetase deficiency but without mutations in the exons of the GSS gene. *Human Mutatations*, *22*, 497.

66. Shi, Z.Z., Habib, G.M., Rhead, W.J., Gahl, W.A., He, X., Sazer, S., Lieberman, M.W. (1996). Mutations in the glutathione synthetase gene cause 5-oxoprolinuria. *Nature Genetics*, *14*, 361–365.

67. Erasmus, E., Mienie, L.J., de Vries, W.N., de Wet, W.J., Carlsson, B., Larsson, A. (1993). Prenatal analysis in two suspected cases of glutathione synthetase deficiency. *Journal of Inherited Metabolic Disorders*, *16*, 837–843.

68. Manning, N.J., Davies, N.P., Olpin, S.E., Carpenter, K.H., Smith, M.F., Pollitt, R.J., Duncan, S.L., Larsson, A., Carlsson, B. (1994). Prenatal diagnosis of glutathione synthase deficiency. *Prenatal Diagnosis*, *14*, 475–478.

69. Jain, A., Buist, N.R., Kennaway, N.G., Powell, B.R., Auld, P.A., Martensson, J. (1994). Effect of ascorbate or N-acetylcysteine treatment in a patient with hereditary glutathione synthetase deficiency. *Journal of Pediatrics*, *124*, 229–233.

70. Baehner, R.L., Boxer, L.A. (1979). Role of membrane vitamin E and cytoplasmic glutathione in the regulation of phagocytic functions of neutrophils and monocytes. *American Journal of Pediatric Hematology/Oncology*, *1*, 71–76.

71. Martensson, J., Meister, A. (1991). Glutathione deficiency decreases tissue ascorbate levels in newborn rats: Ascorbate spares glutathione and protects. *Proceedings of the National Academy of Sciences USA*, *88*, 4656–4660. (Published erratum appears in *Proceedings of the National Academy of Sciences USA* 88, no. 15(1991): 6898.)

72. Janaky, R., Varga, V., Hermann, A., Saransaari, P., Oja, S.S. (2000). Mechanisms of L-cysteine neurotoxicity. *Neurochemistry Research*, *25*, 1397–1405.

73. Anderson, M.E., Levy, E.J., Meister, A. (1994). Preparation and use of glutathione monoesters. *Methods in Enzymology*, *234*, 492–499.

74. O'Daley, S. (1968). An abnormal sulphydryl compound in urine. *Irish Journal of Medical Science*, *7*, 578–579.

75. Goodman, S.I., Mace, J.W., Pollack, S. (1971). Serum γ-glutamyl transpeptidase deficiency. *Lancet*, *1*, 234–235.

76. Schulman, J.D., Goodman, S.I., Mace, J.W., Patrick, A.D., Tietze, F., Butler, E.J. (1975). Glutathionuria: Inborn error of metabolism due to tissue deficiency of γ-glutamyl transpeptidase. *Biochemical and Biophysical Research Communications*, *65*, 68–74.

77. Wright, E.C., Stern, J., Ersser, R., Patrick, A.D. (1980). Glutathionuria: γ-glutamyl transpeptidase deficiency. *Journal of Inherited Metabolic Diseases*, *2*, 3–7.

78. Hammond, J.W., Potter, M., Wilcken, B., Truscott, R. (1995). Siblings with γ-glutamyl-transferase deficiency. *Journal of Inherited Metabolic Diseases 18*, 82–83.

79. Iida, M., Yasuhara, T., Mochizuki, H., Takakura, H., Yanagisawa, T., Kubo, H. (2005). Two Japanese brothers with hereditary γ-glutamyl transpeptidase deficiency. *Journal of Inherited Metabolic Diseases*, *28*, 49–55.

80. Mayatepek, E., Okun, J.G., Meissner, T., Assmann, B., Hammond, J., Zschocke, J., Lehmann, W.D. (2004). Synthesis and metabolism of leukotrienes in γ-glutamyl trans-peptidase deficiency. *Journal of Lipid Research, 45*, 900–904.

81. Kumar, T.R., Wiseman, A.L., Kala, G., Kala, S.V., Matzuk, M.M., Lieberman, M.W. (2000). Reproductive defects in γ-glutamyl transpeptidase- deficient mice. *Endocrinology, 141*, 4270–4277.

82. Larsson, A., Mattsson, B., Wauters, E.A., van Gool, J.D., Duran, M., Wadman, S.K. (1981). 5-oxoprolinuria due to hereditary 5-oxoprolinase deficiency in two brothers: A new inborn error of the γ-glutamyl cycle. *Acta Paediatrica Scandinavica, 70*, 301–308.

83. Roesel, R.A., Hommes, F.A., Samper, L. (1981). Pyroglutamic aciduria (5-oxoprolinuria) without glutathione synthetase deficiency and with decreased pyroglutamate hydrolase activity. *Journal of Inherited Metabolic Diseases, 4*, 89–90.

84. Henderson, M.J., Larsson, A., Carlsson, B., Dear, P.R. (1993). 5-Oxoprolinuria associated with 5-oxoprolinase deficiency: Further evidence that this is a benign disorder. *Journal of Inherited Metabolic Diseases, 16*, 1051–1052.

85. Mayatepek, E., Hoffmann, G.F., Larsson, A., Becker, K., Bremer, H.J. (1995). 5-Oxoprolinase deficiency associated with severe psychomotor developmental delay, failure to thrive, microcephaly and microcytic anaemia. *Journal of Inherited Metabolic Diseases, 18*, 83–84.

86. Bernier, F.P., Snyder, F.F., McLeod, D.R. (1996). Deficiency of 5-oxoprolinase in an 8-year-old with developmental delay. *Journal of Inherited Metabolic Diseases, 19*, 367–368.

87. Cohen, L.H., Vamos, E., Heinrichs, C., Toppet, M., Courtens, W., Kumps, A., Mardens, Y., Carlsson, B., Grillner, L., Larsson, A. (1997). Growth failure, encephalopathy, and endocrine dysfunctions in two siblings, one with 5-oxoprolinase deficiency. *European Journal of Pediatrics, 156*, 935–938.

88. Nitanai, Y., Satow, Y., Adachi, H., Tsujimoto, M. (2002). Crystal structure of human renal dipeptidase involved in beta-lactam hydrolysis. *Journal of Molecular Biology, 321*, 177–184.

89. Nakagawa, H., Inazawa, J., Inoue, K., Misawa, S., Kashima, K., Adachi, H., Nakazato, H., Abe, T. (1992). Assignment of the human renal dipeptidase gene (DPEP1) to band q24 of chromosome 16. *Cytogenetics and Cell Genetics, 59*, 258–260.

90. Anderson, M.E., Allison, R.D., Meister, A. (1982). Interconversion of leukotrienes cata-lyzed by purified γ-glutamyl transpeptidase: Concomitant formation of leukotriene D4 and γ-glutamyl amino acids. *Proceedings of the National Academy of Sciences USA, 79*, 1088–1091.

91. Littlewood, G.M., Hooper, N.M., Turner, A.J. (1989). Ectoenzymes of the kidney micro-villar membrane. Affinity purification, characterization and localization of the phospho-lipase C-solubilized form of renal dipeptidase. *Biochemical Journal, 257*, 361–367.

92. Mayatepek, E. (1999). 5-Oxoprolinuria in patients with and without defects in the γ-glutamyl cycle. *European Journal of Pediatrics, 158*, 221–225.

93. Oberholzer, V.G., Wood, C.B., Palmer, T., Harrison, B.M. (1975). Increased pyrogluta-mic acid levels in patients on artificial diets. *Clinica Chimica Acta, 62*, 299–304.

94. Tham, R., Nystrom, L., Holmstedt, B. (1968). Identification by mass spectrometry of pyr-oglutamic acid as a peak in the gas chromatography of human urine. *Biochemical Pharmacology, 17*, 1735–1738.

95. Stokke, O., Marstein, S., Jellum, E., Lie, S.O. (1982). Accumulation of pyroglutamic acid (5-oxoproline) in homocystinuria. *Scandinavian Journal of Clinical and Laboratory Investigation*, *42*, 361–369.

96. Pitt, J.J., Brown, G.K., Clift, V., Christodoulou, J. (1990). Atypical pyroglutamic aciduria: Possible role of paracetamol. *Journal of Inherited Metabolic Diseases*, *13*, 755–756.

97. Bonham, J.R., Rattenbury, J.M., Meeks, A., Pollitt, R.J. (1989). Pyroglutamicaciduria from vigabatrin. *Lancet*, *1*, 1452–1453.

98. Croal, B.L., Glen, A.C., Kelly, C.J., Logan, R.W. (1998). Transient 5-oxoprolinuria (pyroglutamic aciduria) with systemic acidosis in an adult receiving antibiotic therapy. *Clinical Chemistry*, *44*, 336–340.

99. Ghauri, F.Y., McLean, A.E., Beales, D., Wilson, I.D., Nicholson, J.K. (1993). Induction of 5-oxoprolinuria in the rat following chronic feeding with N-acetyl 4-aminophenol (paracetamol). *Biochemical Pharmacology*, *46*, 953–957.

100. Jackson, A.A., Persaud, C., Hall, M., Smith, S., Evans, N., Rutter, N. (1997). Urinary excretion of 5-L-oxoproline (pyroglutamic acid) during early life in term and preterm infants. *Archives of Disease in Childhood. Fetal and Neonatal Edition*, *76*, F152–F157.

101. Jackson, A.A., Badaloo, A.V., Forrester, T., Hibbert, J.M., Persaud, C. (1987). Urinary excretion of 5-oxoproline (pyroglutamic aciduria) as an index of glycine insufficiency in normal man. *British Journal of Nutrition*, *58*, 207–214.

102. Rizzo, C., Ribes, A., Pastore, A., Dionisi-Vici, C., Greco, M., Rizzoni, G., Federici, G. (1999). Pyroglutamic aciduria and nephropathic cystinosis. *Journal of Inherited Metabolic Diseases*, *22*, 224–226.

103. Griffith, O.W., Meister, A. (1979). Glutathione: Interorgan translocation, turnover, and metabolism. *Proceedings of the National Academy of Sciences USA*, *76*, 5606–5610.

104. Shi, Z.Z., Osei-Frimpong, J., Kala, G., Kala, S.V., Barrios, R.J., Habib, G.M., Lukin, D.J., Danney, C.M., Matzuk, M.M., Lieberman, M.W. (2000). Glutathione synthesis is essential for mouse development but not for cell growth in culture. *Proceedings of the National Academy of Sciences USA*, *97*, 5101–5106.

105. Dalton, T.P., Dieter, M.Z., Yang, Y., Shertzer, H.G., Nebert, D.W. (2000). Knockout of the mouse glutamate cysteine ligase catalytic subunit (Gclc) gene: Embryonic lethal when homozygous, and proposed model for moderate glutathione deficiency when heterozygous. *Biochemical and Biophysical Research Communications*, *279*, 324–329.

106. Yang, Y., Dieter, M.Z., Chen, Y., Shertzer, H.G., Nebert, D.W., Dalton, T.P. (2002). Initial characterization of the glutamate-cysteine ligase modifier subunit Gclm(−/−) knockout mouse. Novel model system for a severely compromised oxidative stress response. *Journal of Biological Chemistry*, *277*, 49446–49452.

107. Harding, C.O., Williams, P., Wagner, E., Chang, D.S., Wild, K., Colwell, R.E., Wolff, J.A. (1997). Mice with genetic γ-glutamyl transpeptidase deficiency exhibit glutathionuria, severe growth failure, reduced life spans, and infertility. *Journal of Biological Chemistry*, *272*, 12560–12567.

108. Meister, A. (1983). Selective modification of glutathione metabolism. *Science*, *220*, 472–477.

CHAPTER 16

HOMOCYSTEINE METABOLISM AND PATHOLOGICAL IMPLICATIONS: THE HOMOCYSTEINE THIOLACTONE HYPOTHESIS OF VASCULAR DISEASE

HIERONIM JAKUBOWSKI

16.1 INTRODUCTION

Early animal studies have suggested that high protein diets can be harmful. Subsequent examinations of individual dietary amino acids have led to the conclusion that methionine, ingested in excess, is the most toxic amino acid [1–3]. For example, in female rats fed diets containing 5% methionine there were no successful pregnancies [4]. In other studies animals fed high protein or high methionine diets for 2 years developed hyperhomocysteinemia and evidence of vascular disease [5, 6]. On the other hand, methionine-restricted diet increases life span in rats [7] and inhibits age-related disease processes [8], including cancer [9]. Excess methionine is toxic because it leads to elevation of homocysteine (Hcy) in body tissues, particularly when intake of folate, vitamin B12, or vitamin B6 is inadequate [10].

Severe hyperhomocysteinemia secondary to mutations in the cystathionine β-synthase (CBS), methylenetetrahydrofolate reductase (MTHFR), or methionine synthase (MS) genes (Fig. 16.1) causes pathological changes in multiple organs, including the cardiovascular system and the brain, and leads to premature death due to vascular complications, usually thromboembolism in affected arteries and veins [10–14]. McCully observed advanced arterial lesions in children with inborn errors in Hcy metabolism and proposed that Hcy causes vascular disease [15]. Although severe hyperhomocysteinemia is rare, mild hyperhomocysteinemia is quite prevalent in the general population and is also associated with an increased risk of several common diseases [16], such as cardiovascular disease and mortality [17, 18], pregnancy complications and birth defects [19, 20], Alzheimer's disease and other

Glutathione and Sulfur Amino Acids in Human Health and Disease. Edited by R. Masella and G. Mazza
Copyright © 2009 John Wiley & Sons, Inc.

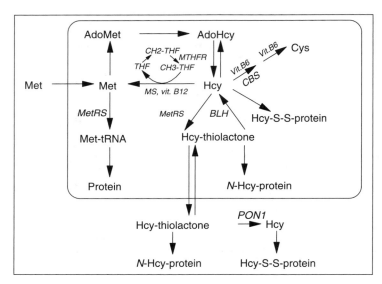

Figure 16.1 Schematic representation of human homocysteine metabolism. Abbreviations: Met, methionine; Cys, cysteine; MS, methionine synthase; THF, tetrahydrofolate; MTHFR, 5,10-methylene-THF reductase; CBS, cystathionine β-synthase; Hcy, homocysteine; AdoMet, S-adenosylmethionine; AdoHcy, S-adenosylhomocysteine; MetRS, methionyl-tRNA synthetase; BLH, bleomycin hydrolase; PON1, paraoxonase 1.

neurological complications [21, 22], osteoporosis and hip fracture [23–25]. Although associations alone do not prove causality, accumulating experimental evidence suggests that it is biologically plausible that excess Hcy can damage and impair normal cellular and physiological function and cause disease [26].

Atherosclerosis, a disease of the vascular wall, is initiated by endothelial damage [27]. Endothelial dysfunction, immune activation, and thrombosis, characteristic features of vascular disease [27], are all observed in hyperhomocysteinemic humans [10] and animals [28, 29]. The degree of impairment in endothelial function during hyperhomocysteinemia is similar to that observed with hypercholesterolemia or hypertension [28]. The strongest evidence that excess Hcy plays a causal role in atherothrombosis comes from the studies of severe genetic hyperhomocysteinemia in humans and the finding that Hcy lowering by vitamin B supplementation greatly improves vascular outcomes in CBS-deficient patients [10–12]. For example, whereas untreated CBS-deficient patients suffered one vascular event per 25 patient-years [30], treated CBS-deficient patients suffered only one vascular event per 263 patient-years (relative risk 0.091, $p < 0.001$) [12]. Hcy-lowering therapy started early in life also prevents brain disease from severe MTHFR deficiency [13, 31]. Furthermore, studies of genetic and nutritional hyperhomocysteinemia in animal models also provide strong support for a causative role of Hcy [28, 32]. In humans, lowering plasma Hcy by vitamin B supplementation improves cognitive function in the general population [33] and leads to a 21% to 24% reduction of vascular outcomes in high risk stroke patients [34, 35], but not in myocardial infarction (MI) patients [35, 36]. A recent meta-analysis of Hcy-lowering trials provides evidence that folic acid supplementation can significantly reduce the risk of stroke in primary prevention, provided that the intervention lasts more than 3 years and results in total Hcy (tHcy) lowering >20% [37].

Although Hcy is a ubiquitous intermediary metabolite in the three domains of life, its excess can be extremely toxic to human [38–41], animal [42], yeast [43–45], and bacterial cells [46]. Why Hcy is toxic is not entirely clear and is a subject of intense studies, particularly in the context of human pathophysiology [26, 28, 32, 47–52]. Hcy is one of the most reactive amino acids and participates in at least seven reactions in biological systems [47]. In addition to its elimination by remethylation to methionine or transsulfuration to cysteine (via cystathionine) and oxidation to disulfides, Hcy can also be converted to potentially toxic metabolites, such as Hcy-thiolactone, S-adenosylhomocysteine (AdoHcy), homocysteic acid, or S-nitroso-Hcy. Protein biosynthesis-related pathways of Hcy metabolism, involving Hcy-thiolactone, have been elucidated in various organisms, including human, and provided molecular basis for the Hcy-thiolactone hypothesis to account for Hcy-induced pathology [47, 48, 53–55]. In this chapter, I will summarize the fundamental biochemistry of Hcy-thiolactone and discuss mechanisms by which it can contribute to human vascular disease.

16.2 AN OVERVIEW OF HCY METABOLISM

In mammals, Hcy is formed from dietary methionine (Met) as a result of cellular methylation reactions [10] (Fig. 16.1). Dietary Met is first taken up by cells and then activated by ATP to yield S-adenosylmethionine (AdoMet), a universal methyl donor. As a result of the transfer of its methyl group to an acceptor, AdoMet is converted to S-adenosylhomocysteine (AdoHcy). The reversible enzymatic hydrolysis of AdoHcy is the only known source of Hcy in the human body. Levels of Hcy are regulated by remethylation to Met, catalyzed by the enzyme Met synthase (MS), and transsulfuration to cysteine, the first step of which is catalyzed by the enzyme cystathionine β-synthase (CBS). The remethylation requires vitamin B12 and 5,10-methyl-tetrahydrofolate (CH$_3$-THF), generated by 5,10-methylene-THF reductase (MTHFR) [13] (Fig. 16.1). An alternative remethylation pathway is catalyzed by betaine : Hcy methyltransferase [10] (not shown). The transsulfuration requires vitamin B6. Hcy formation is ubiquitous and occurs in all human organs, as does Hcy remethylation catalyzed by MS. However, Hcy remethylation catalyzed by betaine : Hcy methyltransferase and the transsulfuration occurs largely in the liver and kidneys and is absent from vascular tissues [56]. Hcy also forms disulfides, mostly with proteins (Hcy-S-S-protein) [57–59]. A fraction of Hcy is also metabolized by methionyl-tRNA synthetase (MetRS) to a thioester, Hcy-thiolactone [47, 48, 54, 55]. The flow through the Hcy-thiolactone pathway is increased in hyperhomocysteinemia secondary to a high Met diet, inadequate supply of CH$_3$-THF, or impairment of remethylation or transsulfuration reactions by genetic alterations of enzymes, such as CBS, MS, or

MTHFR. The conversion to Hcy-thiolactone has been suggested [60] to contribute to Hcy efflux observed in cultured human cells [61]. Hcy-thiolactone is hydrolyzed to Hcy by intracellular and extracellular Hcy-thiolactonases, otherwise known as bleomycin hydrolase (BLH) [62] and paraoxonase 1 (PON1) [58], respectively, which allow its reutilization in the transmethylation and transsulfuration reactions. Another pathway of Hcy-thiolactone metabolism involves protein N-homocysteinylation, that is, chemical modification of protein amino groups resulting in the formation of N-Hcy-protein [57–60] (Fig. 16.1).

In addition to its thiol form (i.e., Hcy as a chemical), oxidized forms such as the disulfide homocystine (Hcy-S-S-Hcy), mixed disulfides with cysteine (Hcy-S-S-Cys) [63] and plasma proteins (Hcy-S-S-protein) (mainly with albumin [63] and globulins [59]), occur in the human blood; the sum of these Hcy species is called "total" Hcy (tHcy) and used as a marker in clinical studies of human disease [64]. However, because alkaline pH used in the standard methods of tHcy determination leads to hydrolysis of Hcy-thiolactone, the tHcy pool could also include Hcy-thiolactone. Hcy-S-S-protein accounts for ~80% of tHcy, Hcy-S-S-Hcy and Hcy-S-S-Cys account for 20%, whereas the thiol Hcy accounts for only ~1% of tHcy [63]. In healthy humans, tHcy concentration in plasma (~10 μM) is approximately twofold higher than in urine [65]. In mice, however, plasma tHcy (3.5 μM) is 15-fold lower than urinary tHcy [66]. While in humans urinary tHcy clearance is insignificant (~1%), in mice a significant fraction of tHcy (38%) is eliminated by urinary excretion [66].

In rodents, concentrations of intracellular tHcy are similar to the plasma concentrations. Like in rodent plasma, a significant pool of Hcy bound to intracellular proteins by disulfide linkages (Fig. 16.1) exists in rodent tissues [67]. For example, protein-S-S-Hcy accounts for ~42% of tHcy in rat liver, kidney, heart, and lung. In rat cerebrum and cerebellum protein-S-S-Hcy accounts for 30.4% and 5.3%, respectively, of tHcy [67]. It remains to be demonstrated whether human intracellular proteins also carry disulfide-bound Hcy.

AdoHcy, an immediate precursor of Hcy (Fig. 16.1), occurs in human cells and plasma at micromolar and nanomolar concentrations, respectively [68, 69]. Ado Hcy concentrations are 33-fold higher in human urine than in plasma, consistent with its significant fractional excretion (39%) [69].

Two novel Hcy metabolites, Hcy-thiolactone [44, 65, 66, 70, 71] and protein N-linked Hcy (N-Hcy-protein) [59, 70, 72], have been discovered recently in humans and mice and mechanisms of their biosynthesis elucidated [47, 48] (Fig. 16.1). In normal humans and mice, plasma Hcy-thiolactone occurs at nanomolar concentrations, whereas urinary Hcy-thiolactone is ~100-fold higher [65, 66, 71]; >95% of the filtered plasma Hcy-thiolactone is cleared by the kidney [65, 66]. In normal human blood, N-Hcy-protein occurs at micromolar concentrations [59].

16.3 TOXICITY OF HCY AND ITS METABOLITES

Numerous clinical studies have established that elevated plasma tHcy is associated with vascular disease [16–18]. However, as discussed above, tHcy is a composite marker, comprised of at least five different Hcy species, each of which could exert a distinct biological effect. Moreover, tHcy does not encompass other Hcy metabolites present in the human blood, such as AdoHcy, Hcy-thiolactone, and protein N-linked Hcy [47]. Thus, a contribution of individual Hcy species to cardiovascular risk or mortality is likely to be obscured by using tHcy as a marker [73]. Indeed, in a few studies that addressed this issue, plasma AdoMet [68] and anti-*N*-Hcy-protein autoantibodies [53, 74] turned out to be much more sensitive indicators of human cardiovascular disease than plasma tHcy.

The presence of multiple molecular Hcy species raises a question regarding whether any of those species could be more harmful than the other. Available evidence suggests that the thiol Hcy is more harmful than the oxidized (disulfide) Hcy species. In a few studies that directly addressed the toxicity of different Hcy species, the thiol Hcy was associated with endothelial dysfunction, whereas much more abundant disulfide Hcy species were not [75, 76]. The thiol Hcy can be harmful because it is metabolized to a toxic metabolite, Hcy-thiolactone [47, 60, 77–79], which occurs in humans [44, 65, 70, 71] and mice [66]. That the conversion to Hcy-thiolactone is responsible for the thiol Hcy toxicity has been demonstrated in a rat embryo model, in which both L- and D-Hcy-thiolactone were found to be toxic [80]. However, only the metabolically active L-enantiomer, but not the inactive D-enantiomer, of the thiol Hcy is toxic to rat embryos [80]. Plasma levels of the thiol Hcy are maintained low because of its elimination in reactions with blood proteins [58], mainly albumin and globulins [59].

Although it has been suggested that the formation of Hcy-*S*-*S*-protein disulfides may explain mechanistically the toxicity of elevated Hcy levels [52], there is no convincing evidence that any of the disulfide species of Hcy occurring in the plasma is harmful to the human body [75, 76]. Whether the formation of intracellular Hcy-*S*-*S*-protein mixed disulfides (Fig. 16.1) in humans could be harmful has recently been addressed in an ex vivo study, which suggests that Hcy binding to metallothionein causes increase in intracellular free zinc and oxidative stress in cultured human endothelial cells treated with exogenous Hcy [81]. However, whether Hcy binding can be replicated with purified metallothionein has not been reported. Although these effects were ascribed to the formation of a putative Hcy-*S*-*S*-metallothionein disulfide, the authors' observations that Hcy binding was not affected by 10 mM glutathione and that cysteine did not form a disulfide with metallothionein [81] suggest that Hcy may bind to metallothionein by another mechanism, possibly N-homocysteinylation. In fact, Hcy-thiolactone and protein N-linked Hcy are major Hcy species formed by human endothelial cells [82]. Like other proteins [57], metallothionein is expected to be a target for N-homocysteinylation by Hcy-thiolactone as well.

Experimental evidence suggests that AdoHcy can be harmful. For example, the intracellular accumulation of AdoHcy inhibits endothelial cell growth [83] and exerts epigenetic effects on gene expression by interfering with cellular methylation reactions and changing DNA methylation patterns [84, 85]. In humans, plasma AdoHcy is highly correlated with plasma tHcy, whereas increased plasma and lymphocyte AdoHcy levels are associated with decreased DNA methylation [84, 86]. Furthermore, an increase in plasma AdoHcy is a much more sensitive indicator of human cardiovascular disease than an increase in plasma tHcy [68]. However, the effects of elevated AdoHcy on DNA methylation appear to be tissue dependent. For example, in hyperhomocysteinemic mice, plasma tHcy correlates positively with AdoHcy in most tissues, except the kidney [87], and negatively with DNA methylation, as expected, in the liver. On the other hand, paradoxical increases in DNA methylation occur in the brain and the aorta of hyperhomocysteinemic animals [85]. These findings suggest that factors other than the methylation capacity can influence DNA methylation patterns.

It has been known since 1974 that chronic treatments of animals with Hcy-thiolactone cause pathophysiological changes similar to those observed in human genetic hyperhomocysteinemia [88]. For example, Hcy-thiolactone [88] infusions in baboons for up to 3 months produce atherosclerotic changes, such as patchy desquamation of vascular endothelium and arterial thrombosis [89, 90]. Recent studies show that Hcy-thiolactone-supplemented diet produces atherosclerosis in rats [91], whereas treatments with Hcy-thiolactone cause developmental abnormalities in chick embryos, including neural tube defects [92–94]. Remarkably, optic lens dislocation, a characteristic diagnostic feature present in the CBS-deficient human patients [10–12], has also been observed in Hcy-thiolactone-treated chick embryos [95]. However, rabbits, which have ∼10-fold higher levels of serum Hcy-thiolactonase/PON1 than humans or other animals, and thus efficiently detoxify Hcy-thiolactone [58, 96, 97], are resistant to the detrimental effects of Hcy-thiolactone infusions [98, 99]. Indeed, Hcy-thiolactone infused into rabbits is cleared from the blood within <15 min [98]. A report that Hcy-thiolactone infusions cause atherosclerosis in rabbits [100] could not be reproduced by other investigators [98, 99]. Efficient elimination of Hcy-thiolactone may also account for the lack of any changes in vascular morphology in pigs infused for up to 60 days with Hcy-thiolactone [101]. Like other harmful products of normal metabolism, Hcy-thiolactone is also eliminated by urinary excretion, as demonstrated in humans and mice [65, 66].

Hcy-thiolactone is also known to be acutely toxic in experimental animal models. For example, acute infusions of Hcy-thiolactone into mice or rats cause seizures and death within minutes [102–104]. Exposure of rat embryos to Hcy-thiolactone causes lethality, growth retardation, and developmental abnormalities [80]. Hcy-thiolactone is also toxic to mouse embryos but does not cause neural tube defects [105]. In one study Hcy-thiolactone was reported to be nonteratogenic in mouse embryos [106], but the maximum dose used in that study was lower than those used in other studies, so that an embryotoxic dose had not been reached. An additional factor that could have contributed to the negative outcome of the Hansen et al. study [106], was the inclusion in the embryo culture media of the antibiotic streptomycine (not used in the Van Aerts et al. [80] and Greene et al. [105] studies), which inactivates Hcy-thiolactone [82].

Hcy-thiolactone has also been shown to be more toxic than Hcy to cultured animal and human cells. For example, in early studies with adult bovine aortic endothelial cells, treatments with Hcy-thiolactone caused gross morphological changes and cell lysis during a 16 h incubation, whereas treatments with Hcy were ineffective [107]. Recent studies show that treatments with Hcy-thiolactone induce endoplasmic reticulum (ER) stress and unfolded protein response (UPR) in retinal epithelial cells [40], as well as apoptotic death in cultured human vascular endothelial cells [41, 108], promyeloid cells [109], and placental trophoblasts [110]. Although exogenous Hcy also induces apoptosis, much higher concentrations are required [38, 41], suggesting that Hcy-thiolactone is more potent than Hcy in causing apoptotic cell death [40, 41, 108]. Furthermore, exogenous Hcy-thiolactone inhibits insulin signaling in rat hepatoma cells [111].

Accumulating evidence suggests that *N*-Hcy-protein is harmful to the human body. For example, plasma protein N-linked Hcy levels are elevated in patients with coronary artery disease (CAD), compared with apparently healthy individuals [112]. As will be discussed in greater detail in the following sections of this chapter, *N*-Hcy-protein is detrimental because of its ability to induce cell death [113], an autoimmune response [53, 74, 114, 115], and to interfere with blood clotting [116, 117].

16.4 PHYSICAL-CHEMICAL PROPERTIES OF HCY-THIOLACTONE

Hcy-thiolactone, a cyclic thioester of Hcy, is prepared chemically by intramolecular condensation of methionine or Hcy. For example, boiling with hydriodic acid for 4 h, a procedure originally developed for the determination of protein methionine [118], quantitatively converts L-methionine to D,L-Hcy-thiolactone with the liberation of methyl iodide (Scheme 16.1). The hydriodic acid digestion procedure is a convenient method for the preparation of D,L-^{35}S-Hcy-thiolactone for biological studies [119]. Racemic D,L-^{35}S-Hcy-thiolactone is resolved to L-^{35}S-Hcy and D-^{35}S-Hcy-thiolactone by treatment with bleomycin hydrolase (BLH) [62, 119].

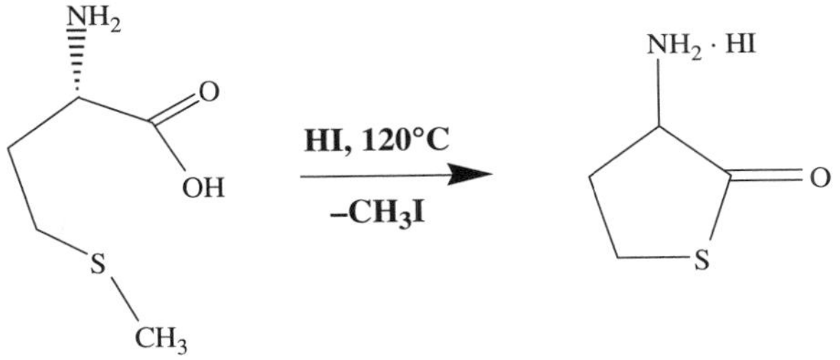

Scheme 16.1 The hydriodic acid-dependent conversion of methionine to Hcy-thiolactone. Reprinted with permission from Reference 47.

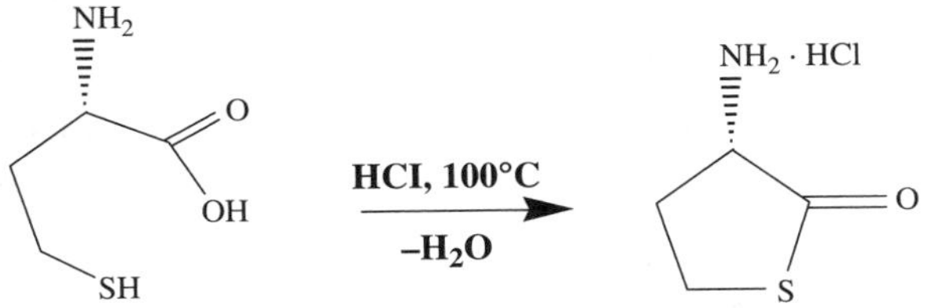

Scheme 16.2 The hydrochloric acid-dependent conversion of Hcy to Hcy-thiolactone. Reprinted with permission from Reference 47.

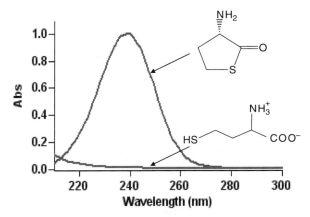

Figure 16.2   Absorption spectra of L-Hcy-thiolactone · HCl (0.2 mM in water, 25°C). D,L-Hcy (0.2 mM), shown for comparison, does not appreciably absorb UV light above 220 nm. Reprinted with permission from Reference 47.

TABLE 16.1   Physical-Chemical Properties of L-Hcy-Thiolactone and L-Hcy

Property	L-Hcy-Thiolactone	L-Hcy
Chemical character	Aminoacyl-thioester	Mercaptoamino acid
UV spectrum	Yes, $\lambda_{max} = 240$ nm, $\varepsilon = 5{,}000\ M^{-1}\ cm^{-1}$	No significant absorption at $\lambda > 220$ nm
Stability at 37°C, $t_{0.5}$		
Phosphate-saline	∼30 h	2 h
Human serum	∼1 h	2 h
pK_a of amino group	6.67[a]	9.04, 9.71[b] 9.02, 9.69 (thiol group)[b]
Chemical reactivity	−Acylates amino groups of protein lysine residues[c] −Reacts with aldehydes to afford tetrahydrothiazines[a] −Resistant to oxidation −Base hydrolyzed to Hcy	−Condenses to Hcy-thiolactone −Reacts with aldehydes to afford tetrahydrothiazines[a] −Oxidized to disulfides −Reacts with nitric oxide to afford S-nitroso-Hcy[d]

[a]Data from Reference 123.
[b]Data from Reference 125.
[c]Data from References 57 and 60.
[d]Data from References 70, 79, and 128.
Source: from Reference 47.

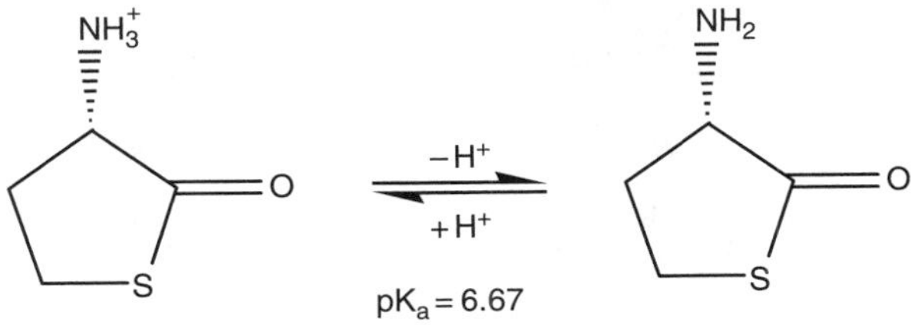

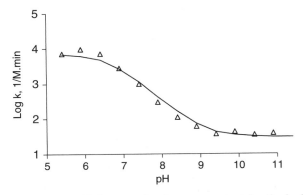

Scheme 16.3 Acid and base forms of Hcy-thiolactone. Reprinted with permission from Reference 123.

Intramolecular condensation of L-Hcy to L-Hcy-thiolactone occurs in the presence of hydrochloric acid (Scheme 16.2) [47]. The rate of the reaction depends on the acid concentration and temperature. For example, in 0.6 N or 6 N hydrochloric acid at 100°C, 50% condensation occurs in 15 min or <5 min, respectively. Because Hcy-thiolactone, in contrast to Hcy, absorbs ultraviolet light (Fig. 16.2), the acid-dependent conversion to Hcy-thiolactone is a convenient procedure for the determination of Hcy in biological samples [44, 59, 65, 66, 71, 120].

Differences in physical-chemical properties of Hcy-thiolactone and Hcy are highlighted in Table 16.1. Hcy-thiolactone, like other thioesters, absorbs ultraviolet light with a maximum at 240 nm and $\varepsilon \sim 5000 \, M^{-1} cm^{-1}$ in water (Fig. 16.2) [47], which allows its facile detection in biological samples [44, 120–122]. The pK_a of its α-amino group is unusually low at 6.67 [123]. Thus, under physiological conditions, Hcy-thiolactone exists as a neutral base form (Scheme 16.3) and freely diffuses through cell membranes [43, 44, 60, 77, 82, 120–122, 124]. In contrast, under physiological conditions the α-amino group of Hcy ($pK_a = 9.04$ or 9.71) (Table 16.1) [125] exists in a positively charged acid form.

Figure 16.3 pH dependence of the second-order rate constant for the hydrolysis of Hcy-thiolactone (HTL) ($k = k_{obs}/[OH^-]$). The solid line is theoretical line for the reactions of acid and base HTL forms calculated from the equation $k = (k_{HTL^+})(1 - \alpha) + (k_{HTL^0})\alpha$ in which α is the fraction of HTL as the base form, based on a pK_a of 6.67. Reprinted with permission from Reference 123.

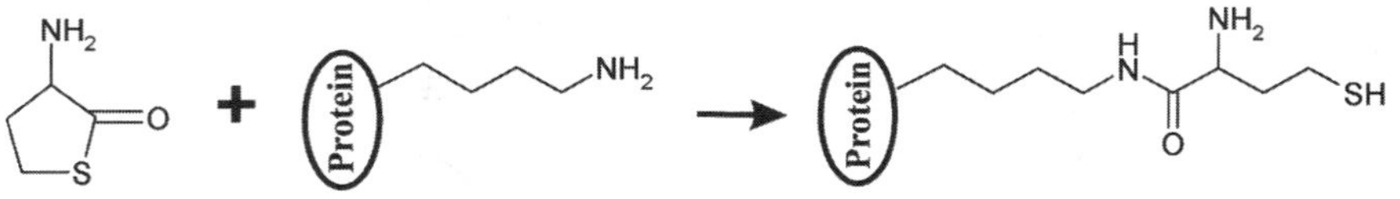

Scheme 16.4 Chemical modification of a protein lysine residue by Hcy-thiolactone. Reprinted with permission from Reference 65.

The hydrochloric acid salt of Hcy-thiolactone is stable indefinitely at room temperature. Under physiological conditions of pH and temperature, Hcy-thiolactone (half-life of ~25 h [60, 126]) is more stable than intermolecular aminoacyl-thioesters (e.g., methionyl-S-CoA hydrolyzes with a half-life of 2.25 h [127]). In alkaline solutions Hcy-thiolactone quickly hydrolyzes to Hcy (Table 16.1). For example, in

TABLE 16.2 Second-Order Rate Constants, k, for Reactions of Hcy-Thiolactone with Proteins and Other Compounds*

Protein (kDa) or Other Compound	k at 25°C, $M^{-1}h^{-1}$	k at 37°C, $M^{-1}h^{-1}$
α_2-Macroglobulin (725)	400	
Low density lipoprotein (500)	150	
Fibrinogen (340)	101	
γ-Globuline (140)	112	
Transferrin (80)	150	560
Albumin (68)	128	466
Hemoglobin (64)	84	600
MetRS (64)	60	
α-Crystalline (40)	10	
DNase I (37)	9	
Trypsin (24)	9	
Myoglobin (16)	40	
Cytochrome c (12.5)	36	150
RNase A (12.5)	3	
Poly-Lys (150)		6700
LysLys		26
LysAla		3
Lysine	1	5
α-N-acetyl-lysine		3.8
ε-N-acetyl-lysine		1.2
Formaldehyde[a]	8648	
Acetaldehyde[a]	2496	
Streptomycin[b]	1200	2000

*Except as noted, linear kinetics with respect to the concentrations of Hcy-thiolactone and listed compounds, are observed.
[a]Nonlinear kinetics, suggesting the formation of an intermediate, are observed. Data recalculated from Reference 123.
[b]H. Jakubowski, unpublished data.
Source: Data compiled from References 57 and 123.

0.1 M NaOH, hydrolysis of Hcy-thiolactone is completed in 15 min at room temperature [119, 128]. The rate of hydroxide-catalyzed hydrolysis of Hcy-thiolactone depends on the ionization status of its amino group. The positively charged acid form is hydrolyzed 186 times faster than the neutral base form (Fig. 16.3) [123].

The thioester bond of Hcy-thiolactone is highly susceptible to reactions with nucleophiles (Table 16.1). For example, under physiological conditions of pH and temperature, Hcy-thiolactone modifies proteins by forming N-Hcy-protein adducts, in which Hcy is N-linked to the ε-amino group of protein lysine residues, as shown in Scheme 16.4 [47, 57, 60]. Other amino acid side-chain groups in protein do not react appreciably with Hcy-thiolactone [57, 72, 117, 129]. The ε-amino group of lysine exhibits threefold greater reactivity than the α-amino group with Hcy-thiolactone (second-order rate constants $3.8\,M^{-1}h^{-1}$ and $1.2\,M^{-1}h^{-1}$, respectively; Table 16.2 [57]).

The α-amino group of Hcy thiolactone is highly reactive towards electrophiles (Table 16.1), such as formaldehyde, acetaldehyde, pyridoxal phosphate, o-phthalaldehyde, or streptomycin [47, 123]. Corresponding 1,3-tetrahydrothiazine-4-carboxylic acids are formed as products of these reactions (Scheme 16.5) [123].

The reactivity of Hcy-thiolactone with aldehydes depends on the ionization status of its α-amino group. For example, the positively charged acid form of

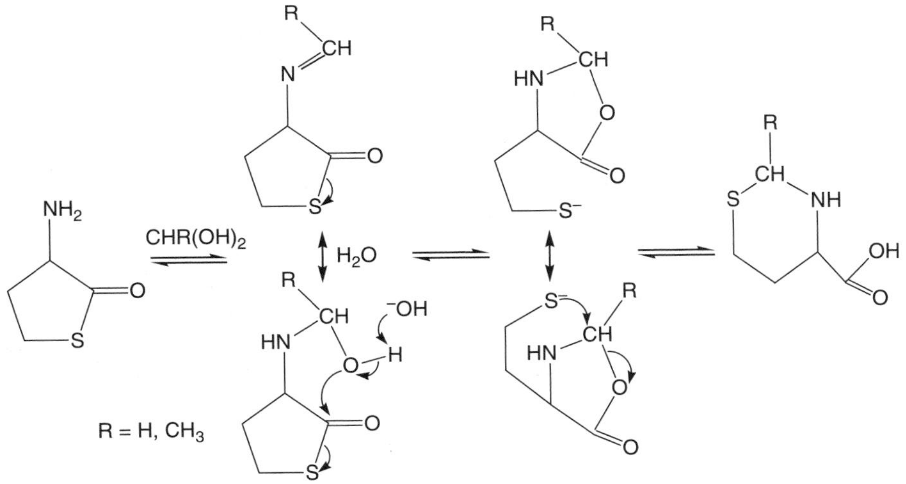

Scheme 16.5 1,4-Tetrahydrothiazine formation. The mechanism for the formation of 1,4-tetrahydrothiazine from Hcy-thiolactone and formaldehyde (R = H) or acetaldehyde (R = CH$_3$). The initial product of the reaction of Hcy-thiolactone with aldehydes is carbinolamine in a chemical equilibrium with imine. The formation of the carbinolamine greatly destabilizes the thioester bond by facilitating anchimeric assistance by the carbinolamine group, which makes possible an intramolecular attack of the oxygen on the thioester bond to form a five-membered lactone. This leads to the liberation of the thiolate group. Subsequent attack of the thiolate on an aldehyde-derived carbon leads to rapid formation of the six-membered ring of the tetrahydrothiazine and lysis of the lactone. Reprinted with permission from Reference 123.

Hcy-thiolactone (Scheme 16.3) reacts with formaldehyde or acetaldehyde 79 or 73 times faster, respectively, than the neutral base form [123]. At physiological pH, second-order rate constants for the reaction with aldehydes are 1200 to 8400 $M^{-1}h^{-1}$, more than 200 times faster than for the reaction of Hcy-thiolactone with lysine (Table 16.2). The reaction of Hcy-thiolactone with o-phthalaldehyde, generating a fluorescent adduct, offers a sensitive method for the determination of Hcy-thiolactone [65, 66, 71, 130].

16.5 THE MECHANISM OF HCY-THIOLACTONE BIOSYNTHESIS

Although Hcy-thiolactone was obtained by chemical synthesis in the 1930s, the first indication of its biological significance came almost 50 years later with the discovery of the enzymatic conversion of Hcy to Hcy-thiolactone in error editing reactions of some aminoacyl-tRNA synthetases [131]. Because of its similarity to the protein amino acids methionine, leucine, and isoleucine, the nonprotein amino acid Hcy poses an accuracy problem for the protein biosynthetic apparatus [54, 55, 70, 132]. For example, during protein biosynthesis Hcy is often mistakenly selected in place of Met by methionyl-tRNA synthetase (MetRS) and activated with ATP to form Hcy-AMP. However, the misactivated Hcy is not transferred to tRNA, but instead converted to Hcy-thiolactone in an error-editing reaction (Scheme 16.6) [131].

Similar reactions occur with leucyl-tRNA and isoleucyl-tRNA synthetases, both in vitro [131] and in vivo [121, 132]. Cell culture and whole organism studies have shown that the formation of Hcy-thiolactone is universal; it occurs in all organisms and cell types investigated, from bacteria [44, 121, 122, 124], yeast [43, 44], and plants [120] to mice [66] and humans [44, 65, 66, 71].

The involvement of MetRS in the biosynthesis of Hcy-thiolactone in vivo has been originally documented in microorganisms, such as *Escherichia coli* [124] and the yeast *Saccharomyces cerevisiae* [43]. The evidence that MetRS is involved in Hcy-thiolactone biosynthesis in mammals, including humans, came with the findings that Hcy-thiolactone is synthesized by cultured human cervical carcinoma (HeLa), mouse adenocarcinoma (RAG), and Chinese hamster ovary (CHO) cells [77], and that a temperature-sensitive MetRS mutant of CHO cells fails to synthesize Hcy-thiolactone at the nonpermissive temperature [77]. Subsequent work has demonstrated that MetRS is also involved in Hcy-thiolactone biosynthesis in plants [120].

Although studied in several biological systems, the molecular mechanism of Hcy editing is best understood for *E. coli* MetRS. The Hcy editing reaction occurs in the synthetic/editing active site [133], whose major function is to carry out the synthesis of Met-tRNA [134]. Whether methionine or Hcy completes the synthetic or editing

$$MetRS + Hcy + ATP \overset{-PP_i}{\Leftrightarrow} MetRS \cdot Hcy\text{~}AMP \overset{-AMP}{\Rightarrow} Hcy\text{-thiolactone} + MetRS$$

Scheme 16.6 The formation of Hcy-thiolactone catalyzed by methionyl-tRNA synthetase. MetRS, methionyl-tRNA synthetase.

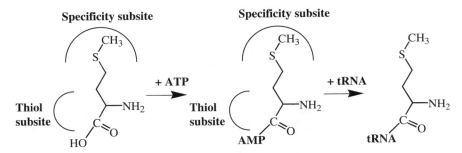

Figure 16.4   The aminoacylation of tRNA with Met catalyzed by methionyl-tRNA synthetase. Reprinted with permission from Reference 132.

pathway, respectively, is determined by the partitioning of its side chain between the specificity and thiol-binding subsites of the synthetic/editing active site [135]. A subsite that binds carboxyl and α-amino groups of methionine or Hcy does not appear to contribute to specificity [133]. Methionine completes the synthetic pathway because its side chain is firmly bound by the hydrophobic and hydrogen bonding interactions with the specificity subsite (Fig. 16.4). The crystal structure of the MetRS · Met complex [134] reveals that hydrophobic interactions involve side chains of Tyr[15], Trp[253], Pro[257], and Tyr[260]; Trp[305] closes the bottom of the hydrophobic pocket, but is not in contact with the methyl group of the substrate methionine (Fig. 16.5). The sulfur atom of the substrate methionine makes two hydrogen bonds: one with the hydroxyl of Tyr[260] and the other with the backbone amide of Leu[13].

The noncognate substrate Hcy, missing the methyl group of methionine, cannot interact with the specificity subsite as effectively as cognate methionine does. This allows the side chain of Hcy to move to the thiol-binding subsite, which promotes the synthesis of the thioester bond during editing (Fig. 16.6). Mutations of Tyr[15] and Trp[305] affect Hcy/Met discrimination by MetRS [133]. Asp[52], which forms a hydrogen bond with the α-amino group of the substrate methionine, deduced from the crystal structure of the MetRS · Met complex [134], is involved in the catalysis of both synthetic and editing reactions, but does not contribute to substrate specificity of the enzyme. The substitution Asp52Ala inactivates the synthetic and editing functions of MetRS [128, 133, 135].

Furthermore, the thiol-binding subsite also supports the ability of MetRS to edit in *trans*, that is, to catalyze thioester bond formation between a thiol and the cognate methionine (Fig. 16.7). With CoA-SH or cysteine as a thiol substrate, MetRS catalyzes the formation of Met-*S*-CoA thioesters [127] and Met-Cys di-peptides [135], respectively. The formation of Met-Cys di-peptide proceeds via a Met-*S*-Cys thioester intermediate, which spontaneously rearranges to the Met-Cys dipeptide. Remarkably, the formation of the Met-Cys dipeptide as a result of editing in *trans* is as fast as the formation of Hcy-thiolactone during Hcy editing.

Because the lack of efficient interactions of the side chain of Hcy with the specificity subsite is responsible for Hcy editing, keeping the side chain of Hcy in the

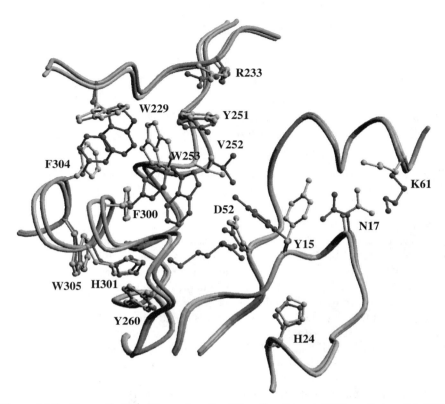

Figure 16.5 The synthetic/editing active site of *E. coli* methionyl-tRNA synthetase (MetRS). Hydrophobic and hydrogen bonding interactions provide specificity for the cognate substrate L-methionine. Superimposition of a-carbon chain backbones for the MetRS · Met complex (burly-wood) and free MetRS (light gray), solved at 1.8 Å resolution, shows movements of active site residues upon binding of methionine. Residue colors are red in the MetRS · Met complex and green in free MetRS, and L-methionine is magenta. Reprinted with permission from Reference 134. (See color insert.)

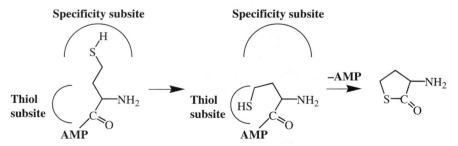

Figure 16.6 The synthesis of Hcy-thiolactone during Hcy editing catalyzed by methionyl-tRNA synthetase. Reprinted with permission from Reference 70.

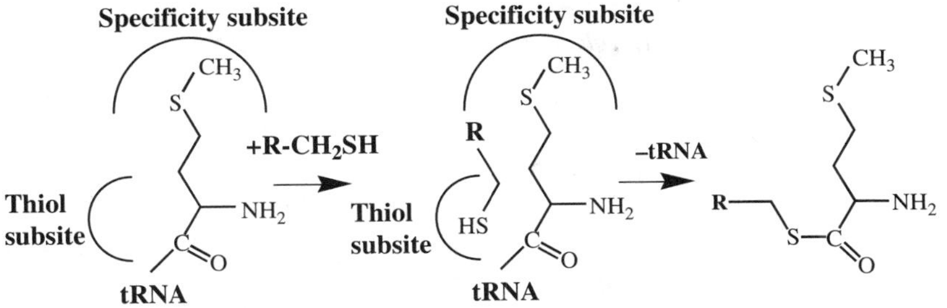

Figure 16.7   Editing in *trans*: synthesis of methionyl thioesters catalyzed by methionyl-tRNA synthetase. Reprinted with permission from Reference 70.

specificity subsite is expected to prevent editing and facilitate the transfer to tRNA[Met]. This can be achieved by utilizing nitrosothiol chemistry. Indeed, S-nitrosylation of Hcy prevents binding of its S-nitrosylated side chain to the editing subsite and enhances the binding to the specificity subsite, which in turn prevents editing of S-nitroso-Hcy and leads to the formation of S-nitroso-Hcy-tRNA[Met] (Fig. 16.8; Table 16.3). Active site mutations in MetRS that have detrimental effects on tRNA aminoacylation with Met have similar detrimental effects on tRNA aminoacylation with S-nitroso-Hcy, consistent with the binding of S-nitroso-Hcy and Met to the same active site [128].

Whereas S-nitroso-Hcy-tRNA[Met] (half-life 26 min) is as stable as Met-tRNA[Met], Hcy-tRNA[Met] (prepared by denitrosylation of S-nitroso-Hcy-tRNA[Met]) is the least stable aminoacyl-tRNA known (a half-life of 15 s), converting to Hcy-thiolactone and free tRNA. As expected, S-nitroso-Hcy-tRNA[Met] is a substrate for protein synthesis [128]. For example, when cultures of E. coli metE mutant cells expressing mouse dihydrofolate reductase (DHFR) protein were supplemented with S-nitroso-Hcy, the synthesized DHFR protein was found to contain Hcy. Globin and luciferase, produced in an in vitro mRNA-programmed rabbit reticulocyte protein synthesis system supplemented with S-nitroso-Hcy-tRNA[Met], contain Hcy at positions normally occupied by Met. Translationally incorporated Hcy is also present in proteins from

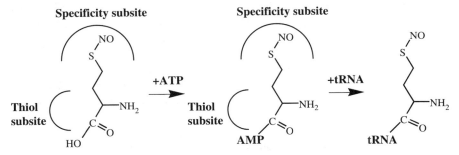

Figure 16.8   The aminoacylation of tRNA with S-nitroso-Hcy catalyzed by MetRS. Reprinted with permission from Reference 70.

TABLE 16.3 Relative Binding, Editing, and tRNA Aminoacylation under Steady-State Conditions by _E. coli_ Methionyl-tRNA Synthetase

Amino Acid	Binding $\times 10^4$	Rate of Editing	Rate of tRNA Aminoacylation $\times 10^6$
Methionine	10,000	1	10^6
Homocysteine	54	60	$<1^a$
S-nitroso-Hcy	8	<1	12,000

[a]Hcy is not incorporated directly into tRNA.

Source: Compiled from References 45, 128, and 131.

cultured human vascular endothelial cells [70], which are known to produce nitric oxide and S-nitroso-Hcy [136]. Thus, Hcy can gain access to the genetic code by S-nitrosylation-mediated invasion of the methionine-coding pathway. Whether translational incorporation of Hcy occurs in the human or animal body remains to be investigated.

16.6 STRUCTURAL AND FUNCTIONAL CONSEQUENCES OF PROTEIN MODIFICATION BY HCY-THIOLACTONE

In proteins, only the side-chain amino groups of lysine residues, but not any other amino acid residues, are modified by Hcy-thiolactone [57, 78, 97]. Moreover, the N-terminal α-amino groups in proteins do not appear to react with Hcy-thiolactone. Using proteomic approaches only internal lysine residues were identified as targets for Hcy-thiolactone modification in human serum albumin, hemoglobin, cytochrome c, and fibrinogen [72, 117, 129, 137].

Protein N-homocysteinylation goes to completion within a few hours at physiological conditions of pH and temperature [57, 58, 78]. Second-order rate constants for reactions of Hcy-thiolactone with individual purified proteins (Table 16.2) indicate that lysine content is a major determinant of the reactivity of most proteins with Hcy-thiolactone. For proteins that vary in size from 104 to 698 amino acid residues there is a very good correlation ($r = 0.97$) between a protein's lysine content and its reactivity with Hcy-thiolactone [57]. Larger proteins, such as fibrinogen (3588 amino acid residues) and low-density lipoproteins (LDL) ($\sim$5000 amino acid residues), react with Hcy-thiolactone approximately sixfold less efficiently than expected from their lysine contents (Table 16.2). Of many lysine residues present in a protein only a few are predominant sites for modification by Hcy-thiolactone, as has been shown for albumin [72, 137], hemoglobin (R. Glowacki, H. Jakubowski, unpublished data), fibrinogen [117], and cytochrome c [129]. Specific N-Hcy-peptides of N-Hcy-albumin, containing N-homocysteinylated Lys4 and Lys525, are easily detected in tryptic digests of human serum samples by using proteomic approaches [137]. Assaying these N-Hcy peptides in serum samples provides a new diagnostic tool for monitoring protein damage caused by Hcy-thiolactone.

That protein N-linked Hcy is present in human plasma proteins was first reported in 2000 [78]. Subsequent studies have confirmed this finding [59, 138, 139]. As all known proteins contain lysine residues, each protein is a target for modification by Hcy-thiolactone. Indeed, when [^{35}S]Hcy-thiolactone is added to human or animal serum, each individual serum protein becomes N-homocysteinylated in proportion to its abundance [57]. Protein N-linked Hcy occurs in purified serum albumin from various organisms, such as human, sheep, pig, rabbit, rat, mouse, and chicken [59]. Examination of individual purified blood proteins demonstrates that 0.36% to 0.60% of protein N-linked Hcy is present in normal human hemoglobin, serum albumin, and γ-globulins. Other serum proteins, such as fibrinogen, LDL, HDL, transferrin, and antitrypsin, contain 0.04% to 0.1% of protein N-linked Hcy [59]. Recalculation of these values (by taking into account normal levels of individual blood proteins) shows that the concentration of N-linked Hcy carried on hemoglobin in erythrocytes is 27.8 μM (Table 16.4), greater than the concentration of plasma tHcy. Albumin and γ-globulin carry micromolar concentrations of N-linked Hcy, whereas fibrinogen, transferrin, antitrypsin, HDL, and LDL carry nanomolar concentrations of protein N-linked Hcy (Table 16.4). Interestingly, hemoglobin and γ-globulin also carry significant concentrations of S-linked Hcy (Table 16.4), which represent about 22% and 48%, respectively, of S-linked Hcy carried on albumin. The inability to detect protein-N-linked Hcy in transthyretin reported in Reference 140 is most likely due to inadequate sensitivity of the methods used.

N-Hcy-proteins are novel examples of modified proteins that expand the known repertoire of protein modifications by other metabolites, such as glucose, products of lipid peroxidation, or certain drugs, such as penicillin or aspirin [57]. These protein modification reactions share two common aspects: (1) each involves protein lysine residues as sites of modifications, and (2) they are linked to human pathological conditions, such as diabetes, vascular disease, Alzheimer's disease, or drug allergy or intolerance [57]. As discussed elsewhere in this chapter, each type of protein modification is disease specific, for example, modifications of fibrinogen by

TABLE 16.4 Concentrations of Hcy Carried on Proteins in Normal Human Blood

Protein	Protein N-Linked Hcy μM	Protein S-Linked Hcy μM
Hemoglobin[a]	27.8	3.3
Albumin[b]	2.8	7.3
γ-Globulin[b]	0.7	3.5
Fibrinogen[b]	0.014	<0.019
Transferrin[b]	0.028	<0.005
Antitrypsin[b]	0.024	0.007
HDL[b]	0.023	0.047
LDL[b]	0.017	0.009

[a]Concentrations in erythrocytes.
[b]Plasma concentrations.
Source: Data recalculated from data in Reference 59.

Hcy-thiolactone, glucose, or products of lipid peroxidation affect fibrin clot structure specifically in hyperhomocysteinemia, diabetes, or hypercholesterolemia, respectively.

The immediate result of protein N-homocysteinylation is substitution of the ε-amino group of a protein lysine residue with an Hcy residue containing a free thiol group. This leads to a decrease of the net positive charge on a protein, due to the fact that the highly basic ε-amino group of a protein lysine residue ($pK_a = 10.5$) is replaced by a less basic α-amino group of N-linked Hcy (estimated $pK_a \sim 7$). Such structural alterations affect biological function of Hcy-thiolactone-modified proteins.

The first detailed studies of structural alterations in a protein caused by N-homocysteinylation have been carried out with human serum albumin [72], a known target for N-homocysteinylation in the human body [59]. These studies have led to a discovery of a novel molecular form of albumin and provided a paradigm illustrating how the function of a protein thiol can be affected by N-homocysteinylation. Of the two major physiological forms of human albumin (Fig. 16.9), albumin-Cys^{34}-S-S-Cys (containing cysteine in a disulfide linkage with Cys^{34} of albumin) is N-homocysteinylated faster than albumin-Cys^{34}-SH (mercaptoalbumin, containing Cys^{34} with a free thiol). The reactivity of Lys^{525}, a predominant site of N-homocysteinylation, is about twofold greater in albumin-Cys^{34}-S-S-Cys than in mercaptoalbumin. The different susceptibilities of albumin-Cys^{34}-S-S-Cys and albumin-Cys^{34}-SH to the modification by Hcy-thiolactone are consistent with a structural transition in albumin dependent on the status of the Cys^{34} residue [141]. N-homocysteinylations of albumin-Cys^{34}-S-S-Cys and albumin-Cys^{34}-SH yield two different primary products, N-(Hcy-SH)-albumin-Cys^{34}-SH and N-(Hcy-SH)-albumin-Cys^{34}-S-S-Cys, respectively (Fig. 16.9). However, subsequent thiol-disulfide exchange reactions result in the formation of a single product, N-(Hcy-S-S-Cys)-albumin-Cys^{34}-SH (Fig. 16.9), which is more sensitive to proteolysis than the N-homocysteinylated mercaptoalbumin, N-(Hcy-SH)-albumin-Cys^{34}-SH. Among many possible sites in albumin, Lys^{525} is a predominant site of N-homocysteinylation in vitro and in vivo. Taken together, these results provide evidence for a novel form of albumin,

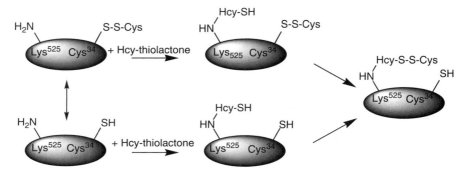

Figure 16.9   N-Homocysteinylation of Lys^{525}. N-Homocysteinylation of Lys^{525} prevents the structural transition in albumin dependent on the status of the conserved Cys^{34} residue. Albumin molecule is rendered as an oval. Reprinted with permission from Reference 48.

N-(Hcy-S-S-Cys)-albumin-Cys^{34}-SH, and suggest that a disulfide at Cys^{34}, a conserved residue in albumins from various organisms, promotes the conversion of N-(Hcy-SH)-albumin-Cys^{34}-SH to a more proteolytically sensitive form N-(Hcy-S-S-Cys)-albumin-Cys^{34}-SH. These data also suggest that, by rendering Cys^{34} reduced, N-homocysteinylation prevents the structural transition in albumin dependent on the status of the conserved Cys^{34} residue (Fig. 16.9).

Studies of the modification of cytochrome c by Hcy-thiolactone provide a paradigm illustrating how the function of a heme-containing protein can be affected by N-homocysteinylation [129]. Four lysine residues of cytochrome c, Lys^8 or Lys^{13}, Lys^{86} or Lys^{87}, Lys^{99} and Lys^{100}, are preferential sites for the modification by Hcy-thiolactone in vitro. N-homocysteinylation of ferricytochrome c results in its conversion to a ferrous form, which is manifested as a change in the color of the solution from red to green (Fig. 16.10). Experimental data are consistent with the following mechanism (Fig. 16.10). Reaction of Hcy-thiolactone with any of the four susceptible lysine residues of ferricytochrome c affords N-(Hcy-SH)-Cyt c(Fe^{3+}). The heme iron in the product undergoes reduction by the thiolate of N-linked Hcy, to afford modified ferrocytochrome c, N-(Hcy-S$^{\cdot}$)-Cyt c(Fe^{2+}). The reduction occurs in *trans* between different molecules of N-(Hcy-SH)-Cyt c(Fe^{3+}), and can also occur with other N-Hcy proteins. For example, a similar reduction of heme-Fe^{3+} was also observed during incubation of ferricytochrome c with N-(Hcy-SH)-albumin. An intramolecular reduction is unlikely, because the sites of N-homocysteinylation are located too far from the heme iron. Dimerization of the tiyl radicals in different molecules of the Hcy-modified ferrocytochrome c, N-(Hcy-S$^{\cdot}$)-Cyt c(Fe^{+2}), leads to the formation of

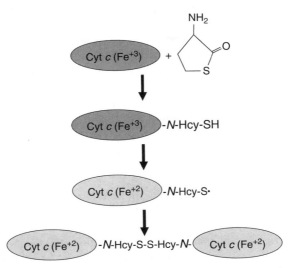

Figure 16.10 Cytochrome c N-Homocysteinylation. N-Homocysteinylation of cytochrome c renders it reduced and leads to oligomerization. Oxidized and reduced forms of cytochrome c are shown as dark- and light-grey ovals, respectively. Reprinted with permission from Reference 129.

multimeric forms of N-homocysteinylated cytochrome c (Fig. 16.10) that are observed on nonreducing SDS-PAGE gels [57]. Furthermore, N-Hcy-cytochrome c becomes more resistant than the native cytochrome c to proteolytic degradation. Thus, N-homocysteinylation of susceptible lysine residues in cytochrome c has important structural and functional consequences, manifested by increased resistance to proteolysis and change in iron redox state. A thiol of the N-linked Hcy introduced by N-homocysteinylation changes the redox state of the heme ligand of cytochrome c by rendering it reduced (Fig. 16.10) [129].

As will be discussed in greater detail elsewhere in this chapter, the modification by Hcy-thiolactone also interferes with the function of a major blood clotting protein, fibrinogen.

16.7 THE HCY-THIOLACTONE HYPOTHESIS OF VASCULAR DISEASE

The findings that Hcy is metabolized to the thioester Hcy-thiolactone, which has the ability to chemically modify proteins in human cells, provided the basis for the Hcy-thiolactone hypothesis, originally formulated in 1997 [60]. The hypothesis states that the metabolic conversion of Hcy to Hcy-thiolactone followed by the nonenzymatic protein modification by Hcy-thiolactone, which impairs or alters biological function, is an underlying mechanism that contributes to the deleterious effects of hyperhomocysteinemia, such as observed in vascular disease (Fig. 16.11) [48, 53, 57, 60, 82]. The thioester chemistry of Hcy-thiolactone (Table 16.1) underlies its ability to form stable isopeptide bonds with protein lysine residues (Scheme 16.4). Hcy-thiolactone-mediated incorporation of Hcy into protein impacts cellular physiology through many routes. Major pathophysiologic consequences of Hcy-thiolactone-dependent protein N-homocysteinylation identified thus far include activation of an adaptive immune response, manifested by an enhanced synthesis of autoantibodies against N-Hcy-proteins [53, 74, 114, 115], and enhanced thrombosis, caused by N-homocysteinylation of fibrinogen [116, 117] (Fig. 16.11). Evidence supporting the Hcy-thiolactone hypothesis is discussed in greater detail in the following sections.

16.7.1 Hcy-Thiolactone Levels Are Elevated in Genetic or Dietary Hyperhomocysteinemia

In order to verify predictions of the Hcy-thiolactone hypothesis in humans and animals, we have developed highly sensitive and reproducible Hcy-thiolactone assays. Our cation-exchange HPLC method exploits unique physicochemical properties of Hcy-thiolactone to achieve its separation, identification, and quantification by fluorescence after post-column derivatization with o-phthalaldehyde [44, 65, 66, 71]. This method is highly selective and sensitive, and has a detection limit of 0.36 nM. As little as 25 fmol Hcy-thiolactone in a sample can be detected and quantified [65, 71]. Examples of HPLC analyses of human plasma and urinary Hcy-thiolactone are shown in Figs. 16.12 and 16.13, respectively.

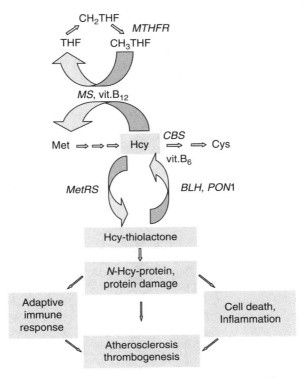

Figure 16.11 The hypothesis of Hcy-thiolactone-mediated vascular disease. Abbreviations: Met, methionine; Cys, cysteine; MS, methionine synthase; THF, tetrahydrofolate; MTHFR, 5,10-methylene-THF reductase; CBS, cystathionine β-synthase; Hcy, homocysteine; MetRS, methionyl-tRNA synthetase; BLH, bleomycin hydrolase; PON1, paraoxonase 1. Adapted with permission from Reference 66.

The Hcy-thiolactone hypothesis predicts that Hcy-thiolactone will be elevated under conditions predisposing to vascular disease, such as hyperhomocysteinemia. This prediction has been confirmed in vivo in humans and mice. Indeed, we found that the CBS deficiency in humans results in elevation of Hcy-thiolactone levels; mean plasma Hcy-thiolactone concentration in CBS-deficient patients (14.4 nM) was 72-fold higher than in normal subjects (Table 16.5) [66]. This finding is consistent with previous ex vivo observations that cultured human CBS-deficient fibroblasts synthesize much more Hcy-thiolactone than normal fibroblasts [60].

We also found that 5-methyltetrahydrofolate deficiency, secondary to a mutation in the *MTHFR* gene, leads to elevation of Hcy-thiolactone levels in humans: plasma Hcy-thiolactone in MTHFR-deficient patients (11.8 nM) was 24- or 59-fold higher than in *MTHFR* heterozygous or normal individuals, respectively (Table 16.5) [66]. This in vivo finding is consistent with our previous ex vivo observations showing that limited availability of folic acid greatly enhances Hcy-thiolactone synthesis in human fibroblasts [60] and vascular endothelial cells [82]. It should be noted that, because

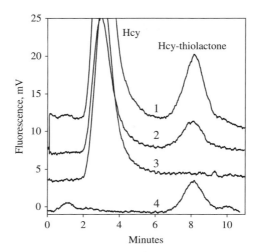

Figure 16.12 Determination of plasma Hcy-thiolactone by cation exchange HPLC. Hcy-thiolactone standard (100 fmol) elutes at 8 min (trace 4). Analyses of samples prepared from human plasma containing 6.7 nM and 2.8 nM Hcy-thiolactone are illustrated by trace 1 and trace 2, respectively. Hcy-thiolactone is absent in plasma samples treated with NaOH before HPLC analysis (trace 3). A peak eluting in a void volume is due to Hcy present in plasma samples. Detection is by fluorescence emission at 480 nm (excitation at 370 nm) after post-column derivatization with o-phthalaldidehyde. Reprinted with permission from Reference 71.

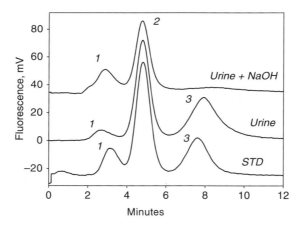

Figure 16.13 Cation exchange HPLC determination of Hcy-thiolactone in human urine. Samples prepared from human urine (determined to contain 538 nM Hcy-thiolactone) before (middle trace) and after 5 min treatment with 0.1 M NaOH (top trace). Lower trace (labeled STD) was obtained with a standard sample containing 0.5 pmol Hcy (peak 1), 200 pmol histidine (peak 2), 1 pmol Hcy-thiolactone (peak 3). Detection is by fluorescence emission at 480 nm (excitation at 370 nm) after post-column derivatization with o-phthalaldidehyde. Reprinted with permission from Reference 65.

TABLE 16.5 Plasma Hcy-Thiolactone and tHcy Concentrations in Control Humans and Subjects with Genetic Deficiencies in Hcy Metabolism

Genotype	No. of Subjects	Hcy-Thiolactone (nM)			tHcy (μM)		
		Mean ± SD	Median	Range	Mean ± SD	Median	Range
MTHFR −/−	4[a]	11.8 ± 8.8	6.8	2.9–22.2	50.1 ± 15.1	44.9	23–68
MTHFR +/−	4	0.5 ± 0.29	0.5	0.1–1.0	7.8 ± 2.8	7.0	5.2–12.2
MTHFR +/+	9	0.2 ± 0.14	0.15	0.1–0.4	7.2 ± 0.9	7.2	6.0–8.6
CBS −/−	14[a]	14.4 ± 30.4	2.8	0.1–100.8	36.1 ± 25.8	25.5	15–93

[a]*MTHFR* −/− and *CBS* −/− patients were on Hcy-lowering therapy.

Source: Reprinted with permission from Reference 66.

TABLE 16.6 Mean ± SD Urinary and Plasma Hcy-Thiolactone and tHcy Concentrations in Mice Fed a Control or Hyperhomocysteinemic Diet[*]

Diet (6 weeks)	Urinary HTL nM	Urinary tHcy μM	Plasma HTL nM	Plasma tHcy μM	Urinary HTL/ Plasma HTL	Urinary tHcy/ Plasma tHcy
Control	136 ± 22	45 ± 14	3.7 ± 2.1	3.0 ± 1.5	37	15
High Met	3490 ± 3780	1360 ± 840	13.8 ± 4.8	51.8 ± 22.7	252	26
High Hcy	496 ± 151	338 ± 146	3.2 ± 0.5	21.4 ± 10.2	155	16

[*]Each diet group contained eight mice.

Source: Reprinted with permission from Reference 66.

MTHFR-deficient patients, like CBS-deficient patients, were on Hcy-lowering therapy, their Hcy-thiolactone concentrations represent minimal values. In one patient for whom samples were obtained before therapy, the therapy resulted in lowering plasma Hcy-thiolactone from 47.3 nM to 16.6 nM (tHcy was lowered from 208 μM before therapy to 66.2 μM after therapy) [66].

A high-Met or high-Hcy diet leads to elevation in body Hcy levels both in humans and animals and is often used as a model of experimental hyperhomocysteinemia [28, 32]. We found that a high Met diet fed to mice for 6 weeks increases plasma and urinary Hcy-thiolactone 3.7-fold and 25-fold, respectively, compared to mice fed a normal chow diet. Normal plasma and urinary Hcy-thiolactone levels in mice are 3.7 nM and 140 nM, respectively (Table 16.6) [66]. Plasma and urinary tHcy levels are elevated 17-fold and 30-fold, respectively, by a high Met diet. A high Hcy diet was somewhat less effective than a high Met diet in increasing plasma or urinary Hcy-thiolactone and tHcy levels in mice (Table 16.6).

Taken together, these findings show that genetic or dietary hyperhomocysteinemia increases not only tHcy but also Hcy-thiolactone levels in human and mice, as predicted by the Hcy-thiolactone hypothesis (Fig. 16.11).

16.7.2 Protein N-Linked Hcy Is Elevated in Hyperhomocysteinemia and Is Associated with CAD in Humans

The Hcy-thiolactone hypothesis [66] predicts that protein N-homocysteinylation will be elevated under conditions conducive to atherosclerosis, such as hyperhomocysteinemia. The verification of this prediction became possible with the development of sensitive chemical [59] and immunological assays [112] for measurements of protein N-linked Hcy in humans. Indeed, as predicted by the Hcy-thiolactone hypothesis, protein N-linked Hcy is elevated in subjects with genetic hyperhomocysteinemia (Table 16.7) [59, 70, 72, 78].

Hyperhomocysteinemia and higher cardiovascular risk and mortality are also observed in uremic patients [142]. As predicted, significantly higher protein N-linked Hcy levels are observed in hyperhomocysteinemic uremic patients on hemodialysis than in control subjects (Table 16.7) [138, 139]. Interestingly, the ratio of protein

TABLE 16.7   Mean $\pm$ SD Plasma N-Hcy-Protein and tHcy Concentrations in Control and Hyperhomocysteinemic Subjects

Subjects (n)	N-Hcy-Protein, μM	tHcy, μM
Control (6)[a]	0.18 ± 0.17	7.1 ± 3.1
Hyperhomocysteinemic (6)[a]	4.9 ± 2.4	70.2 ± 42.8
	$P = 0.003$	$P = 0.005$
Control (14)[b]	0.35 ± 0.13	11.4 ± 1.0
Uremic on hemodialysis (28)[b]	0.68 ± 0.10	57.8 ± 9.2
	$P < 0.05$	$P < 0.001$

[a]H. Jakubowski, unpublished data. N-Hcy-protein was assayed according to Reference 59.
[b]Data from Reference 139.

N-linked Hcy to tHcy is lower in hemodialysis patients than in control subjects [138, 139]. Similarly, the ratio of protein N-linked Hcy to tHcy in patients with high plasma tHcy (50 to 120 μM) is lower than in patients with low plasma tHcy (5 to 40 μM) [59]. The lower protein N-linked Hcy/tHcy ratios suggest that the Hcy-thiolactone clearance is more effective at high plasma tHcy levels. This suggestion is supported by a finding that in mice fed a hyperhomocysteinemic high Met or Hcy diet urinary/plasma Hcy-thiolactone is seven- or fourfold higher, respectively, compared to mice fed a normal diet [66].

Hyperhomocysteinemia is linked with increased mortality in CAD patients [18]. In a clinical study that examined a relationship between Hcy and CAD, plasma protein N-linked Hcy, like plasma tHcy, levels were significantly higher in coronary heart disease patients than in controls [112]. Furthermore, there was a weak but significant positive correlation between protein N-linked Hcy level and the number of diseased coronary arteries: the higher the protein N-linked Hcy level the greater the number of afflicted arteries.

Using polyclonal rabbit anti-N-Hcy-protein IgG antibodies [143], we have demonstrated that N-Hcy-protein is present in diseased human cardiac tissues [144]. We observed positive immunohistochemical staining of myocardium and aorta samples from cardiac surgery patients. Control experiments have demonstrated that the staining was specific for N-Hcy-protein. No immunostaining was observed with rabbit preimmune IgG, with iodoacetamide-treated tissues (which destroys the $N\varepsilon$-Hcy-Lys epitope), or with the antibody pre-adsorbed with N-Hcy-albumin [144].

16.8   PATHOPHYSIOLOGIC CONSEQUENCES OF PROTEIN N-HOMOCYSTEINYLATION

The sensitivity of mammalian cells and organisms to Hcy-thiolactone raises a broader question of the mechanistic basis underlying this sensitivity. Hcy-thiolactone-mediated incorporation of Hcy into protein (Scheme 16.4) can impact cellular physiology through many routes. Protein modification by Hcy-thiolactone can disrupt protein folding, and create altered proteins with newly acquired interactions, or can lead to induction of autoimmune responses. In the following sections, recently recognized pathophysiological effects of protein N-homocysteinylation are discussed.

During the folding process, proteins form their globular native states in a manner determined by their primary amino acid sequence [145, 146]. Thus, small changes in amino acid sequence caused by Hcy incorporation have the potential to create misfolded protein aggregates. Indeed, as I have shown, N-Hcy-proteins have a propensity to form protein aggregates [57, 78]. The appearance of misfolded/aggregated proteins in the endoplasmic reticulum (ER) activates a signaling pathway, the unfolded protein response (UPR), that, when overwhelmed, leads to cell death via apoptosis. Protein aggregates are known to be inherently toxic [147]. The findings that N-Hcy-LDL, like other N-Hcy-proteins [57, 78, 97], has the propensity to aggregate [148] and induces cell death in cultured human endothelial cells [113], is consistent with this concept (Fig. 16.11). Other investigators have shown that ER stress and UPR can be induced in cultured endothelial cells and in mice by elevating Hcy [38, 39, 149, 150], which, as we have shown, also elevates Hcy-thiolactone [44, 66, 82]. Furthermore, treatments with Hcy-thiolactone induce ER stress and UPR in retinal epithelial cells [40], as well as apoptotic death in cultured human vascular endothelial cells [41, 108]. In this scenario, protein modification by Hcy-thiolactone causing the formation of N-Hcy-proteins leads to the UPR and induction of the apoptotic pathway. Consistent with this scenario, we have recently found that cellular levels of N-Hcy-proteins are elevated under conditions of Hcy- or Hcy-thiolactone-induced ER stress (J. Perła-Kajan, H. Jakubowski, unpublished data). Proteolytic degradation of N-Hcy-proteins can generate potentially antigenic peptides, which can be displayed on the cell surface and induce an adaptive immune response [48, 53].

16.8.1 N-Homocysteinylation of Fibrinogen Contributes to Thrombosis in Humans

Fibrinogen is a dimer of three polypeptides, Aα, Bβ, Cγ, linked by 29 disulfide bonds. During coagulation fibrinogen is converted to an insoluble fibrin by thrombin-catalyzed removal of fibrinopeptides from the Aα and Bβ chains. Although fibrinogen does not have a free thiol, and thus cannot bind Hcy by a disulfide linkage, the protein is known to undergo facile N-homocysteinylation by Hcy-thiolactone in vitro [57, 78], and, like other circulating proteins, carry N-linked Hcy in vivo in human blood (Table 16.4) [59]. Because lysine residues are important for the binding of fibrinolytic enzymes to fibrin, their modification by Hcy-thiolactone is likely to impair fibrinolysis.

Recent data suggest that N-homocysteinylation of fibrinogen by Hcy-thiolactone can lead to increased thrombogenesis. For example, clots formed from Hcy-thiolactone-treated normal human plasma or fibrinogen lyse slower than clots from untreated controls [117]. Some of the 12 lysine residues susceptible to N-homocysteinylation, located in the D and αC domains of fibrinogen, are close to tPA and plasminogen binding or plasmin cleavage sites, which can explain abnormal characteristics of clots formed from N-Hcy-fibrinogen [117]. The in vitro prothrombotic effects of N-Hcy-fibrinogen are similar to the prothrombotic effects of fibrinogen mutations in humans, which introduce a cysteine thiol group, for example, Aα Arg$^{16} \rightarrow$ Cys,

$Arg^{554} \rightarrow Cys$, $Ser^{532} \rightarrow Cys$; $B\beta \ Arg^{14} \rightarrow Cys$, $Arg^{44} \rightarrow Cys$, $Arg^{255} \rightarrow Cys$; $C\gamma$ $Arg^{275} \rightarrow Cys$, $Tyr^{354} \rightarrow Cys$ [151–154] (human fibrinogen database is available at http://www.geht.org).

The presence of N-Hcy-fibrinogen in the circulation [59] is consistent with a hypothesis that the modified fibrinogen can impair fibrinolysis in vivo. The in vivo relevance of fibrinogen N-homocysteinylation in humans is further supported by our findings that elevated plasma tHcy decreases permeability, and increases resistance to lysis, of fibrin clots from plasma of CAD patients and healthy subjects [116]. Moreover, fibrin clot structure is more compact and less permeable in CAD patients than in controls. These detrimental effects of elevated plasma tHcy on fibrin clot structure are consistent with a mechanism involving fibrinogen modification by Hcy-thiolactone (Fig. 16.14) [116].

Furthermore, in patients with diabetes and hypercholesterolemia, clot structure is more thrombogenic than in CAD patients or healthy subjects. However, the influence of Hcy on clot structure in patients with diabetes or hypercholesterolemia is obscured by the dominant effects of glucose or cholesterol, respectively [116]. These findings suggest that fibrinogen modifications by glucose or products of lipid oxidation, like the modification by Hcy-thiolactone, are detrimental or that these modifications predominate over the modification by Hcy-thiolactone in patients with diabetes or hypercholesterolemia (Fig. 16.14).

We also found that lowering plasma tHcy by folic acid supplementation improves clot structure (increases permeability and susceptibility to lysis) in asymptomatic human subjects. This finding suggests that Hcy-lowering therapy by vitamin supplementation can have beneficial antithrombotic effects [116]. Taken together, these results support a hypothesis that fibrinogen N-homocysteinylation by Hcy-thiolactone leads to abnormal resistance of fibrin clots to lysis in vivo and thus contributes to increased risk of thrombogenesis [116, 117] (Fig. 16.11). In addition, other fibrinogen modifications, such as those occurring in hypercholesterolemia or hyperglycemia, can also increase the risk of thrombogenesis (Fig. 16.14) [116].

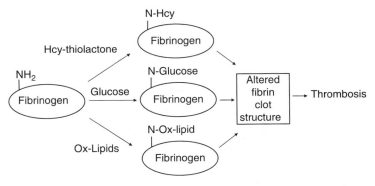

Figure 16.14 Fibrinogen modifications affect fibrin clot structure and lead to enhanced thrombosis [116].

16.8.2   An Adaptive Autoimmune Response to *N*-Hcy-Proteins Is Associated with Atherosclerosis in Humans

Atherosclerosis is now widely recognized as a chronic inflammatory disease that involves innate and adaptive immunity [155–157]. That inflammation is important is supported by studies showing that increased plasma concentration of markers of inflammation, such as C-reactive protein (CRP), interleukin-1, serum amyloid A, and soluble adhesion molecules are independent predictors of vascular events [158]. Autoantibodies against modified LDL were found to be elevated in vascular disease patients in some, but not all studies [159]. Lipid peroxidation is thought to play a central role in the initiation of both cellular and humoral responses. Reactive aldehydes resulting from phospholipid peroxidation, such as malondialdehyde, 4-hydroxynonenal, and 1-palmitoyl-2-(5-oxovaleroyl)-*sn*-glycero-3-phosphocholine can modify lysine residues in LDL and in other proteins. The resulting oxidized lipids-protein adducts, for example, malondialdehyde-LDL, carry neo-self epitopes, which are recognized by specific innate and adaptive immune responses. As discussed in the following paragraphs, protein N-homocysteinylation by Hcy-thiolactone also leads to corresponding autoimmune responses.

The details of the mechanism underlying the role of Hcy in adaptive immune response are beginning to emerge. The modification by Hcy-thiolactone [160], like other chemical modifications, such as glycation, acetylation, methylation, ethylation, and carbamylation [157], renders LDL highly immunogenic. Furthermore, immunization of rabbits with Hcy-thiolactone-modified keyhole limpet hemocyanin (KHL) leads to generation of antibodies binding to *N*-Hcy-LDL (Fig. 16.15) [114, 143]. Of considerable interest are the observations that antisera from such immunizations bound not only to the *N*-Hcy-LDL but to a variety of other proteins on which the N-linked Hcy epitope was present, such as *N*-Hcy-albumin, *N*-Hcy-hemoglobin, *N*-Hcy-transferrin, and *N*-Hcy-antitrypsin. These data suggest that autoantibodies, once formed in vivo in response to *N*-Hcy-LDL or any other *N*-Hcy-protein, would be capable of binding to other endogenous *N*-Hcy-proteins.

Hcy incorporation into proteins triggers an adaptive immune response, manifested by the induction of autoantibodies against *N*ε-Hcy-Lys epitopes on *N*-Hcy-proteins in humans, such as *N*-Hcy-hemoglobin, *N*-Hcy-albumin, *N*-Hcy-transferrin, and *N*-Hcy-antitrypsin [114]. The antigen specificity of human autoantibodies (Fig. 16.15) is essentially identical to the specificity of rabbit anti-*N*-Hcy-protein antibodies generated by inoculations with *N*-Hcy-LDL or *N*-Hcy-KLH [114]. In humans, the plasma levels of anti-*N*-Hcy-protein autoantibodies [74, 114, 115, 143] and protein *N*-linked Hcy [59, 70, 72, 78] vary considerably among individuals and are strongly correlated with plasma Hcy (Fig. 16.16), but not with Cys or Met [114]. Such a relationship is consistent with the Hcy-thiolactone hypothesis (Fig. 16.11): elevation in Hcy leads to inadvertent elevation in Hcy-thiolactone, observed ex vivo in human fibroblasts [60] and endothelial cells [44, 82], and in vivo in humans and mice [44, 65, 66, 71]. Hcy-Thiolactone mediates Hcy incorporation into proteins and the formation of neo-self antigens *N*ε-Hcy-Lys on proteins (Scheme 16.4). Raising levels of the neo-self *N*ε-Hcy-Lys epitopes trigger an autoimmune response (Fig. 16.11). Furthermore, plasma levels of anti-*N*-Hcy-protein autoantibodies, like

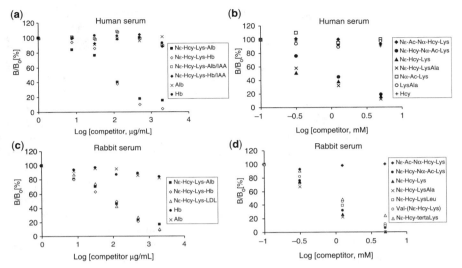

Figure 16.15 Human autoantibody binding to N-Hcy-hemoglobin. Specificity of binding to N-Hcy-hemoglobin of human autoantibody (a, b) and rabbit antibody (c, d). Microtiter wells were coated with 10 µg/mL human N-Hcy-hemoglobin and incubated with a 40-fold dilution of a human serum (a, b) or 200-fold dilution of rabbit antiserum (c, d) with or without indicated competitor. Rabbit antiserum was obtained from animals inoculated with N-Hcy-Keyhole limpet hemocyanine (KLH). Results are expressed as B/B_o, where B is the amount of IgG bound in the presence of competitor and B_o that without competitor. Reprinted with permission from Reference 114.

the levels of plasma tHcy, are higher in groups of male stroke or CAD patients than in control groups. These observations suggest that an autoimmune response against N-Hcy-proteins is a general feature of atherosclerosis in man [48, 53].

To examine the clinical usefulness of anti-N-Hcy-protein IgG autoantibodies, we analyzed their predictive value in CAD, and compared it to the predictive value of tHcy and other risk factors [74]. We found that an age-adjusted risk for early CAD in men <50 years old, related to seropositivity for anti-N-Hcy-protein IgG

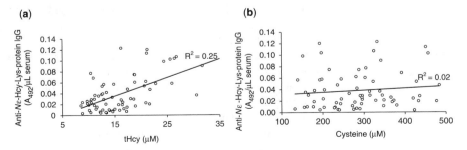

Figure 16.16 Relationships between serum anti-N-Hcy-protein IgG and tHcy (a) or cysteine (b) in healthy human subjects. Reprinted with permission from Reference 114.

autoantibodies, is 9.87 (95% CI 4.50–21.59, $p < 10^{-5}$). In multivariate logistic regression analysis, only seropositivity to anti-N-Hcy-protein IgG autoantibodies (OR 14.92; 95% CI 4.47–49.19; $p = 0.00002$), smoking (OR 8.84; 95% CI 2.46–31.72; $p = 0.001$), hypertension (OR 43.45; 95% CI 7.91–238.7), and HDL cholesterol (OR 0.015; 95% CI 0.002–0.098; $p = 0.00002$) were independent predictors of early CAD. Interestingly, anti-N-Hcy-protein IgG autoantibodies are more sensitive than tHcy as a predictor of early CAD in men. A risk for premature CAD is almost 15-fold higher in subjects seropositive for anti-N-Hcy-protein IgG autoantibodies, when adjusted for coronary risk factors, Hcy and CRP. These analyses show that elevated levels of anti-N-Hcy-protein autoantibodies significantly contribute to the risk of CAD in male patients [74].

The findings that the levels of N-Hcy-protein are elevated in uremic patients on hemodialysis [138, 139] suggest that an autoimmune response against N-Hcy-protein might also be enhanced in these patients. This possibility was examined in a group of 43 patients (58.8 years old) who were on maintenance hemodialysis for an average of 50 months and an age- and sex-matched group of 31 apparently healthy individuals [161]. Significantly higher levels of anti-N-Hcy-protein IgG autoantibodies were found in the hemodialysis patients, compared with controls. Like in our previous studies with stroke patients [114], the levels of anti-N-Hcy-protein IgG autoantibodies were strongly correlated with plasma tHcy, both in hemodialysis patients and in controls. Furthermore, a subgroup of hemodialysis patients who survived MI ($n = 14$) had significantly higher levels of anti-N-Hcy-protein IgG autoantibodies than a subgroup of hemodialysis patients without a history of CAD ($n = 29$) [161]. Taken together, these data suggest that an autoimmune response against N-Hcy-proteins contributes to the development of CAD in hemodialysis patients.

In general, antibodies protect against exogenous pathogens and endogenous altered neo-self molecules to maintain homeostasis by neutralization and clearance. Like other autoantibodies [157], the anti-N-Hcy-protein autoantibodies can be beneficial or deleterious. For example, the clearing of N-Hcy-proteins from circulation by the autoantibodies would be beneficial. On the other hand, binding of the autoantibodies to N-Hcy-proteins [53, 114, 143] in tissues may contribute to the deleterious effects of hyperhomocysteinemia on many organs [10–12]. For instance, if the neo-self $N\varepsilon$-Hcy-Lys epitopes were present on endothelial cell membrane proteins, anti-N-Hcy-protein autoantibodies would form antigen-antibody complexes on the surface of the vascular wall. Endothelial cells coated with anti-N-Hcy-protein autoantibodies would be taken up by the macrophage via the Fc receptor, resulting in injury to the vascular surface. Under chronic exposures to excess Hcy the neo-self epitopes $N\varepsilon$-Hcy-Lys, which initiate the injury, are formed continuously, and the repeating attempts to repair the damaged vascular wall would lead to an atherosclerotic lesion (Fig. 16.11) [48, 53].

The involvement of an autoimmune response in CAD is consistent with our findings that lowering plasma tHcy by folic acid supplementation for 3 and 6 months lowers anti-N-Hcy-protein autoantibodies levels in control subjects but not in patients with CAD [115]. These findings show that the production of anti-N-Hcy-protein IgG autoantibodies is modifiable by lowering plasma tHcy as quickly as 3 months, but only in healthy subjects. These findings also suggest that while primary Hcy-lowering intervention by vitamin supplementation is beneficial, secondary intervention may be ineffective, and may explain at least in part the failure of vitamin therapy [35, 36] to lower cardiovascular events in MI patients.

16.8.3 Hyperhomocysteinemia, N-Hcy-Protein, and Innate Immune Responses

We also found that the levels of anti-N-Hcy-protein autoantibodies are weakly, but significantly, correlated with plasma CRP levels ($r = 0.24$, $p = 0.002$) [74]. Other evidence also suggests that Hcy contributes to innate immune responses. Indeed, many human studies, although not all [162–165], have reported associations between Hcy and markers of inflammation. For example, significant associations between plasma tHcy and CRP were observed in the Framingham Heart Study [166] and in the Physician's Health Study [167]. In another study, hyperhomocysteinemia is associated with increased levels of both CRP and interleukin-6 in humans [168]. A similar positive association between Hcy and interleukin-6 was reported in patients with diabetic nephropathy [169]. Importantly, in the Holven et al. study [168], elevated levels of interleukin-6 were observed in hyperhomocysteinemic individuals in the absence of hypercholesterolemia. Plasma Hcy was positively associated with soluble tumor necrosis factor (TNF) receptor in the Nurses' Health Study [170]. A positive correlation is observed between plasma tHcy and neopterin (a marker of Th1 type immune response) in Parkinson's disease patients [171].

Furthermore, dietary hyperhomocysteinemia is known to trigger an innate immune response and enhance vascular inflammation in mice, manifested by increased activation of nuclear factor (NF)-κB in the aorta and kidney, enhanced expression of vascular cell adhesion molecule (VCAM)-1 and receptor for advanced glycation end products (RAGE) in the aorta and TNF-α in plasma [29]. Elevated Hcy is associated with elevated monocyte chemotactic protein-1 and increased expression of vascular adhesion molecules in humans [172, 173] and rats [174–176].

How Hcy triggers an innate immune response and whether N-Hcy-proteins are involved is unknown. However, given that hyperhomocysteinemia causes elevation of Hcy-thiolactone and N-Hcy-protein levels in humans and mice [66], these responses are likely to be caused by N-Hcy-protein, particularly by N-Hcy-LDL. Consistent with this suggestion are the observations that N-Hcy-LDL is highly immunogenic [160], is present in human blood [59], and is taken up by macrophages faster than unmodified LDL [148]. Further studies are needed to elucidate the mechanism of Hcy-induced innate immune responses.

16.9 URINARY ELIMINATION OF HCY-THIOLACTONE

As noted above, Hcy-thiolactone is a toxic Hcy metabolite that inadvertently modifies protein lysine residues, and in the process, impairs or alters the biological function of the protein. Thus, it may not be surprising that the ability to detoxify Hcy-thiolactone has evolved in mammals. Indeed, we found that Hcy-thiolactone is detoxified by urinary excretion [65]. Normal human urinary concentrations of Hcy-thiolactone vary from 11 nM to 485 nM and are $\sim$100-fold higher than those found in plasma [71]. Urinary Hcy-thiolactone accounts for 2.5% to 28% of urinary tHcy. Calculations based on a normal human glomerular filtration rate of 180 L/day and a free plasma Hcy concentration of 3 μM indicate that 99% of filtered tHcy is reabsorbed [177]. A similar calculation for Hcy-thiolactone (0.12 to 2.4 nM in plasma and 286 to 415 nmol/day eliminated with urine) indicates that only 0.4% to 3.8% is reabsorbed and >95% of filtered Hcy-thiolactone was excreted in humans [65]. Efficient urinary elimination of Hcy-thiolactone is typical for the waste or toxic products of normal human metabolism.

Whereas relative renal clearance of tHcy is only about 0.001 to 0.003, the clearance of Hcy-thiolactone is 0.2 to 7.0 of creatinine clearance [65]. This suggests that in some individuals Hcy-thiolactone is not only filtered in the glomeruli, but also secreted into the tubular lumen. On the other hand, high local intrarenal synthesis of Hcy-thiolactone cannot be excluded. However, this is unlikely given a significant positive correlation between urinary and plasma Hcy-thiolactone concentrations. Interestingly, urinary Hcy-thiolactone correlates negatively with urinary pH, whereas there is no correlation between urinary tHcy and urinary pH (Fig. 16.17). This suggests that the ionization status of the α-amino group of Hcy-thiolactone (pK = 6.67) [123] affects its urinary excretion. An uncharged form of Hcy-thiolactone is excreted in the urine, where it gains a positive charge due to acidification. The positively charged form of Hcy-thiolactone is not reabsorbed in the tubules. Urinary acidification apparently maintains low fractional concentration of the uncharged Hcy-thiolactone inside the tubular lumen, thus enabling continuous diffusion of the uncharged form of Hcy-thiolactone from the tubular cells into the lumen.

Although it contributes relatively little to the daily flux of tHcy in a healthy individual [178], renal excretion removes a large fraction of Hcy-thiolactone [65], which would otherwise cause protein N-homocysteinylation. Thus, urinary excretion is an important route of Hcy-thiolactone elimination from the human body and intact renal function is important for Hcy-thiolactone detoxification.

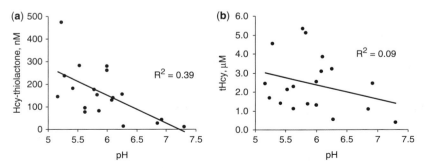

Figure 16.17 Urinary concentrations of Hcy-thiolactone (a), but not total Hcy (tHcy) (b) are negatively correlated with urinary pH. Reprinted with permission from Reference 65.

In addition to humans, mice have also been shown to eliminate Hcy-thiolactone by urinary excretion. Urinary Hcy-thiolactone in mice fed a normal chow diet is 140 nM [66], similar to urinary Hcy-thiolactone in humans [65]. In mice fed a hyper-homocysteinemic high methionine or high Hcy diet, urinary Hcy-thiolactone increases 25-fold or 3.6-fold, compared to mice fed a normal diet (Table 16.6). The distributions of Hcy-thiolactone between plasma and urine in mice fed a normal diet and humans are similar: much higher Hcy-thiolactone concentrations accumulate in urine than in plasma (urinary : plasma Hcy-thiolactone is 37 in mice [66] and 100 in humans [65]). This shows that urinary clearances of Hcy-thiolactone in mice and humans are similar, and that in mice, like in humans [65], >95% of the filtered Hcy-thiolactone is excreted in the urine. Furthermore, significantly higher urinary : plasma Hcy-thiolactone ratios are found in mice fed hyperhomocysteinemic high methionine or high Hcy diet than in the animals fed a normal diet (Table 16.6). This finding suggests that urinary clearance of Hcy-thiolactone is much more efficient in hyperhomocysteinemic mice, compared to animals with normal tHcy levels.

16.10 ENZYMATIC ELIMINATION OF HCY-THIOLACTONE

Studies of Hcy-thiolactone detoxification mechanisms have also led to discoveries of two major enzymes that hydrolyze Hcy-thiolactone in humans (Fig. 16.1): extracellular calcium-dependent Hcy-thiolactonase identical to serum paraoxonase 1 (PON1) [58] and intracellular thiol-dependent Hcy-thiolactonase identical to bleomycin hydrolase (BLH) present ubiquitously in human tissues [62]. Enzymatic hydrolysis of Hcy-thiolactone to Hcy allows its clearance by reutilization in the transmethylation and transsulfuration pathways (Fig. 16.1). Because they participate in the elimination of the atherogenic metabolite Hcy-thiolactone, PON1 and BLH are likely to play protective roles (Fig. 16.11). The in vitro catalytic efficiency of the enzymatic hydrolysis of Hcy-thiolactone by human intracellular BLH is greater than the efficiency of human extracellular PON1. Thus, BLH is expected to hydrolyze most of the Hcy-thiolactone produced in the human body. Hcy thiolactone that escapes intracellular hydrolysis by BLH passes into the circulation. Once in the circulation, Hcy-thiolactone is cleared by the kidney and mopped up by PON1.

PON1, named for its ability to hydrolyze the organophosphate paraoxon, is synthesized exclusively in the liver and carried on high-density lipoproteins (HDL) in the circulation. PON1-deficient mice are more sensitive to organophosphate toxicity and to a high-fat diet-induced atherosclerosis than wild-type littermates [179, 180]. In vitro studies indicate that HDL from PON1-deficient animals is unable to prevent LDL oxidation. PON1-deficient mice may be useful in studies related to factors regulating susceptibility to atherosclerosis.

Our lab has found that PON1 is an Hcy-thiolactonase which protects against protein modification by Hcy-thiolactone in cultured human cells [58] and serum in vitro [96], and that PON1-deficient mice lack serum Hcy-thiolactonase activity [58, 97]. Human *PON1* has genetic polymorphisms, for example, *PON1-M55L*, *PON1-R192Q*, which affect PON1 function [181, 182], including Hcy-thiolactonase activity

[96, 183]. However, the PON1 phenotype (Hcy-thiolactonase or paraoxonase activity) is a better predictor of cardiovascular disease than are the *PON1-M55L* or *PON1-R192Q* genotypes [181, 182, 184, 185]. Furthermore, Hcy is a negative regulator of PON1 expression in the mouse [186], whereas Hcy-thiolactonase activity of PON1 is negatively correlated with plasma Hcy in humans [183]. Its negative effects on PON1 expression or activity may contribute to the proatherogenic role of Hcy. PON1 is the only enzyme that metabolizes Hcy-thiolactone in human or other mammalian sera. However, Hcy-thiolactonase activity is not present in chicken serum [58, 97], which makes chicken embryos particularly sensitive to Hcy-thiolactone toxicity [92, 95].

BLH, named for its ability to hydrolyze the anticancer drug bleomycin, was studied in the context of cancer therapy [187, 188]. BLH-deficient mice are more sensitive to bleomycin toxicity than wild type and prone to tail dermatitis [189]. Human BLH has been implicated in Alzheimer's disease and is considered as a target for a drug that can prevent or slow the progression of the disease. A genetic polymorphism of human *BLH*, Ile443→Val, is associated with an increased risk for Alzheimer's disease [190]. Immunochemical staining suggests that higher BLH levels accumulate in diseased brains from Alzheimer's patients than in controls [191]. Furthermore, BLH has the ability to process amyloid precursor protein and amyloid-β in vitro [192–194].

BLH, in contrast to PON1, is ubiquitous in various mammalian tissues, but its expression level (activity, protein, and mRNA) can vary between tissues, as shown in mice [189, 195], rats [196, 197], rabbits [195, 198, 199], and humans [187], and is also present in other species [200, 201]. Vascular lesions, predominantly located in the endothelium, that are observed in cancer patients following perfusion with bleomycin [202] are most likely due to very low BLH expression, as determined by the absence of any detectable Hcy-thiolactonase activity in endothelial cells [82]. Human and yeast BLH have almost identical molecular structures, similar to the 20S proteasome, and belong to a family of self-compartmentalizing intracellular cysteine proteases [200, 203]. Its evolutionary conservation and wide distribution suggests that BLH has a conserved cellular function.

The function of BLH was elucidated in 2006, when we found that BLH is a major intracellular Hcy-thiolactonase in humans and yeast [62]. In an attempt to answer a question whether Hcy-thiolactone is detoxified intracellularly, we purified intracellular Hcy-thiolactone-hydrolyzing enzymes from human placenta and the yeast *Saccharomyces cerevisiae*. Proteomic analyses have identified these enzymes as human and yeast BLH, respectively. We also found that recombinant human and yeast BLH, expressed in *E. coli*, exhibit Hcy-thiolactonase activities similar to those of native enzymes and that active site mutations, C73A for human BLH and H369A for yeast BLH, inactivate the Hcy-thiolactonase activity. Furthermore, we demonstrated that yeast *blh1* mutants are deficient in Hcy-thiolactonase activity in vitro and in vivo, produce more Hcy-thiolactone and exhibit greater sensitivity to Hcy toxicity than wild-type yeast cells. Taken together, these data show that BLH is in fact a Hcy-thiolactonase that protects cells against Hcy toxicity by hydrolyzing intracellular Hcy-thiolactone [62].

16.11 CONCLUSIONS

In this chapter, I have described fundamental aspects of Hcy-thiolactone biochemistry, summarized the evidence supporting the Hcy-thiolactone hypothesis of vascular disease, in particular emphasizing the importance of Hcy-thiolactone-mediated protein N-homocysteinylation in two aspects of Hcy pathobiology, adaptive immune response and thrombogensies. Of many known naturally occurring Hcy species, only the thioester Hcy-thiolactone can mediate the incorporation of Hcy into proteins via stable isopeptide bonds, which creates altered proteins with newly acquired interactions. With the development of novel analytical methods, studies testing the predictions of the Hcy-thiolactone hypothesis in humans and experimental animals became possible. These studies show that genetic or dietary hyperhomocysteinemia greatly elevates levels of Hcy-thiolactone and protein N-linked Hcy in humans and mice. Other studies provide evidence that N-Hcy-proteins are immunogenic in rabbits and humans. In humans, protein N-homocysteinylation causes the formation of neo-self protein N-linked Hcy epitopes, which induce an adaptive immune response, manifested by the formation of anti-N-Hcy-protein IgG autoantibodies. Levels of these autoantibodies are elevated in stroke and CAD patients and thus could play an important role in atherosclerosis. Other data show that N-homocysteinylation of fibrinogen by Hcy-thiolactone explains thrombogenic effects of elevated plasma tHcy levels in humans. Furthermore, primary Hcy-lowering vitamin therapy is beneficial in that it improves fibrin clot properties and lowers the levels of anti-N-Hcy-protein autoantibodies in healthy subjects. In contrast, secondary vitamin intervention appears to be ineffective: it lowers plasma tHcy, but not anti-N-Hcy-protein autoantibodies in CAD patients. Finally, the roles of Hcy-thiolactone-detoxifying enzymes, PON1 and BLH, as well as urinary Hcy-thiolactone elimination were discussed. Although some progress has been made, we are only at the beginning of our study of the importance of protein N-homocysteinylation. Along with other aspects of protein N-homocysteinylation, further studies of the roles of anti-N-Hcy-protein autoantibodies and Hcy-thiolactone elimination in health and disease are likely to yield an understanding of the fundamental mechanisms that evolved to deal with the consequences of Hcy-thiolactone formation.

REFERENCES

1. Benevenga, N.J. (1974). Toxicities of methionine and other amino acids. *Journal of Agricultural and Food Chemistry, 22*, 2–9.

2. Benevenga, N.J., Steele, R.D. (1984). Adverse effects of excessive consumption of amino acids. *Annual Review of Nutrition, 4*, 157–181.

3. Harper, A.E., Benevenga, N.J., Wohlhueter, R.M. (1970). Effects of ingestion of disproportionate amounts of amino acids. *Physiological Reviews, 50*, 428–558.

4. Matsueda, S., Niiyama, Y. (1982). The effects of excess amino acids on maintenance of pregnancy and fetal growth in rats. *Journal of Nutritional Science and Vitaminology, 28*, 557–573.

5. Osborne-Pellegrin, M.J., Fau, D. (1992). Effects of chronic absorption of dietary supplements of methionine and cystine on arterial morphology in the rat. *Experimental and Molecular Pathology, 56,* 49–59.

6. Fau, D., Peret, J., Hadjiisky, P. (1988). Effects of ingestion of high protein or excess methionine diets by rats for two years. *Journal of Nutrition, 118,* 128–133.

7. Richie, J.P., Jr., Leutzinger, Y., Parthasarathy, S., Malloy, V., Orentreich, N., Zimmerman, J.A. (1994). Methionine restriction increases blood glutathione and longevity in F344 rats. *FASEB Journal, 8,* 1302–1307.

8. Sanz, A., Caro, P., Ayala, V., Portero-Otin, M., Pamplona, R., Barja, G. (2006). Methionine restriction decreases mitochondrial oxygen radical generation and leak as well as oxidative damage to mitochondrial DNA and proteins. *FASEB Journal, 20,* 1064–1073.

9. Komninou, D., Leutzinger, Y., Reddy, B.S., Richie, J.P., Jr. (2006). Methionine restriction inhibits colon carcinogenesis. *Nutrition and Cancer, 54,* 202–208.

10. Mudd, S.H., Levy, H.L., Krauss, J.P. (2001). Disorders of transsulfuration. In Scriver, C.R., Beaudet, A.L., Sly, W.S., Valle, D., Childs, B., Kinzler, K.W., Vogelstein, B., Eds., *The Metabolic and Molecular Bases of Inherited Disease,* pp. 2007–2056. New York: McGraw-Hill.

11. Kluijtmans, L.A., Boers, G.H., Kraus, J.P., van den Heuvel, L.P., Cruysberg, J.R., Trijbels, F.J., Blom, H.J. (1999). The molecular basis of cystathionine beta-synthase deficiency in Dutch patients with homocystinuria: Effect of CBS genotype on biochemical and clinical phenotype and on response to treatment. *American Journal of Human Genetics, 65,* 59–67.

12. Yap, S., Boers, G.H., Wilcken, B., Wilcken, D.E., Brenton, D.P., Lee, P.J., Walter, J.H., Howard, P.M., Naughten, E.R. (2001). Vascular outcome in patients with homocystinuria due to cystathionine beta-synthase deficiency treated chronically: A multicenter observational study. *Arteriosclerosis, Thrombosis and Vascular Biology, 21,* 2080–2085.

13. Rosenblatt, D., Fenton, W. (2001). Disorders of transsulfuration. In Scriver, C., Beaudet, A., Sly, W., Valle, D., Childs, B., Kinzler, K.W., Vogelstein, B., Eds., *The Metabolic and Molecular Bases of Inherited Disease,* pp. 3897–3933. New York: McGraw-Hill.

14. Visy, J.M., Le Coz, P., Chadefaux, B., Fressinaud, C., Woimant, F., Marquet, J., Zittoun, J., Visy, J., Vallat, J.M., Haguenau, M. (1991). Homocystinuria due to 5,10-methylenetetrahydrofolate reductase deficiency revealed by stroke in adult siblings. *Neurology, 41,* 1313–1315.

15. McCully, K.S. (1969). Vascular pathology of homocysteinemia: Implications for the pathogenesis of arteriosclerosis. *American Journal of Pathology, 56,* 111–128.

16. Refsum, H., Nurk, E., Smith, A.D., Ueland, P.M., Gjesdal, C.G., Bjelland, I., Tverdal, A., Tell, G.S., Nygard, O., Vollset, S.E. (2006). The Hordaland Homocysteine Study: A community-based study of homocysteine, its determinants, and associations with disease. *Journal of Nutrition, 136,* 1731S–1740S.

17. Wald, D.S., Law, M., Morris, J.K. (2002). Homocysteine and cardiovascular disease: Evidence on causality from a meta-analysis. *British Medical Journal, 325,* 1202.

18. Anderson, J.L., Muhlestein, J.B., Horne, B.D., Carlquist, J.F., Bair, T.L., Madsen, T.E., Pearson, R.R. (2000). Plasma homocysteine predicts mortality independently of traditional risk factors and C-reactive protein in patients with angiographically defined coronary artery disease. *Circulation, 102,* 1227–1232.

19. Vollset, S.E., Refsum, H., Irgens, L.M., Emblem, B.M., Tverdal, A., Gjessing, H.K., Monsen, A.L., Ueland, P.M. (2000). Plasma total homocysteine, pregnancy complications, and adverse pregnancy outcomes: The Hordaland Homocysteine study. *American Journal of Clinical Nutrition, 71*, 962–968.

20. Daly, S., Cotter, A., Molloy, A.E., Scott, J. (2005). Homocysteine and folic acid: Implications for pregnancy. *Seminars in Vascular Medicine, 5*, 190–200.

21. Clarke, R., Smith, A.D., Jobst, K.A., Refsum, H., Sutton, L., Ueland, P.M. (1998). Folate, vitamin B12, and serum total homocysteine levels in confirmed Alzheimer disease. *Archives of Neurology, 55*, 1449–1455.

22. Seshadri, S., Beiser, A., Selhub, J., Jacques, P.F., Rosenberg, I.H., D'Agostino, R.B., Wilson, P.W., Wolf, P.A. (2002). Plasma homocysteine as a risk factor for dementia and Alzheimer's disease. *New England Journal of Medicine, 346*, 476–483.

23. McLean, R.R., Jacques, P.F., Selhub, J., Tucker, K.L., Samelson, E.J., Broe, K.E., Hannan, M.T., Cupples, L.A., Kiel, D.P. (2004). Homocysteine as a predictive factor for hip fracture in older persons. *New England Journal of Medicine, 350*, 2042–2049.

24. van Meurs, J.B., Dhonukshe-Rutten, R.A., Pluijm, S.M., van der Klift, M., de Jonge, R., Lindemans, J., de Groot, L.C., Hofman, A., Witteman, J.C., van Leeuwen, J.P., Breteler, M.M., Lips, P., Pols, H.A., Uitterlinden, A.G. (2004). Homocysteine levels and the risk of osteoporotic fracture. *New England Journal of Medicine, 350*, 2033–2041.

25. Gjesdal, C.G., Vollset, S.E., Ueland, P.M., Refsum, H., Drevon, C.A., Gjessing, H.K., Tell, G.S. (2006). Plasma total homocysteine level and bone mineral density: The Hordaland Homocysteine Study. *Archives of Internal Medicine, 166*, 88–94.

26. Perla-Kajan, J., Twardowski, T., Jakubowski, H. (2007). Mechanisms of homocysteine toxicity in humans. *Amino Acids, 32*, 561–572.

27. Lusis, A.J. (2000). Atherosclerosis. *Nature, 407*, 233–241.

28. Lentz, S.R. (2005). Mechanisms of homocysteine-induced atherothrombosis. *Journal of Thrombosis and Haemostasis, 3*, 1646–1654.

29. Hofmann, M.A., Lalla, E., Lu, Y., Gleason, M.R., Wolf, B.M., Tanji, N., Ferran, L.J., Jr., Kohl, B., Rao, V., Kisiel, W., Stern, D.M., Schmidt, A.M. (2001). Hyperhomocysteinemia enhances vascular inflammation and accelerates atherosclerosis in a murine model. *Journal of Clinical Investigation, 107*, 675–683.

30. Mudd, S.H., Skovby, F., Levy, H.L., Pettigrew, K.D., Wilcken, B., Pyeritz, R.E., Andria, G., Boers, G.H., Bromberg, I.L., Cerone, R., Fowler, B., Gröbe, H., Schmidt, H., Schweitzer, L. (1985). The natural history of homocystinuria due to cystathionine beta-synthase deficiency. *American Journal of Human Genetics, 37*, 1–31.

31. Strauss, K.A., Morton, D.H., Puffenberger, E.G., Hendrickson, C., Robinson, D.L., Wagner, C., Stabler, S.P., Allen, R.H., Chwatko, G., Jakubowski, H., Niculescu, M.D., Mudd, S.H. (2007). Prevention of brain disease from severe 5,10-methylenetetrahydro-folate reductase deficiency. *Molecular Genetics and Metabolism, 91*, 165–175.

32. Lawrence de Koning, A.B., Werstuck, G.H., Zhou, J., Austin, R.C. (2003). Hyperhomocysteinemia and its role in the development of atherosclerosis. *Clinical Biochemistry, 36*, 431–441.

33. Durga, J., van Boxtel, M.P., Schouten, E.G., Kok, F.J., Jolles, J., Katan, M.B., Verhoef, P. (2007). Effect of 3-year folic acid supplementation on cognitive function in older adults in the FACIT trial: A randomised, double blind, controlled trial. *Lancet, 369*, 208–216.

34. Spence, J.D., Bang, H., Chambless, L.E., Stampfer, M.J. (2005). Vitamin Intervention For Stroke Prevention trial: An efficacy analysis. *Stroke, 36*, 2404–2409.

35. Lonn, E., Yusuf, S., Arnold, M.J., Sheridan, P., Pogue, J., Micks, M., McQueen, M.J., Probstfield, J., Fodor, G., Held, C., Genest, J., Jr. (2006). Homocysteine lowering with folic acid and B vitamins in vascular disease. *New England Journal of Medicine, 354*, 1567–1577.

36. Bonaa, K.H., Njolstad, I., Ueland, P.M., Schirmer, H., Tverdal, A., Steigen, T., Wang, H., Nordrehaug, J.E., Arnesen, E., Rasmussen, K. (2006). Homocysteine lowering and cardiovascular events after acute myocardial infarction. *New England Journal of Medicine, 354*, 1578–1588.

37. Wang, X., Qin, X., Demirtas, H., Li, J., Mao, G., Huo, Y., Sun, N., Liu, L., Xu, X. (2007). Efficacy of folic acid supplementation in stroke prevention: A meta-analysis. *Lancet, 369*, 1876–1882.

38. Zhang, C., Cai, Y., Adachi, M.T., Oshiro, S., Aso, T., Kaufman, R.J., Kitajima, S. (2001). Homocysteine induces programmed cell death in human vascular endothelial cells through activation of the unfolded protein response. *Journal of Biological Chemistry, 276*, 35867–35874.

39. Hossain, G.S., van Thienen, J.V., Werstuck, G.H., Zhou, J., Sood, S.K., Dickhout, J.G., de Koning, A.B., Tang, D., Wu, D., Falk, E., Poddar, R., Jacobsen, D.W., Zhang, K., Kaufman, R.J., Austin, R.C. (2003). TDAG51 is induced by homocysteine, promotes detachment-mediated programmed cell death, and contributes to the development of atherosclerosis in hyperhomocysteinemia. *Journal of Biological Chemistry, 278*, 30317–30327.

40. Roybal, C.N., Yang, S., Sun, C.W., Hurtado, D., Vander Jagt, D.L., Townes, T.M., Abcouwer, S.F. (2004). Homocysteine increases the expression of vascular endothelial growth factor by a mechanism involving endoplasmic reticulum stress and transcription factor ATF4. *Journal of Biological Chemistry, 279*, 14844–14852.

41. Kerkeni, M., Tnani, M., Chuniaud, L., Miled, A., Maaroufi, K., Trivin, F. (2006). Comparative study on in vitro effects of homocysteine thiolactone and homocysteine on HUVEC cells: Evidence for a stronger proapoptotic and proinflammative homocysteine thiolactone. *Molecular and Cellular Biochemistry, 291*, 119–126.

42. Mattson, M.P., Shea, T.B. (2003). Folate and homocysteine metabolism in neural plasticity and neurodegenerative disorders. *Trends in Neurosciences, 26*, 137–146.

43. Jakubowski, H. (1991). Proofreading in vivo: Editing of homocysteine by methionyl-tRNA synthetase in the yeast *Saccharomyces cerevisiae. EMBO Journal, 10*, 593–598.

44. Jakubowski, H. (2002). The determination of homocysteine-thiolactone in biological samples. *Analytical Biochemistry, 308*, 112–119.

45. Jakubowski, H., Goldman, E. (1992). Editing of errors in selection of amino acids for protein synthesis. *Microbiological Reviews, 56*, 412–429.

46. Tuite, N.L., Fraser, K.R., O'Byrne, C.P. (2005). Homocysteine toxicity in *Escherichia coli* is caused by a perturbation of branched-chain amino acid biosynthesis. *Journal of Bacteriology, 187*, 4362–4371.

47. Jakubowski, H. (2004). Molecular basis of homocysteine toxicity in humans. *Cellular and Molecular Life Science, 61*, 470–487.

48. Jakubowski, H. (2006). Pathophysiological consequences of homocysteine excess. *Journal of Nutrition, 136*, 1741S–1749S.

49. Jacobsen, D.W. (2006). Homocysteine targeting of plasma proteins in hemodialysis patients. *Kidney International, 69*, 787–789.

50. Jacobsen, D.W., Catanescu, O., Dibello, P.M., Barbato, J.C. (2005). Molecular targeting by homocysteine: A mechanism for vascular pathogenesis. *Clinical Chemistry and Laboratory Medicine, 43*, 1076–1083.

51. Carmel, R., Jacobsen, D.W. (2001). *Homocysteine in Health and Disease*. Cambridge, UK: Cambridge University Press.

52. Glushchenko, A.V., Jacobsen, D.W. (2007). Molecular targeting of proteins by L-homocysteine: Mechanistic implications for vascular disease. *Antioxidants and Redox Signaling, 9*, 1883–1898.

53. Jakubowski, H. (2005). Anti-N-homocysteinylated protein autoantibodies and cardiovascular disease. *Clinical Chemistry and Laboratory Medicine, 43*, 1011–1014.

54. Jakubowski, H. (2005). tRNA synthetase editing of amino acids. In *Encyclopedia of Life Sciences*. http://www.els.net/doi:10.1038/npg.els.0003933. Chichester: Wiley.

55. Jakubowski, H. (2005). Accuracy of aminoacyl-tRNA synthetases: Proofreading of amino acids. In Ibba, M., Francklyn, C., Cusack, S., Eds., *The Aminoacyl-tRNA Synthetases*, pp. 384–396. Georgetown, TX: Landes Bioscience/Eurekah.com.

56. Chen, P., Poddar, R., Tipa, E.V., Dibello, P.M., Moravec, C.D., Robinson, K., Green, R., Kruger, W.D., Garrow, T.A., Jacobsen, D.W. (1999). Homocysteine metabolism in cardiovascular cells and tissues: Implications for hyperhomocysteinemia and cardiovascular disease. *Advances in Enzyme Regulation, 39*, 93–109.

57. Jakubowski, H. (1999). Protein homocysteinylation: Possible mechanism underlying pathological consequences of elevated homocysteine levels. *FASEB Journal, 13*, 2277–2283.

58. Jakubowski, H. (2000). Calcium-dependent human serum homocysteine thiolactone hydrolase. A protective mechanism against protein N-homocysteinylation. *Journal of Biological Chemistry, 275*, 3957–3962.

59. Jakubowski, H. (2002). Homocysteine is a protein amino acid in humans. Implications for homocysteine-linked disease. *Journal of Biological Chemistry, 277*, 30425–30428.

60. Jakubowski, H. (1997). Metabolism of homocysteine thiolactone in human cell cultures. Possible mechanism for pathological consequences of elevated homocysteine levels. *Journal of Biological Chemistry, 272*, 1935–1942.

61. Christensen, B., Refsum, H., Vintermyr, O., Ueland, P.M. (1991). Homocysteine export from cells cultured in the presence of physiological or superfluous levels of methionine: Methionine loading of non-transformed, transformed, proliferating, and quiescent cells in culture. *Journal of Cellular Physiology, 146*, 52–62.

62. Zimny, J., Sikora, M., Guranowski, A., Jakubowski, H. (2006). Protective mechanisms against homocysteine toxicity: The role of bleomycin hydrolase. *Journal of Biological Chemistry, 281*, 22485–22492.

63. Refsum, H., Smith, A.D., Ueland, P.M., Nexo, E., Clarke, R., McPartlin, J., Johnston, C., Engbaek, F., Schneede, J., McPartlin, C., Scott, J.M. (2004). Facts and recommendations about total homocysteine determinations: An expert opinion. *Clinical Chemistry, 50*, 3–32.

64. Mudd, S.H., Finkelstein, J.D., Refsum, H., Ueland, P.M., Malinow, M.R., Lentz, S.R., Jacobsen, D.W., Brattstrom, L., Wilcken, B., Wilcken, D.E., Blom, H.J., Stabler, S.P., Allen, R.H., Selhub, J., Rosenberg, I.H. (2000). Homocysteine and its disulfide

derivatives: A suggested consensus terminology. *Arteriosclerosis, Thrombosis and Vascular Biology, 20*, 1704–1706.

65. Chwatko, G., Jakubowski, H. (2005). Urinary excretion of homocysteine-thiolactone in humans. *Clinical Chemistry, 51*, 408–415.

66. Chwatko, G., Boers, G.H., Strauss, K.A., Shih, D.M., Jakubowski, H. (2007). Mutations in methylenetetrahydrofolate reductase or cystathionine beta-synthase gene, or a high-methionine diet, increase homocysteine thiolactone levels in humans and mice. *FASEB Journal, 21*, 1707–1713.

67. Svardal, A., Refsum, H., Ueland, P.M. (1986). Determination of in vivo protein binding of homocysteine and its relation to free homocysteine in the liver and other tissues of the rat. *Journal of Biological Chemistry, 261*, 3156–3163.

68. Kerins, D.M., Koury, M.J., Capdevila, A., Rana, S., Wagner, C. (2001). Plasma S-adenosylhomocysteine is a more sensitive indicator of cardiovascular disease than plasma homocysteine. *American Journal of Clinical Nutrition, 74*, 723–729.

69. Stabler, S.P., Allen, R.H. (2004). Quantification of serum and urinary S-adenosylmethionine and S-adenosylhomocysteine by stable-isotope-dilution liquid chromatography-mass spectrometry. *Clinical Chemistry, 50*, 365–372.

70. Jakubowski, H. (2001). Translational accuracy of aminoacyl-tRNA synthetases: Implications for atherosclerosis. *Journal of Nutrition, 131*, 2983S–2987S.

71. Chwatko, G., Jakubowski, H. (2005). The determination of homocysteine-thiolactone in human plasma. *Analytical Biochemistry, 337*, 271–277.

72. Glowacki, R., Jakubowski, H. (2004). Cross-talk between Cys34 and lysine residues in human serum albumin revealed by N-homocysteinylation. *Journal of Biological Chemistry, 279*, 10864–10871.

73. Undas, A., Jakubowski, H. (2006). Letter by Undas and Jakubowski regarding article, "Relationship between homocysteine and mortality in chronic kidney disease." *Circulation, 114*, e547; author reply e548.

74. Undas, A., Jankowski, M., Twardowska, M., Padjas, A., Jakubowski, H., Szczeklik, A. (2005). Antibodies to N-homocysteinylated albumin as a marker for early-onset coronary artery disease in men. *Thrombosis and Haemostasis, 93*, 346–350.

75. Chambers, J.C., Obeid, O.A., Kooner, J.S. (1999). Physiological increments in plasma homocysteine induce vascular endothelial dysfunction in normal human subjects. *Arteriosclerosis, Thrombosis and Vascular Biology, 19*, 2922–2927.

76. Chambers, J.C., Ueland, P.M., Wright, M., Dore, C.J., Refsum, H., Kooner, J.S. (2001). Investigation of relationship between reduced, oxidized, and protein-bound homocysteine and vascular endothelial function in healthy human subjects. *Circulation Research, 89*, 187–192.

77. Jakubowski, H., Goldman, E. (1993). Synthesis of homocysteine thiolactone by methionyl-tRNA synthetase in cultured mammalian cells. *FEBS Letters, 317*, 237–240.

78. Jakubowski, H. (2000). Homocysteine thiolactone: Metabolic origin and protein homocysteinylation in humans. *Journal of Nutrition, 130*, 377S–381S.

79. Jakubowski, H. (2003). Homocysteine-thiolactone and S-nitroso-homocysteine mediate incorporation of homocysteine into protein in humans. *Clinical Chemistry and Laboratory Medicine, 41*, 1462–1466.

80. Van Aerts, L.A., Klaasboer, H.H., Postma, N.S., Pertijs, J.C., Peereboom, J.H., Eskes, T.K., Noordhoek, J. (1993). Stereospecific in vitro embryotoxicity of L-homocysteine in pre- and post-implantation rodent embryos. *Toxicology in Vitro, 7*, 743–749.

81. Barbato, J.C., Catanescu, O., Murray, K., DiBello, P.M., Jacobsen, D.W. (2007). Targeting of metallothionein by L-homocysteine: A novel mechanism for disruption of zinc and redox homeostasis. *Arteriosclerosis, Thrombosis and Vascular Biology*, 27, 49–54.

82. Jakubowski, H., Zhang, L., Bardeguez, A., Aviv, A. (2000). Homocysteine thiolactone and protein homocysteinylation in human endothelial cells: Implications for atherosclerosis. *Circulation Research*, 87, 45–51.

83. Wang, H., Yoshizumi, M., Lai, K., Tsai, J.C., Perrella, M.A., Haber, E., Lee, M.E. (1997). Inhibition of growth and p21ras methylation in vascular endothelial cells by homocysteine but not cysteine. *Journal of Biological Chemistry*, 272, 25380–25385.

84. Ingrosso, D., Cimmino, A., Perna, A.F., Masella, L., De Santo, N.G., De Bonis, M.L., Vacca, M., D'Esposito, M., D'Urso, M., Galletti, P., Zappia, V. (2003). Folate treatment and unbalanced methylation and changes of allelic expression induced by hyperhomocysteinaemia in patients with uraemia. *Lancet*, 361, 1693–1699.

85. Devlin, A.M., Bottiglieri, T., Domann, F.E., Lentz, S.R. (2005). Tissue-specific changes in H19 methylation and expression in mice with hyperhomocysteinemia. *Journal of Biological Chemistry*, 280, 25506–25511.

86. Yi, P., Melnyk, S., Pogribna, M., Pogribny, I.P., Hine, R.J., James, S.J. (2000). Increase in plasma homocysteine associated with parallel increases in plasma S-adenosylhomocysteine and lymphocyte DNA hypomethylation. *Journal of Biological Chemistry*, 275, 29318–29323.

87. Caudill, M.A., Wang, J.C., Melnyk, S., Pogribny, I.P., Jernigan, S., Collins, M.D., Santos-Guzman, J., Swendseid, M.E., Cogger, E.A., James, S.J. (2001). Intracellular S-adenosylhomocysteine concentrations predict global DNA hypomethylation in tissues of methyl-deficient cystathionine beta-synthase heterozygous mice. *Journal of Nutrition*, 131, 2811–2818.

88. Mudd, S., Levy, H., Skovby, F. (1989). Disorders of transsulfuration. In Scriver, C.R., Beaudet, A.L., Sly, W.S., Vale, D., Eds., *The Metabolic Basis of Inherited Disease*, pp. 693–734. New York: McGraw-Hill.

89. Harker, L.A., Slichter, S.J., Scott, C.R., Ross, R. (1974). Homocystinemia. Vascular injury and arterial thrombosis. *New England Journal of Medicine*, 291, 537–543.

90. Harker, L.A., Harlan, J.M., Ross, R. (1983). Effect of sulfinpyrazone on homocysteine-induced endothelial injury and arteriosclerosis in baboons. *Circulation Research*, 53, 731–739.

91. Endo, N., Nishiyama, K., Otsuka, A., Kanouchi, H., Taga, M., Oka, T. (2006). Antioxidant activity of vitamin B6 delays homocysteine-induced atherosclerosis in rats. *British Journal of Nutrition*, 95, 1088–1093.

92. Rosenquist, T.H., Ratashak, S.A., Selhub, J. (1996). Homocysteine induces congenital defects of the heart and neural tube: Effect of folic acid. *Proceedings of the National Academy of Sciences USA*, 93, 15227–15232.

93. Boot, M.J., Steegers-Theunissen, R.P., Poelmann, R.E., van Iperen, L., Gittenberger-de Groot, A.C. (2004). Homocysteine induces endothelial cell detachment and vessel wall thickening during chick embryonic development. *Circulation Research*, 94, 542–549.

94. Brouns, M.R., Afman, L.A., Vanhauten, B.A., Hekking, J.W., Kohler, E.S., van Straaten, H.W. (2005). Morphogenetic movements during cranial neural tube closure in the chick embryo and the effect of homocysteine. *Anatomy and Embryology (Berlin)*, 210, 81–90.

95. Maestro de las Casas, C., Epeldegui, M., Tudela, C., Varela-Moreiras, G., Perez-Miguelsanz, J. (2003). High exogenous homocysteine modifies eye development in early chick embryos. *Birth Defects Research. Part A, Clinical and Molecular Teratology*, *67*, 35–40.

96. Jakubowski, H., Ambrosius, W.T., Pratt, J.H. (2001). Genetic determinants of homocysteine thiolactonase activity in humans: Implications for atherosclerosis. *FEBS Letters*, *491*, 35–39.

97. Jakubowski, H. (2001). Biosynthesis and reactions of homocysteine thiolactone. In Jacobson, D., Carmel, R., Eds., *Homocysteine in Health and Disease*, pp. 21–31. Cambridge, UK: Cambridge University Press.

98. Donahue, S., Struman, J.A., Gaull, G. (1974). Arteriosclerosis due to homocyst(e)inemia. Failure to reproduce the model in weanling rabbits. *American Journal of Pathology*, *77*, 167–163.

99. Makheja, A.N., Bombard, A.T., Randazzo, R.L., Bailey, J.M. (1978). Anti-inflammatory drugs in experimental atherosclerosis. Part 3. Evaluation of the atherogenicity of homocystine in rabbits. *Atherosclerosis*, *29*, 105–112.

100. McCully, K.S., Ragsdale, B.D. (1970). Production of arteriosclerosis by homocysteinemia. *American Journal of Pathology*, *61*, 1–11.

101. Reddy, G.S., Wilcken, D.E. (1982). Experimental homocysteinemia in pigs: Comparison with studies in sixteen homocystinuric patients. *Metabolism*, *31*, 778–783.

102. Spence, A.M., Rasey, J.S., Dwyer-Hansen, L., Grunbaum, Z., Livesey, J., Chin, L., Nelson, N., Stein, D., Krohn, K.A., Ali-Osman, F. (1995). Toxicity, biodistribution and radioprotective capacity of L-homocysteine thiolactone in CNS tissues and tumors in rodents: Comparison with prior results with phosphorothioates. *Radiotherapy and Oncology*, *35*, 216–226.

103. Folbergrova, J. (1997). Anticonvulsant action of both NMDA and non-NMDA receptor antagonists against seizures induced by homocysteine in immature rats. *Experimental Neurology*, *145*, 442–450.

104. Langmeier, M., Folbergrova, J., Haugvicova, R., Pokorny, J., Mares, P. (2003). Neuronal cell death in hippocampus induced by homocysteic acid in immature rats. *Epilepsia*, *44*, 299–304.

105. Greene, N.D., Dunlevy, L.E., Copp, A.J. (2003). Homocysteine is embryotoxic but does not cause neural tube defects in mouse embryos. *Anatomy and Embryology (Berlin)*, *206*, 185–191.

106. Hansen, D.K., Grafton, T.F., Melnyk, S., James, S.J. (2001). Lack of embryotoxicity of homocysteine thiolactone in mouse embryos in vitro. *Reproductive Toxicology*, *15*, 239–244.

107. Rodgers, G.M., Kane, W.H. (1986). Activation of endogenous factor V by a homocysteine-induced vascular endothelial cell activator. *Journal of Clinical Investigations*, *77*, 1909–1916.

108. Mercie, P., Garnier, O., Lascoste, L., Renard, M., Closse, C., Durrieu, F., Marit, G., Boisseau, R.M., Belloc, F. (2000). Homocysteine-thiolactone induces caspase-independent vascular endothelial cell death with apoptotic features. *Apoptosis*, *5*, 403–411.

109. Huang, R.F., Huang, S.M., Lin, B.S., Wei, J.S., Liu, T.Z. (2001). Homocysteine thiolactone induces apoptotic DNA damage mediated by increased intracellular hydrogen peroxide and caspase 3 activation in HL-60 cells. *Life Sciences*, *68*, 2799–2811.

110. Kamudhamas, A., Pang, L., Smith, S.D., Sadovsky, Y., Nelson, D.M. (2004). Homocysteine thiolactone induces apoptosis in cultured human trophoblasts: A mechanism for homocysteine-mediated placental dysfunction? *American Journal of Obstetrics and Gynecology*, *191*, 563–571.

111. Najib, S., Sanchez-Margalet, V. (2005). Homocysteine thiolactone inhibits insulin-stimulated DNA and protein synthesis: Possible role of mitogen-activated protein kinase (MAPK), glycogen synthase kinase-3 (GSK-3) and p70 S6K phosphorylation. *Journal of Molecular Endocrinology*, *34*, 119–126.

112. Yang, X., Gao, Y., Zhou, J., Zhen, Y., Yang, Y., Wang, J., Song, L., Liu, Y., Xu, H., Chen, Z., Hui, R. (2006). Plasma homocysteine thiolactone adducts associated with risk of coronary heart disease. *Clinica Chimica Acta*, *364*, 230–234.

113. Ferretti, G., Bacchetti, T., Moroni, C., Vignini, A., Nanetti, L., Curatola, G. (2004). Effect of homocysteinylation of low density lipoproteins on lipid peroxidation of human endothelial cells. *Journal Cell Biochemistry*, *92*, 351–360.

114. Undas, A., Perla, J., Lacinski, M., Trzeciak, W., Kazmierski, R., Jakubowski, H. (2004). Autoantibodies against N-homocysteinylated proteins in humans: Implications for atherosclerosis. *Stroke*, *35*, 1299–1304.

115. Undas, A., Stepien, E., Glowacki, R., Tisonczyk, J., Tracz, W., Jakubowski, H. (2006). Folic acid administration and antibodies against homocysteinylated proteins in subjects with hyperhomocysteinemia. *Thrombosis and Haemostasis*, *96*, 342–347.

116. Undas, A., Brozek, J., Jankowski, M., Siudak, Z., Szczeklik, A., Jakubowski, H. (2006). Plasma homocysteine affects fibrin clot permeability and resistance to lysis in human subjects. *Arteriosclerosis, Thrombosis and Vascular Biology*, *26*, 1397–1404.

117. Sauls, D.L., Lockhart, E., Warren, M.E., Lenkowski, A., Wilhelm, S.E., Hoffman, M. (2006). Modification of fibrinogen by homocysteine thiolactone increases resistance to fibrinolysis: A potential mechanism of the thrombotic tendency in hyperhomocysteinemia. *Biochemistry*, *45*, 2480–2487.

118. Baernstein, H.D. (1934). A modification of the method for determining methionine in proteins. *Journal of Biological Chemistry*, *106*, 451–456.

119. Jakubowski, H. (2007). Facile syntheses of (35)S-homocysteine-thiolactone, (35)S.homocystine, (35)S-homocysteine, and S-nitroso-(35)S-homocysteine. *Analytical Biochemistry*, *370*, 124–126.

120. Jakubowski, H., Guranowski, A. (2003). Metabolism of homocysteine-thiolactone in plants. *Journal of Biological Chemistry*, *278*, 6765–6770.

121. Jakubowski, H. (1995). Proofreading in vivo. Editing of homocysteine by aminoacyl-tRNA synthetases in *Escherichia coli*. *Journal of Biological Chemistry*, *270*, 17672–17673.

122. Gao, W., Goldman, E., Jakubowski, H. (1994). Role of carboxy-terminal region in proofreading function of methionyl-tRNA synthetase in *Escherichia coli*. *Biochemistry*, *33*, 11528–11535.

123. Jakubowski, H. (2006). Mechanism of the condensation of homocysteine thiolactone with aldehydes. *Chemistry*, *12*, 8039–8043.

124. Jakubowski, H. (1990). Proofreading in vivo: Editing of homocysteine by methionyl-tRNA synthetase in *Escherichia coli*. *Proceedings of the National Academy of Sciences USA*, *87*, 4504–4508.

125. Reuben, D.M., Bruice, T.C. (1976). Reaction of thiol anions with benzene oxide and malachite green. *Journal of the American Chemistry Society, 98*, 114–121.

126. Dudman, N.P., Hicks, C., Lynch, J.F., Wilcken, D.E., Wang, J. (1991). Homocysteine thiolactone disposal by human arterial endothelial cells and serum in vitro. *Arteriosclerosis and Thrombosis, 11*, 663–670.

127. Jakubowski, H. (1998). Aminoacylation of coenzyme A and pantetheine by aminoacyl-tRNA synthetases: Possible link between noncoded and coded peptide synthesis. *Biochemistry, 37*, 5147–5153.

128. Jakubowski, H. (2000). Translational incorporation of S-nitrosohomocysteine into protein. *Journal of Biological Chemistry, 275*, 21813–21816.

129. Perla-Kajan, J., Marczak, L., Kajan, L., Skowronek, P., Twardowski, T., Jakubowski, H. (2007). Modification by homocysteine thiolactone affects redox status of cytochrome c. *Biochemistry, 46*, 6225–6231.

130. Mukai, Y., Togawa, T., Suzuki, T., Ohata, K., Tanabe, S. (2002). Determination of homocysteine thiolactone and homocysteine in cell cultures using high-performance liquid chromatography with fluorescence detection. *Journal of Chromatography B Analytical Technologies in the Biomedical and Life Sciences, 767*, 263–268.

131. Jakubowski, H., Fersht, A.R. (1981). Alternative pathways for editing non-cognate amino acids by aminoacyl-tRNA synthetases. *Nucleic Acids Research, 9*, 3105–3117.

132. Jakubowski, H. (2002). From accuracy of protein synthesis to cardiovascular disease: The role of homocysteine. *Biotechnologia (Poznan), 58*, 11–24.

133. Kim, H.Y., Ghosh, G., Schulman, L.H., Brunie, S., Jakubowski, H. (1993). The relationship between synthetic and editing functions of the active site of an aminoacyl-tRNA synthetase. *Proceedings of the National Academy of Sciences USA, 90*, 11553–11557.

134. Serre, L., Verdon, G., Choinowski, T., Hervouet, N., Risler, J.L., Zelwer, C. (2001). How methionyl-tRNA synthetase creates its amino acid recognition pocket upon L-methionine binding. *Journal of Molecular Biology, 306*, 863–876.

135. Jakubowski, H. (1996). The synthetic/editing active site of an aminoacyl-tRNA synthetase: Evidence for binding of thiols in the editing subsite. *Biochemistry, 35*, 8252–8259.

136. Stamler, J.S., Osborne, J.A., Jaraki, O., Rabbani, L.E., Mullins, M., Singel, D., Loscalzo, J. (1993). Adverse vascular effects of homocysteine are modulated by endothelium-derived relaxing factor and related oxides of nitrogen. *Journal of Clinical Investigations, 91*, 308–318.

137. Sikora, M., Marczak, L., Stobiecki, M., Twardowski, T., Jakubowski, H. (2007). Determination of N-homocysteinylated albumin in human serum. *Clinical Chemistry and Laboratory Medicine, 45*, A35.

138. Uji, Y., Motomiya, Y., Hanyu, N., Ukaji, F., Okabe, H. (2002). Protein-bound homocystamide measured in human plasma by HPLC. *Clinical Chemistry, 48*, 941–944.

139. Perna, A.F., Satta, E., Acanfora, F., Lombardi, C., Ingrosso, D., De Santo, N.G. (2006). Increased plasma protein homocysteinylation in hemodialysis patients. *Kidney International, 69*, 869–876.

140. Sass, J.O., Nakanishi, T., Sato, T., Sperl, W., Shimizu, A. (2003). S-homocysteinylation of transthyretin is detected in plasma and serum of humans with different types of hyperhomocysteinemia. *Biochemical and Biophysical Research Communications, 310*, 242–246.

141. Christodoulou, J., Sadler, P.J., Tucker, A. (1994). A new structural transition of serum albumin dependent on the state of Cys34. Detection by 1H-NMR spectroscopy. *European Journal of Biochemistry/FEBS*, *225*, 363–368.

142. Mallamaci, F., Zoccali, C., Tripepi, G., Fermo, I., Benedetto, F.A., Cataliotti, A., Bellanuova, I., Malatino, L.S., Soldarini, A. (2002). Hyperhomocysteinemia predicts cardiovascular outcomes in hemodialysis patients. *Kidney International*, *61*, 609–614.

143. Perla, J., Undas, A., Twardowski, T., Jakubowski, H. (2004). Purification of antibodies against N-homocysteinylated proteins by affinity chromatography on N-omega-homocysteinyl-aminohexyl-agarose. *Journal of Chromatography B Analytical Technologies in the Biomedical and Life Sciences*, *807*, 257–261.

144. Perła-Kaján, J., Stanger, O., Ziółkowska, A., Melandowicz, L.K., Twardowski, T., Jakubowski, H. (2007). Immunohistochemical detection of N-homocysteinylated proteins in cardiac surgery patients. *Clinical Chemistry and Laboratory Medicine*, *45*, A36.

145. Anfinsen, C.B. (1973). Principles that govern the folding of protein chains. *Science*, *181*, 223–230.

146. Fersht, A. (2000). *Structure and Mechanism in Protein Science*. New York: W.H. Freeman and Company.

147. Stefani, M. (2004). Protein misfolding and aggregation: New examples in medicine and biology of the dark side of the protein world. *Biochimica et Biophysica Acta*, *1739*, 5–25.

148. Naruszewicz, M., Olszewski, A.J., Mirkiewicz, E., McCully, K.S. (1994). Thiolation of low density lipoproteins by homocysteine thiolactone causes increased aggregation and altered interaction with cultured macrophages. *Nutrition, Metabolism and Cardiovascular Diseases*, *4*, 70–77.

149. Werstuck, G.H., Lentz, S.R., Dayal, S., Hossain, G.S., Sood, S.K., Shi, Y.Y., Zhou, J., Maeda, N., Krisans, S.K., Malinow, M.R., Austin, R.C. (2001). Homocysteine-induced endoplasmic reticulum stress causes dysregulation of the cholesterol and triglyceride biosynthetic pathways. *Journal of Clinical Investigations*, *107*, 1263–1273.

150. Zhou, J., Moller, J., Danielsen, C.C., Bentzon, J., Ravn, H.B., Austin, R.C., Falk, E. (2001). Dietary supplementation with methionine and homocysteine promotes early atherosclerosis but not plaque rupture in ApoE-deficient mice. *Arteriosclerosis, Thrombosis and Vascular Biology*, *21*, 1470–1476.

151. Koopman, J., Haverkate, F., Grimbergen, J., Engesser, L., Novakova, I., Kerst, A.F., Lord, S.T. (1992). Abnormal fibrinogens IJmuiden (B beta Arg14–Cys) and Nijmegen (B beta Arg44–Cys) form disulfide-linked fibrinogen-albumin complexes. *Proceedings of the National Academy of Sciences USA*, *89*, 3478–3482.

152. Koopman, J., Haverkate, F., Grimbergen, J., Lord, S.T., Mosesson, M.W., DiOrio, J.P., Siebenlist, K.S., Legrand, C., Soria, J., Soria, C., Caen, J.P. (1993). Molecular basis for fibrinogen Dusart (A alpha 554 Arg $\longrightarrow$ Cys) and its association with abnormal fibrin polymerization and thrombophilia. *Journal of Clinical Investigations*, *91*, 1637–1643.

153. Marchi, R., Lundberg, U., Grimbergen, J., Koopman, J., Torres, A., de Bosch, N.B., Haverkate, F., Arocha Pinango, C.L. (2000). Fibrinogen Caracas V, an abnormal fibrinogen with an alpha 532 Ser $\longrightarrow$ Cys substitution associated with thrombosis. *Thrombosis and Haemostasis*, *84*, 263–270.

154. Hanss, M., Biot, F. (2001). A database for human fibrinogen variants. *Annals of the NewYork Academy of Sciences*, *936*, 89–90.

155. Libby, P. (2006). Inflammation and cardiovascular disease mechanisms. *American Journal of Clinical Nutrition, 83*, 456S–460S.

156. Forrester, J.S., Libby, P. (2007). The inflammation hypothesis and its potential relevance to statin therapy. *American Journal of Cardiology, 99*, 732–738.

157. Binder, C.J., Shaw, P.X., Chang, M.K., Boullier, A., Hartvigsen, K., Horkko, S., Miller, Y.I., Woelkers, D.A., Corr, M., Witztum, J.L. (2005). The role of natural antibodies in atherogenesis. *Journal of Lipid Research, 46*, 1353–1363.

158. Libby, P., Ridker, P.M., Maseri, A. (2002). Inflammation and atherosclerosis. *Circulation, 105*, 1135–1143.

159. Lopes-Virella, M.F., Thorpe, S.R., Derrick, M.B., Chassereau, C., Virella, G. (2005). The immunogenicity of modified lipoproteins. *Annals of the New York Academy of Sciences, 1043*, 367–378.

160. Ferguson, E., Parthasarathy, S., Joseph, J., Kalyanaraman, B. (1998). Generation and initial characterization of a novel polyclonal antibody directed against homocysteine thiolactone-modified low density lipoprotein. *Journal of Lipid Research, 39*, 925–933.

161. Undas, A., Kolarz, M., Kopec, G., Glowacki, R., Placzkiewicz-Jankowska, E., Tracz, W. (2007). Autoantibodies against N-homocysteinylated proteins in patients on long-term haemodialysis. *Nephrology, Dialysis, Transplantation, 22*, 1685–1689.

162. Durga, J., van Tits, L.J., Schouten, E.G., Kok, F.J., Verhoef, P. (2005). Effect of lowering of homocysteine levels on inflammatory markers: A randomized controlled trial. *Archives of Internal Medicine, 165*, 1388–1394.

163. Folsom, A.R., Desvarieux, M., Nieto, F.J., Boland, L.L., Ballantyne, C.M., Chambless, L.E. (2003). B vitamin status and inflammatory markers. *Atherosclerosis, 169*, 169–174.

164. Ravaglia, G., Forti, P., Maioli, F., Servadei, L., Martelli, M., Arnone, G., Talerico, T., Zoli, M., Mariani, E. (2004). Plasma homocysteine and inflammation in elderly patients with cardiovascular disease and dementia. *Experimental Gerontology, 39*, 443–450.

165. Peeters, A.C., van Aken, B.E., Blom, H.J., Reitsma, P.H., den Heijer, M. (2007). The effect of homocysteine reduction by B-vitamin supplementation on inflammatory markers. *Clinical Chemistry and Laboratory Medicine, 45*, 54–58.

166. Friso, S., Jacques, P.F., Wilson, P.W., Rosenberg, I.H., Selhub, J. (2001). Low circulating vitamin B(6) is associated with elevation of the inflammation marker C-reactive protein independently of plasma homocysteine levels. *Circulation, 103*, 2788–2791.

167. Rohde, L.E., Hennekens, C.H., Ridker, P.M. (1999). Survey of C-reactive protein and cardiovascular risk factors in apparently healthy men. *American Journal of Cardiology, 84*, 1018–1022.

168. Holven, K.B., Aukrust, P., Retterstol, K., Hagve, T.A., Morkrid, L., Ose, L., Nenseter, M.S. (2006). Increased levels of C-reactive protein and interleukin-6 in hyperhomocysteinemic subjects. *Scandinavian Journal of Clinical and Laboratory Investigation, 66*, 45–54.

169. Aso, Y., Yoshida, N., Okumura, K., Wakabayashi, S., Matsutomo, R., Takebayashi, K., Inukai, T. (2004). Coagulation and inflammation in overt diabetic nephropathy: Association with hyperhomocysteinemia. *Clinica Chimica Acta, 348*, 139–145.

170. Shai, I., Stampfer, M.J., Ma, J., Manson, J.E., Hankinson, S.E., Cannuscio, C., Selhub, J., Curhan, G., Rimm, E.B. (2004). Homocysteine as a risk factor for coronary heart diseases and its association with inflammatory biomarkers, lipids and dietary factors. *Atherosclerosis, 177*, 375–381.

171. Widner, B., Leblhuber, F., Frick, B., Laich, A., Artner-Dworzak, E., Fuchs, D. (2002). Moderate hyperhomocysteinaemia and immune activation in Parkinson's disease. *Journal of Neural Transmission, 109*, 1445–1452.

172. Powers, R.W., Majors, A.K., Cerula, S.L., Huber, H.A., Schmidt, B.P., Roberts, J.M. (2003). Changes in markers of vascular injury in response to transient hyperhomocysteinemia. *Metabolism, 52*, 501–507.

173. Holven, K.B., Scholz, H., Halvorsen, B., Aukrust, P., Ose, L., Nenseter, M.S. (2003). Hyperhomocysteinemic subjects have enhanced expression of lectin-like oxidized LDL receptor-1 in mononuclear cells. *Journal of Nutrition, 133*, 3588–3591.

174. Wang, G., Woo, C.W., Sung, F.L., Siow, Y.L., O, K. (2002). Increased monocyte adhesion to aortic endothelium in rats with hyperhomocysteinemia: Role of chemokine and adhesion molecules. *Arteriosclerosis, Thrombosis and Vascular Biology, 22*, 1777–1783.

175. Zhang, R., Ma, J., Xia, M., Zhu, H., Ling, W. (2004). Mild hyperhomocysteinemia induced by feeding rats diets rich in methionine or deficient in folate promotes early atherosclerotic inflammatory processes. *Journal of Nutrition, 134*, 825–830.

176. Lee, H., Kim, J.M., Kim, H.J., Lee, I., Chang, N. (2005). Folic acid supplementation can reduce the endothelial damage in rat brain microvasculature due to hyperhomocysteinemia. *Journal of Nutrition, 135*, 544–548.

177. van Guldener, C., Stehouwer, C.D. (2003). Homocysteine metabolism in renal disease. *Clinical Chemistry and Laboratory Medicine, 41*, 1412–1417.

178. Guttormsen, A.B., Mansoor, A.M., Fiskerstrand, T., Ueland, P.M., Refsum, H. (1993). Kinetics of plasma homocysteine in healthy subjects after peroral homocysteine loading. *Clinical Chemistry 39*, 1390–1397.

179. Shih, D.M., Gu, L., Xia, Y.R., Navab, M., Li, W.F., Hama, S., Castellani, L.W., Furlong, C.E., Costa, L.G., Fogelman, A.M., Lusis, A.J. (1998). Mice lacking serum paraoxonase are susceptible to organophosphate toxicity and atherosclerosis. *Nature, 394*, 284–287.

180. Shih, D.M., Xia, Y.R., Wang, X.P., Miller, E., Castellani, L.W., Subbanagounder, G., Cheroutre, H., Faull, K.F., Berliner, J.A., Witztum, J.L., Lusis, A.J. (2000). Combined serum paraoxonase knockout/apolipoprotein E knockout mice exhibit increased lipoprotein oxidation and atherosclerosis. *Journal of Biological Chemistry, 275*, 17527–17535.

181. Jarvik, G.P., Hatsukami, T.S., Carlson, C., Richter, R.J., Jampsa, R., Brophy, V.H., Margolin, S., Rieder, M., Nickerson, D., Schellenberg, G.D., Heagerty, P.J., Furlong, C.E. (2003). Paraoxonase activity, but not haplotype utilizing the linkage disequilibrium structure, predicts vascular disease. *Arteriosclerosis, Thrombosis and Vascular Biology, 23*, 1465–1471.

182. Jarvik, G.P., Rozek, L.S., Brophy, V.H., Hatsukami, T.S., Richter, R.J., Schellenberg, G.D., Furlong, C.E. (2000). Paraoxonase (PON1) phenotype is a better predictor of vascular disease than is PON1(192) or PON1(55) genotype. *Arteriosclerosis, Thrombosis and Vascular Biology, 20*, 2441–2447.

183. Lacinski, M., Skorupski, W., Cieslinski, A., Sokolowska, J., Trzeciak, W.H., Jakubowski, H. (2004). Determinants of homocysteine-thiolactonase activity of the paraoxonase-1 (PON1) protein in humans. *Cellular and Molecular Biology (Noisy-le-grand), 50*, 885–893.

184. Mackness, B., Davies, G.K., Turkie, W., Lee, E., Roberts, D.H., Hill, E., Roberts, C., Durrington, P.N., Mackness, M.I. (2001). Paraoxonase status in coronary heart disease: Are activity and concentration more important than genotype? *Arteriosclerosis, Thrombosis and Vascular Biology, 21*, 1451–1457.

185. Domagała, T.B., Łacinski, M., Trzeciak, W.H., Mackness, B., Mackness, M.I., Jakubowski, H. (2006). The correlation of homocysteine-thiolactonase activity of the paraoxonase (PON1) protein with coronary heart disease status. *Cellular and Molecular Biology (Noisy-le-grand), 52*, 4–10.

186. Robert, K., Chasse, J.F., Santiard-Baron, D., Vayssettes, C., Chabli, A., Aupetit, J., Maeda, N., Kamoun, P., London, J., Janel, N. (2003). Altered gene expression in liver from a murine model of hyperhomocysteinemia. *Journal of Biological Chemistry, 278*, 31504–31511.

187. Bromme, D., Rossi, A.B., Smeekens, S.P., Anderson, D.C., Payan, D.G. (1996). Human bleomycin hydrolase: Molecular cloning, sequencing, functional expression, and enzymatic characterization. *Biochemistry, 35*, 6706–6714.

188. Wang, H., Ramotar, D. (2002). Cellular resistance to bleomycin in *Saccharomyces cerevisiae* is not affected by changes in bleomycin hydrolase levels. *Biochemistry and Cell Biology, 80*, 789–796.

189. Schwartz, D.R., Homanics, G.E., Hoyt, D.G., Klein, E., Abernethy, J., Lazo, J.S. (1999). The neutral cysteine protease bleomycin hydrolase is essential for epidermal integrity and bleomycin resistance. *Proceedings of the National Academy of Sciences USA, 96*, 4680–4685.

190. Papassotiropoulos, A., Bagli, M., Jessen, F., Frahnert, C., Rao, M.L., Maier, W., Heun, R. (2000). Confirmation of the association between bleomycin hydrolase genotype and Alzheimer's disease. *Molecular Psychiatry, 5*, 213–215.

191. Namba, Y., Ouchi, Y., Takeda, A., Ueki, A., Ikeda, K. (1999). Bleomycin hydrolase immunoreactivity in senile plaque in the brains of patients with Alzheimer's disease. *Brain Research, 830*, 200–202.

192. Lefterov, I.M., Koldamova, R.P., Lazo, J.S. (2000). Human bleomycin hydrolase regulates the secretion of amyloid precursor protein. *FASEB Journal, 14*, 1837–1847.

193. Lefterov, I.M., Koldamova, R.P., Lefterova, M.I., Schwartz, D.R., Lazo, J.S. (2001). Cysteine 73 in bleomycin hydrolase is critical for amyloid precursor protein processing. *Biochemical and Biophysical Research Communications, 283*, 994–999.

194. Kajiya, A., Kaji, H., Isobe, T., Takeda, A. (2006). Processing of amyloid beta-peptides by neutral cysteine protease bleomycin hydrolase. *Protein and Peptide Letters, 13*, 119–123.

195. Lazo, J.S., Humphreys, C.J. (1983). Lack of metabolism as the biochemical basis of bleomycin-induced pulmonary toxicity. *Proceedings of the National Academy of Sciences USA, 80*, 3064–3068.

196. Takeda, A., Higuchi, D., Yamamoto, T., Nakamura, Y., Masuda, Y., Hirabayashi, T., Nakaya, K. (1996). Purification and characterization of bleomycin hydrolase, which represents a new family of cysteine proteases, from rat skin. *Journal of Biochemistry (Tokyo), 119*, 29–36.

197. Kamata, Y., Itoh, Y., Kajiya, A., Karasawa, S., Sakatani, C., Takekoshi, S., Osamura, R.Y., Takeda, A. (2007). Quantification of neutral cysteine protease bleomycin hydrolase and its localization in rat tissues. *Journal of Biochemistry (Tokyo), 141*, 69–76.

198. Nishimura, C., Tanaka, N., Suzuki, H., Tanaka, N. (1987). Purification of bleomycin hydrolase with a monoclonal antibody and its characterization. *Biochemistry*, *26*, 1574–1578.

199. Sebti, S.M., Mignano, J.E., Jani, J.P., Srimatkandada, S., Lazo, J.S. (1989). Bleomycin hydrolase: Molecular cloning, sequencing, and biochemical studies reveal membership in the cysteine proteinase family. *Biochemistry*, *28*, 6544–6548.

200. Zheng, W., Johnston, S.A., Joshua-Tor, L. (1998). The unusual active site of Gal6/bleomycin hydrolase can act as a carboxypeptidase, aminopeptidase, and peptide ligase. *Cell*, *93*, 103–109.

201. Niemer, I., Muller, G., Strobel, G., Bandlow, W. (1997). Bleomycin hydrolase (Blh1p), a multi-sited thiol protease in search of a distinct physiological role. *Current Genetics*, *32*, 41–51.

202. Burkhardt, A., Holtje, W.J., Gebbers, J.O. (1976). Vascular lesions following perfusion with bleomycin. Electron-microscopic observations. *Virchows Archives*, *372*, 227–236.

203. O'Farrell, P.A., Gonzalez, F., Zheng, W., Johnston, S.A., Joshua-Tor, L. (1999). Crystal structure of human bleomycin hydrolase, a self-compartmentalizing cysteine protease. *Structure*, *7*, 619–627.

CHAPTER 17

HOMOCYSTEINE AND CARDIOVASCULAR DISEASE

JAYANTA R. DAS and SANJAY KAUL

17.1 INTRODUCTION

Cardiovascular disease is impacted by a multitude of risk factors, both acquired and inherent. This complex interaction has been the focus of many years of investigation, and the results have helped us to shape both therapy and prevention. The recognition of traditional risk factors such as age, gender, hypertension, hypercholesterolemia, family history, diabetes mellitus, and tobacco use, has made a significant mark on how clinicians treat patients. Even though the traditional risk factors remain the bedrock of cardiovascular risk prediction, our ability to forecast future clinical events remains inexact [1]. Consequently, the medical community continues to search out novel indicators of cardiovascular risk to refine risk stratification, illuminate the pathogenesis of atherosclerosis, and to identify new targets for therapy.

Homocysteine has been proposed as an additional risk factor related to cardiovascular illness. It is a sulfur amino acid that is produced during the metabolism of the essential amino acid methionine. The theory of a relationship between the sulfur moiety and cardiovascular disease has been present since the late 1960s [2]. At that time McCully noted that children with homocystinuria, a disease caused by an inborn error of methionine metabolism, presented with atherothrombosis of the peripheral, coronary, and cerebral vasculature. Homocystinuria patients commonly present with homocysteine levels greater than 50-fold their normal values. A few years after McCully's revelation, Wilcken and Wilcken provided the first evidence of a relationship between abnormal homocysteine metabolism and coronary artery disease in the general population [3]. In the wake of such findings, a significant amount of research and investigation has been performed in recent years in order to elucidate the role of homocysteine in atherothrombotic cardiovascular disease.

Glutathione and Sulfur Amino Acids in Human Health and Disease. Edited by R. Masella and G. Mazza
Copyright © 2009 John Wiley & Sons, Inc.

There are three prerequisites to declaring homocysteine as a pathogenic risk factor in the development of cardiovascular disease [4]. First, robust epidemiologic evidence is necessary to establish a strong, consistent, and independent association between elevated homocysteine levels and adverse cardiovascular outcomes. Second, biologic plausibility must be demonstrated, by the elucidation of a coherent mechanism by which homocysteine directly promotes atherothrombosis. Third, modification of cardiovascular risk should be illustrated by prospective, randomized intervention trials aimed at reducing homocysteine levels. Only by a valid demonstration of data that meet these essential criteria can homocysteine be justified to belong in the pantheon of the traditional cardiovascular risk factors.

17.2 HOMOCYSTEINE METABOLISM

Homocysteine (Hcy) is a sulfur amino acid formed during the metabolism of methionine, an essential amino acid found in the diet [5]. Homocysteine is metabolized through two separate vitamin-dependent pathways, remethylation or transsulfuration (Fig. 17.1). Remethylation is a salvage pathway whereby Hcy acquires a methyl group from 5-methyl tetrahydrofolate through the enzyme methionine synthase. Vitamin B12 is required to catalyze this reaction. In addition folate is required to create 5-methyl tetrahydrofolate, during a cycle catalyzed by methylene tetrahydrofolate reductase (MTHFR). Another method of remethylation is catalyzed by betaine in

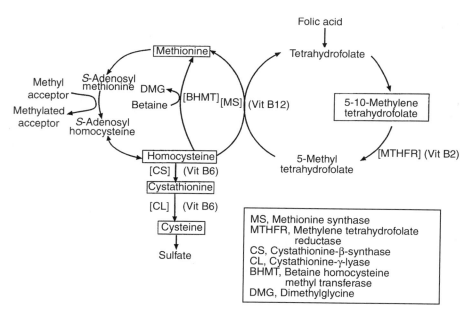

Figure 17.1 Homocysteine metabolism. Homocysteine is metabolized through two separate vitamin-dependent pathways, remethylation or transsulfuration.

the liver. Transsulfuration is an alternate pathway that is activated during periods of cysteine depletion or methionine surplus. In this vitamin B6-dependent reaction, cystathionine-β-synthase (CBS) catalyzes the combination of serine and homocysteine to form cystathionine.

Cystathionine can then undergo hydrolysis to cysteine and sulfate through another vitamin B6-dependent reaction catalyzed by cystathionine-γ-lyase. Lastly, cysteine can be degraded to glutathionine and sulfate.

17.3 HOMOCYSTEINE FORMS IN VIVO

Homocysteine is a four-carbon thiol amino acid that exists in various forms within human plasma depending on the redox status of its sulfhydryl group [6]. It circulates in the plasma in two forms—the free sulfhydryl form (reduced Hcy and the disulfide Hcy where two molecules of Hcy are bound symmetrically by disulfide), and protein bound (albumin being the most common protein substrate). The protein bound form of Hcy represents around 70% of the total found in human plasma [7]. The term "total" homocysteine (tHcy) refers to the sum of all Hcy species in serum (free and protein bound) [6].

Only very high levels of total homocysteine (homocystinuric range >100 µmol) result in saturation of plasma protein binding sites [8]. Thus, the relatively large differences in measured tHcy between individuals in the general population (on the order of 5 µmol/L) represent very small changes in circulating reduced homocysteine. Albumin and tHcy concentrations seem to affect each other, consistent with the finding that a large proportion of tHcy is protein bound [9].

17.4 HOMOCYSTEINE MEASUREMENT

Laboratory measurements of Hcy depend on proper collection, storage, and analysis to ensure accurate testing. To prevent a protein-rich meal from causing transient elevation in Hcy, a fasting sample is generally recommended for measurement [10]. This elevation is most likely secondary to an added increase in the dietary amino acid methionine to circulation. It has been shown that patients tested when fasting have relatively stable Hcy levels over time [11]. Another important aspect of measurement is the period between sample collection and storage. It is of upmost importance to process and refrigerate the sample as soon as possible. Homocysteine synthesis and release continues to occur in the red blood cell at room temperature. Unless the plasma or serum is separated from the cells, Hcy concentration will rise at a rate of 10% per hour in stored blood even with additives such as EDTA [12, 13]. Separation of plasma from cells and refrigeration should occur within the first hour of collection.

There are a number of different methods used in the measurement of Hcy [13]. High performance liquid chromatography (HPLC), gas chromatography-mass spectrometry, and immunoassays are common methods of analysis. It appears that each of these methods is reliable for clinical use [14–18]. Study choice is often guided by issues of cost, technician skill, and equipment available. It appears that clinical labs seem to prefer using routine chemistry analyzers rather than HPLC or spectrometry at this time [13].

Reference ranges for Hcy are necessary for a clinician to separate normal and pathologic values. The precise definition is somewhat difficult to discern, since studies have shown that the relationship between total Hcy and cardiovascular risk is a graded phenomenon. Many studies that show a correlation between risk and total Hcy derive this relationship by comparing a given cohort's highest and lowest interquartile levels as opposed to absolute levels. In addition, a number of different variables can affect levels [19]. One obvious influence is the dietary practice of a population. Reference ranges for Hcy decreased by 15% in North America following the mandatory supplementation of flour with folate in 1998 [13]. Age is a factor, as is gender. There is a progressive increase of Hcy levels with age. Mean values tend to double as one ages from childhood to an octogenarian. Males average 1 to 2 μmol/L higher than females. In patients who live in a region where food is folate fortified, the upper limit of normal (ULN) of tHcy levels is 12 μmol/L in adults <65 years old, and 16 μmol/L in adults >65 years old. In regions where food is not folate fortified the ULN of total Hcy levels is 15 μmol/L in adults <65 years old, and 20 μmol/L in adults >65 years old. Elevations of 16 to 30 μmol/L, 31 to 100 μmol/L, and >100 μmol/L have been classified as mild, moderate, and severe hyperhomocysteinemia, respectively [20].

A confounding variable to Hcy measurement may be the clinical status of the patient itself. During acute atherothrombotic events, patients develop an acute inflammatory response resulting in a decrease in albumin. Since the preponderance of Hcy in plasma is bound to albumin, levels are altered. Studies show that during the first two days following an acute coronary syndrome; Hcy levels slightly decrease or remain the same [21]. However, the levels rise sharply thereafter and may remain elevated for as long as six months [22, 23]. These findings illustrate the impact of timing of Hcy measurement. For example, elevated levels after an initial acute event may result in overestimation of a correlate between Hcy and risk. Thus, it is important to measure steady-state Hcy levels.

17.4.1 Oral Methionine Loading

The oral methionine load test is much like the oral glucose tolerance test; its purpose is to evaluate patients with a normal fasting plasma Hcy level to determine whether or not they may be at higher risk for an atherothrombotic event. The test is performed by giving patients oral methionine dissolved in orange juice at a dose of 100 mg/kg of body weight [24]. Blood is drawn before and after the test, and it has been shown that the post-load draw at two hours has been validated [25]. It is thought that methionine loading could uncover up to 39% of patients with Hcy-related cardiovascular risk but with normal fasting Hcy levels [26]. As stated before, the remethylation pathway is thought to be active when there is a lack of methionine, while the transsulfuration process appears to be active during periods of methionine excess. An abnormal response to a methionine load would primarily reflect a defect in the transsulfuration pathway, but would be insensitive to defects in the remethylation pathway.

17.5 CAUSES OF HYPERHOMOCYSTEINEMIA

Plasma Hcy concentration is dependent on several factors. Genetics, nutrition, disease states, and environment all play a role in the basal Hcy level of a patient (Table 17.1).

Homocystinuria and severe hyperhomocysteinemia are caused by rare inborn errors of metabolism resulting in marked elevations of plasma and urine Hcy concentrations [27]. These inborn errors represent mutations in the metabolic pathways of methionine synthesis. Rare defects include dysfunction or deficiency of the methionine synthase enzyme and other flaws in the metabolic cycle. The most significant of these mutations is marked by a homozygous deficiency in CBS, resulting in the disorder homocystinuria. It is estimated that approximately 50% of untreated patients with homocystinuria will have an atherothromboembolic event before the age of 30 [28, 29]. Only 1% of patients presenting with coronary artery disease and hyperhomocystinemia are found to be heterozygous for CBS deficiency, making it an insensitive marker for cardiac risk.

The most common genetic mutation responsible for hyperhomocysteinemia results in a thermolabile variant of MTHFR with poor enzymatic activity. Five to fourteen percent of the population is homozygous for this C677T mutation [4, 30]. The variant is formed when a point mutation (substitution of valine to alanine) occurs in the coding region of the MTHFR binding site [28]. Homozygotes with this defect are found to have up to a 25% (2.6 μmol/L) higher total homocysteine level than wild types.

Homocysteine metabolism is a vitamin-dependent process. The absence of these cofactors (vitamin B6, vitamin B12, and folate) may result in elevated Hcy levels. Clinically it appears that up to two-thirds of cases of hyperhomocysteinemia in the elderly are thought to be secondary to vitamin deficiency [30]. Examination of the Framingham cohort reveals a strong inverse correlation between serum folate and fasting Hcy level and a weaker yet still significant inverse correlation between vitamin B12 and fasting Hcy [31].

There are a number of other etiologies known to be responsible for hyperhomocysteinemia, including a number of disease states. Hyperhomocysteinemia has been associated with both hypothyroidism and pernicious anemia [28]. As mentioned before, serum Hcy levels appear to be closely related to elevations in creatinine. In addition, several forms of cancer have been found to have an increased incidence of hyperhomocysteinemia. These carcinomas include breast, ovarian, and pancreatic [28, 32].

TABLE 17.1 Causes of Hyperhomocysteinemia

Genetic enzyme polymorphisms: methylene-tetrahydrofolate reductase, methionine synthase, cystathionine β-synthase.
Dietary deficiency: folic acid, vitamin B12, vitamin B6, methionine
Lifestyle factors: chronic alcoholism, smoking, high coffee intake
Medications: methotrexate, sulfonamides, antacids, niacin
Renal failure
Severe diabetes
Systemic lupus erythematosus
Hyperproliferative disorders

A large number of drugs and toxins appear to increase homocysteine levels. Methotrexate and phenytoin are both known to impair folate metabolism resulting in elevated Hcy in plasma. It has also been reported that both smoking and theophylline interfere with vitamin B6 synthesis, also resulting in augmented Hcy values [28].

Other causes include chronic alcohol use, high coffee intake (more than five cups daily), end stage diabetes, systemic lupus erythematosus (SLE), sulfonamides, antacids, and niacin.

17.6 THERAPEUTIC OPTIONS FOR LOWERING ELEVATED HOMOCYSTEINE

Treatment options for hyperhomocysteinemia are shown in Table 17.2. Folic acid treatment lowers tHcy by an average of 25% in patients with or without a prior history of cardiovascular diseases (CVD). Folic acid treatment appears to be more efficacious in patients with high serum tHcy and lower serum folate levels [33]. The addition of vitamin B12 produces an additional reduction in tHcy of 7%. Although vitamin B6 supplementation does not affect fasting tHcy levels, it may have a role in the treatment of post-methionine load tHcy elevation. Vitamin B6 is essential in its role as a cofactor in the transsulfuration pathway converting homocysteine to cysteine [33]. Methionine loading results in an increase in the activity of this reaction, thus augmenting the importance of vitamin B6. Betaine (trimethylglycine) is a source of remethylation of homocysteine to methionine in the liver. In patients suffering from homocystinuria, betaine supplementation can be quite effective in lowering tHcy levels [34]. However, in normal patients the efficacy in betaine treatment is much less than that of folate [35]. Betaine reduces fasting homocysteine by 12% to 20% without affecting folate levels. Choline is a precursor to betaine, and may be used as an alternative treatment for decreasing fasting or post-methionine load tHcy [36]. Fortification of foods with folate has shown mild reductions in homocysteine values in the United States [33, 37–39].

17.7 EPIDEMIOLOGIC EVIDENCE LINKING HOMOCYSTEINE AND ATHEROTHROMBOTIC VASCULAR DISEASE

Case control and prospective studies appear to demonstrate a graded association between tHcy and cardiovascular risk. Because tHcy is associated with traditional cardiac risk factors such as age, smoking, high cholesterol, hypertension, renal failure, and sedentary lifestyle, it is important to demonstrate that tHcy is an independent risk factor for cardiovascular disease.

17.7.1 Retrospective Analysis

Retrospective case-control studies consistently show an association between homocysteine and coronary artery disease (CAD). In 1995, Boushey et al. reviewed 15 cross-sectional and case-control studies examining a relationship between Hcy and ischemic heart disease. They estimated that a 5 μmol/L increase in fasting Hcy was associated with an increase in CAD of 60% in men and 80% in women [40]. The same study

TABLE 17.2   **Therapeutic Options to Lower Homocysteine**

Folic acid, 500 to 5000 μg (25% reduction in tHcy)
Vitamin B12, 1000 to 3000 μg (addition to folate adds 7% to reduction in tHcy)
Vitamin B6, 10 to 500 mg (reduction in post-methionine tHcy)
Trimethylglycine (TMG), 500 to 9000 mg (reduces fasting tHcy 20%)
Choline, 250 to 3000 mg (reduces both fasting and post-methionine tHcy)
Inositol, 250 to 1000 mg
Zinc, 30 to 90 mg
S-adenosyl-methionine, 200 to 800 mg

demonstrated a risk for peripheral vascular disease (OR 6.8, 95% CI, 2.9–15.8), and cerebrovascular disease (OR 2.5, 95% CI, 2.0–3.0) associated with elevated tHcy.

Surrogate markers also seem to be affected by hyperhomocysteinemia in retrospective studies. Elderly patients with increased Hcy concentrations were evaluated in the Framingham cohort. These patients exhibited a greater than 25% risk of having extracranial artery stenosis [41]. When patients with highest Hcy levels (>14.4 μmol/L) were compared to patients with the lowest (<9.1 μmol/L), their risk of extracranial artery stenosis was doubled. Carotid intimal-medial wall thickness also appears to increase with elevations of Hcy [42].

Elevated Hcy levels also appear to be associated with increased risk of venous thrombosis. A retrospective meta-analysis was performed which showed that for patients with homocysteine levels above the 95th percentile, an odds ratio for harm could be seen (OR 2.5, 95% CI 1.8–3.5). This phenomenon was also seen in those with elevated post-methionine load Hcy levels (OR 2.6, 95% CI 1.6–4.4) [43].

In 2002, two large independent meta-analyses were published detailing the findings of multiple retrospective studies (Table 17.3). One, the Homocysteine Studies Collaboration [44] reviewed eighteen retrospective investigations performed between 1966 and 1999. The analysis revealed that in a sample size of 7761 healthy patients, those with a 25% increase (3 μmol/L ↑) in serum Hcy were at a 49% greater risk of developing ischemic heart disease. Risk of stroke in the same set of patients also trended towards harm but was not significant (RR 1.16, 95% CI 0.99–1.37). Wald et al. presented another meta-analysis looking at 72 retrospective studies [45]. In their investigation they looked at the clinical differences between patients who were homozygous for the MTHFR gene mutation versus those who were homozygous for the normal gene. Out of the pool of 16,849 patients it was found that those with the MTHFR mutation had a 21% increased risk (RR 1.21, 95% CI 1.06–1.39) of ischemic heart disease, and a nonsignificant 31% increased risk for stroke (RR 1.31, 95% CI 0.80–2.15). For those patients with 5 μmol/L or greater elevation in Hcy, risk for ischemic heart disease (IHD) was increased by 43% (RR 1.43, 95% CI 1.11–1.84), and for stroke by 65% (RR 1.65, 95% CI 0.66–4.13).

17.7.2 Prospective Analysis

As shown above there is strong retrospective evidence of a link between Hcy levels and cardiovascular disease. Prospective studies, however, have been less robust in their ability to demonstrate such a relationship.

TABLE 17.3 Epidemiologic Evidence Linking Homocysteine and Atherothrombotic Vascular Disease

Source	Study Type (No. of Studies)	Sample Size	Variable[a]	Ischemic Heart Disease (Rate Ratio, 95% CI)	Stroke (Rate Ratio, 95% CI)
Homocysteine Studies Collaboration [44]	Retrospective (18)	7,761	+3 μmol/L tHcy	1.49 (1.41–1.61)	1.16 (0.99–1.37)
	Prospective (12)	9,025	+3 μmol/L tHcy	1.20 (1.12–1.30)	1.30 (1.11–1.52)
Wald et al. [45]				1.12 (1.04–1.20)[b]	1.23 (1.05–1.45)[b]
	Retrospective (72)	16,849	MTHFR (TT vs. wild type)	1.21 (1.06–1.39)	1.31 (0.80–2.15)
			+5 μmol/L tHcy	1.43 (1.11–1.84)	1.65 (0.66–4.13)
	Prospective (20)	3,820	+5 μmol/L tHcy	1.19 (1.12–1.25)[b]	1.32 (1.18–1.49)[b]

[a]Denotes an increase in serum homocysteine between study groups (data modified to demonstrate higher risk with higher homocysteine).
[b]Adjusted for traditional cardiovascular risk factors such as hypertension, hypercholesterolemia, diabetes, etc., and regression dilution bias.
MTHFR = Methylene-tetrahydrofolate reductase.

There have been a number of studies that have not shown consistent evidence of a connection between Hcy and CVD. For instance, the Multiple Risk Factor Intervention Trial and the Atherosclerosis Risk in Communities Study were two prospective trials that failed to show an increased risk of CVD in a hyperhomocysteinemic population [46, 47]. After adjusting for confounding variables such as traditional risk factors, no statistically significant association was observed. The Kuopio Ischemic Heart Disease Risk Factor Study followed a healthy cohort of patients and found no association between increased Hcy and coronary outcomes [48]. The Physicians' Health Study attributed increased cardiac risk to elevated Hcy, but its findings did not hold up at long-term follow up [49]. A number of studies have called into question the association between hyperhomocysteinemia and cerebrovascular disease as well. Verhoef et al. failed to show a link between elevated Hcy and ischemic stroke in their study [50]. This was also the case with a Finnish study of patients between the ages of 40 and 64 that found no association between increased Hcy values and cerebrovascular disease [51].

In contrast, several prospective studies do support the association of hyperhomocysteinemia and cardiovascular disease. The prospective Tromsø study reported a graded relationship between Hcy levels and death [52]. In 1997, Nygård et al. published a prospective study that demonstrated a mortality risk ratio of 1.6 for subjects with tHcy >15 µmol/L compared to those with tHcy at 10 µmol/L [53]. The British Regional Heart Study was a nested case control study that followed patients from 24 towns in England ranging from ages 40 to 59 with no prior history of CVA. At the end of the study it appeared that the risk of ischemic stroke paralleled a graded increase in Hcy. When comparing those patients who fell into the highest quartile of tHcy with those in the lowest, the odds ratio of stroke was 2.8 [54]. A prospective study of elderly patients followed over 9.9 years in the Framingham cohort presented data showing that patients with tHcy levels in the highest quartile had a relative risk of 1.82 (95% CI, 1.14–1.92) compared to those in the lowest quartile [55]. Two cohort studies have also shown a connection between stroke and hyperhomocysteinemia. One of the studies found that normotensive patients with higher baseline levels of Hcy were at higher risk to develop stroke [56], while the other study used a Cox regression analysis in elderly patients to show that the risk ratio for new stroke increased for each micromole of Hcy elevation. The risk ratio per micromole was 1.079 (95% CI, 1.038–1.121) [57].

Perhaps the strongest prospective data regarding homocysteine and cardiovascular disease comes from two large meta-analyses. The Homocysteine Studies Collaboration examined 9025 patients in 12 prospective studies [44]. Compared to a 49% increase in the risk of IHD associated with 25% elevation in serum homocysteine levels observed in the retrospective studies, a 20% increase (RR 1.20, 95% CI 1.12–1.30) was reported in the prospective studies. In contrast, a stronger association was reported for stroke in the prospective studies, consistent with the findings of the retrospective studies (30% increase in risk of harm [RR 95% CI 1.11–1.52] versus 16%) [4, 44] (Table 17.3). Adjustment for traditional risk factors and regression dilution bias further attenuated the association. Wald et al. [45] looked at 20 prospective trials, evaluating 3820 patients. This population of patients differed between the two groups by 5 μmol/L of Hcy value. The results of this trial when adjusted for traditional risk factors showed a risk ratio of 1.19 (95% CI 1.12–1.25) for IHD, and a risk ratio of 1.32 (95% CI 1.18–1.49) for stroke [4, 45]. The results for both outcomes were attenuated in comparison to the retrospective data.

Based on the totality of evidence, it appears that there is a graded and independent relationship between homocysteine and atherothrombotic vascular risk [4]. Stronger associations between tHcy and CVD are observed in retrospective studies, while weaker evidence is reported in more robust prospective studies. There are a number of possible reasons for this discrepancy. Confounding variables may be a factor. Homocysteine has been associated with a number of traditional risk factors that may actually be responsible for a predilection to CVD outcomes [19]. It is also associated with vitamin deficiencies and renal failure, which also may be causal factors. For example, the Kuopio Ischemic Heart Disease Risk Factor study suggested an association between CAD outcomes and folate deficiency [4, 58]. Sampling bias may also be an issue. As mentioned earlier, homocysteine concentrations have been found to rise by as much as 40% during a post-CVD event period. This being the case, retrospective studies may be sampling during a period of transient tHcy elevation, thus overestimating the association. In addition, the rise in homocysteine after a cardiovascular event may be part of an inflammatory response to tissue damage or repair [4]. This suggests that tHcy may perhaps be more a consequence than a cause of cardiovascular disease [59].

17.8   HOMOCYSTEINE AND ATHEROTHROMBOSIS: PATHOPHYSIOLOGIC MECHANISMS

In order to define Hcy as a legitimate cardiovascular risk factor, a coherent pathophysiologic mechanism(s) by which serum tHcy leads to disease needs to be established. Some of the potential mechanisms are listed in Table 17.4.

17.8.1   Endothelial Dysfunction

Laboratory investigation suggests a strong relationship between Hcy and impairment of vascular endothelial function. Aortic rings of mice in which the gene that encodes CBS was knocked out (leading to elevated Hcy levels) demonstrate impaired acetylcholine-induced endothelium-dependent vasodilator responses compared to wild-type controls [60]. Human studies have been performed examining the connection between serum Hcy and vascular physiology. Endothelium-dependent flow-mediated vasodilation has been found to vary in a number of human populations [61]. Patients found to have moderate hyperhomocystinemia or those found to be homozygous for homocystinuria, or given an oral methionine load, all exhibited impaired vasodilatation in comparison to age- and gender-matched controls [61].

A major mechanism by which hyperhomocysteinemia can impair endothelial function is related to reduced production or increased elimination of nitric oxide (NO). Studies have shown that when endothelium is either exposed to Hcy for

TABLE 17.4   Homocysteine and Atherothrombosis: Pathophysiologic Mechanisms

Atherogenesis	Thrombogenesis
• Induces vascular inflammation via expression of TNFα and iNOS • Increase oxidative strees • Induces DNA hypomethylation and gene expression for cell growth and differentiation • Promotes the oxidation of low density lipoprotein • Enhances uptake of modified lipoproteins by macrophages • Induces endothelial dysfunction 　↑ oxidant stress, ↑ asymmetric dimethylarginine (ADMA), 　↑ inflammation, ↓ bioavailability of NO • Promotes lipid accumulation via induction of HMG-CoA reductase • Stimulates vascular smooth muscle cell DNA synthesis and proliferation • Directly toxic to endothelial cells	• Induces tissue factor activity • Promotes leukocyte-endothelial interactions via MCP-1 and IL-8 • Enhances endothelial-cell associated factor V activity • Impairs inactivation of factor Va by activated protein C • Inhibits the binding of antithrombin III to the endothelium • Reduces endothelial binding sites for tissue plasminogen activator • Enhances binding of lipopoprotein (a) to fibrin • Decreases cell surface thrombomodulin and protein C activation • Increases platelet aggregation

long periods [62], or exposed to high Hcy levels [63], NO production is reduced. One proposed mechanism by which homocysteine may reduce NO levels stems from its chemical properties. Sulfhydryl compounds, such as Hcy, can form reactive oxygen species by autooxidation. Reactive oxygen (O_2^-) combines with NO, leading to the formation of peroxynitrite ($ONOO^-$), a reactive intermediate that is toxic to the endothelial cells, resulting in endothelial dysfunction. Another mechanism may be related to reduction of glutathionine peroxidase activity. This enzyme catalyzes the reduction of hydrogen and lipid peroxides to their corresponding alcohols, allowing cells to neutralize free radicals and prevent oxidative inactivation of cell components, such as NO [64]. One study exposed bovine aortic endothelial cells to serum containing high levels of Hcy [65]. When glutathione peroxidase activity was recorded, an 81% reduction was seen. Loss of NO activity may also promote atherosclerosis due to its activity in impairing platelet aggregation and leukocyte adhesion [66].

17.8.2 Endothelial Damage

Homocysteine may directly damage vascular tissues [61]. Monolayers of human umbilical vein endothelial cells have been studied noting cell detachment and loss of radiolabeled chromium as markers of cell damage [67]. The magnitude of injury increased relative to the dose of Hcy in the serum. Elevated Hcy concentration also appears to result in reactive oxygen species secondary to oxidative stress. Heterozygous CBS knockout mice fed a high methionine diet exhibited an increase in carotid artery staining for superoxide [68]. Gross pathological evidence of Hcy-related toxicity has also been demonstrated. In one study, baboons treated with intravenous doses of Hcy developed intimal lesions and vessel damage [69]. Another mechanism of injury was discovered when endothelial cell components were studied. Endothelial cells exposed to hyperhomocysteinemic serum exhibited both DNA degradation and a loss of nicotinamide adenine dinucleotide (NAD^+) consistent with exposure to free radicals [70, 71].

17.8.3 Atherothrombosis

Laboratory investigation suggests an association between hyperhomocysteinemia and both atherosclerosis and thrombosis. Experimental studies suggest that hyperhomocysteinemic mice develop atherosclerotic lesions more quickly than controls [66]. In 2001, Hofmann et al. published a study looking at the effects of a hyperhomocysteinemic diet on atherosclerosis-prone [apolipoprotein-E (apo-E)-deficient] mice [72]. At the end of the study, the aortic rings of the treated subjects had developed atherosclerotic plaques of larger size and greater complexity than those of the controls [66, 72]. When apo-E-deficient mice were crossbred with CBS-deficient mice to create a double "knockout" model, the animals developed severe hyperhomocysteinemia, and large cholesterol-rich atherosclerotic lesions [66, 73].

Elevated levels of Hcy appear to affect multiple mechanisms of coagulation and thrombosis. One in vitro study found that homocysteine helped to induce an endothelial protease that enhances factor V activity [61, 74]. Patients with hyperhomocystinuria have been found to have a higher prevalence of dysfunctional antithrombin III (reduced activity) [75]. In another study, human endothelial cells were exposed to elevated Hcy in serum, resulting in poor protein C activity. The mechanism of this finding appeared to be competitive inhibition of thrombin binding to thrombomodulin, an action necessary for the protein C pathway to function [76]. Homocysteine also appears to decrease fibrinolysis. Activation of plasminogen requires fibrin binding, this can be competitively blocked by lipoprotein(a). Hyperhomocysteinemia also promotes competitive inhibition of fibrin binding [77]. Lastly, Hcy has been shown to play a role in platelet activation. One study looked at endothelial cells exposed to Hcy in serum. The cells in culture displayed a loss of nitric oxide bioavailability resulting in platelet aggregation [78].

In conclusion, these and other investigations have provided a coherent and biologically plausible basis for homocysteine to exert a direct role in the promotion of cardiovascular disease.

17.9 IMPACT OF HOMOCYSTEINE-LOWERING THERAPY ON ATHEROTHROMBOTIC VASCULAR DISEASE

The last step in declaring Hcy as a causal risk factor for cardiovascular disease is the demonstration of risk modification based on prospective randomized trials evaluating the effects of Hcy treatment. Folic acid and vitamin B12 and B12 supplementation have been investigated in a number of randomized studies. Both surrogate markers such as restenosis, plaque area, and positive stress tests, and hard outcomes such as stroke, myocardial infarction, and death have been evaluated.

17.9.1 Surrogate Outcomes

A number of studies of Hcy treatment have proven benefit in regards to surrogate outcomes (Table 17.5). One study revealed that healthy siblings of CVD patients had a reduced incidence of positive stress electrocardiograms if they had received pre-test treatment for moderate hyperhomocysteinemia [79]. Another study of patients with mild hyperhomocysteinemia revealed that combination therapy using folate, vitamin B12, and vitamin B6 resulted in significant regression in carotid plaques [80]. Other studies have also shown Hcy treatment resulting in modification of vascular anatomy. In a population of renal transplant recipients, Hcy treatment was shown to decrease carotid intima media thickness by 32% [81]. Patients in the placebo arm actually showed a 23% increase in intima media thickness at 6 months follow up. In contrast to these studies, a recent trial examing homocysteine-lowering therapy revealed that treatment had no effect on inflammatory markers associated with atherothrombosis such as C-reactive protein, soluble intercellular adhesion molecule-1, oxidized low density lipoprotein, and autoantibodies against oxidized low density lipoprotein [82].

17.9.2 Clinical Outcomes: Impact on Vascular Restenosis

Two major trials have addressed the impact of vitamin therapy on coronary artery restenosis in hyperhomocysteinemic patients. In 2001, Schynder et al. published a prospective, double-blinded, randomized clinical trial evaluating 205 patients with baseline normal to mild hyperhomocysteinemia (11 μmol/L). A statistically significant reduction in angiographic restenosis was demonstrated with homocysteine lowering [83]. Subgroup analysis revealed that the restenosis benefit occurred in patients who underwent angioplasty (10.3% versus 41.9%, $p = 0.001$), but not in those who underwent bare-metal stenting (20.6% versus 29.9%, $p = 0.32$). The trial was extended to 533 patients to examine the effect of homocysteine-lowering therapy on major adverse cardiac events (MACE). A statistically significant reduction in MACE compared to the placebo arm was seen [84]. When each component of the composite endpoint was examined separately, the reduction in MACE could be attributed primarily to a reduction in target lesion revascularization (restenosis) but not to nonfatal myocardial infarction (MI) or death. In 2004, Lange et al. published the second study in which 636 patients were randomized to either vitamin therapy or placebo after angiography and bare metal stent placement [85]. The results showed that even in the face of successful Hcy lowering, restenosis was not reduced, but on the contrary, both MACE and restenosis were increased. Subset analysis showed that harm occurred in patients who previously had Hcy levels in the normal range (15 μmol/L) (36.2% versus 25.3%, $p = 0.02$), whereas slight but not significant benefit was observed in patients with tHcy levels >15 μmol/L (27.2% versus 31.7%, $p = $ NS). No significant effect was seen on the outcomes of death or nonfatal MI. A number of factors may help

TABLE 17.5 **Summary of Randomized Controlled Trials Investigating the Impact of Homocysteine-Lowering Therapy on Cardiovascular Outcomes**

Study	Duration	Sample Size	Treatment Groups	Outcomes Rate Ratio (95% CI)
Surrogate Outcomes				
Vermeulen et al. [79] (volunteers)	24 Months	78 80	5 mg FA, 250 mg B6 Placebo	0.4 (0.2–0.9): stress ECG 0.9 (0.6–1.3): ABI 1.0 (0.3–4.1): PAD 0.9 (0.5–1.6): carotid stenosis
Marcucci et al. [81] (post-renal transplant)	6 Months	25 28	5 mg FA, 50 mg B6, 4 mg B12 Placebo	32 ± 13% decrease in carotid intima media thickness 23 ± 21% increase in carotid intima media thickness
Clinical Outcomes: Restenosis				
Schnyder et al. [83] (post-PTCA/ stenting)	6 Months	105 100	1 mg FA, 10 mg B6, 0.4 mg B12 Placebo	0.46 (0.28–0.73): restenosis 0.52 (0.28–0.98): MACE 0.48 (0.25–0.94): TLR
Swiss Heart Study, Schnyder et al. [84] (post-PTCA/stenting)	12 Months	272 281	1 mg FA, 10 mg B6, 0.4 mg B12 Placebo (×6 months)	0.68 (0.48–0.96): MACE 0.62 (0.40-0.97): TLR 0.60 (0.24–1.51): nonfatal MI 0.52 (0.13–2.04): cardiac death 0.54 (0.16–1.70): mortality

Study	Duration	N	Intervention	Results
Lange et al. [85] (post-stenting)	6 Months	316 320	1.2 mg FA, 48 mg B6, 60 μg B12 Placebo	1.30 (1.0–1.69): restenosis 1.53 (1.03–2.28): MACE

Clinical Outcomes: Hard Endpoints

Study	Duration	N	Intervention	Results
VISP trial [88] (post-stroke)	24 Months	1,827 (high-dose) 1,853 (low-dose)	2.5 mg FA, 25 mg B6, 0.4 mg B12 0.02 mg FA, 0.2 mg B6, 6 μg B12	1.0 (0.8–1.3): recurrent stroke 0.9 (0.7–1.2): MACE 0.9 (0.7–1.1): mortality
NORVIT trial [89] (post MI)	40 Months	937 935 934 943	0.8 mg FA, 40 mg B6, 0.4 mg B12 (group A) 0.8 mg FA, 0.4 mg B12 (group B) 40 mg B6 (group C) Placebo (group D)	[Results Groups A + B vs Groups C + D] 1.08 (0.93–1.25) MI, stroke, SCD 1.02 (0.83–1.26): death 1.06 (0.91–1.24): MI 1.02 (0.68–1.51): stroke 1.22 (0.88–1.70): cancer [Results: Group A vs. Group D] 1.22 (1.00–1.50): MI, stroke, SCD 1.21 (0.91–1.61): death 1.23 (0.99–1.52): MI 0.83 (0.47–1.47): stroke 1.02 (0.65–1.58): cancer
HOPE-2 trial [90] (vascular disease, diabetes)	60 Months	2,758 2,764	2.5 mg FA, 50 mg B6, 1.0 mg B12 Placebo	0.95 (0.84–1.07): CV death, MI, stroke 0.96 (0.81–1.13): CV death 0.98 (0.85–1.14): MI 0.75 (0.59–0.97): stroke

Abbreviations: ABI: atherothrombotic brain infarction; CV: cardiovascular; ECG: electrocardiogram; FA: folic acid; MACE: major adverse cardiac events; MI; myocardial infarction; PAD: peripheral arterial disease; PTCA: percutaneous transluminal coronary angioplasty; SCD: sudden cardiovascular death; TLR: target lesion revascularization.

427

explain the divergent findings of this study in comparison to the previously reported study. For instance, the Lange trial employed a higher treatment dose of folate and vitamins, especially vitamin B6 (including intravenous loading). Other factors include the widespread use of bare-metal stents in the Lange trial (100% versus 50% in past studies), longer average coronary lesion length in comparison to earlier studies, higher risk patients in earlier studies (participants in prior studies had a higher proportion of smokers, diabetics, and prior known CAD); higher serum Hcy levels; and limited angiographic follow-up (76% compared with 100%).

17.9.3   Clinical Outcomes: Impact on Hard Vascular Events

Recently, several randomized controlled trials have been published evaluating the effects of supplemental folic acid and B vitamins on the risk of cardiovascular disease. Two of the initial studies failed to show any benefit in regards to cardiovascular events when adding folic acid to statin therapy. The studies were small open label trials, the FOLARDA study (Folic Acid on Risk Diminishment after Acute Myocardial Infarction) looked at a population of post-acute MI patients [86], while the Goes study looked at those diagnosed with stable CAD [87].

More data have been recently compiled with the completion of three large, multi-center, double-blind, randomized controlled trials. Each trial looked at the impact of Hcy-lowering therapy on cardiovascular events in high risk patients.

The VISP (Vitamin Intervention for Stroke Prevention) study was the first large-scale randomized interventional trial to report hard endpoints [88]. The trial evaluated the difference in Hcy treatment when using high versus low dose vitamin B therapy in patients with ischemic stroke. The high dose formulation appeared to have no significant effect on the outcomes of recurrent stroke, coronary events, or death. These results were in contrast to what investigators had expected, and suggested that though elevated Hcy and CVD risk may be associated, therapy could be inconsequential. Kaul et al. have noted a number of limitations of the VISP trial [4]. For one, the difference in Hcy concentration (2 μmol/L) between treatment arms was minimal. The patient population studied had very mild hyperhomocysteinemia above baseline (possibly reflecting the effects of widespread folic acid fortification in North America); this may have masked the effect of therapy on stroke events. In addition, patients in both arms were treated with a low dose vitamin supplementation during the 1-month run-in phase; possibly normalizing vitamin status in both groups, making further therapy overkill. There were also a number of issues with results and design. The recurrent stroke rate was lower than anticipated, follow-up period was short (2 years), and the trial was not placebo-controlled, but rather a comparison of two treatment doses (high versus low). All of these factors limited the statistical power of the VISP trial to reliably identify or exclude a modest but clinically important therapeutic effect of vitamin therapy.

The NORVIT (Norwegian Vitamin Trial) tested the hypothesis that long-term (median follow-up of 40 months) treatment with B vitamins would lower the incidence of MI, stroke, and sudden cardiac death in patients with acute MI [89]. One difference from the VISP trial was the treatment of patients from a region without folate fortification. Nearly 3750 Norwegian patients were enrolled and randomized into four groups. Plasma Hcy levels decreased by about 27% in patients taking folic acid (whether or not they were also taking vitamin B6) compared with vitamin B6- and placebo-treated patients. Plasma folate levels rose six- to sevenfold with folic acid treatment [4]. The primary endpoint occurred in approximately 18% of each of the placebo, folic acid vitamin B12, and vitamin B6 groups [89]. In the group that received combination therapy (folic acid, vitamin B12,vitamin B6), however, there was a nominally significant relative increase in the primary endpoint by 22% ($p = 0.05$) and nonfatal MI by 30% ($p = 0.05$), and a nonsignificant 17% decrease ($p = 0.52$) in stroke versus placebo. The cumulative hazard ratio for the combination therapy group, as compared with the other three groups, was 1.20 (95% CI 1.02–1.41). Event rates, including individual components of the primary endpoint, tended to be higher in the folic acid, vitamin B12 group versus vitamin B6 and the placebo group. Subgroup analyses showed no suggestion of benefit in any subgroup.

The HOPE-2 (Heart Outcomes Prevention Evaluation-2) trial examined the effects of folate and vitamin therapy in a group of patients 55 or older with prior histories of vascular disease or diabetes [90]. The 5 year study enrolled 5522 patients, 70% of whom were from countries with folate-fortified diets. The two arms of the study included subjects randomized to daily treatment with a combined pill containing 2.5 mg of folic acid, 50 mg of vitamin B6, and 1 mg of vitamin B12, and subjects randomized to placebo. The primary composite outcome was cardiac death, MI, and stroke. Treatment led to a mean decrease in Hcy of 2.4 μmol/L (0.3 mg/L) versus a slight increase of 0.8 μmol/L in those receiving placebo. Despite effective reduction in homocysteine levels no significant effect was seen on the primary outcome or the individual components except for a 25% reduction in stroke [4, 90]. An increase in the number of patients hospitalized for unstable angina was observed with active treatment. Subgroup analysis showed no evidence of benefit in any group, regardless of initial Hcy level or country of origin (issue of folate fortification).

A large meta-analysis was performed by Bazzano et al. looking at trial data regarding the effect of Hcy therapy on clinical outcomes (Table 17.6) [91]. The investigators

TABLE 17.6   The Impact of Folate Theraphy on Clinical Outcomes

Endpoint (No. of Trials)	Sample Size	Summary RR (95% CI)	P Value	Heterogeneity P Value	I^2 Statistic
Cardiovascular disease[a] (10)	14,440	0.95 (0.88–1.03)	0.18	0.33	12%
Coronary heart disease[a] (11)	16,877	1.04 (0.92–1.17)	0.57	0.15	31%
Stroke[a] (8)	13,806	0.86 (0.71–1.04)	0.11	0.27	20%
Mortality, all causes[a] (10)	14,995	0.96 (0.88–1.04)	0.32	0.87	0%
Stroke[b] (8)	16,841	0.82 (0.68–1)	0.05	0.22	26%

[a]Data from Bazzano et al. [91].
[b]Data from Wang et al. [98].

felt that the published results seemed inconsistent, and that individually they had insufficient statistical power on their own. Trials felt to meet eligibility needed to be randomized and controlled, record all CVD events as well as death, use folic acid in the intervention arm, and have a follow-up of 6 months or more. Twelve trials were included representing data from 16,958 participants [84–90, 92–97]. Dosage of folic acid in the intervention groups ranged from 0.5 to 15 mg/d, and duration of follow-up ranged from 6 months to 5 years. Homocysteine reduction ranged from 1.5 to 26 μmol/L. No statistically significant benefit of vitamin therapy was seen on a random effects meta-analysis (CVD, RR 0.95, 95% CI 0.88–1.03; coronary heart disease [CHD], RR 1.04, 95% CI 0.92–1.17; stroke, RR 0.86, 95% CI 0.71–1.04; mortality, all causes, RR 0.96, 95% CI 0.88–1.04). Heterogeneity appeared to be minimal among the trials. The authors felt that their analysis was more robust than others performed in the past, because of a lack of confounding and bias (only randomized controlled trials included), and the absence of heterogeneity. The authors did state, however, that even with their large sample size they only reached 84% power to detect a 10% reduction in CVD risk and 64% power to detect a 10% reduction in total mortality. They felt that only after all of the ongoing multicenter trials are finished could an analysis be performed with sufficient power to determine if a 25% reduction in homocysteine could reduce CHD risk by 10%.

The most recent meta-analysis addressing Hcy-lowering therapy and cardiovascular endpoints was reported by Wang et al. [98]. This review looked at many of the same studies included in the meta-analysis performed by Bazzano et al. [91]; however, one trial by Liem et al. [87] was excluded since it derived its results from the same study population as another report [94], and another study was added [99]. The additional study was the Linxian Nutrition Intervention, a trial performed in China evaluating the benefits of folic acid supplementation over a follow-up of 72 months. Once the results of the trial were pooled, it appeared that folic acid supplementation (with or without other B vitamins) did in fact significantly reduce risk of stroke (RR 0.82, 95% CI 0.68–1.00). In addition, on the basis of subgroup analysis, the authors speculated that the stroke benefit of folate treatment would be greatest in regions where one would expect the largest reduction in Hcy (non folate-fortified regions). They also theorized that since atherosclerosis is a long and insidious disease, perhaps the beneficial effects of folic acid therapy also needed time to come to light. Trials with an intervention duration of >36 months were found to have a greater, but not statistically significant, risk reduction of stroke than those with a shorter duration of follow-up (RR 0.89, 95% CI 0.55–1.42 versus RR 0.75, 95% CI 0.62–0.91).

The data from the three largest completed trials of Hcy lowering with folic acid and vitamin B12 with or without vitamin B6 (VISP [88], NORVIT [89], and HOPE-2 [90]) consistently demonstrate no treatment benefit in patients with established vascular disease. These trials primarily evaluated white, middle-aged patients exposed to folate-fortified food (70% in HOPE-2, 100% in VISP) with only mild increases in Hcy levels (<15 μmol/L). It is possible that homocysteine-lowering therapy might potentially still prove to be beneficial in populations other than those studied—for example, in Southeast Asian patients where homocysteine levels typically exceed 15 μmol/L related to genetic or dietary factors. However, subgroup analyses of the

NORVIT and HOPE-2 trials provide useful insights. In 40% of patients in the NORVIT trial with a baseline Hcy level above 13 μmol/L (mean homocysteine level was 17.4 μmol/L in this subgroup), homocysteine-lowering therapy provided no benefit. Similarly, no treatment benefit was observed among patients in the upper fifth of the baseline homocysteine distribution ($\geq$19.7 μmol/L) in HOPE-2. It is quite possible that this lack of benefit may be related to inadequate statistical power in these subgroups. Thus, whether homocysteine-lowering therapy is going to be beneficial cannot be answered definitively until prospective, randomized trials are conducted in these populations. Ongoing large trials that are currently exploring these issues and the planned meta-analyses of all trials (12 trials involving about 52,000 participants with adequate statistical power, 7 in populations without fortification, and 5 in populations with fortification) [100] might help answer remaining relevant clinical questions.

17.10 CONCLUSIONS

Severe elevation of Hcy concentration in patients with homocystinuria leads to a high incidence of premature atherothrombotic events. In vitro and in vivo studies have demonstrated a myriad of biologically plausible mechanisms whereby Hcy may promote atherosclerotic and thrombotic vascular disease. Multiple observational studies have also provided evidence that mild to moderately elevated Hcy levels enhance vascular risk in both the general population and in those with a history of CAD. The overall risk for vascular disease is small, with prospective studies reporting weaker association compared to retrospective studies. Lastly, the evidence base has failed to prove thus far that homocysteine-lowering therapy makes a consistent and significant impact on hard clinical outcomes. After a comprehensive review of each of these issues, it appears prudent to conclude that the role of Hcy as either a mediator or marker of cardiovascular risk remains unclear at this time.

Even though the clinical uses of Hcy remain indefinite, physicians can implement the current knowledge to make valid decisions regarding its utility. A structured approach based on recommendations of a number of expert panels is summarized in Table 17.7.

With regards to screening, routine examination of Hcy levels is not yet recommended. However, screening may be advisable for individuals who manifest atherothrombotic disease that is out of proportion to their traditional risk factors or who have a family history of premature atherosclerotic disease. Proper measurement may be performed using one of two methods. Clinicians may draw either fasting Hcy concentrations or post-methionine load levels. It is important that blood samples be processed quickly to ensure accurate results, and that standardization is enacted to minimize variation among laboratories. A uniform normal range should be established, with separate limits based on presence of folate fortification (without folate [upper limit of normal of 15 μmol/L] and with folate [12 μmol/L]). Vitamin supplementation with folate, B6, and B12 has been shown to significantly lower homocysteine concentration and benefit surrogate cardiovascular outcomes.

TABLE 17.7   Summary of Recommendation for Screening and Treatment of Elevated Homocysteine

Screening	• Routine screening not yet recommended
	• Screening may be advisable in individuals who:
	- Manifest disease out of proportion to traditional risk factors
	- Have a family history of premature atherosclerotic disease
Measurement	• Plasma (or serum) total homocysteine, fasting or post-methionine load (more sensitive)
	• Blood samples must be processed quickly (<1 h at room temperature, <8 h on ice)
	• Enzymatic or immunologic assays more practical than chromatographic assays
	• Standardization required to minimize variation among laboratories
	• Normal range 5 to 15 μmol/L (12 μmol/L as upper limit with folate fortification)
Treatment	• Routine treatment with vitamin supplements not yet recommended
	• Diet rich in folate and B vitamins encouraged
	• Treatment with folate (0.5 to 5 mg) and vitamin B12 (0.5–1 mg) may be beneficial in high risk patients
	• Therapeutic target in high risk individuals <10 μmol/L (U.S.), <13–15 μmol/L (EU)
	• Vitamin B12 status should be determined before starting therapy

The recommendations are based on a European Expert Panel, the American Heart Association Science Advisory Statement, the U.S. Preventive Services Task Force, and the American College of Cardiology Foundation Complementary Medicine Expert Consensus Document.

Currently, however, there is no evidence that vitamin B supplementation reduces cardiovascular risk, and there may even be a suggestion of potential harm with treatment with high-dose vitamin B. Given these findings there has been a renewed scrutiny of homocysteine's role in atherothrombotic vascular disease. Whether Hcy is causative in the pathogenesis of atherothrombotic vascular disease will have to await the completion of a number of large, randomized controlled trials currently studying the effect of homocysteine-lowering vitamins on cardiovascular endpoints. Until then, the elevation of Hcy to the pantheon of risk factors for vascular disease remains an elusive goal.

REFERENCES

1. Von Eckardstein, A. (2004). Is there a need for novel cardiovascular risk factors? *Nephrology, Dialysis, Transplantation*, *19*, 761–765.
2. McCully, K.S. (1969). Vascular pathology of homocysteinemia: Implications for the pathogenesis of arteriosclerosis. *American Journal of Pathology*, *56*, 111–128.

3. Wilcken, D.E., Wilcken, B. (1976). The pathogenesis of coronary artery disease: A possible role for methionine metabolism. *Journal of Clinical Investigation, 57,* 1079–1082.

4. Kaul, S., Zadeh, A.A., Shah, P.K. (2006). Homocysteine hypothesis for atherothrombotic cardiovascular disease, not validated. *Journal of the American College of Cardiology, 48,* 914–923.

5. Selhub, J. (1999). Homocysteine metabolism. *Annual Review of Nutrition, 19,* 217–246.

6. Ueland, P.M., Refsum, H., Stabler, S., Manilow, M.R., Andersson, A., Allen, R.H. (1993). Total homocysteine in plasma or serum: Methods and clinical applications. *Clinical Chemistry, 39*(9), 1764–1779.

7. Refsum, H., Helland, S., Ueland, P.M. (1985). Radioenzymic determination of homocysteine in plasma and urine. *Clinical Chemistry, 31,* 624–628.

8. Mansoor, M.A., Ueland, P.M., Aarsland, A., Svardal, A.M. (1993). Redox status and protein binding of plasma homocysteine and other aminothiols in patients with homocystinuria. *Metabolism, 42,* 1481–1485.

9. Tzakas, P.A.N., Langman, L.J., Evrosky, J., Cole, D.E.C. (2000). The importance of serum proteins in the interpretation of total homocysteine. *Clinical Biochemistry, 33,* 240–241.

10. Guttormsen, A.B., Schneede, J., Finkerstrand, T., Ueland, P.M., Refsum, H.M. (1994). Plasma concentrations of homocysteine and other aminothiol compounds are related to food intake in healthy human subjects. *Journal of Nutrition, 124,* 1934–1941.

11. McKinley, M.C., Strain, J.J., McPartlin, J., Scott, J.M., McNulty, H. (2001). Plasma homocysteine is not subject to seasonal variation. *Clinical Chemistry, 47,* 1430–1436.

12. Andersson, A., Isaksson, A., Hultberg, B. (1992). Homocysteine export from erythrocytes and its implication for plasma sampling. *Clinical Chemistry, 38,* 1311–1315.

13. Hortin, G.L. (2006). Homocysteine: Clinical significance and laboratory measurement. *Laboratory Medicine, 37*(9), 551–553.

14. Nexo, E., Engbaek, F., Ueland, P.M., Westby, C., O'Gorman, P., Johnston, C., Kase, B.F., Guttormsen, A.B., Alfheim, I., McPartlin, J., Smith, D., Møller, J., Rasmussen, K., Clarke, R., Scott, J.M., Refsum, H. (2000). Evaluation of novel assays in clinical chemistry: Quantification of plasma total homocysteine. *Clinical Chemistry, 46,* 1150–1156.

15. Roberts, R.F., Roberts, W.L. (2004). Performance characteristics of a recombinant enzymatic cycling assay for quantification of total homocysteine in serum or plasma. *Clinica Chimica Acta, 344,* 95–99.

16. Tan, Y., Sun, X., Tang, L., Zhang, N., Han, Q., Xu, M., Tan, X., Hoffman, R.M. (2003). Automated enzymatic assay for homocysteine. *Clinical Chemistry, 49,* 1029–1030.

17. Dou, C., Xia, D., Zhang, L., Chen, X., Flores, P., Datta, A., Yuan, C. (2005). Development of a novel enzymatic cycling assay for total homocysteine. *Clinical Chemistry, 51,* 1987–1989.

18. Tuschl, K., Bodamer, O.A., Erwa, W., Muhl, A. (2005). Rapid analysis of total plasma homocysteine by tandem mass spectrometry. *Clinica Chimica Acta, 351,* 139–141.

19. Nygard, O., Vollset, S.E., Refsum, H., Stensvold, I., Tverdal, A., Nordrehaug, J.E., Ueland, M., Kvale, G. (1995). Total plasma homocysteine and cardiovascular risk profile. The Hordaland Homocysteine Study. *JAMA, 274,* 1526–1533.

20. Refsum, H., Smith, A.D., Ueland, P.M., Nexo, E., Clarke, R., McPartlin, J., Johnston, C., Engbaek, F., Schneede, J., McPartlin, C., Scott J.M. (2004). Facts and recommendations

about total homocysteine determinations: An expert opinion. *Clinical Chemistry*, *50*, 3–32.

21. Auer, J., Eber, B. (1999). Homocysteine and fibrinolysis in acute occlusive coronary events. *Lancet*, *354*, 1474–1475.

22. Egerton, W., Silberberg, J., Crooks, R., Ray, C., Xie, L., Dudman, N. (1996). Serial measures of plasma homocysteine after acute myocardial infarction. *American Journal of Cardiology*, *77*, 759–761.

23. Landgren, F., Israelsson, B., Lindgren, A., Hultberg, B., Andersson, A., Brattstrom, L. (1995). Plasma homocysteine in acute myocardial infarction: Homocysteine-lowering effect of folic acid. *Journal of Internal Medicine*, *237*, 381–388.

24. Malinow, M.R., Bostom, A.G., Krauss, R.M. (1999). Homocysteine, diet, and cardiovascular diseases. a statement for healthcare professionals from the Nutrition Committee, American Heart Association. *Circulation*, *99*, 178–182.

25. Bostom, A.G., Roubenoff, R., Dellaripa, P., Nadeau, M.R., Sutherland, P., Wilson, P.W., Jacques, P.F., Selhub, J., Rosenberg, I.H. (1995). Validation of abbreviated oral methionine-loading test. *Clinical Chemistry*, *41*, 948–949.

26. Bostom, A.G., Jacques, P.F., Nadeau, M.R., Williams, R.R., Ellison, R.C., Selhub, J. (1995). Post-methionine load hyperhomocysteinemia in persons with normal fasting total plasma homocysteine: Initial results from the NHLBI Family Heart Study. *Atherosclerosis*, *116*, 147–151.

27. Mudd, S.H., Levy, H.L., Skovby, F. (1995). Disorders of transsulfuration. In Scriver, C.R., Beaudet, A.L., Sly, W.S., Valle, D., Eds., *The Metabolic and Molecular Basis of Inherited Disease*, 7th ed., Vol. 1, pp. 1279–1327. New York: McGraw-Hill.

28. Welch, G.N., Loscalzo, J. (1998). Homocysteine and atherothrombosis. *New England Journal of Medicine*, *338*, 1042–1050.

29. Klerk, M., Verhoef, P., Clarke, R., Blom, H.J., Schouten, E.G. (2002). MTHFR Studies Collaboration Group. MTHFR 677C→T polymorphism and risk of coronary heart disease: A meta-analysis. *JAMA*, *288*, 2023–2031.

30. Selub, J., Jacques, P.F., Wilson, P.W., Rush, D., Rosenberg, I.H. (1993). Vitamin status and intake as primary determinants of homocysteinemia in an elderly population. *JAMA*, *270*, 2693–2698.

31. Tsai, M.Y., Welge, B.G., Hanson, N.Q., Bignell, M.K., Vessey, J., Schwichtenberg, K., Yang, F., Bullemer, F.E., Rasmussen, R., Graham, K.J. (1999). Genetic causes of mild hyperhomocysteinemia in patients with premature occlusive coronary artery diseases. *Atherosclerosis*, *143*, 163–170.

32. Ueland, P.M., Refsum, H. (1989). Plasma homocysteine, a risk factor for vascular disease: Plasma levels in health, disease, and drug therapy. *Journal of Laboratory and Clinical Medicine*, *114*, 473–501.

33. Booth, G.L., Wang, E.E.L., with the Canadian Task Force on Preventive Health Care. (2000). Preventive health care, 2000 update: Screening and management of hyperhomocysteinemia for the prevention of coronary artery disease events. *Canadian Medical Association Journal*, *163*(1), 21–29.

34. Wilcken, D.E. (1997). The natural history of vascular disease in homocystinuria and the effects of treatment. *Journal of Inherited Metabolic Diseases*, *20*, 295–300.

35. Brouwer, I.A., Verhoef, P., Urgert, R. (2000). Betaine supplementation and plasma homocysteine in healthy volunteers. *Archives of Internal Medicine*, *160*, 2546–2547.

36. Olthof, M.R., Brink, E.J., Katan, M.B., Verhoef, P. (2005). Choline supplemented as phosphatidylcholine decreases fasting and postmethionine-loading plasma homocysteine concentrations in healthy men. *American Journal of Clinical Nutrition, 82,* 111–117.

37. Schorah, C.J., Devitt, H., Lucock, M., Dowell, A.C. (1998). The responsiveness of plasma homocysteine to small increases in dietary folic acid: A primary care study. *European Journal of Clinical Nutrition, 52,* 407–411.

38. Jacques, P.F., Selhub, J., Bostom, A.G., Wilson, P.W.F., Rosenberg, I.H. (1999). The effect of folic acid fortification on plasma folate and total homocysteine concentrations. *New England Journal of Medicine, 340,* 1449–1454.

39. Malinow, M.R., Duell, P.B., Hess, D.L., Anderson, P.H., Kruger, W.D., Phillipson, B.E., Gluckman, R.A. (1998). Reduction of plasma homocyst(e)ine levels by breakfast cereal fortified with folic acid in patients with coronary heart disease. *New England Journal of Medicine, 338,* 1009–1015.

40. Boushey, C.J., Beresford, S.A., Omenn, G.S., Motulsky, A.G. (1995). A quantitative assessment of plasma homocysteine as a risk factor for vascular disease. Probable benefits of increasing folic acid intakes. *JAMA, 274,* 1049–1057.

41. Selhub, J., Jacques, P.F., Bostom, A.G., D'Agostino, R.B., Wilson, P.W.F., Belanger, A.J., O'Leary, D.H., Wolf, P.A., Schaefer, E.J., Rosenberg, I.H. (1995). Association between plasma homocysteine concentrations and extracranial carotid artery stenosis. *New England Journal of Medicine, 332,* 286–291.

42. Tsai, M.Y., Arnett, D.K., Eckfeldt, J.H., Williams, R.R., Ellison, R.C. (2000). Plasma homocysteine and its association with carotid intimal-medial wall thickness and prevalent coronary heart disease: NHLBI Family Heart Study. *Atherosclerosis, 151,* 519–524.

43. den Heijer, M., Rosendaal, F.R., Blom, H.J., Gerrit, W.B., Bos, G.M. (1998). Hyperhomocysteinemia and venous thrombosis: A meta-analysis. *Thrombosis and Haemostasis, 80,* 874–877.

44. Homocysteine Studies Collaboration. (2002). Homocysteine and risk of ischemic heart disease and stroke: A meta-analysis. *JAMA, 288,* 2015–2022.

45. Wald, D.S., Law, M., Morris, J.K. (2002). Homocysteine and cardiovascular disease: Evidence on causality from a meta-analysis. *British Medical Journal, 325,* 1202–1206.

46. Evans, R.W., Shaten, B.J., Hempel, J.D., Cutler, J.A., Kuller, L.H. (1997). Homocysteine and risk of cardiovascular disease in the Multiple Risk Factor Intervention Trial. *Arteriosclerosis, Thrombosis, and Vascular Biology, 17,* 1947–1953.

47. Folsom, A.R., Nieto, F.J., McGovern, P.G., Tsai, M.Y., Malinow, M.R., Eckfeldt, J.H., Hess, D.L., Davis, D.E. (1998). Prospective study of coronary heart disease incidence in relation to fasting total homocysteine, related genetic polymorphisms, and B vitamins: The Atherosclerosis Risk in Communities (ARIC) study. *Circulation, 98,* 204–210.

48. Voutilainen, S., Lakka, T.A., Hamelahti, P., Lehtimaki, T., Poulsen, H.E., Salonen, J.T. (2000). Plasma total homocysteine concentration and the risk of acute coronary events: The Kuopio Ischaemic Heart Disease Risk Factor Study. *Journal of Internal Medicine, 248,* 217–222.

49. Stampfer, M.J., Malinow, M.R., Willett, W.C., Newcomer, L.M., Upson, B., Ullmann, D., Tishler, P.V., Hennekens, C.H. (1992). A prospective study of plasma homocyst(e)ine and risk of myocardial infarction in US physicians. *JAMA, 268,* 877–881.

50. Verhoef, P., Hennekens, C.H., Malinow, M.R., Kok, F.J., Willett, W.C., Stampfer, M.J. (1994). A prospective study of plasma homocyst(e)ine and risk of ischemic stroke. *Stroke*, *25*, 1924–1930.

51. Alfthan, G., Pekkanen, J., Jauhiainen, M., Pitkaniemi, J., Karvonen, M., Tuomilehto, J., Salonen, J.T., Ehnholm, C. (1994). Relation of serum homocysteine and lipoprotein(a) concentrations to atherosclerotic disease in a prospective Finnish population based study. *Atherosclerosis*, *106*, 9–19.

52. Arnesen, E., Refsum, H., Bonaa, K.H., Ueland, P.M., Forde, O.H., Nordrehaug, J.E. (1995). Serum total homocysteine and coronary heart disease. *International Journal of Epidemiology*, *24*, 704–709.

53. Nygård, O., Nordrehaug, J.E., Refsum, H., Ueland, P.M., Farstad, M., Vollset, S.E. (1997). Plasma homocysteine levels and mortality in patients with coronary artery disease. *New England Journal of Medicine*, *337*, 230–236.

54. Perry, I.J., Refsum, H., Morris, R.W., Ebrahim, S.B., Ueland, P.M., Shaper, A.G. (1995). Prospective study of serum total homocysteine concentration and risk of stroke in middle aged British men. *Lancet*, *346*, 1395–1398.

55. Bostom, A.G., Rosenberg, I.H., Silbershatz, H., Jacques, P.F., Selhub, J., D'Agostino, R.B., Wilson, P.W.F. (1999). Nonfasting plasma total homocysteine levels and stroke incidence in elderly persons: The Framingham study. *Annals of Internal Medicine*, *131*, 352–355.

56. Stewhouwer, C.D., Weijenberg, M.P., van den Berg, M., Jakobs, C., Feskens, E.J.M., Kromhout, D. (1998). Serum homocysteine and risk of coronary heart disease and cerebrovascular disease in elderly men: A 10 year follow up. *Arteriosclerosis, Thrombosis, and Vascular Biology*, *18*, 1895–1901.

57. Aronow, W.S., Ahn, C., Gutstein, H. (2000). Increased plasma homocysteine is an independent predictor of new atherothrombotic brain infarction in older persons. *American Journal of Cardiology*, *86*, 585–586.

58. Voutilainen, S., Virtanen, J.K., Rissanen, T.H., Alfthan, G., Laukkanen, J., Nyyssönen, K., Mursu, J., Valkonen, V., Tuomainen, T., Kaplan, G.A., Salonen, J.T. (2004). Serum folate and homocysteine and the incidence of acute coronary events: The Kuopio Ischaemic Heart Disease Risk Factor Study. *American Journal of Clinical Nutrition*, *80*, 317–323.

59. Dudman, N.P. (1999). An alternative view of homocysteine. *Lancet*, *354*, 2072–2074.

60. Dayal, S., Bottiglieri, T., Aming, E. (2001). Endothelial dysfunction and elevation of S-adenosylhomocysteine in cystathionine β-synthase-deficient mice. *Circulation Research*, *88*, 1203–1209.

61. Thambyrajah, J., Townend, J.N. (2000). Homocysteine and atherothrombosis: Mechanisms for injury. *European Heart Journal*, *21*, 967–974.

62. Stamler, J.S., Osborne, J.A., Jaraki, O., Rabbani, L.E., Mullins, M., Singel, D., Loscalzo, J. (1993). Adverse vascular effects of homocysteine are modulated by endothelium derived relaxing factor and related oxides of nitrogen. *Journal of Clinical Investigation*, *91*, 308–318.

63. Upchurch, G.R., Jr., Welch, G.N., Loscalzo, J. (1996). Homocysteine, EDRF and endothelial function. *Journal of Nutrition*, *126*(4 Suppl), 1290S–1294S.

64. Loscalzo, J. (1996). The oxidant stress of hyperhomocysteinemia. *Journal of Clinical Investigation*, *98*, 5–7.

65. Upchurch, G.R., Jr., Welch, G.N., Fabian, A.J., Freedman, J.E., Johnson, J.L., Keaney, J.L., Jr., Loscalzo, J. (1997). Homocysteine decreases bioavailable nitric oxide by a mechanism involving glutathione peroxidase. *Journal of Biological Chemistry*, *272*, 17012–17017.

66. Lentz, S.R. (2005). Mechanisms of homocysteine-induced athrerothrombosis. *Journal of Thrombosis and Haemostasis*, *3*, 1646–1654.

67. Wall, R.T., Harlan, J.M., Harker, L.A., Striker, G.E. (1980). Homocysteine induced endothelial cell injury in vitro: A model for the study of vascular injury. *Thrombosis Research*, *18*, 113–121.

68. Dayal, S., Arning, E., Bottiglieri, T., Böger, R.H., Sigmund, C.D., Faraci, F.M., and Lentz, S.R. (2004). Cerebral vascular dysfunction mediated by superoxide in hyperhomocysteinemic mice. *Stroke*, *35*, 1957–1962.

69. Harker, L.A., Ross, R., Slichter, S.J., Scott, C.R. (1976). Homocysteine induced arteriosclerosis. The role of endothelial cell injury and platelet response in its genesis. *Journal of Clinical Investigation*, *58*, 731–741.

70. Blundell, G., Jones, B.G., Rose, F.A., Tudball, N. (1996). Homocysteine mediated endothelial cell toxicity and its amelioration. *Atherosclerosis*, *122*, 163–172.

71. Kirkland, J.B. (1991). Lipid peroxidation, protein thiol oxidation and DNA damage in hydrogen peroxide induced injury to endothelial cells: Role of activation of poly(ADP-ribose)polymerase. *Biochimica et Biophysica Acta*, *1092*, 319–325.

72. Hofmann, M.A., Lalla, E., Lu, Y., Gleason, M.R., Wolf, B.M., Tanji, N., Ferran, L.J., Kohl, B., Rao,V., Kisiel, W., Stern, D.M., Schmidt, A.M. (2001). Hyperhomocysteinemia enhances vascular inflammation and accelerates atherosclerosis in a murine model. *Journal of Clinical Investigation*, *107*, 675–683.

73. Wang, H., Jiang, X., Yang, F., Gaubatz, J.W., Ma, L., Magera, M.J., Yang, X.F., Berger, X.F., Durante, W., Pownall, H.J., Schafer, A.I. (2003). Hyperhomocysteinemia accelerates atherosclerosis in cystathionine beta-synthase and apolipoprotein E double knock-out mice with and without dietary perturbation. *Blood*, *101*, 3901–3907.

74. Rodgers, G.M., Kane, W.H. (1986). Activation of endogenous factor V by a homocysteine induced vascular endothelial cell activator. *Journal of Clinical Investigation*, *77*, 1909–1916.

75. Palareti, G., Salardi, S., Piazzi, S., Legnani, C., Poggi, M., Grauso, F., Caniato, A., Coccheri, S., Cacciari, E. (1986). Blood coagulation changes in homocystinuria: Effects of pyridoxine and other specific therapy. *Journal of Pediatrics*, *109*, 1001–1006.

76. Rodgers, G.M., Conn, M.T. (1990). Homocysteine, an atherogenic stimulus, reduces protein C activation by arterial and venous endothelial cells. *Blood*, *75*, 895–901.

77. Harpel, P.C., Chang, V.T., Borth, W. (1992). Homocysteine and other sulfhydryl compounds enhance the binding of lipoprotein(a) to fibrin: A potential biochemical link between thrombosis, atherogenesis, and sulfhydryl compound metabolism. *Proceedings of the National Academy of Sciences USA*, *89*, 10193–10197.

78. Stamler, J.S., Osborne, J.A., Jaraki, O., Rabbani, L.E., Mullins, M., Singel, D., Loscalzo, J. (1993). Adverse vascular effects of homocysteine are modulated by endothelium derived relaxing factor and related oxides of nitrogen. *Journal of Clinical Investigation*, *91*, 308–318.

79. Vermeulen, E.G., Stehouwer, C.D., Twisk, J.W., van den Berg, M., de Jong, S.C., Mackaay, A.J., van Campen, C.M., Visser, F.C., Jakobs, C.A., Bulterjis, E.J.,

Rauwerda, J.A. (2000). Effect of homocysteine lowering treatment with folic acid plus vitamin B6 on progression of subclinical atherosclerosis: A randomized, placebo controlled trial. *Lancet, 355*, 517–522.

80. Hackam, D.G., Peterson, J.C., Spence, J.D. (2000). What level of plasma homocyst(e)ine should be treated? Effects of vitamin therapy on progression of carotid atherosclerosis in patients with homocyst(e)ine levels above and below 14 micromol/L. *American Journal of Hypertension, 13*, 105–110.

81. Marcucci, R., Zanazzi, M., Bertoni, E., Rosati, A., Fedi, S., Lenti, M., Prisco, D., Castellani, S., Abbate, R., Salvadori, M. (2003). Vitamin supplementation reduces the progression of atherosclerosis in hyperhomocysteinemic renal-transplant recipients. *Transplantation, 75*, 1551–1555.

82. Durga, J., van Tits, L.J., Schouten, E.G., Kok, F.J., Verhoef, P. (2005). Effect of lowering of homocysteine levels on inflammatory markers: A randomized controlled trial. *Archives of Internal Medicine, 165*, 1388–1394.

83. Schnyder, G., Roffi, M., Pin, R., Flammer, Y., Lange, H., Eberli, F.R., Meier, B., Turi, Z.G., Hess, O.M. (2001). Decreased rate of coronary restenosis after lowering of plasma homocysteine levels. *New England Journal of Medicine, 345*, 1593–1600.

84. Schnyder, G., Roffi, M., Flammer, Y., Pin, R., Hess, O.M. (2002). Effect of homocysteine-lowering therapy with folic acid, vitamin B12, and vitamin B6 on clinical outcome after percutaneous coronary intervention: The Swiss Heart study: A randomized controlled trial. *JAMA, 288*, 973–979.

85. Lange, H., Suryapranata, H., De Luca, G., Börner, C., Dille, J., Kallmayer, K., Pasalary, M.N., Scherer, E., Dambrink, J.H.E. (2004). Folate therapy and in-stent restenosis after coronary stenting. *New England Journal of Medicine, 350*, 2673–2681.

86. Liem, A.H., van Boven, A.J., Veeger, N.J., Withagen, A.J., de Medina, R.M.R., Tijssen, J.G.P., van Veldhuisen, D.J. (2004). Folic Acid on Risk Diminishment after Acute Myocardial Infarction Study Group. Efficacy of folic acid when added to statin therapy in patients with hypercholesterolemia following acute myocardial infarction: A randomized pilot trial. *International Journal of Cardiology, 93*, 175–179.

87. Liem, A.H., Reynierse-Buitenwerf, G.H., Zwinderman, A.H., Jukema, J., van Veldhuisen, D.J. (2003). Secondary prevention with folic acid: Effects on clinical outcomes. *Journal of the American College of Cardiology, 41*, 2105–2113.

88. Toole, J.F., Malinow, M.R., Chambless, L.E., Spence, J.D., Pettigrew, L.C., Howard, V.J., Sides, E.J., Wang, C.H., Stampfer, M. (2004). Lowering homocysteine in patients with ischemic stroke to prevent recurrent stroke, myocardial infarction, and death: The Vitamin Intervention for Stroke Prevention (VISP) randomized controlled trial. *JAMA, 291*, 565–575.

89. Bønaa, K.H., Njølstad, I., Ueland, P.M., Schirmer, H., Tverdal, A., Steigen, T., Wang, H., Nordrehaug, J.E., Arnesen, E., Rasmussen, K., NORVIT Trial Investigators. (2006). Homocysteine lowering and cardiovascular events after acute myocardial infarction. *New England Journal of Medicine, 354*, 1578–1588.

90. Lonn, E., Yusuf, S., Arnold, M.J., Sheridan, P., Pogue, J., Micks, M., McQueen, M.J., Probstfield, J., Fodor, G., Held, C., Genest, J., Jr., Heart Outcomes Prevention Evaluation (HOPE)-2 Investigators. (2006). Homocysteine lowering with folic acid and B vitamins in vascular disease. *New England Journal of Medicine, 354*, 1567–1577.

91. Bazzano, L.A., Reynolds, K., Holder, K., He, J. (2006). Effect of folic acid supplementation on risk of cardiovascular diseases: A meta-analysis of randomized controlled trials. *JAMA, 296*, 2720–2726.

92. Righetti, M., Serbelloni, P., Milani, S., Ferrario, G.M. (2006). Homocysteine-lowering vitamin B treatment decreases cardiovascular events in hemodialysis patients. *Blood Purification, 24*, 379–386.

93. Zoungas, S., McGrath, B.P., Branley, P., Kerr, P.G., Muske, C., Wolfe, R., Atkins, R.C., Nicholls, K., Fraenkel, M., Hutchison, B.G., Walker, R., McNeil, J.J. (2006). Cardiovascular morbidity and mortality in the Atherosclerosis and Folic Acid Supplementation Trial (ASFAST) in chronic renal failure: A multicenter, randomized controlled trial. *Journal of the American College of Cardiology, 47*, 1108–1116.

94. Liem, A., Reynierse-Buitenwerf, G.H., Zwinderman, A.H., Jukema, J.W., van Veldhuisen, D.J. (2005). Secondary prevention with folic acid: Results of the Goes extension study. *Heart, 91*, 1213–1214.

95. Wrone, E.M., Hornberger, J.M., Zehnder, J.L., McCann, L.M., Coplon, N.S., Fortmann, S.P. (2004). Randomized trial of folic acid for prevention of cardiovascular events in end-stage renal disease. *Journal of the American Society of Nephrology, 15*, 420–426.

96. Righetti, M., Ferrario, G.M., Dilani, S., Serbelloni, P., La Rosa, L., Uccellini, M., Sessa, A. (2003). Effects of folic acid treatment on homocysteine levels and vascular disease in hemodialysis patients. *Medical Science Monitor, 9*, 19–24.

97. Baker, F., Picton, D., Blackwood, S., Hunt, J., Erskine, M., Dyas, M. (2002). Blinded comparison of folic acid and placebo in patients with ischemic heart disease: An outcome trial. *Circulation, 106*(Suppl 2), 741S.

98. Wang, X., Qin, X., Demirtas, H., Li, J., Mao, G., Huo, Y., Sun, N., Liu, L., Xu, X. (2007). Efficacy of folic acid supplementation in stroke prevention: A meta-analysis. *Lancet, 369*, 1876–1882.

99. Mark, S.D., Wang, W., Fraumeni, J.F., Jr., Li, J.Y., Taylor, P.R., Wang, G.Q., Guo, W., Dawsey, S.M., Li, B., Blot, W.J. (1996). Lowered risks of hypertension and cerebrovascular disease after vitamin/mineral supplementation: The Linxian Nutrition Intervention. *American Journal of Epidemiology, 143*, 658–664.

100. B-Vitamin Treatment Trialists' Collaboration. (2006). Homocysteine-lowering trials for prevention of cardiovascular events: A review of the design and power of the large randomized trials. *American Heart Journal, 151*, 282–287.

CHAPTER 18

HOMOCYSTEINE AND NEUROLOGICAL DISORDERS

RODICA E. PETREA and SUDHA SESHADRI

18.1 INTRODUCTION

Homocysteine is a sulfur-containing amino acid that is not synthesized de novo in humans, but is formed in the organism during the metabolism of the essential amino acid methionine and another sulfur-containing amino-acid, cysteine [1]. Once formed, homocysteine is metabolized further through one of two pathways, a remethylation pathway and a transsulfuration pathway (see Fig. 4.1). The remethylation pathway is catalyzed by the enzymes methionine synthase and N5,N10-methylenetetrahydrofolate reductase (MTHFR); requires cobalamin (vitamin B12), as a cofactor, and folate as cosubstrate. The transsulfuration pathway is stimulated either by an excess of methionine or by requirements for cystathionine and cysteine synthesis. The latter pathway requires that homocysteine condenses with serine to form cystathionine, which is eventually metabolized to cysteine through a reaction catalyzed by the vitamin B6-dependent enzyme, cystathionine β-synthase. Thus, circulating and tissue concentrations of homocysteine are intimately related not only to the function of these enzymes, but also to the concentrations of folate, vitamin B12, and vitamin B6 in the body. Hence, subsequent discussions regarding the role of homocysteine in neurological health and disease will, of necessity, digress at times into discussions of the role that these vitamins play in determining brain health. We will advance the argument that elevated plasma homocysteine levels are associated with dysfunction in the vascular supply to the brain manifested as carotid artery dysfunction and an increased propensity to various types of stroke. Further we will show that elevated plasma homocysteine levels have been associated both cross-sectionally, and on prospective follow-up, with an increased risk of developing both vascular dementia and Alzheimer's disease (AD). Finally, there is evidence to suggest that plasma homocysteine levels affect subclinical measures of baseline brain function (and accelerate

Glutathione and Sulfur Amino Acids in Human Health and Disease. Edited by R. Masella and G. Mazza
Copyright © 2009 John Wiley & Sons, Inc.

age-related decline in brain function) as assessed using brain magnetic resonance imaging (MRI) and cognitive function tests in middle-aged adults who are free of clinical stroke and dementia. It is less certain whether the observed associations are incidental (risk markers) or causal (risk factors) [2]. On the one hand, there are many studies describing various cellular and biochemical pathways through which excess homocysteine could directly impair macrovascular and microvascular, neuronal and glial function. On the other hand, clinical trials of folate or multivitamin therapy to prevent stroke and cognitive decline have been disappointing. We will briefly discuss possible explanations for this discrepancy. The role of monitoring and treating elevated plasma homocysteine levels in persons with clinical neurological diseases such as transient ischemic attacks, stroke, mild cognitive impairment, dementia and AD will be discussed. Finally, we will emphasize that the potentially adverse effects of hyperhomocystemia on the brain are important not only in the primary and secondary prevention of stroke, cognitive impairment, and dementia but also because some of the medications routinely used by neurologists have been shown to cause an elevation of homocysteine levels. This is true for instance in patients with Parkinson's disease (PD) who are treated with levodopa, as well as in patients treated with first generation antiepileptic drugs.

Brain damage, as a consequence of elevated plasma homocysteine (tHcy) levels, was first described in children with an inherited metabolic disorder, "homocystinuria" by two independent groups of investigators from the United States and Ireland [3, 4]. These children had a defect in the function of the enzyme cystathionine β-synthase resulting in very high circulating concentrations of homocysteine (100 to 450 µmol/L) [5] and presented with ectopia lentis, myopia, osteoporosis, mental retardation, and early death due to thromboembolic events such as stroke and myocardial infarction. It has been shown subsequently that correcting the elevated plasma homocysteine levels and increasing the availability of cystathionine in the brain through the administration of pyridoxine (in a subset of pyridoxine responsive subjects) or with a low methionine, cystine-enhanced diet supplemented with pyridoxine, vitamin B12 and folate, could lower plasma tHcy levels and prevent all the classic manifestations of homocystinuria, including the risks of mental retardation and stroke [6].

In 1969, McCully reported a frequent association of various congenital enzymatic defects with severe early atherosclerosis; the common feature underlying these conditions was hyperhomocysteinemia. McCully extrapolated from the premature atherosclerotic changes seen in these children to suggest that a modestly elevated plasma homocysteine level might be one of the factors responsible for the development of atherosclerosis in the general population [7]. Whereas hyperhomocysteinemia attributable solely to a genetic enzymatic defect was admittedly rare [6], subsequent studies found that hyperhomocysteinemia as a result of environmental factors and of gene-nutrient interactions was common [8, 9]. As described in earlier chapters, a multitude of causes can increase circulating concentrations of homocysteine, either transiently or chronically (see Table 17.1). The recognition that several causes of hyperhomocysteinemia were potentially preventable spurred case control and prospective epidemiological studies exploring the relationship between hyperhomocysteinemia of different etiologies and premature atherosclerosis. As a result hyperhomocysteinemia emerged in the early 1990s as an independent potentially modifiable risk factor for cardiovascular disease, coronary artery disease, carotid atherosclerosis, and stroke [10].

18.2 WHAT IS AN "ABNORMAL" PLASMA HOMOCYSTEINE LEVEL IN CLINICAL STUDIES OF NEUROLOGICAL DISEASE?

The reference to plasma homocysteine levels in this and other articles in the neurology literature refers to *total plasma homocysteine* (tHcy), a term used to describe a combined pool of free (0.2%) and protein-bound (80%) homocysteine, homocystine, and homocysteine-cysteine mixed disulfides (20%). The reference limits for circulating tHcy concentrations are conventionally acknowledged to be in the range of 5 to 14 μmol/L. Hyperhomocysteinemia has been classified as moderate (15 to 30 μmol/L), intermediate (30 to 100 μmol/L), or severe (>100 μmol/L) [11] and the prevalence of moderate, intermediate, and severe hyperhomocysteinemia using this definition has been estimated at 10%, 1%, and 0.02%, respectively [9]. Using a population sample of healthy, young controls, Joosten et al. found that the $\geq$14 μmol/L value was >2 standard deviations above the mean [12]. Similarly, in the Framingham Heart study cohort 90% of persons with apparently adequate levels of folate and vitamins B12 and B6 had a plasma tHcy <14 μmol/L [13]. However, for most neurological conditions it appears that the adverse effects of elevated plasma tHcy levels extend along a continuum across the range of observed values without a definite threshold. The concept of how high a homocysteine level is "abnormal" has been evolving and it appears clear that "average" may not be optimal in terms of disease risk. In 1997, the United States mandated dietary folate fortification; all cereal grain flour products such as bread and breakfast cereals were fortified with physiological amounts of folate (140 mg/100 g of flour). Since then average plasma tHcy levels have fallen by 50% [14], but there is data to suggest that even levels as low as 9 μg/dL may increase the risk of stroke and other neurological disease. Conversely, in subgroups such as the elderly and those with renal disease, a significant

TABLE 18.1 Distribution of Baseline Homocysteine within Sex-Pooled, 5-Year Age Groups[*]

Age (Years)	No. of Subjects	Mean[a]	SD	Range[a]	75th Percentile[a]
65–69	46	11.5	3.9	5.4–25.5	13.2
70–74	457	12.1	5.9	4.1–66.7	13.8
75–79	315	12.6	5.9	3.5–66.9	14.5
80–84	179	14.2	7.3	4.5–56.1	16.5
85–89	66	15.3	8.0	5.5–59.6	19.3
90–94	29	22.3	12.6	5.4–61.6	26.6[a]

[*]Difference in mean values between men and women was not significant.
[a]Values of plasma total homocysteine (tHcy) are recorded in μmol/L.
Source: Adapted from Seshadri et al. [121]. Used with permission.

minority or even a majority of subjects may have tHcy levels above those conventionally considered normal; analyses examining the effect of elevated plasma tHcy in these
populations have to account for this distribution. The age-sex distribution of plasma
tHcy levels in a Framingham study sample is shown in Table 18.1.

18.3 ELEVATED PLASMA HOMOCYSTEINE AND THE RISK OF CAROTID ATHEROSCLEROSIS

The presence or absence of subclinical carotid artery dysfunction and atherosclerotic
disease can be assessed using several measures. Carotid artery stiffness can be
assessed by tonometry [15]. The earliest atherosclerotic change detectable may be a
change in intimo-medial thickness; subsequently discernable atherosclerotic plaque
burden may be quantified using measures of plaque area or degree of carotid stenosis.
An elevated plasma homocysteine level has been associated with each of these indices.
An acute increase in plasma tHcy following oral methionine loading has been shown
to acutely increase carotid arterial stiffness in 18 healthy middle-aged subjects [16]. A
cross-sectional study of Framingham Heart Study participants ($n = 1962$, mean age
61 years) showed that concurrent plasma tHcy levels were associated with an increased
carotid-femoral pulse wave velocity in men [17]. Elevated plasma tHcy, even in an
apparently normal range of $<14 \mu mol/L$, appears to be weakly related to increases
in carotid intimal-medial thickness (IMT) [18–21]. Lowering plasma tHcy by administration of vitamins has been reported to decrease carotid IMT in case control studies,
particularly in patients with chronic renal disease [22, 23]. However, in most population-based studies this association between plasma tHcy and carotid IMT disappeared after adjusting for other known cardiovascular risk factors [24, 25].

An elevated plasma tHcy has been associated with a greater prevalence of extracranial carotid stenosis (documented by B-mode ultrasound) among healthy middle-
aged participants in the Rotterdam and Framingham studies [26, 27]. For example, in
the Framingham study, when subjects with a tHcy level in the highest quartile (≥ 14.4
$\mu mol/L$) were compared to subjects with a tHcy in the lowest quartile ($\leq 9.1 \mu mol/$
L), the odds ratio of a subject in the former group having carotid stenosis $\geq 25\%$ were
doubled. There is insufficient data on the role, if any, of plasma tHcy levels in determining restenosis risk after carotid endarterectomy and angioplasty [28, 29], although
trials examining the effect of tHcy lowering on restenosis after coronary angioplasty
have suggested some possible benefit [30–34]. An elevated plasma tHcy is also
more likely to be documented in persons with carotid or other cervical artery dissec-
tions [35–37].

18.4 HYPERHOMOCYSTEINEMIA AND THE RISK OF STROKE

Stroke is the leading cause of disability, second among leading causes of mortality in
developing countries and third in the United States. Community-based data from a

North American sample of European descent describe a lifetime risk of stroke in a middle-aged woman of 1 in 5, with the corresponding risk in a man of 1 in 6 [38]. Therefore the identification of preventable risk factors for stroke is of paramount importance. A stroke is a sudden focal neurological deficit due to a disturbance in the blood supply to the brain. It commonly results from arterial occlusion which may be atherothrombotic (stroke due to an occlusion of one of the arteries supplying a portion of the brain), or embolic (stroke due to a clot forming in the heart, aorta, or a large artery and traveling distally to occlude an artery supplying the brain). Approximately 20% of strokes are due to brain hemorrhage and a tiny fraction result from thrombosis in the large cerebral veins and dural venous sinuses. Elevated plasma tHcy levels have been associated with an increased risk of ischemic stroke. This seems particularly true of atherothrombotic strokes and remains true whether one considers large artery infarcts or smaller lacunar (<20 mm in size, due to occlusion of deep, end arterioles) strokes. A similar association has been shown with transient ischemic attacks (deficit lasting less than 24 hours) [39]. Since elevated plasma tHcy levels have also been related to an increased risk of coronary artery disease, heart failure, and atrial fibrillation, all of which cause embolic stroke, an association between tHcy levels and cardioembolic stroke is also observed [40–42]. An elevated plasma tHcy appears to increase stroke risk in both men and women, among infants and children [43, 44], as well as the elderly, in all racial and ethnic groups studied to date [45, 46] and in some subgroups at an increased a priori risk of stroke, such as persons with systemic lupus erythematosus [47], sickle cell anemia [48], and chronic renal disease [49].

Data from initial case control studies [50, 51] have been summarized in several excellent reviews [52, 53]. Prospective epidemiological studies have also largely (but not invariably) [54, 55] confirmed such an association, and again these data have been collated in several meta-analyses [52, 53, 56–58]. The results of these meta-analyses vary based on the selection of studies, with one meta-analysis describing an increased risk of 400% among persons in the top 5% of plasma tHcy levels, whereas another meta-analysis by the Homocysteine Studies Collaboration suggested that a 25% decline in plasma tHcy levels, a decrease of approximately 3 μmol/L from a level of 11 μmol/L, was associated with no more than a modest, nonsignificant (19%) lowering of stroke risk [10]. Based on a review of the numerous studies, however, the most convincing estimates are of an approximately 50% increase in the odds ratio (OR) of prevalent stroke for every 5 μmol/L increase in plasma tHcy and a 40% increased risk of incident stroke among persons with hyperhomocysteinemia (>14 μmol/L) [52, 56]. Are the higher risks noted in case control studies due to acute elevations of plasma tHcy in the post-stroke period? On the contrary, Meiklejohn et al., who measured fasting plasma Hcy concentrations in cases and controls within the first 24 hours and at three months after an atherothrombotic stroke, observed that plasma tHcy concentrations were not higher in cases than in controls immediately after the event [59].

The most reliable data available from a single, prospective study may be data from the Framingham study, which has reliable pre-event measures of plasma tHcy levels and meticulous ascertainment of all stroke events. Among 1947 Framingham participants (mean age 70 ± 7 years), 165 incident strokes were documented over a 10-year follow-up. Using multivariable Cox proportional hazards models, adjusted for known stroke risk factors, there was a linear increase in the risk of stroke across quartiles of plasma tHcy ($p < 0.001$) [60]. The risk of cardiovascular disease (CVD) mortality doubled among persons with hyperhomocysteinemia (RR: 2.2; 95% CI, 1.7–2.8) [61]. Iso et al. used a nested, case control study design to examine the association of circulating tHcy levels with risk of all stroke and various stroke subtypes in 11,846 Japanese men and women. The multivariate OR associated with a 5 μmol/L increase in tHcy was 1.40 (1.09–1.80) for total strokes, 1.52 (1.07–2.14) for ischemic strokes, 1.48 (1.01–2.18) for lacunar strokes, and 1.10 (0.76–1.59) for hemorrhagic strokes [46].

Knowing that individuals homozygous for the T allele of the MTHFR C677T polymorphism have higher plasma homocysteine concentrations than those with CC genotype Casas et al. [62] predicted that individuals homozygous for the T allele of the MTHFR C677T polymorphism would be at an increased risk of stroke. They compared the expected OR for stroke among TT homozygotes, extrapolated from genotype-phenotype and phenotype-disease studies, and the observed OR from a meta-analysis of 111 genotype-disease association studies. In a total of 15,635 people without prevalent cardiovascular disease the weighted mean difference in homocysteine concentration between TT and CC homozygotes was 1.93 μmol/L (95% CI, 1.38–2.47) and the expected OR for incident stroke corresponding to this difference in plasma tHcy levels, based on previous observational studies, was 1.20 (1.10–1.31). The observed OR for incident stroke in 13,928 persons included in the genetic meta-analysis was 1.26 (1.14–1.40) for TT versus CC homozygotes, similar to the expected OR ($p = 0.029$). The concordance between the observed increased risk of stroke among the TT homozygous and the predicted risk of stroke corresponding to the difference in homocysteine concentration between the two genotypes was argued to be suggestive of a causal relation between plasma tHcy concentrations and risk of stroke [62].

Despite the wealth of clinical and epidemiological evidence relating elevated plasma tHcy levels to an increased risk of ischemic stroke and all CVD endpoints, recent secondary prevention trials have failed to show a beneficial effect of tHcy-lowering vitamin therapy on reducing CVD risk [63–65], although a benefit was observed for the secondary prevention of stroke as compared to all CVD [66]. Further, it has been suggested that administration of vitamin therapy to persons with mild hyperhomocysteinemia could have an adverse effect on CVD risk (perhaps because unmetabolized folate increases oxidative stress) [67], although this effect was not noted for the specific endpoint of stroke [68]. These studies do document that an improvement in folate status has a direct effect on lowering plasma tHcy levels, but the latter has not been shown to significantly decrease the risk of coronary heart disease and stroke [69–71]. The Vitamins in Stroke Prevention (VISP) trial did not find any benefit overall from high dose vitamin therapy but in subgroup analysis the lowest stroke risk was observed in the subgroup of participants with B12 levels above the sample median who were also on high dose vitamin therapy, whereas the highest stroke risk was observed in subjects with circulating B12 levels below the median, who were also on the lower dose of vitamins. Groups with high baseline B12 and low dose vitamin supplementation and with low baseline B12 and high dose vitamin supplementation had intermediate risk. The negative overall results could therefore be attributed to variation in underlying B12 levels [64] The NORVIT study compared four groups of subjects: persons on placebo, on vitamin B6 alone, on B12 + folate, and on all three vitamins. The investigators observed a barely 22% increased risk in the all three vitamin treatment groups, compared to placebo, for the combined myocardial infarction (MI), stroke, and coronary sudden death endpoint (1.22, 95%CI 1.00–1.50) but not for stroke alone (RR 0.88, 95% CI 0.74–1.05) [65]. The HOPE-2 trial did not find a benefit of vitamin therapy overall but did observe a benefit for the specific endpoint of stroke [66–70]. One way to reconcile the results from the various observational studies with the disappointing results of clinical trials would be to conclude that vitamin administration to lower plasma tHcy levels may be effective in primary prevention but not in the secondary prevention of stroke. A biologically plausible explanation might be that the effect of an elevated plasma tHcy level accrues over a prolonged period of time (the VISP study had a follow-up period of only 2 years versus the 8-year follow-up in the observational Framingham study), and that tHcy may play a less important role in increasing the risk of an occlusive thrombus or embolus that precipitates an acute stroke. However, this explanation remains unsubstantiated and is only one of several possible explanations. It has been argued that the response to folic acid supplementation might vary by vitamin B12 status and by concomitant dietary intake of polyunsaturated fatty acids; perhaps high-dose B12 supplementation and polyunsaturated fatty acids should be administered along with folic acid in future clinical trials [71]. There have been no primary prevention trials addressing the role of tHcy-lowering interventions; detailed observational data could help with the optimal design of such a study.

Elevated plasma tHcy levels have a prothrombotic and procoagulant effect and may promote venous thrombosis [72]. Pregnancy has been associated, especially in developing countries with limited antenatal care, with folate deficiency and elevated circulating tHcy levels [73, 74]. This may be one of the factors responsible for the increased risk of cerebral venous sinus thrombosis observed in pregnant women in their third trimester and postpartum.

18.5 ELEVATED PLASMA HOMOCYSTEINE LEVELS ARE ASSOCIATED WITH THE RISK OF DEMENTIA AND ALZHEIMER'S DISEASE

Dementia is defined as a clinical syndrome characterized by the acquired loss of cognitive abilities severe enough to interfere with work or usual social activities and family obligations. It requires the documentation of a decline from a prior level of cognitive function and persistence of the condition, the duration being defined in months and years rather than days or weeks. Usually, though not always, the condition is progressive. Dementia affects multiple domains of intellectual function. The *Diagnostic and Statistical Manual of Mental Disorders-IV* (DSM-IV) criteria require involvement of short-term and long-term memory and at least one of the following spheres of mental activity: language, praxis, executive function (abstract thought, judgment, and problem solving), and cortical perception [75]. Finally, the diagnosis presupposes an alert patient, thus excluding persons with acute confusional states. The two commonest causes of dementia are AD and vascular dementia (VaD). Criteria for the diagnosis of AD are well established but it remains a diagnosis best made by careful clinical observation over time and ideally confirmation after death with a detailed brain autopsy [76]. Criteria for VaD still vary widely although consensus criteria are emerging [77–79]. All definitions require the presence of cognitive or behavioral problems amounting to dementia, disease affecting blood vessels or blood flow to part or all of the brain, and evidence by history, clinical examination, or on imaging of damage to part or all of brain due to vascular factors. Elevated tHcy levels have not been linked to the rarer causes of dementia (such as dementia with Lewy bodies or progressive supranuclear palsy) so these etiologies will not be discussed further.

Cobalamin deficiency has been long acknowledged to be associated with a range of neuropyschiatric manifestations and with cognitive impairment; symptoms described have ranged from depression and delirium to frank dementia, although this was thought to occur in the setting of a pernicious anemia [80]. Since mild cobalamin deficiency is common in the elderly (prevalence of 12% to 25%) [12, 81–83], the association between mild cobalamin deficiency and cognitive decline has been assessed using elevated plasma tHcy concentrations and elevated plasma methylmalonic acid (MMA) as indices of mild cobalamin deficiency in otherwise apparently healthy elderly people; Nilsson et al., and others, argue that tHcy is the better index [84–88].

In the 1980s, several investigators who were studying the effects of Vitamin B12 (cobalamin) deficiency on the brain observed that elevated levels of homocysteine, initially evaluated as a marker of subclinical B12 deficiency, correlated better with the prevalence of cognitive deficits and neuropsychiatric abnormalities than did serum levels of vitamin B12 itself [89, 90]. Further studies over the next two decades have repeatedly linked plasma tHcy levels to cognitive function in unselected populations. This association has not only been observed cross-sectionally, but baseline plasma homocysteine levels have also been related to cognitive decline on follow-up. This was true in both men and women and in Caucasian, Hispanic, and African American samples. While the effects were noted in persons both over and under the age of 65 years, the effects were more pronounced in older persons [91, 92]. Some studies observed an interaction with the apolipoprotein E $\varepsilon 4$ genotype while others did not.

A total of 70 male participants (aged 54 to 81 years) in the Normative Aging Study were assessed with a cognitive test battery. Lower concentrations of vitamin B12 and folate ($p = 0.003$) and higher concentrations of plasma tHcy ($p = 0.0009$) were each associated with poorer spatial copying skills ($p = 0.04$, 0.003, and 0.0009, respectively). The association of plasma tHcy levels with performance on a spatial copying task persisted after adjustment for a clinical diagnosis of vascular disease [93]. Miller and colleagues studied a large population-based cohort of older Latinos residing in California using a linguistically and culturally validated cognitive test battery.

In this study, the Sacramento Area Latino Study on Aging (SALSA), which evaluated 1789 subjects aged ≥ 60 years, plasma tHcy levels showed modest inverse associations with the overall Mini-Mental State Examination (MMSE) score and with tests of attention, abstraction, and visuospatial organization (the picture-association, verbal attention-span, and pattern-recognition tests; $p \leq 0.05$) even after adjustment for age, sex, education, acculturation, red blood cell folate, plasma B12 and serum creatinine levels and presence or absence of depression [94]. In Framingham Offspring participants who were free of clinical stroke and dementia, elevated plasma tHcy levels were associated with poorer cognitive performance on an extensive battery of neuro-psychological tests [91]; there was a continuous, inverse linear relation between plasma tHcy concentrations and cognitive performance in older persons free of dementia and stroke [95]. In the Rotterdam study of 1077 persons aged 60 to 90 years without demential, persons in the top quintile of plasma tHcy levels (>14 μmol/L) had significantly lower scores on tests of global function, psychomotor speed, and memory function [96]. Hyperhomocysteinemia in the top two deciles of the distribution (>13.7 μmol/L) was associated with poor verbal memory performance among over 1200 older Americans (age 70 ± 0.5 years) enrolled in the Third National Health and Nutrition Examination Survey (NHANES) study; this was independent of folate levels [97]. However, few studies have related baseline plasma tHcy levels to cognitive decline. McCaddon and colleagues, in a small study of 32 elderly persons tested twice (at baseline and after a 5 year follow-up period), observed that higher baseline plasma tHcy levels were related to a greater decline in MMSE scores ($p < 0.001$) and to the rate of decline in cognitive performance tests assessing word recall ($p = 0.01$), orientation ($p = 0.02$), and constructional praxis ($p < 0.0001$) [98]. However, the Rotterdam study failed to relate baseline tHcy levels to decline in MMSE scores over a 2 year period [99]. This discrepancy is probably explained by the longer follow-up in the former study. In the Framingham cohort, we observed that among 604 subjects with biennial MMSE testing, baseline plasma tHcy levels did not predict a decline in MMSE scores after a 2 year follow-up period, but did predict decline after a 4 year period (decline of 0.09 points per SD rise in baseline tHcy; $p = 0.006$; unpublished observations). In the Baltimore Study of Aging, an increase in plasma tHcy concentrations from the 25th to the 75th percentile, despite all values falling within a generally accepted normal range, was associated with a decline in mean neurocognitive test scores equivalent to 4.2 years of aging [100]. These and other studies (and meta-analyses) suggest that elevated plasma tHcy levels are associated with lower baseline cognitive performance and with greater decline in cognition over time [84, 92, 100–114]. Diabetes mellitus may potentiate the adverse effects of elevated plasma tHcy levels [113].

Simultaneously, in the 1990s, several epidemiological studies of cardiovascular disease in the elderly, such as the Rotterdam study, were demonstrating that persons at a high risk of vascular disease also appeared to have a high risk of developing AD [115]. Further, persons with a stroke were not only at risk of developing (not surprisingly) vascular dementia, but also at an increased risk of developing AD [116]. Based on the fact that homocysteine is a risk factor for vascular disease and the observed direct association between elevated plasma homocysteine levels and cognitive impairment, Clarke, McCaddon and others postulated that elevated plasma homocysteine levels might play a pathophysiological role in the development of dementia and AD [117, 118]. Clarke et al. [117] utilized data from the Oxford Project to Investigate Memory and Ageing (OPTIMA). Plasma tHcy levels were compared in 164 patients with AD (76 with autopsy-confirmed AD, 88 with clinically diagnosed AD) and 108 dementia-free controls. Persons with AD were twice as likely (OR 2.0; 95% CI 1.1–3.4) to have a tHcy >14 µmol/L compared to controls after adjusting for age, sex, cigarette smoking, social class, and APOE genotype [117]. Conversely, patients with AD were more likely to have elevated plasma tHcy levels and low serum vitamin B12 levels than control subjects. Other case control studies have also related elevated plasma tHcy levels with stroke, VaD and AD. McIlroy et al. [119] compared fasting levels of plasma tHcy in four groups: subjects with AD, VaD, nondemented stroke survivors (NDS), and controls free of neurological disease. The odds ratio for having a plasma tHcy ≥13.3 µmol/L (the 75th percentile value in the control group) was significantly increased in all three patient groups [119]. However, one vexing question remained unanswered by these cross-sectional observations: was the observed association causal or secondary to poor nutrition in subjects with mild cognitive impairment and early, undiagnosed, AD? Did the observed hyperhomocystenemia truly precede the onset of dementia?

The Bradford–Hill criteria for deciding if an observed association is likely to be causal require the documentation of a temporal relationship (the risk factor being present before the onset of the disease), a strong association, a dose-response effect so that higher levels of risk factor exposure are associated with greater risk, consistent results despite several ways of asking the question and in various ethnic and geographically discrete study samples, and finally biological plausibility [120].

A consistent temporal association between elevated plasma tHcy levels at baseline and the risk of incident AD over 8 years of follow-up could be demonstrated in the Framingham study. Seshadri et al. [121] prospectively evaluated 1092 persons from the Framingham original cohort who were documented to be free of dementia at the time of enrollment and plasma tHcy measurement. The observed association was strong and there was a clear dose-response relationship; a tHcy level in the highest age- and sex-specific quartile doubled the risk of developing dementia or AD, after adjustment for age, gender, APOE ε4 genotype, and serum levels of folate, vitamins B6 and B12. The risk was continuous; for every one SD increase in the log-transformed baseline value of plasma tHcy there was a 30% increase in the relative risk of dementia and 40% increase in the relative risk of AD [121] (Fig. 18.1, Table 18.2).

Over the past five years, there have been only a few additional prospective studies relating the elevated baseline plasma tHcy levels to the risk of incident dementia and AD. The Conselice Study of Brain Aging, which followed 816 subjects over four years, did find an association equal in magnitude to the Framingham study report with a relative risk of 2.1 (95% CI 1.2–3.8) for developing AD in persons with a baseline tHcy >15 µmol/L, compared to all other subjects [122]. However, the Washington-Heights Inwood Columbia Aging Project did not find a significant

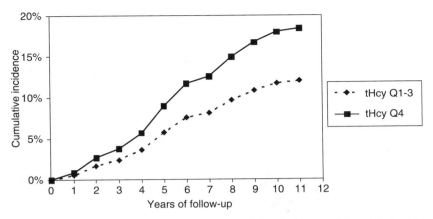

Figure 18.1 Kaplan-Meier plots showing the cumulative incidence of dementia in subjects with baseline plasma homocysteine levels in the highest age-specific quartile (tHcy Q4) compared to subjects with plasma homocysteine in the first, second, or third age-specific quartile (tHcy Q1-3). Adapted from Seshadri et al. [121]. Used with permission.

association between tHcy levels and incident AD. The relative risk of AD associated with a plasma tHcy in the highest versus the lowest quartile was 1.4 (95% CI 0.8–2.4). The failure to find an association can perhaps be explained by the high levels of plasma tHcy noted among the control subjects since over 60% of all study participants had a plasma tHcy >14 μmol/L [123].

Elevated plasma tHcy levels have also been associated, in persons free of clinical disease, with a greater prevalence of measures of subclinical ischemic injury (abnormal white matter hyperintensities and silent cerebral infarcts), and with measures of subclinical brain aging (lower total and regional brain volumes, greater brain atrophy, and lower hippocampal volumes). Recently, a study of 1965 Framingham Offspring Study participants (1050 women; age 62 ± 9 years) who were free of clinical stroke, dementia, or other neurological disease related concurrent plasma tHcy levels, as well as prior levels obtained 3 to 10 years earlier, to these brain MRI measures. On multivariable regression both measures of tHcy were related to total brain volume; participants with a plasma tHcy level in the highest age-, sex-specific quartile had a smaller total brain/intracranial cavity ratio (by −0.37% and −0.48%; $p = 0.01$ and <0.001, respectively), compared to participants with lower levels. Prior tHcy levels were associated with an increased prevalence of silent brain infarcts (RR: 1.5; 95% CI 1.1–2.1; $p = 0.02$) and concurrent tHcy levels with smaller frontal and temporal lobar volumes (−0.14% and −0.10%; $p = 0.001$ and 0.04, respectively) [124]. The observed association with smaller total brain volumes confirms the results of smaller studies that used semiquantitative MRI techniques [125–127]. The increased risk of subclinical infarcts has also been shown in prior studies [128, 129]. In addition,

TABLE 18.2 Multivariable Cox Proportional-Hazards Regression Models Examining the Relation of Plasma Total Homocysteine (as a Continuous Variable) to the Risk of Incident Dementia and Alzheimer's Disease

Model with	Variables Adjusted for in Analysis	All-Cause Dementia				Alzheime	
		Cases/N	HR[a]	95% CI[a]	P	Cases/N	HR
Baseline homocysteine[b]	Age & sex	111/1092	1.28	1.07–1.52	0.007	83/1092	1.36
	Age, sex *and APOE genotype*	105/1012	1.30	1.09–1.56	0.003	79/1012	1.40
	Age, sex, APOE genotype *and plasma levels of folate, vitamins B12 and B6*[c]	77/789	1.45	1.14–1.84	0.002	54/789	1.62
	Age, sex, APOE genotype, plasma B vitamins *and additional covariates*[d]	60/680	1.45	1.09–1.92	0.009	44/680	1.78
Remote homocysteine[b]	Age & sex	88/935	1.35	1.06–1.73	0.016	67/935	1.43
	Age, sex *and APOE genotype*	82/864	1.33	1.03–1.71	0.031	63/864	1.39
	Age, sex, APOE genotype *and additional covariates*[d]	72/771	1.43	1.08–1.89	0.013	56/771	1.57

[a]HR denotes hazard ratio and CI denotes confidence interval. Hazard ratios are per increment of 1 SD (0.4) in og-tHcy.

[b]Baseline homocysteine was estimated on nonfasting plasma samples collected at the 20th biennial examination (1986–1990); remote homocysteine was estimated on nonfasting plasma samples collected at the 16th biennial examination (1979–1982).

[c]Log-transformed values of plasma folate and vitamin B6 were used in the model.

[d]Additional covariates included in model are education status, prevalent stroke, smoking, alcohol intake, diabetes mellitus, body-mass index, and systolic blood pressure as recorded at the baseline examination in which plasma total homocysteine was measured.

Source: Adapted from Seshadri et al. [121]. Used with permission.

three studies have described a cross-sectional association of plasma tHcy levels with smaller hippocampal volumes [127, 130, 131]. The Framingham study and the Cardiovascular Health study did not observe a significant association between plasma tHcy levels and the prevalence and severity of white matter hyperintensity (WMH) on brain MRI. A Japanese study observed that whereas plasma tHcy levels or the MTHFR TT genotype were related to the combined risk of SBI and WMH, they were not related to WMH alone [132, 133]. However, several other groups have found an association between plasma tHcy levels and WMH. These latter studies often included older patients with clinical stroke or dementia [134], and a greater prevalence of CVD risk factors [128, 135, 136].

Kado and colleagues studied decline in physical performance over a three year period (1988 to 1991) using measures of physical function (balance, gait, lower body strength, and coordination) in 499 men and women aged 70 to 79 years who were enrolled in the MacArthur Studies of Successful Aging [137]. They found that for every one standard deviation increase in plasma tHcy (mean 11.6 ± 4.3 μmol/L) there was a 50% increase in the odds that the subject would be in the worst quartile of decline in physical function, even after adjusting for age, sex, baseline physical performance, smoking, vitamin status, and incident stroke. The Epidemiology of Vascular Aging (EVA) study examined the relationship between tHcy, white matter hyperintensities, and cognitive decline in 1241 healthy elderly people followed up over four years. Cross-sectional analyses found that the OR of cognitive decline was 2.8-fold ($p < 0.05$) higher in subjects with tHcy levels >15 μmol/L compared to participants with a tHcy level <10 μmol/L, where "cognitive decline" was defined as a decrease in the Mini-Mental State Examination score of three points or more between the baseline and two year follow-up examinations [106].

18.5.1 Biological Plausibility

There are several potential biological pathways that could mediate the observed association between plasma tHcy and the development of AD; these include cellular and vascular pathways. Homocysteine is an essential intermediary in the metabolism of methionine through a methylation cycle that requires vitamin B12, folate, and B$_6$ (pyridoxine) and generates an activated methyl group in the compound S-adenosyl-methionine (SAM) which in turn serves as the methyl donor for methylation reactions within the neuron, including the methylation of nucleic acids, phospholipids, proteins, myelin, and catecholamines. Homocysteine promotes ischemic damage by altering LDL receptor function and promoting atherosclerotic plaque formation within large arteries. It binds to N-methyl-D-aspartate (NMDA) receptors in the arterial wall and has been shown to reduce endothelial reactivity to the vasodilatory effects of nitrous oxide and to stimulate vascular smooth muscle proliferation. Elevated plasma tHcy levels have prothrombotic and procoagulant effects [138]. Circulating tHcy has also been shown to increase blood–brain barrier permeability. At a microscopic level, altered cerebrocortical capillary structure has been demonstrated in folate-deficient rats [139]. Elevated plasma tHcy levels have been shown to accelerate aging. Homocysteine treatment of cell cultures doubles the rate of telomere shortening and reduces the number of population doublings [140]. Methionine- and cysteine-deficient diets which lower tissue and circulating tHcy extend the mean lifespan in rats. Polymorphisms in the MTHFR gene associated with lower plasma tHcy have been linked to longevity in select human populations [141]. A metabolite, homocysteic acid, promotes excitotoxic damage by activating glutamatergic NMDA receptors [142, 143]; hence homocysteine may be directly neurotoxic. In cell cultures, it promotes calcium influx and the generation of free oxygen radicals, accelerates DNA damage, and promotes apoptosis in hippocampal neurons [144, 145]. Elevated plasma tHcy promotes the homocysteinylation of proteins (which can alter their structural and enzymatic functions) [146, 147] and inhibits Na^+/K^+ ATPase activity [148]. Exogenous administration of homocysteine to Wistar rats impairs hippocampal energy metabolism as measured by $^{14}CO_2$ production and glucose uptake [149]. Homocysteine directly interacts with both the amyloid and tau pathways implicated in the pathophysiology of AD. It induces a homocysteine-responsive endoplasmic reticulum stress protein, Herp, that interacts with Presenilin (PS) 1 and 2 to increase β-amyloid (Aβ) generation [150] and also sensitizes cultured hippocampal neurons to the neurotoxicity of insoluble β-amyloid deposits [145, 151]. Homocysteine promotes tau hyperphosphorylation by inhibiting protein phosphatase 2 A (PP2A) [152].

Despite the arguments earlier that the relationship between elevated plasma tHcy levels and an increased risk of brain aging, stroke, and dementia meets the Bradford–Hill criteria suggesting a causal relationship and despite the wealth of biological data supporting a role for homocysteine in the pathogenesis of dementia and AD, it has been suggested that an elevated plasma tHcy level may not play an etiological role (be a true risk factor) in the development of stroke or dementia but may be merely a risk marker of oxidative stress, vitamin B12 or B6 deficiency, impaired renal function, or overall atherosclerotic burden [153]. McCaddon et al. [90] proposed that the hyperhomocysteinemia preceding AD is merely a marker of functional B12 deficiency due to increased brain oxidative stress. Oxidative stress can convert vitamin B12 to an inactive form impairing methinonine synthase activity and thus causing accumulation of homocysteine [90]. One reason we remain uncertain as to which, if any, of the many putative biological pathways are physiologically and pathologically important is that most cell culture and animal studies have used supraphysiological concentrations of homocysteine. Studies of endogenous homocysteine concentrations in animal models of AD would help clarify these issues, and a few such studies have recently been published. Transgenic and doubly transgenic mice models of AD, that is, strains overexpressing the mutant APP gene (Thy1-APP$_{751}$SL), the human tau isoform (TG32), or the human FAD mutant presenilin 1 (PS1M146L) did not develop higher levels of plasma tHcy than wild-type mice, showing that the mutations causing AD do not necessarily lead to hyperhomocystinemia and that hyperhomocysteinemia is not essential for the deposition of β-amyloid [154]. On the other hand if a genetically hyperhomocysteinemic mouse strain (carrying a cystathionine β-synthase mutation) is mated with an APP*/PS1* mouse model of amyloidosis, the progeny not only have hyperhomocysteinemia but also greater than expected deposition of β-amyloid that is directly correlated with serum tHcy levels [155].

18.5.2 Clinical Trials of Homocysteine Lowering to Prevent the Development and Progression of Cognitive Impairment and Dementia

There have been no large studies addressing the role of homocysteine-lowering treatments in preserving cognition and preventing dementia. Cognitive tests were appended to the Vitamins in Stroke Prevention (VISP) and the Vitamins to Prevent Stroke (VITATOPS) trials [156–158]. Most ongoing studies are designed to evaluate the effect of homocysteine-lowering therapies such as high dose vitamins, betaine, or phosphatidylcholine on the rate of cognitive decline in persons already diagnosed with mild to moderate dementia [159, 160], whereas the most interesting group to study would be persons with mild cognitive impairment (MCI), who have a high rate of conversion to clinical AD but in whom the disease process might be more easily modified [161, 162]. In a small observational study, Annerbo and colleagues noted that a low-normal plasma tHcy level reduced the risk of progression of MCI to AD but data from randomized, clinical trials is very limited [163]. The VITAL (VITamins to slow Alzheimer's) study included a few patients with MCI but the number was too small ($n = 43$) and the follow-up period too short (12 weeks) to permit a definitive answer [164]. A two-center randomized, double-blind trial of folate and B12 in 185 persons with ischemic vascular disease included subjects with an MMSE in the 19 to 26 range; at one year follow-up subjects on folate and B12 had lower plasma tHcy levels but did not differ in their cognitive performance. Again, the results are inconclusive since the cognitive assessment tools and period of follow-up were limited and results for the MCI subgroup were not studied separately [165]. Two recently initiated randomized controlled studies (FACT and VITACOG) will study the effect of homocysteine-lowering vitamin therapy on cognitive test scores ($n = 170$ and 350, respectively) in persons with MCI [166]. Future studies should address the effect of varied homocysteine-lowering interventions, including lifestyle modifications such as diet, reduced caffeine intake, and cessation of smoking, as well as evaluating drug treatments. Age, sex, and genotype interactions (for example with the APOE ε4 and the MTHFR 677T genotypes) should be carefully evaluated.

18.6 PARKINSON'S DISEASE

Elevated plasma tHcy levels have been observed in persons with Parkinson's disease, as compared to controls [167–172]. Further, a study of 369 subjects enrolled in the Washington Height's Inwood area observed a cross-sectional relationship between elevated plasma tHcy levels and the presence of mild Parkinsonian signs on examination [173]. However, the frequency of the C677T allele of the MTHFR gene did not differ between persons with Parkinson's disease and control subjects; hence it has been suggested that the observed hyperhomocysteinemia is *secondary* to levodopa treatment [167]. Homocysteine is produced by the *O*-methylation of levodopa, an action facilitated by the enzyme catechol *O*-methyl transferase (COMT). As discussed earlier, homocysteic acid causes excitotoxic neuronal injury, increases oxidative stress, and may result in neuronal loss in the substantia nigra [174]. Hence the observation that exogenous levodopa administration (as treatment for the symptoms of PD) raises plasma tHcy levels causes concern and raises the possibility that this may be one mechanism accelerating the pathological process in Parkinsonian patients on levodopa therapy [175]. Two approaches have been tried to lower plasma tHcy levels in these subjects, administration of the COMT inhibitors tolcapone or entcapone and administration of folate and vitamin B12 [169, 170, 176]. The clinical significance of the observed hyperhomocystinemia and the benefit of lowering tHcy levels (if any) need to be studied in clinical trials.

18.7   EPILEPSY

Homocysteine can be epileptogenic but this has only been documented at supraphysiological doses [177, 178]. It is established that several of the first-generation anti- epileptic agents can elevate plasma tHcy levels. The resulting hyperhomocysteinemia may partly mediate well-known side effects of anticonvulsants such as bone loss [72, 179]. Concomitant administration of folic acid may mitigate the risk of hyperhomocysteinemia.

18.8   CONCLUSIONS

In summary, elevated plasma tHcy levels have been associated with a variety of common neurological diseases such as stroke and Alzheimer's disease. Furthermore, it has been associated with brain imaging, cognitive and physical function measures of subclinical brain aging among persons free of clinical disease. There are several biologically plausible mechanisms that may explain a causal association but it remains possible that an elevated plasma tHcy level is merely a biomarker of an underlying pathological process. Since an elevated tHcy level can be reduced by changes in diet and vitamin intake, the observed associations, their biological underpinnings, and the value or futility of homocysteine-lowering therapy in the primary and secondary prevention of stroke are areas that deserve urgent and thoughtful scrutiny.

ACKNOWLEDGMENTS

Sudha Seshadri is supported by grants 5R01-AG08122, R01-AG033193 and 5R01-AG16495 from the National Institute on Aging and grant 5R01-NS17950-19 from the National Institute of Neurological Disorders and Stroke.

REFERENCES

1. Mangoni, A.A., Jackson, S.H. (2002). Homocysteine and cardiovascular disease: Current evidence and future prospects. *American Journal of Medicine*, *112*(7), 556–565.

2. Seshadri, S. 2006. Elevated plasma homocysteine levels: Risk factor or risk marker for the development of Alzheimer's disease? *Journal of Alzheimer's Disease*, 9, 393–398.

3. Gerritsen, T., Vaughn, J.G., Waisman, H.A. (1962). The identification of homocystine in the urine. *Biochemical and Biophysical Research Communications*, 9, 493–496.

4. Carson, N.A., Cusworth, D.C., Dent, C.E, Field, C.M., Neill, D.W., Westall, R.G. (1963). Homocystinuria: A new inborn error of metabolism associated with mental deficiency. *Archives of Disease in Childhood*, 38, 425–436.

5. Mudd, S.H., Finkelstein, J.D., Irreverre, F., Laster, L. (1964). Homocystinuria: An enzymatic defect. *Science*, 143, 1443–1445.

6. Yap, S., Naughten, E. (1998). Homocystinuria due to cystathionine ± synthase deficiency in Ireland: 25 years' experience of a newborn screened and treated population with reference to clinical outcome and biochemical control. *Journal of Inherited Metabolic Diseases*, 21(7), 738–747.

7. McCully, K.S. (1969). Vascular pathology of homocysteinemia: Implications for the pathogenesis of arteriosclerosis. *American Journal of Pathology*, 56(1), 111–128.

8. Kang, S.S., Zhou, J., Wong, P.W., Kowalisyn, J., Strokosch, G. (1988). Intermediate homocysteinemia: A thermolabile variant of methylenetetrahydrofolate reductase. *American Journal of Human Genetics*, 43(4), 414–421.

9. Nygard, O., Refsum, H., Ueland, P.M., Vollset, S.E. (1998). Major lifestyle determinants of plasma total homocysteine distribution: The Hordaland Homocysteine Study. *American Journal of Clinical Nutrition*, 67(2), 263–270.

10. Homocysteine Studies Collaboration. (2002). Homocysteine and risk of ischemic heart disease and stroke: A meta-analysis. *JAMA*, 288(16), 2015–2022.

11. Kang, S.S., Wong, P.W., Malinow, M.R. (1992). Hyperhomocyst(e)inemia as a risk factor for occlusive vascular disease. *Annual Review of Nutrition*, 12, 279–298.

12. Joosten, E., van den Berg, A., Riezler, R., Naurath, H.J., Lindenbaum, J., Stabler, S.P., Allen, R.H. (1993). Metabolic evidence that deficiencies of vitamin B-12 (cobalamin), folate, and vitamin B-6 occur commonly in elderly people. *American Journal of Clinical Nutrition*, 58(4), 468–476.

13. Selhub, J., Jacques, P.F., Wilson, P.W.F., Rush, D., Rosenberg, I.H. (1993). Vitamin status and intake as primary determinants of homocysteinemia in an elderly population. *JAMA*, 270(22), 2693–2698.

14. Jacques, P.F., Selhub, J., Bostom, A.G., Wilson, P.W.F., Rosenberg, I.H. (1999). The effect of folic acid fortification on plasma folate and total homocysteine concentrations. *New England Journal of Medicine*, 340(19), 1449–1454.

15. Mitchell, G.F., Parise, H., Benjamin, E.J., Larson, M.G., Keyes, M.J., Vita, J.A., Vasan, R.S., Levy, D. (2004). Changes in arterial stiffness and wave reflection with advancing age in healthy men and women: The Framingham Heart Study. *Hypertension*, 43(6), 1239–1245.

16. Nestel, P.J., Chronopoulos, A., Cehun, M. (2003). Arterial stiffness is rapidly induced by raising the plasma homocysteine concentration with methionine. *Atherosclerosis*, 171(1), 83–86.

17. Levy, D., Hwang, S.J., Kayalar, A., Benjamin, E.J., Vasan, R.S., Parise, H., Larson, M.G., Wang, T.J., Selhub, J., Jacques, P.F., Vita, J.A., Keyes, M.J., Mitchell, G.F. (2007). Associations of plasma natriuretic peptide, adrenomedullin, and homocysteine levels

with alterations in arterial stiffness: The Framingham Heart Study. *Circulation, 115*(24), 3079–3085.

18. Voutilainen, S., Alfthan, G., Nyyssonen, K., Salonen, R., Salonen, J.T. (1998). Association between elevated plasma total homocysteine and increased common carotid artery wall thickness. *Annals of Medicine, 30*(3), 300–306.

19. Willinek, W.A., Ludwig, M., Lennarz, M., Holler, T., Stumpe, K.O. (2000). High-normal serum homocysteine concentrations are associated with an increased risk of early atherosclerotic carotid artery wall lesions in healthy subjects. *Journal of Hypertension, 18*(4), 425–430.

20. Aronow, W.S., Ahn, C., Schoenfeld, M.R. (1997). Association between plasma homocysteine and extracranial carotid arterial disease in older persons. *American Journal of Cardiology, 79*(10), 1432–1433.

21. Durga, J., Verhoef, P., Bots, M.L., Schouten, E. (2004). Homocysteine and carotid intima-media thickness: A critical appraisal of the evidence. *Atherosclerosis, 176*(1), 1–19.

22. Nanayakkara, P.W., van Guldener, C., ter Wee, P.M., Scheffer P.G., van Ittersum, F.J., Twisk, J.W., Teelink, T., van Dorp, W., Stehouwer, C.D. (2007). Effect of a treatment strategy consisting of pravastatin, vitamin E, and homocysteine lowering on carotid intima-media thickness, endothelial function, and renal function in patients with mild to moderate chronic kidney disease: Results from the Anti-Oxidant Therapy in Chronic Renal Insufficiency (ATIC) Study. *Archives of Internal Medicine, 167*(12), 1262–1270.

23. Till, U., Rohl, P., Jentsch, A., Till, H., Muller, A., Bellstedt, K., Plonne, D., Fink, H.S., Vollandt, R., Sliwka, U., Herrmann, F.H., Petermann, H., Riezler, R. (2005). Decrease of carotid intima-media thickness in patients at risk to cerebral ischemia after supplementation with folic acid, vitamins B6 and B12. *Atherosclerosis, 181*(1), 131–135.

24. Nakhai-Pour, H.R., Grobbee, D.E., Bots, M.L., Muller, M., van der Schouw, Y.T. (2007). Circulating homocysteine and large arterial stiffness and thickness in a population-based sample of middle-aged and elderly men. *Journal of Human Hypertension, 21*(12), 942–948.

25. de Bree, A., Mennen, L.I., Zureik, M., Ducros, V., Guilland, J.C., Nicolas, J.P., Emery-Fillon, N., Blacher, J., Hercberg, S., Galan, P. (2006). Homocysteine is not associated with arterial thickness and stiffness in healthy middle-aged French volunteers. *International Journal of Cardiology, 113*(3), 332–340.

26. Bots, M.L., Launer, L.J., Lindemans, J., Hofman, A., Grobbee, D.E. (1997). Homocysteine, atherosclerosis, and prevalent cardiovascular disease in the elderly: The Rotterdam Study. *Journal of Internal Medicine, 242*(4), 339–347.

27. Selhub, J., Jacques, P.F., Bostom, A.G., D'Agostino, R.B., Wilson, P.W., Belanger, A.J., O'Leary, D.H., Wolf, P.A., Rush, D., Schaefer, E.J., Rosenberg, I.H. (1996). Relationship between plasma homocysteine, vitamin status and extracranial carotid-artery stenosis in the Framingham Study population. *Journal of Nutrition, 126*(4 Suppl), 1258S–1265S.

28. Hillenbrand, R., Hillenbrand, A., Liewald, F., Zimmermann, J. (2008). Hyperhomocysteinemia and recurrent carotid stenosis. *BMC Cardiovascular Disorders, 8*, 1.

29. Samson, R.H., Yungst, Z., Showalter, D.P. (2004). Homocysteine, a risk factor for carotid atherosclerosis, is not a risk factor for early recurrent carotid stenosis following carotid endarterectomy. *Vascular and Endovascular Surgery, 38*(4), 345–348.

30. Kojoglanian, S.A., Jorgensen, M.B., Wolde-Tsadik, G., Burchette, R.J., Aharonian, V.J. (2003). Restenosis in intervened coronaries with hyperhomocysteinemia (RICH). *American Heart Journal*, *146*(6), 1077–1081.

31. Schnyder, G., Rouvinez, G. (2003). Total plasma homocysteine and restenosis after percutaneous coronary angioplasty: Current evidence. *Annals of Medicine*, *35*(3), 156–163.

32. Schnyder, G., Roffi, M., Flammer, Y., Pin, R., Hess, O.M. (2002). Effect of homocysteine-lowering therapy with folic acid, vitamin B12, and vitamin B6 on clinical outcome after percutaneous coronary intervention: The Swiss Heart study: A randomized controlled trial. *JAMA*, *288*(8), 973–979.

33. Ambrosi, P. (2003). Homocysteine and post-angioplasty restenosis. *Nutrition, Metabolism, and Cardiovascular Diseases*, *13*(6), 391–397.

34. Schnyder, G., Roffi, M., Pin, R., Flammer, Y., Lange, H., Eberli, F.R., Meier, B., Turi, Z.G., Hess, O.M. (2001). Decreased rate of coronary restenosis after lowering of plasma homocysteine levels. *New England Journal of Medicine*, *345*(22), 1593–1600.

35. Galbussera, A., Tremolizzo, L., Longoni, M., Facheris, M., Tagliabue, E., Appollonio, I., Ferrarese, C. (2006). Is elevated post-methionine load homocysteinaemia a risk factor for cervical artery dissection? *Neurological Science*, *27*(1), 78–79.

36. Arauz, A., Hoyos, L., Cantu, C., Jara, A., Martinez, L., Garcia, I., Fernandez, M.L., Alonso, E. (2007). Mild hyperhomocysteinemia and low folate concentrations as risk factors for cervical arterial dissection. *Cerebrovascular Diseases*, *24*(2–3), 210–214.

37. Rubinstein, S.M., Peerdeman, S.M., van Tulder, M.W., Riphagen, I., Haldeman, S. (2005). A systematic review of the risk factors for cervical artery dissection. *Stroke*, *36*(7), 1575–1580.

38. Seshadri, S., Wolf, P.A. (2007). Lifetime risk of stroke and dementia: Current concepts, and estimates from the Framingham Study. *Lancet Neurology*, *6*(12), 1106–1114.

39. Bos, M.J., van Goor, M.L., Koudstaal, P.J., Dippel, D.W. (2005). Plasma homocysteine is a risk factor for recurrent vascular events in young patients with an ischaemic stroke or TIA. *Journal of Neurology*, *252*(3), 332–337.

40. Bostom, A.G., Silbershatz, H., Jacques, P.F., Selhub, J., D'Agostino, R.B., Wolf, P.A., Rosenberg, I.H., Wilson, P.W.F. (1998). Serum total homocysteine levels predict all cause and cardiovascular disease mortality in elderly Framingham men and women. *Circulation*, *97*(8), 818.

41. Marcucci, R., Betti, I., Cecchi, E., Poli, D., Giusti, B., Fedi, S., Lapini, I., Abbate, R., Gensini, G.F., Prisco, D. (2004). Hyperhomocysteinemia and vitamin B6 deficiency: New risk markers for nonvalvular atrial fibrillation? *American Heart Journal*, *148*(3), 456–461.

42. Vasan, R.S., Beiser, A., D'Agostino, R.B., Levy, D., Selhub, J., Jacques, P.F., Rosenberg, I.H., Wilson, P.W. (2003). Plasma homocysteine and risk for congestive heart failure in adults without prior myocardial infarction. *JAMA*, *289*(10), 1251–1257.

43. Hogeveen, M., Blom, H.J., Van Amerongen, M., Boogmans, B., Van Beynum, I.M., Van de Bor, M. (2002). Hyperhomocysteinemia as risk factor for ischemic and hemorrhagic stroke in newborn infants. *Journal of Pediatrics*, *141*(3), 429–431.

44. Van Beynum, I.M., Smeitink, J.A., den Heijer, M., te Poele Pothoff, M.T., Blom, H.J. (1999). Hyperhomocysteinemia: A risk factor for ischemic stroke in children. *Circulation*, *99*(16), 2070–2072.

45. Kittner, S.J., Giles, W.H., Macko, R.F., Hebel, J.R., Wozniak, M.A., Wityk, R.J., Stolley, P.D., Stern, B.J., Sloan, M.A., Sherwin, R., Price, T.R., McCarter, R.J., Johnson, C.J., Earley, C.J., Buchholz, D.W., Malinow, M.R. (1999). Homocyst(e)ine and risk of cerebral infarction in a biracial population: The stroke prevention in young women study. *Stroke, 30*(8), 1554–1560.

46. Iso, H., Moriyama, Y., Sato, S., Kitamura, A., Tanigawa, T., Yamagishi, K., Imano, H., Ohira, T., Okamura, T., Naito, Y., Shimamoto, T. (2004). Serum total homocysteine concentrations and risk of stroke and its subtypes in Japanese. *Circulation, 109*(22), 2766–2772.

47. Petri, M., Roubenoff, R., Dallal, G.E., Nadeau, M.R., Selhub, J., Rosenberg, I.H. (1996). Plasma homocysteine as a risk factor for atherothrombotic events in systemic lupus erythematosus. *Lancet, 348*(9035), 1120–1124.

48. Houston, P.E., Rana, S., Sekhsaria, S., Perlin, E., Kim, K.S., Castro, O.L. (1997). Homocysteine in sickle cell disease: Relationship to stroke. *American Journal of Medicine, 103*(3), 192–196.

49. Bostom, A.G., Shemin, D., Verhoef, P., Nadeau, M.R., Jacques, P.F., Selhub, J., Dworkin, L., Rosenberg, I.H. (1997). Elevated fasting total plasma homocysteine levels and cardiovascular disease outcomes in maintenance dialysis patients: A prospective study. *Arteriosclerosis Thrombosis and Vascular Biology, 17*(11), 2554–2558.

50. Clarke, R., Daly, L., Robinson, K., Naughten, E., Cahalane, S., Fowler, B., Graham, I. (1991). Hyperhomocysteinemia: An independent risk factor for vascular disease. *New England Journal of Medicine, 324*(17), 1149–1155.

51. Brattstrom, L., Lindgren, A., Israelsson, B., Malinow, M.R., Norrving, B., Upson, B., Hamfelt, A. (1992). Hyperhomocysteinaemia in stroke: Prevalence, cause, and relationships to type of stroke and stroke risk factors. *European Journal of Clinical Investigations, 22*(3), 214–221.

52. Boushey, C.J., Beresford, S.A., Omenn, G.S., Motulsky, A.G. (1995). A quantitative assessment of plasma homocysteine as a risk factor for vascular disease: Probable benefits of increasing folic acid intakes. *JAMA, 274*(13), 1049–1057.

53. Clarke, R., Collins, R., Lewington, S., Donald, A., Alfthan, G., Tuomilehto, J., Arnesen, E., Bonaa, K., Blacher, J., Boers, G.H.J., Bostom, A., Bots, M.L., Grobee, D.E., Brattstrom, L., Breteler, M.M.B., Hofman, A., Chambers, J.C., Kooner, J.S., Coull, B.M., Evans, R.W., Kuller, L.H., Evers, S., Folsom, A.R., Freyburger, G., Parrot, F., Genst, J., Dalery, K., Graham, I.M., Daly, L., Hoogeveen, E.K., Kostense, P.J., Stehouwer, C.D.A., Hopknis, P.N., Jacques, P., Selhub, J., Luft, F.C., Jungers, P., Lindgren, A., Lolin, Y.I., Loehrer, F., Fowler, B., Mansoor, M.A., Malinow, M.R., Ducimetiere, P., Nygard, O., Refsum, H., Vollset, S.E., Ueland, P.M., Omenn, G.S., Beresford, S.A.A., Roseman, J.M., Parving, H.H., Gall, M.A., Perry, I.J., Ebraham, S.B., Shaper, A.G., Robinson, K., Jacobsen, D.W., Schwartz, S.M., Siscovick, D.S., Stampfer, M.J., Henekens, C.H., Feskens, E.J.M., Kromhout, D., Ubbink, J., Elwood, P., Pickering, J., Verhoef, P., von Eckardstein, A., Schulte, H., Assmann, G., Wald, N., Law, M.R., Whincup, P.H., Wilcken, D.E.L., Sherliker, P., Linksted, P., Smith, G.D., Witteman, J.C.M., Israelsson, B., Sexton, G., Wu, L.L., Joubran, R., Norrving, B., Hultberg, B., Andersson, A., Johansson, B.B., Bergmark, C., Svardal, A.M., Evans, A.E., Pancharuniti, N., Lewis, C.A., Holman, R., Stratton, I., Johnston, C., Morris, J. (2002). Homocysteine and risk of ischemic heart disease and stroke: a meta-analysis. *JAMA, 288*(16), 2015–2022.

54. Alfthan, G., Pekkanen, J., Jauhiainen, M., Pitkaniemi, J., Karvonen, M., Tuomilehto, J., Salonen, J.T., Ehnholm, C. (1994). Relation of serum homocysteine and lipoprotein(a) concentrations to atherosclerotic disease in a prospective Finnish population based study. *Atherosclerosis*, *106*(1), 9–19.

55. Verhoef, P., Hennekens, C.H., Malinow, M.R., Kok, F.J., Willett, W.C., Stampfer, M.J. (1994). A prospective study of plasma homocyst(e)ine and risk of ischemic stroke. *Stroke*, *25*(10), 1924–1930.

56. Bautista, L.E., Arenas, I.A., Penuela, A., Martinez, L.X. (2002). Total plasma homocysteine level and risk of cardiovascular disease: A meta-analysis of prospective cohort studies. *Journal of Clinical Epidemiology*, *55*(9), 882–887.

57. Eikelboom, J.W., Hankey, G.J. (2001). Associations of homocysteine, C-reactive protein and cardiovascular disease in patients with renal disease. *Current Opinion in Nephrology and Hypertension*, *10*(3), 377–383.

58. Moller, J., Nielsen, G.M., Tvedegaard, K.C., Andersen, N.T., Jorgensen, P.E. (2000). A meta-analysis of cerebrovascular disease and hyperhomocysteinaemia. *Scandinavian Journal of Clinical and Laboratory Investigation*, *60*(6), 491–499.

59. Meiklejohn, D.J., Vickers, M.A., Dijkhuisen, R., Greaves, M. (2001). Plasma homocysteine concentrations in the acute and convalescent periods of atherothrombotic stroke. *Stroke*, *32*(1), 57–62.

60. Bostom, A.G., Rosenberg, I.H., Silbershatz, H., Jacques, P.F., Selhub, J., D'Agostino, R.B., Wilson, P.W.F., Wolf, P.A. (1999). Nonfasting plasma total homocysteine levels and stroke incidence in elderly persons: The Framingham Study. *Annals of Internal Medicine*, *131*(5), 352–355.

61. Bostom, A.G., Silbershatz, H., Rosenberg, I.H., Selhub, J., D'Agostino, R.B., Wolf, P.A., Jacques, P.F., Wilson, P.W. (1999). Nonfasting plasma total homocysteine levels and all-cause and cardiovascular disease mortality in elderly Framingham men and women. *Archives of Internal Medicine*, *159*(10), 1077–1080.

62. Casas, J.P., Bautista, L.E., Smeeth, L., Sharma, P., Hingorani, A.D. (2005). Homocysteine and stroke: Evidence on a causal link from mendelian randomisation. *Lancet*, *365*(9455), 224–232.

63. Loscalzo, J. (2006). Homocysteine trials: Clear outcomes for complex reasons. *New England Journal of Medicine*, *354*, 1629–1632.

64. Spence, J.D., Bang, H., Chambless, L.E., Stampfer, M.J. (2005). Vitamin Intervention for Stroke Prevention trial: An efficacy analysis. *Stroke*, *36*(11), 2404–2409.

65. Bonaa, K.H., Njolstad, I., Ueland, P.M., Schirmer, H., Tverdal, A., Steigen, T., Wang, H., Nordrehaug, J.E., Arnesen, E., Rasmussen, K. (2006). Homocysteine lowering and cardiovascular events after acute myocardial infarction. *New England Journal of Medicine*, *354*(15), 1578–1588.

66. Mann, J.F., Sheridan, P., McQueen, M.J., Held, C., Arnold, J.M., Fodor, G., Yusuf, S., Lonn, E.M. (2008). Homocysteine lowering with folic acid and B vitamins in people with chronic kidney disease: Results of the renal Hope-2 study. *Nephrology, Dialysis, Transplantation*, *23*(2), 645–653.

67. Strasser, R.H. (2007). Status of homocysteine reduction in prevention of cardiovascular diseases. HOPE–2 study (Heart Outcomes Prevention Evaluation). *Internist (Berlin)*, *48*(3), 327–329.

68. Kullo, I.J. (2006). HOPE 2: Can supplementation with folic acid and B vitamins reduce cardiovascular risk? *Nature Clinical Practice. Cardiovascular Medicine*, *3*(8), 414–415.

69. Lonn, E., Yusuf, S., Arnold, M.J., Sheridan, P., Pogue, J., Micks, M., McQueen, M.J., Probstfield, J., Fodor, G., Held, C., Genest, J., Jr. (2006). Homocysteine lowering with folic acid and B vitamins in vascular disease. *New England Journal of Medicine*, *354*(15), 1567–1577.

70. Lonn, E., Held, C., Arnold, J.M., Probstfield, J., McQueen, M., Micks, M., Pogue, J., Sheridan, P., Bosch, J., Genest, J., Yusuf, S. (2006). Rationale, design and baseline characteristics of a large, simple, randomized trial of combined folic acid and vitamins B6 and B12 in high-risk patients: The Heart Outcomes Prevention Evaluation (HOPE)-2 trial. *Canadian Journal of Cardiology*, *22*(1), 47–53.

71. Cabrini, L., Bochicchio, D., Bordoni, A., Sassi, S., Marchetti, M., Maranesi, M. (2005). Correlation between dietary polyunsaturated fatty acids and plasma homocysteine concentration in vitamin B6-deficient rats. *Nutrition, Metabolism, and Cardiovascular Diseases*, *15*(2), 94–99.

72. den Heijen, M., Koster, T., Blom, H.J., Bos, G.M., Briet, E., Reitsma, P.H., Vandenbroucke, J.P., Rosendaal, F.R. (1996). Hyperhomocysteinemia as a risk factor for deep-vein thrombosis. *New England Journal of Medicine*, *334*(12), 759–762.

73. Aubard, Y., Darodes, N., Cantaloube, M. (2000). Hyperhomocysteinemia and pregnancy: Review of our present understanding and therapeutic implications. *European Journal of Obstetrics, Gynecology, and Reproductive Biology*, *93*(2), 157–165.

74. Lopez-Quesada, E., Vilaseca, M.A., Lailla, J.M. (2003). Plasma total homocysteine in uncomplicated pregnancy and in preeclampsia. *European Journal of Obstetrics, Gynecology, and Reproductive Biology*, *108*(1), 45–49.

75. American Psychiatric Association. (1994). *Diagnostic and Statistical Manual of Mental Disorders (DSM-IV)*. Washington, D.C.: American Psychiatric Association.

76. McKhann, G., Drachman, D., Folstein, M., Katzman, R., Price, D., Stadlan, E.M. (1984). Clinical diagnosis of Alzheimer's disease: Report of the NINCDS-ADRDA Work Group under the auspices of Department of Health and Human Services Task Force on Alzheimer's Disease. *Neurology*, *34*(7), 939–944.

77. Roman, G.C., Tatemichi, T.K., Erkinjuntti, T., Cummings, J.L., Masdeu, J.C., Garcia, J.H., Amaducci, L., Orgogozo, J.M., Brun, A., Hofman, A. (1993). Vascular dementia: Diagnostic criteria for research studies. Report of the NINDS-AIREN International Workshop. *Neurology*, *43*(2), 250–260.

78. Chui, H.C., Victoroff, J.I., Margolin, D., Jagust, W., Shankle, R., Katzman, R. (1992). Criteria for the diagnosis of ischemic vascular dementia proposed by the State of California Alzheimer's Disease Diagnostic and Treatment Centers. *Neurology*, *42*(3 Pt 1), 473–480.

79. Hachinski, V., Iadecola, C., Petersen, R.C., Breteler, M.M., Nyenhuis, D.L., Black, S.E., Powers, W.J., De Carli, C., Merino, J.G., Kalaria, R.N., Vinters, H.V., Holtzman, D.M., Rosenberg, G.A., Wallin, A., Dichgans, M., Marler, J.R., Leblanc, G.G. (2006). National Institute of Neurological Disorders and Stroke-Canadian Stroke Network vascular cognitive impairment harmonization standards. *Stroke*, *37*(9), 2220–2241.

80. Samson, D.C., Swisher, S.N., Christain, R.M., Engel, G.L. (1952). Cerebral metabolic disturbance and delirium in pernicious anemia: Clinical and electroencephalographic studies. *AMA Archives of Internal Medicine*, *90*(1), 4–14.

81. Lindenbaum, J., Rosenberg, I.H., Wilson, P.W., STabler, S.P., Allen, R.H. (1994). Prevalence of cobalamin deficiency in the Framingham elderly population. *American Journal of Clinical Nutrition, 60*(1), 2–11.

82. van Asselt, D.Z., Pasman, J.W., van Lier, H.J., Vingerhoets, D.M., Poels, P.J., Kuin, Y., Blom, H.J., Hoefnagels, W.H. (2001). Cobalamin supplementation improves cognitive and cerebral function in older, cobalamin-deficient persons. *Journal of Gerontology. A Biological Science and Medical Science, 56*(12), M775–M779.

83. Carmel, R. (1996). Prevalence of undiagnosed pernicious anemia in the elderly. *Archives of Internal Medicine, 156*(10), 1097–1100.

84. Goodwin, J.S., Goodwin, J.M., Garry, P.J. (1983). Association between nutritional status and cognitive functioning in a healthy elderly population. *JAMA, 249*(21), 2917–2921.

85. Nilsson, K., Gustafson, L., Hultberg, B. (2001). Improvement of cognitive functions after cobalamin/folate supplementation in elderly patients with dementia and elevated plasma homocysteine. *International Journal of Geriatric Psychiatry, 16*(6), 609–614.

86. Nilsson, K., Gustafson, L., Hultberg, B. (2002). Optimal use of markers for cobalamin and folate status in a psychogeriatric population. *International Journal of Geriatric Psychiatry, 17*(10), 919–925.

87. Budge, M., Johnston, C., Hogervorst, E., de Jager, C., Milwain, E., Iversen, S.D., Barnetson, L., King, E., Smith, A.D. (2000). Plasma total homocysteine and cognitive performance in a volunteer elderly population. *Annals of the New York Academy of Science, 903*, 407–410.

88. Lehmann, M., Gottfries, C.G., Regland, B. (1999). Identification of cognitive impairment in the elderly: Homocysteine is an early marker. *Dementia and Geriatric Cognitive Disorders, 10*(1), 12–20.

89. Lindenbaum, J., Healton, E.B., Savage, D.G., Brust, J.C., Garrett, T.J., Podell, E.R., Marcell, P.D., Stabler, S.P., Allen, R.H. (1988). Neuropsychiatric disorders caused by cobalamin deficiency in the absence of anemia or macrocytosis. *New England Journal of Medicine, 318*(26), 1720–1728.

90. McCaddon, A., Regland, B., Hudson, P., Davies, G. (2002). Functional vitamin B(12) deficiency and Alzheimer disease. *Neurology, 58*(9), 1395–1399.

91. Elias, M.F., Sullivan, L.M., D'Agostino, R.B., Elias, P.K., Jacques, P.F., Selhub, J., Seshadri, S., Au, R., Beiser, A., Wolf, P.A. (2005). Homocysteine and cognitive performance in the Framingham offspring study: Age is important. *American Journal of Epidemiology, 162*(7), 644–653.

92. Wright, C.B., Lee, H.S., Paik, M.C., STabler, S.P., Allen, R.H., Sacco, RL. (2004). Total homocysteine and cognition in a tri-ethnic cohort: The Northern Manhattan Study. *Neurology, 63*(2), 254–260.

93. Riggs, K.M., Spiro, A. III., Tucker, K., Rush, D. (1996). Relations of vitamin B-12, vitamin B-6, folate, and homocysteine to cognitive performance in the Normative Aging Study. *American Journal of Clinical Nutrition, 63*(3), 306–314.

94. Miller, J.W., Green, R., Ramos, M.I., Allen, L.H., Mungas, D.M., Jagust, W.J., Haan, M.N. (2003). Homocysteine and cognitive function in the Sacramento Area Latino Study on Aging. *American Journal of Clinical Nutrition, 78*(3), 441–447.

95. Ravaglia, G., Forti, P., Maioli, F., Scali, R.C., Saccheitti, L., Talerico, T., Mantovani, V., Bianchin, M. (2004). Homocysteine and cognitive performance in healthy elderly subjects. *Archives of Gerontology and Geriatrics, 9*(Suppl), 349–357.

96. Prins, N.D., den Heijer, T., Hofman, A., Koudstaal, P.J., Jolles, J., Clarke, R., Breteler, M.M.B. (2002). Homocysteine and cognitive function in the elderly: The Rotterdam Scan Study. *Neurology*, *59*(9), 1375–1380.

97. Morris, M.S., Jacques, P.F., Rosenberg, I.H., Selhub, J. (2001). Hyperhomocysteinemia associated with poor recall in the third National Health and Nutrition Examination Survey. *American Journal of Clinical Nutrition*, *73*(5), 927–933.

98. McCaddon, A., Hudson, P., Davies, G., Hughes, A., Williams, J.H., Wilkinson, C. (2001). Homocysteine and cognitive decline in healthy elderly. *Dementia and Geriatric Cognitive Disorders*, *12*(5), 309–313.

99. Kalmijn, S., Launer, L.J., Lindemans, J., Bots, M.L., Hofman, A., Breteler, M.M. (1999). Total homocysteine and cognitive decline in a community-based sample of elderly subjects: The Rotterdam Study. *American Journal of Epidemiology*, *150*(3), 283–289.

100. Schafer, J.H., Glass, T.A., Bolla, K.I., Mintz, M., Jedlicka, A.E., Schwartz, B.S. (2005). Homocysteine and cognitive function in a population-based study of older adults. *Journal of the American Geriatrics Society*, *53*(3), 381–388.

101. Adunsky, A., Arinzon, Z., Fidelman, Z., Krasniansky, I., Arad, M., Gepstein, R. (2005). Plasma homocysteine levels and cognitive status in long-term stay geriatric patients: A cross-sectional study. *Archives of Gerontology and Geriatrics*, *40*(2), 129–138.

102. Almeida, O.P., Lautenschlager, N., Flicker, L., Leedman, P., Vasikaran, S., Gelavis, A., Ludlow, J. (2004). Association between homocysteine, depression, and cognitive function in community-dwelling older women from Australia. *Journal of the American Geriatrics Society*, *52*(2), 327–328.

103. Barbaux, S., Plomin, R., Whitehead, A.S. (2000). Polymorphisms of genes controlling homocysteine/folate metabolism and cognitive function. *Neuroreport*, *11*(5), 1133–1136.

104. Budge, M.M., de Jager, C., Hogervorst, E., Smith, A.D. (2002). Total plasma homocysteine, age, systolic blood pressure, and cognitive performance in older people. *Journal of the American Geriatrics Society*, *50*(12), 2014–2018.

105. de Luis, D.A., Fernandez, N., Arranz, M., Aller, R., Izaola, O. (2002). Total homocysteine and cognitive deterioration in people with type 2 diabetes. *Diabetes Research and Clinical Practice*, *55*(3), 185–190.

106. Dufouil, C., Alperovitch, A., Ducros, V., Tzourio, C. (2003). Homocysteine, white matter hyperintensities, and cognition in healthy elderly people. *Annals of Neurology*, *53*(2), 214–221.

107. Duthie, S.J., Whalley, L.J., Collins, A.R., Leaper, S., Berger, K., Deary, I.J. (2002). Homocysteine, B vitamin status, and cognitive function in the elderly. *American Journal of Clinical Nutrition*, *75*(5), 908–913.

108. Flicker, L., Martins, R.N., Thomas, J., Acres, J., Taddei, K., Norman, P., Jamrozik, K., Almeida, O.P. (2004). Homocysteine, Alzheimer genes and proteins, and measures of cognition and depression in older men. *Journal of Alzheimer's Disease*, *6*(3), 329–336.

109. Garcia, A.A., Haron, Y., Evans, L.R., Smith, M.G., Freedman, M., Roman, G.C. (2004). Metabolic markers of cobalamin deficiency and cognitive function in normal older adults. *Journal of the American Geriatrics Society*, *52*(1), 66–71.

110. Lewerin, C., Matousek, M., Steen, G., Johansson, B., Steen, B., Nilsson-Ehle, H. (2005). Significant correlations of plasma homocysteine and serum methylmalonic acid with movement and cognitive performance in elderly subjects but no improvement from

short-term vitamin therapy: A placebo-controlled randomized study. *American Journal of Clinical Nutrition, 81*(5), 1155–1162.

111. Ravaglia, G., Forti, P., Maioli, F., Muscari, A., Sacchetti, L., Arnone, G., Nativio, V., Talerico, T., Mariani, E. (2003). Homocysteine and cognitive function in healthy elderly community dwellers in Italy. *American Journal of Clinical Nutrition, 77*(3), 668–673.

112. Reutens, S., Sachdev, P. (2002). Homocysteine in neuropsychiatric disorders of the elderly. *International Journal of Geriatric Psychiatry, 17*(9), 859–864.

113. Robbins, M.A., Elias, M.F., Budge, M.M., Brennan, S.L., Elias, P.K. (2005). Homocysteine, type 2 diabetes mellitus, and cognitive performance: The Maine-Syracuse Study. *Clinical Chemistry and Laboratory Medicine, 43*(10), 1101–1106.

114. Teunissen, C.E., Blom, A.H., Van Boxtel, M.P., Bosma, H., de Bruijn, C., Jolles, J., Wauters, B.A., Steinbusch, H.W., de Vente, J. (2003). Homocysteine: A marker for cognitive performance? A longitudinal follow-up study. *Journal of Nutrition, Health, and Aging, 7*(3), 153–159.

115. Hofman, A., Ott, A., Breteler, M.M., Bots, M.L., Slooter, A.J., van Harskamp, F., van Duijn, C.N., Van Broeckhoven, C., Grobbee, D.E. (1997). Atherosclerosis, apolipoprotein E, and prevalence of dementia and Alzheimer's disease in the Rotterdam Study. *Lancet, 349*(9046), 151–154.

116. Ivan, C.S., Seshadri, S., Beiser, A., Au, R., Kase, C.S., Kelly-Hayes, M., Wolf, P.A. (2004). Dementia after stroke: The Framingham Study. *Stroke, 35*(6), 1264–1268.

117. Clarke, R., Smith, A.D., Jobst, K.A., Refsum, H., Sutton, L., Ueland, P.M. (1998). Folate, vitamin B12, and serum total homocysteine levels in confirmed Alzheimer disease. *Archives of Neurology, 55*(11), 1449–1455.

118. McCaddon, A., Davies, G., Hudson, P., Tandy, S., Cattell, H. (1998). Total serum homocysteine in senile dementia of Alzheimer type. *International Journal of Geriatric Psychiatry, 13*(4), 235–239.

119. McIlroy, S.P., Dynan, K.B., Lawson, J.T., Patterson, C.C., Passmore, A.P. (2002). Moderately elevated plasma homocysteine, methylenetetrahydrofolate reductase genotype, and risk for stroke, vascular dementia, and Alzheimer disease in Northern Ireland. *Stroke, 33*(10), 2351–2356.

120. Hill, A.B. (1965). The environment and disease: Association or causation? *Proceedings of the Royal Society of Medicine, 58*, 295–300.

121. Seshadri, S., Beiser, A., Selhub, J., Jacques, P.F., Rosenberg, I.H., D'Agostino, R.B., Wilson, P.W.F., Wolf, P.A. (2002). Plasma homocysteine as a risk factor for dementia and Alzheimer's disease. *New England Journal of Medicine, 346*(7), 476–483.

122. Ravaglia, G., Forti, P., Maioli, F., Martelli, M., Servadei, L., Brunetti, N., Porcellini, E., Licastro, F. (2005). Homocysteine and folate as risk factors for dementia and Alzheimer disease. *American Journal of Clinical Nutrition, 82*(3), 636–643.

123. Luchsinger, J.A., Tang, M.X., Shea, S., Miller, J., Green, R., Mayeux, R. (2004). Plasma homocysteine levels and risk of Alzheimer disease. *Neurology, 62*(11), 1972–1976.

124. Seshadri, S., Wolf, P.A., Beiser, A.S., Selhub, J., Au, R., Jacques, P.F., Yoshita, M., Rosenberg, I.H., D'Agostino, R.B., DeCarli, C. (2008). Association of plasma total homocysteine levels with subclinical brain injury: Cerebral volumes, white matter hyperintensity, and silent brain infarcts at volumetric magnetic resonance imaging in the Framingham Offspring Study. *Archives of Neurology, 65*(5), 642–649.

125. Sachdev, P. (2004). Homocysteine, cerebrovascular disease and brain atrophy. *Journal of Neurological Sciences*, *226*(1–2), 25–29.

126. Whalley, L.J., Staff, R.T., Murray, A.D., Duthie, S.J., Collins, A.R., Lemmon, H.A., Starr, J.M., Deary, I.J. (2003). Plasma vitamin C, cholesterol and homocysteine are associated with grey matter volume determined by MRI in non-demented old people. *Neuroscience Letters*, *341*(3), 173–176.

127. Den, H.T., Vermeer, S.E., Clarke, R., Oudkerk, M., Koudstaal, P.J., Hofman, A., Breteler, M.M. (2003). Homocysteine and brain atrophy on MRI of non-demented elderly. *Brain*, *126*(Pt 1), 170–175.

128. Vermeer, S.E., van Dijk, E.J., Koudstaal, P.J., Oudkerk, M., Hofman, A., Clarke, R., Breteler, M.M. (2002). Homocysteine, silent brain infarcts, and white matter lesions: The Rotterdam Scan Study. *Annals of Neurology*, *51*(3), 285–289.

129. Matsui, T., Arai, H., Yuzuriha, T., Yao, H., Miura, M., Hashimoto, S., Higuchi, S., Matsushita, S., Morikawa, M., Kato, A., Sasaki, H. (2001). Elevated plasma homocysteine levels and risk of silent brain infarction in elderly people. *Stroke*, *32*(5), 1116–1119.

130. Bleich, S., Sperling, W., Degner, D., Graesel, E., Bleich, K., Wilhelm, J., Havemann-Reinecke, U., Javaheripour, K., Kornhuber, J. (2003). Lack of association between hippocampal volume reduction and first-onset alcohol withdrawal seizure. A volumetric MRI study. *Alcohol and Alcoholism*, *38*(1), 40–44.

131. Williams, J.H., Pereira, E.A., Budge, M.M., Bradley, K.M. (2002). Minimal hippocampal width relates to plasma homocysteine in community-dwelling older people. *Age Ageing*, *31*(6), 440–444.

132. Longstreth, W.T., Katz, R., Olson, J., Bernick, C., Carr, J.J., Malinow, M.R., Hess, D.L., Cushman, M., Schwartz, S.M. (2004). Plasma total homocysteine levels and cranial magnetic resonance imaging findings in elderly persons: The Cardiovascular Health Study. *Archives of Neurology*, *61*(1), 67–72.

133. Kohara, K., Fujisawa, M., Ando, F., Tabara, Y., Niino, N., Miki, T., Shimokata, H. (2003). MTHFR gene polymorphism as a risk factor for silent brain infarcts and white matter lesions in the Japanese general population: The NILS-LSA Study. *Stroke*, *34*(5), 1130–1135.

134. Hogervorst, E., Ribeiro, H.M., Molyneux, A., Budge, M., Smith, A.D. (2002). Plasma homocysteine levels, cerebrovascular risk factors, and cerebral white matter changes (leukoaraiosis) in patients with Alzheimer disease. *Archives of Neurology*, *59*(5), 787–793.

135. Sachdev, P., Parslow, R., Salonikas, C., Lux, O., Wen, W., Kumar, R., Naidoo, D., Christensen, H., Jorm, A. (2004). Homocysteine and the brain in midadult life: Evidence for an increased risk of leukoaraiosis in men. *Archives of Neurology*, *61*(9), 1369–1376.

136. Wright, C.B., Paik, M.C., Brown, T.R., STabler, S.P., Allen, R.H., Sacco, R.L., DeCarli, C. (2005). Total homocysteine is associated with white matter hyperintensity volume: The Northern Manhattan Study. *Stroke*, *36*(6), 1207–1211.

137. Kado, D.M., Karlamangla, A.S., Huang, M.H., Troen, A., Rowe, J.W., Selhub, J., Seeman, T.E. (2005). Homocysteine versus the vitamins folate, B6, and B12 as predictors of cognitive function and decline in older high-functioning adults: MacArthur Studies of Successful Aging. *American Journal of Medicine*, *118*(2), 161–167.

138. Welch, G.N., Loscalzo, J. (1998). Homocysteine and atherothrombosis. *New England Journal of Medicine, 338*(15), 1042–1050.

139. Kim, J.M., Lee, H., Chang, N. (2002). Hyperhomocysteinemia due to short-term folate deprivation is related to electron microscopic changes in the rat brain. *Journal of Nutrition, 132*(11), 3418–3421.

140. Xu, D., Neville, R., Finkel, T. (2000). Homocysteine accelerates endothelial cell senescence. *FEBS Letters, 470*(1), 20–24.

141. Stessman, J., Maaravi, Y., Hammerman-Rozenberg, R., Cohen, A., Nemanov, L., Gritsenko, I., Gruberman, N., Ebstein, R.P. (2005). Candidate genes associated with ageing and life expectancy in the Jerusalem longitudinal study. *Mechanisms of Ageing and Development, 126*(2), 333–339.

142. Benz, B., Grima, G., Do, K.Q. (2004). Glutamate-induced homocysteic acid release from astrocytes: Possible implication in glia-neuron signaling. *Neuroscience, 124*(2), 377–386.

143. Lehmann, J., Tsai, C., Wood, P.L. (1988). Homocysteic acid as a putative excitatory amino acid neurotransmitter. I. Postsynaptic characteristics at N-methyl-D-aspartate-type receptors on striatal cholinergic interneurons. *Journal of Neurochemistry, 51*(6), 1765–1770.

144. Ho, P.I., Ortiz, D., Rogers, E., Shea, T.B. (2002). Multiple aspects of homocysteine neurotoxicity: Glutamate excitotoxicity, kinase hyperactivation and DNA damage. *Journal of Neuroscience Research, 70*(5), 694–702.

145. Kruman, I.I., Kumaravel, T.S., Lohani, A., Pedersen, W.A., Cutler, R.G., Kruman, Y., Haughey, N., Lee, J., Evans, M., Mattson, M.P. (2002). Folic acid deficiency and homocysteine impair DNA repair in hippocampal neurons and sensitize them to amyloid toxicity in experimental models of Alzheimer's disease. *Journal of Neuroscience, 22*(5), 1752–1762.

146. Jakubowski, H. (1999). Protein homocysteinylation: Possible mechanism underlying pathological consequences of elevated homocysteine levels. *FASEB Journal, 13*(15), 2277–2283.

147. Medina, M., Urdiales, J.L., Mores-Sanchez, M.I. (2001). Roles of homocysteine in cell metabolism: Old and new functions. *European Journal of Biochemistry, 268*(14), 3871–3882.

148. Streck, E.L., Zugno, A.I., Tagliari, B., Wannmacher, C., Wajner, M., Wyse, A.T. (2002). Inhibition of Na^+, K^+-ATPase activity by the metabolites accumulating in homocystinuria. *Metabolism and Brain Diseases, 17*(2), 83–91.

149. Streck, E.L., Matte, C., Vieira, P.S., Calcagnotto, T., Wannmacher, C.M., Wajner, M., Wyse, A.T. (2003). Impairment of energy metabolism in hippocampus of rats subjected to chemically-induced hyperhomocysteinemia. *Biochimica et Biophysica Acta, 1637*(3), 187–192.

150. Sai, X., Kawamura, Y., Kokame, K., Yamaguchi, H., Shiraishi, H., Suzuki, R., Suzuki, T., Kawaichi, M., Miyata, T., Kitamura, T., De Strooper, B., Yanagisawa, K., Komano, H. (2002). Endoplasmic reticulum stress-inducible protein, Herp, enhances presenilin-mediated generation of amyloid beta-protein. *Journal of Biological Chemistry, 277*(15), 12915–21290.

151. White, A.R., Huang, X., Jobling, M.F., Barrow, C.J., Beyreuther, K., Masters, C.L., Bush, A.I., Cappai, R. (2001). Homocysteine potentiates copper- and amyloid beta peptide-mediated toxicity in primary neuronal cultures: Possible risk factors in the Alzheimer's-type neurodegenerative pathways. *Journal of Neurochemistry, 76*(5), 1509–1520.

152. Vafai, S.B., Stock, J.B. (2002). Protein phosphatase 2A methylation: A link between elevated plasma homocysteine and Alzheimer's Disease. *FEBS Letters, 518*(1–3), 1–4.

153. Weiss, N., Hilge, R., Hoffmann, U. (2004). Mild hyperhomocysteinemia: Risk factor or just risk predictor for cardiovascular diseases? *Vasa, 33*(4), 191–203.

154. Santiard-Baron, D., Aupetit, J., Janel, N. (2005). Plasma homocysteine levels are not increased in murine models of Alzheimer's disease. *Neuroscience Research, 53*(4), 447–449.

155. Pacheco-Quinto, J., Rodriguez de Turco, E.B., Derosa, S., Howard, A., Cruz–Sanchez, F., Sambamurti, K., Refolo, L., Petanceska, S., Pappolla, M.A. (2006). Hyperhomocysteinemic Alzheimer's mouse model of amyloidosis shows increased brain amyloid beta peptide levels. *Neurobiology of Diseases, 22*(3), 651–656.

156. Spence, J.D., Howard, V.J., Chambless, L.E., Malinow, M.R., Pettigrew, L.C., Stampfer, M., Toole, J.F. (2001). Vitamin Intervention for Stroke Prevention (VISP) trial: Rationale and design. *Neuroepidemiology, 20*(1), 16–25.

157. Toole, J.F., Malinow, M.R., Chambless, L.E., Spence, J.D., Pettigrew, L.C., Howard, V.J., Sides, E.G., Wang, C.H., Stampfer, M. (2004). Lowering homocysteine in patients with ischemic stroke to prevent recurrent stroke, myocardial infarction, and death: The Vitamin Intervention for Stroke Prevention (VISP) randomized controlled trial. *JAMA, 291*(5), 565–575.

158. VITATOPS Trial Study Group. (2002). The VITATOPS (Vitamins to Prevent Stroke) Trial: Rationale and design of an international, large, simple, randomised trial of homocysteine-lowering multivitamin therapy in patients with recent transient ischaemic attack or stroke. *Cerebrovascular Diseases, 13*(2), 120–126.

159. Aisen, P.S., Egelko, S., Andrews, H., Diaz-Arrastia, R., Weiner, M., DeCarli, C., Jagust, W., Miller, J.W., Green, R., Bell, K., Sano, M. (2003). A pilot study of vitamins to lower plasma homocysteine levels in Alzheimer disease. *American Journal of Geriatric Psychiatry, 11*(2), 246–249.

160. Malouf, M., Grimley, E.J., Areosa, S.A. (2003). Folic acid with or without vitamin B12 for cognition and dementia. *Cochrane Database of Systematic Reviews, 4*, CD004514.

161. Elias, M.F., Beiser, A., Wolf, P.A., Au, R., White, R.F., D'Agostino, R.B. (2000). The preclinical phase of Alzheimer disease: A 22-year prospective study of the Framingham Cohort. *Archives of Neurology, 57*(6), 808–813.

162. Shah, Y., Tangalos, E.G., Petersen, R.C. (2000). Mild cognitive impairment. When is it a precursor to Alzheimer's disease? *Geriatrics, 55*(9), 62, 65–68.

163. Annerbo, S., Wahlund, L.O., Lokk, J. (2005). The relation between homocysteine levels and development of Alzheimer's disease in mild cognitive impairment patients. *Dementia and Geriatric Cognitive Disorders, 20*(4), 209–214.

164. Clarke, R., Harrison, G., Richards, S. (2003). Effect of vitamins and aspirin on markers of platelet activation, oxidative stress and homocysteine in people at high risk of dementia. *Journal of Internal Medicine, 254*(1), 67–75.

165. Stott, D.J., MacIntosh, G., Lowe, G.D., Rumley, A., McMahon, A.D., Langhorne, P., Tait, R.C., O'Reilly, D.S., Spilg, E.G., MacDonald, J.B., MacFarlane, P.W., Westendorp R.G. (2005). Randomized controlled trial of homocysteine-lowering vitamin treatment in elderly patients with vascular disease. *American Journal of Clinical Nutrition, 82*(6), 1320–1326.

166. van Uffelen, J., Hopman-Rock, M., Chin, A.P., van Mechelen, W. (2005). Protocol for Project FACT: A randomised controlled trial on the effect of a walking program and vitamin B supplementation on the rate of cognitive decline and psychosocial wellbeing in older adults with mild cognitive impairment [ISRCTN19227688]. *BMC Geriatrics*, *5*(1), *18*.

167. Religa, D., Czyzewski, K., Styczynska, M., Peplonska, B., Lokk, J., Chodakowska-Zebrowska, M., Stepien, K., Winblad, B., Barcikowska, M. (2006). Hyperhomocysteinemia and methylenetetrahydrofolate reductase polymorphism in patients with Parkinson's disease. *Neuroscience Letters*, *404*(1–2), 56–60.

168. Todorovic, Z., Dzoljic, E., Novakovic, I., Mirkovic, D., Stojanovic, R., Nesic, Z., Krajinovic, M., Prostran, M., Kostic, V. (2006). Homocysteine serum levels and MTHFR C677T genotype in patients with Parkinson's disease, with and without levodopa therapy. *Journal of Neurological Science*, *248*(1–2), 56–61.

169. Valkovic, P., Benetin, J., Blazicek, P., Valkovicova, L., Gmitterova, K., Kukumberg, P. (2005). Reduced plasma homocysteine levels in levodopa/entacapone treated Parkinson patients. *Parkinsonism and Related Disorders*, *11*(4), 253–256.

170. Lamberti, P., Zoccolella, S., Armenise, E., Lamberti, S.V., Fraddosio, A., de Mari, M., Iliceto, G., Livrea, P. (2005). Hyperhomocysteinemia in L-dopa treated Parkinson's disease patients: Effect of cobalamin and folate administration. *European Journal of Neurology*, *12*(5), 365–368.

171. O'Suilleabhain, P.E., Bottiglieri, T., Dewey, R.B., Jr., Sharma, S., Di az-Arrastia, R. (2004). Modest increase in plasma homocysteine follows levodopa initiation in Parkinson's disease. *Movement Disorders*, *19*(12), 1403–1408.

172. Yasui, K., Nakaso, K., Kowa, H., Takeshima, T., Nakashima, K. (2003). Levodopa-induced hyperhomocysteinaemia in Parkinson's disease. *Acta Neurologica Scandinavica*, *108*(1), 66–67.

173. Louis, E.D., Schupf, N., Tang, M.X., Marder, K., Luchsinger, J.A. (2007). Mild parkinsonian signs and plasma homocysteine concentration in community-dwelling elderly individuals. *Archives of Neurology*, *64*(11), 1646–1651.

174. Imamura, K., Takeshima, T., Nakaso, K., Nakashima, K. (2007). Homocysteine is toxic for dopaminergic neurons in primary mesencephalic culture. *Neuroreport*, *18*(13), 1319–1322.

175. Zoccolella, S., Martino, D., Defazio, G., Lamberti, P., Livrea, P. (2006). Hyperhomocysteinemia in movement disorders: Current evidence and hypotheses. *Current Vascular Pharmacology*, *4*(3), 237–243.

176. Muller, T., Kuhn, W. (2006). Tolcapone decreases plasma levels of S-adenosyl-L-homocysteine and homocysteine in treated Parkinson's disease patients. *European Journal of Clinical Pharmacology*, *62*(6), 447–450.

177. Hammond, E.J., Hurd, R.W., Wilder, B.J., Thompson, F.J. (1980). Focal and generalized experimental seizures induced by homocysteine. *Electroencephalography and Clinical Neurophysiology*, *49*(1–2), 184–186.

178. Sprince, H., Parker, C.M., Josephs, J.A., Jr., Magazino, J. (1969). Convulsant activity of homocysteine and other short-chain mercaptoacids: Protection therefrom. *Annals of the New York Academy of Science*, *166*(1), 323–325.

179. Eikelboom, J.W., Baker, R.I. (1998). Venous thrombosis and hyperhomocysteinaemia. *Medical Journal of Australia*, *169*(6), 313–315.

CHAPTER 19

GLUTATHIONE, SULFUR AMINO ACIDS, AND CANCER

JOSÉ M. ESTRELA, JULIAN CARRETERO, and ANGEL ORTEGA

19.1   INTRODUCTION

Glutathione (GSH), the major nonprotein thiol in mammalian cells, is involved in many cellular functions [1]. The GSH content of cancer cells is particularly relevant in regulating (1) carcinogenic mechanisms [2–5]; (2) sensitivity against cytotoxic drugs, ionizing radiation, and some cytokines [6–15]; (3) DNA synthesis [16–18]; and (4) cell proliferation [19–21].

The idea that GSH can protect against oxidation and toxic compounds was developed initially by Barron [22] and others. Hirono found that ascites tumor cells, highly resistant to alkylating agents, had increased levels of nonprotein thiols as compared to cells that were sensitive to these drugs [23]. Since then, the work of many different groups established the concept that GSH is critical for protection against free radicals, reactive oxygen species (ROS), and electrophiles [24].

More than two decades ago, modifications of GSH metabolism were proposed as potentially useful in cancer therapy [25]. Indeed, the introduction of agents that can either increase or decrease GSH concentration in cells opened up the possibility of modulating the cellular response to different anticancer treatments [8, 25, 26]. Nevertheless, approaches to cancer treatment based on modulation of GSH concentrations within the tumor cells must take into consideration the GSH/glutathione disulfide (GSSG) status and the rate of GSH synthesis in these cells [27]. Moreover, some amino acid precursors for GSH synthesis have been shown to be essential in cancer metabolism, for example, glutamine (Gln), which is a major respiratory fuel of tumor cells [28, 29]; methionine (Met), which is essential for tumor growth in vitro as well as in vivo [30, 31] and yields cysteine (Cys) via transulphuration [32, 33]; and Cys, because its bioavailability is rate limiting for GSH synthesis [25], and

Glutathione and Sulfur Amino Acids in Human Health and Disease. Edited by R. Masella and G. Mazza
Copyright © 2009 John Wiley & Sons, Inc.

because different human and murine hematopoietic tumor cell lines are auxotrophic for Cys when compared with nontumor cell lines of different origin [34].

Metastatic spread, not primary tumor burden, is the main cause of cancer-related deaths. For patient prognosis to improve, new systemic therapies capable of effectively inhibiting the outgrowth of seeded tumor cells are necessary. Interaction of metastatic cells with the vascular endothelium activates local release of pro-inflammatory cytokines, which act as signals promoting cancer cell adhesion, extravasation, and proliferation [35]. Recent work in the B16 melanoma (B16M) model shows that metastatic cells display growth-associated changes in their GSH content [36]. Treatment with GSH ester shows that enhanced GSH level by itself increases the metastatic progression in the liver of B16M cells [36]. Moreover, a high percentage of metastatic cells with high GSH levels can survive the combined nitrosative and oxidative stress elicited by the vascular endothelium and, possibly, by macrophages and granulocytes [37]. γ-Glutamyl transpeptidase (GGT) overexpression in the tumor cells and an interorgan flow of GSH (where the liver plays a central role), by increasing Cys availability for tumor GSH synthesis, can function as a metastatic-growth promoting mechanism [38]. Therefore, GSH appears to play a regulatory role in metastatic cell growth and survival.

Resistance to drugs and to ionizing radiation is a major obstacle to the effective treatment of cancer. Multidrug and radiation resistance of many tumors, as compared with normal tissues, appears to be associated with higher GSH levels in the cancer cells [5, 8–11, 17, 26, 36, 37, 39]. Different tumors, including those that exhibit resistance, may be sensitized to chemotherapy and/or radiotherapy by selective GSH depletion [10, 40]. Nevertheless once malignant tumors disseminate systemically, in vivo administration of different GSH-depleting agents (such as, e.g., buthionine sulfoximine [BSO], diethylmaleate, or phorone, which show no selectivity for cancer cells), appears useless against metastatic cell subsets with high GSH content [27].

However, recent work shows that acceleration of GSH efflux facilitates selective GSH depletion in metastatic cells [41], and that this approach can sensitize malignant cells to conventional therapy under in vivo conditions [42].

19.2 CARCINOGENESIS, TUMOR GROWTH, AND CELL DEATH

19.2.1 The Process of Carcinogenesis

Cancer can be conceived as a complex cellular phenotype associated with unlimited replicative potential, independence from growth signals with parallel resistance to growth-inhibitory signaling, evasion of cell death activation, sustained angiogenesis, as well as ability of tissue invasion and metastasis [43]. The process that leads towards malignancy (carcinogenesis) is a long-term multistep process by which carcinogens induce tumor formation [44]. This process typically includes DNA damage and mutagenesis that cause transformation of normal cells into preneoplastic cells (initiation), followed by selective clonal expansion (promotion), and a second mutagenic mechanism responsible for the ability of some malignant cells to acquire more aggressive characteristics (progression). Malignant tumors are invasive, and may metastasize to distant sites through the circulatory system (Fig. 19.1).

Independently of its origin, tumor formation is a genetic disease, where genomic modifications cause loss of cell cycle control and cell differentiation through the activation of oncogenes and/or inactivation of tumor supressor genes [45]. These genetic events can occur with gain or loss of entire chromosomes, as well as specific chromosomal translocations, gene amplifications, deletions, or mutations. Most genetic damage has no serious consequence, is repaired, or may cause cell death [46]. Occasionally, DNA damage and mutation of critical genes, by increasing cell proliferation and/or by decreasing the incidence of cell death, may represent an advantage for tumor survival. Moreover, DNA damage can affect detoxification of chemical carcinogens, and DNA repair [47]. The mutational burden of human cancer is such that around 11,000 mutations per cell were found in a study of colorectal carcinoma [48], although only about 1% of these is expected to affect coding regions [49]. Accordingly, a recent study of various types of human colorectal and breast cancer tumors have identified that individual tumors accumulate an average of

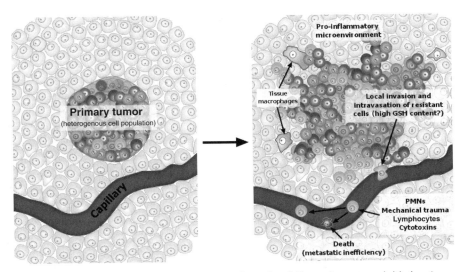

Figure 19.1 Malignant tumor spread. Tumor formation follows three steps: initiation (accumulation of nonlethal mutations), promotion (characteristic clonal expansion of preneoplastic cells, also known as benign tumor), and progression (changes at cellular and molecular levels leading to the typical genomic instability that characterizes the transition from preneoplastic to a neoplastic state). In these stages tumors are surrounded by a continuous basement membrane. Preneoplastic cells suffer metabolic adaptations during the transition to the invasive phenotype. These adaptations facilitate their escape from immune attacks, invasion of local normal tissue, intravasation, and colonization of distant organs. Most circulating cancer cells are eliminated by physiological mechanisms, a fact called "metastatic inefficiency." PMNs, polymorphonuclear cells. (See color insert.)

90 mutated genes, but only about 10% of these seem to play a causal role in carcinogenesis [50].

19.2.2   Reactive Oxygen and Nitrogen Species as Carcinogens

Reactive oxygen species (ROS) are highly reactive molecules that are continuously produced in all aerobic organisms, mostly as a consequence of aerobic respiration. The term covers several types of compounds, including free radicals such as superoxide ($O_2^{\cdot-}$) or hydroxyl ($OH^{\cdot}$), and nonradicals such as hydrogen peroxide (H_2O_2). Similarly, nitrogen-derived free radicals are called reactive nitrogen species (RNS) and their outmost representative precursors are nitric oxide (NO) and peroxynitrite ($ONOO^-$) [51]. Low levels of ROS and RNS are continuously produced in mammalian cells and play important physiological roles [52]. These include processes as diverse as gene expression [53], cell proliferation and survival [54], pathogen clearance by the immune system [13, 55], and blood vessel permeability [56]. However, when the amount of ROS/RNS exceeds the capacity of the antioxidant machinery, the resulting oxidative/nitrosative stress may induce irreversible damages in all cellular macromolecules (proteins, lipids, nucleic acids), including genomic DNA. Therefore, maintenance of redox homeostasis is critical for cell survival and its alteration is involved in the pathophysiology of different diseases, for example, cardiovascular diseases, diabetes, rheumatoid arthritis, neurological disorders, that is, Alzheimer's or Parkinson's disease, and cancer [56–61].

Clinical and epidemiological investigations have provided evidence supporting the role of ROS and RNS in the etiology of cancer due to factors such as solar UV exposure [62, 63], chemical carcinogens, lifestyle, diet and environment, and chronic inflammation conditions where high levels of free radicals are being produced [46, 64, 65]. Free radicals, such as $OH^{\cdot}$, increase DNA mutational rates to comparable levels as those promoted by other well-known carcinogens (i.e., polycyclic aromatic hydrocarbons and aflatoxins), and thus are considered powerful cancer initiators [66]. As we will discuss below, ROS have been shown to promote proliferation of various cell types in vitro [67, 68], which highlights their potential relevance in cancer promotion. Exposure of several cancer cell lines to inflammation- or chemically induced ROS boosts their migratory and invasive behaviors [68–70], thus indicating a possible role of free radicals in promoting the invasive phenotype. It is also known that exposure to free radicals above a certain threshold irreversibly leads to cell death [71, 72]. Furthermore, several cancer chemotherapeutic agents (i.e., cisplatin, arsenic trioxide), as well as radiotherapy, are known to exert their cytotoxic effects through ROS-mediated mechanisms [71]. Moreover, in vivo experiments with animal models also support a causal role of free radicals in cancer. Indeed knockout mice for distinct antioxidant enzymes that regulate ROS levels in vivo (i.e., superoxide dismutase [SOD] and GSH peroxidase [GPx]) not only have higher levels of ROS in their tissues, but also suffer from higher rates of spontaneous tumors [73]. Similarly, mice deficient in *Mth1*, a key enzyme involved in the repair of DNA oxidative lesions, also show higher rates of spontaneous lung, liver, and stomach tumors [74].

19.2.3 Thiol-Containing Molecules and the Initiation of Carcinogenesis

19.2.3.1 GSH and GSH Peroxidases   Due to its reducing thiol-mediated properties, GSH acts as a homeostatic redox buffer [75] and is one of the first cellular defenses against free radicals. Therefore, GSH can inactivate some carcinogens [46], protect against DNA-damaging free radicals [24], preserve the integrity of differents tissues (i.e., the intestinal epithelium) [65], and prevent lipid peroxidation [76]. Directly and indirectly GSH effectively scavenges free radicals and other reactive species (e.g., $OH^\bullet$, $ROO^\bullet$, $ONOO^-$, and H_2O_2) through enzymatic reactions [32], such as those catalyzed by GPx. GPxs (in part selenium-containing enzymes) catalyze the GSH-dependent reduction of H_2O_2 and other peroxides [56]. GSSG is reduced by the glutathione reductase (GR). At present four different selenocysteine-containing GPxs have been characterized from mammalian tissues; in addition, two selenocysteine-independent GPxs are present in mammalian cells. In vitro studies with GPx-overexpressing cells have demostrated the importance of GPxs against H_2O_2-derived damage [77]. However, mice lacking *GPx1* grew normally, showing no sign of decreased H_2O_2 metabolism or increased sensitivity to hyperoxia, suggesting that GPxs only play an important role under oxidative stress conditions [78, 79]. More recently, given the relationship between genomic polymorphisms and increased risk of lung cancer, GPxs have been postulated as candidates for lung cancer susceptibility genes [80].

19.2.3.2 GSH and GSH-S-Transferases   Living organisms are continuously exposed to xenobiotics that may act as carcinogens. These include substances such as aromatic amines, dioxins, and halogenated aromatic hydrocarbons, which normally produce a toxic effect when not disposed properly. Consequently, organisms have developed a sequential two-step detoxification system that is composed of two classes of enzymes: class I and class II detoxification enzymes. Class I includes the cytochrome P450 oxidases [81] that make xenobiotics more soluble by sequentially oxidizing (activating) the xenobiotic at appropriate motifs. Activated xenobiotics are then conjugated by class II enzymes (i.e., GSH-*S*-transferases [GSTs]) with various negatively charged hydrophilic compounds that facilitate their excretion [82].

GSTs catalyze the conjugation of GSH (S-glutathionylation) with different compounds to form mercapturates [83, 84]. This mechanism is involved in the detoxification of electrophilic xenobiotics, such as chemical carcinogens, environmental pollutants, and antitumor agents [32, 85]. GSTs inactivate endogenous-unsaturated aldehydes, quinones, epoxides, and hydroperoxides formed as secondary metabolites during oxidative stress [86]. However S-glutathionylation does not simply facilitates excretion of different compounds, but has been also implicated in stabilization of extracellular proteins, protection of proteins against oxidation of critical Cys residues, and regulation of enzyme activity and/or transcription [87]. Indeed many proteins undergo glutathionylation, for example, some enzymes involved in carbohydrate/energy metabolism, heat shock proteins (e.g., HSP60 and HSP70), enzymes involved in the proteasomal degradation of proteins, some cell death-related proteins, and some cytoskeletal proteins. In addition, many proteins may become glutathionylated under conditions of oxidative and/or nitrosative stress [88], thereby regulating cell responses [89, 90].

GSTs are highly polymorphic and can be divided in six families [91], namely GST alpha, mu, pi, omega, theta, and zeta. Interestingly, five of them (*GSTA1*, *GSTT1*, *GSTM1*, *GSTM2*, and *GSTP1*) have been widely studied as prognostic or risk-modulating factors in human cancer [92–96]. Moreover, reduced activity of some of these enzymes has been found to predispose to some cancer types, which is believed to be accounted for by a general lack of carcinogens detoxification. For instance, the homozygous deletion of the *GSTM1* gene has been shown to predispose to lung, bladder, and colorectal carcinomas [93]. Similarly, reduced GSTP1 activity has been correlated with higher prostate cancer risk [93]. Moreover, GSTs have been associated with multidrug resistance of tumor cells: GSTP1 has been shown to be a prevalent protein in many solid tumors and is normally found overexpressed in drug-resistant cancers [97]. Accordingly, GSTs are currently emerging as new promising targets in cancer therapy [97–99], and several drugs targeting GSTs are being tested in phase II clinical trials [95].

19.2.3.3 *Peroxiredoxins, Thioredoxin, and Metallothioneins*   Peroxiredoxins (Prxs), as GPxs, reduce hydroperoxides and H_2O_2 to the corresponding alcohol or water, and have both peroxidase and cosubstrate activity [100]. Prxs contain one (Prx VI) or two (Prx I-V) Cys in their active site, and are considered important cell redox state regulating enzymes [21]. Moreover, it has been suggested that H_2O_2 could inactivate cytosolic Prxs by hyperoxidation, allowing H_2O_2 to serve as intracellular messenger [101]. Mice lacking *PrxI* show higher ROS levels, and their embryonic fibroblasts showed evidence of *c-Myc* oncogene activation and the ability to be transformed by the *Ras* oncogene alone [102]. Furthermore *PRXI* overexpression has been reported in various human primary tumors, and cancer-specific expression of some Prxs has been detected in different malignancies [35, 103, 104].

Thioredoxins (Trxs), as well as glutaredoxin (Grx), Prxs, and Trx reductases (TR), belong to the thiol-containing antioxidants. The antioxidant function of Trx is based on the reversible oxidation of its catalytic site (Trp-Cys-Gly-Pro-Cys-Lys-) to the Cys disulfide (Trx-S2) [105]. The oxidized form is reduced back to Trx by TR using NADPH. Trx regulates the cell redox state by serving as electron donor to certain Prxs and GPxs [106], is an efficient growth factor, inhibits apoptosis, and offers growth advantages to tumor cells in vivo [107]. A wide variety of human primary tumors overexpresses Trx, which seems to be associated with poor response to anticancer drugs [104, 108, 109].

Metallothioneins (MTs) are low molecular weight and thiol-rich metal binding proteins. The known functions of MTs include antioxidant activity, protection against OH• radicals and heavy metal toxicity, and roles in cell growth and differentiation [110]. Its synthesis is enhanced in rapidly proliferating tissues, thus suggesting a key role in normal and neoplastic cell growth. Recently MTs have been postulated as tumor markers in different carcinomas [111], and have been shown to be involved in resistance to platinum-based therapy [112].

19.2.4 Tumor Growth

Once carcinogenesis initiation has been completed, the second step implies tumor promotion and local growth. The potential role of free radicals in this clonal expansion is based on their ability to mimic the biochemical effects of known tumor promoters. Besides, tumor promoters can also modulate tissue levels of antioxidants and/or anti-free radical cellular defences [113], thus showing a strong inhibitory effects on, for example, SOD and catalase activities [114]. As discussed above, high levels of ROS can induce growth arrest and/or cytotoxicity; although, on the other hand, low levels can stimulate cell proliferation. In this sense, we have to take into account that this dual role of ROS will obviously depend not only on concentration levels, but also on pulse duration, and subcellular localization.

The biological mechanisms regulating proliferation are similar in both normal and tumoral cells. Cancer is a disease that shows excessive cell division due to the aberrant regulation of the process. Cells grow, duplicate their DNA, and each cell segregates the genome into two daughter cells. This complex process is regulated by signaling cascades that modulate gene expression, posttraslational modifications, and protein degradation. The role of intracellular redox state as growth, cell signaling, and/or gene expression regulator is being recognized and is becoming an important issue. In fact alterations in (1) receptor or cytoplasmatic tyrosine kinases, (2) levels of specific growth factors, (3) intracellular processes for conveying membrane signals to the nucleus, (4) portions of the transcription apparatus, (5) genes involved in the cell cycle, or (6) the regulation of DNA replication, all have been shown in neoplastic cells [56].

In the last years the development of molecular biology and cell biology has led to establishment of the concept of a redox cycle within the cell cycle. The presence of redox-sensitive motifs such as metal cofactors in kinases and phosphatases, or Cys residues in cell cycle regulatory proteins and transcription factors, may help to understand the redox cycle and its role in cell division regulation. Redox imbalance leads to activation of a number of transcription and growth factors. In this sense ROS are able to induce overexpression of several growth factors related with tumor proliferation, for example, epidermal growth factor (EGF), vascular endothelial growth factor (VEGF), or platelet-derived growth factor (PDGF) in lung, urinary, or prostate cancers. In addition, several transcription factors are redox-sensitive: AP-1 is a positive regulator of cell division, and inductor or inhibitor of apoptosis (depending on the balance between pro- and anti-apoptotic target genes, and on the duration and type of stimulus); inhibition of NF-κB (a factor related to cell growth, inflammation, and differentiation) [115] blocks cell proliferation, and its upregulation has been observed in blood neoplasms, colon, breast, and pancreas cell lines [114]. Furthermore, the mitogen-activated protein kinase (MAPK) pathway is also regulated by redox changes [100].

GSH and Cys regulate protein turnover [116, 117], DNA synthesis [17, 27], and cellular proliferation in different tissues [27, 118, 119]. GSH levels can fluctuate during the cell cycle [36, 117, 120], and may directly correlate with the tumor growth capacity, for example, rapid GSH synthesis in Ehrlich ascites tumor (EAT) cells is associated with high rates of cellular proliferation [121]. Moreover, in mice inoculated with A549 human lung carcinoma cells [122] or EAT [18], BSO decreased the rate of cancer growth. We found a direct correlation between GSH levels associated with cellular proliferation and metastatic activity [36]. Indeed, intrasplenic inoculation of B16M cells into C57BL/6J syngenic mice induced metastatic foci formation by colonizing different organs; however, the number and size of metastases were much higher when B16M cells with high GSH content were inoculated in vivo [36]. Moreover, when B16M cells with low GSH content were pretreated with GSH ester (which readily enters the cell and delivers free GSH), their metastatic activity increased [36]. Therefore, GSH appears directly involved in regulating tumor growth and metastatic activity.

19.2.5   Cell Death in Cancer

19.2.5.1   Mechanisms   Far from being the end of life, physiological cell death has an essential role in organism surveillance. Regulation of cell death plays a critical role in organism development, morphogenesis, tissue sculpturing, maintenance tissue homeostasis in mature organisms, wound healing, elimination of damaged cells and of infectious pathogen, etc. Physiological cell death without any kind of distinction has been known since the nineteenth century. In 1972, Kerr, Wyllie, and Currie identified the apoptosis as the morphological changes that occur in natural cell death, thus distinguishing this pathway from necrosis which was then linked to acute tissue injury [123]. For years apoptosis has been synonymous with programmed cell death or death under genetic control. The mitochondrion is a key cell death regulation site and the Bcl-2 family of proteins are critical in this process. The Bcl-2 proteins are characterized by the presence of one or several Bcl-2 homology domains and include pro-death and anti-death proteins [124]. Bcl-2 itself is an anti-death protein, and its overexpression has been associated with cancer development, metastatic growth, and chemotherapy resistance [125–128]. On the other hand, expression of pro-death genes, for example, Bax or Bak, is often reduced in cancer cells [129].

Classically necrosis refers to a cell that, in response to a huge damage or physical insult, swells and explodes, then releasing its intracellular content into the surrounding tissue. Thus, necrosis is considered, at the cellular level, an uncontrolled type of cell death. However, on the contrary, there are recent studies suggesting that necrosis is a regulated process involved in multiple developmental, pathological and physiological scenarios [85, 130, 131]. Inhibition of cellular energy production, generation of ROS, imbalance of intracellular Ca^{2+} flux and extracellular cell death signals are able to induce apoptosis and/or necrosis. In this sense, time and intensity of stimulus may determine the type of cell death. Uncoupling the electron chain transport, increasing intracellular Ca^{2+}, inorganic phosphate, alkaline pH, ROS, and/or mitochondrial GSH depletion can cause a transitory loss of the mitochondrial proton gradient and release of mitochondrial proapoptotic molecules through permeability transitory pores (PTP). Nevertheless, a permanent pore opening, usually associated to a mitochondrial bioenergetic failure, leads to necrosis [132–134].

Nowadays, due to the continuous advance of science, another type of classification involving three categories is required, including apoptosis and autophagy (known as PCD I and PCD II, respectively), and necrosis [69]. Moreover even a fourth type of cell death, senescence, must be included if we take into account conditions of long-term or permanent tumor growth arrest often associated with cancer therapy [135].

19.2.5.2 *Role of GSH*
Defective regulation or execution of cell death is widely recognized as the basis of different disorders, including cancer. Many cancer cells avoid death activation, hence increasing survival and therapy resistance. In consequence, different antitumor therapies targeted against cell growth and/or cell death pathways have been developed and assayed in the last decades. However, it must be remarked that conventional and modern therapeutic agents induce cell death by apoptosis and also by nonapoptotic mechanisms [135].

The thiol redox state (controlled by GSH) is one of the endogenous effectors involved in regulating the mitochondrial PTP complex and, in consequence, thiol oxidation may be a causal factor in the mitochondrion-based mechanism that leads to cell death [136, 137]. Mitochondrial GSH is the only defense against peroxides generated from the electron transport chain [138], 1% to 3% of the total O_2 consumed by mitochondria may be accounted for in terms of H_2O_2 production [24]. Moreover, PTP complex opening by itself causes dissipation of the mitochondrial membrane potential (MMP), loss of mitochondrial RNA, cessation of the import of cytosolic proteins, release of Ca^{2+} and GSH from the matrix, mitochondrial uncoupling, increase in ROS generation and, in consequence, GSH oxidation [136].

19.3 INTERCELLULAR AND INTERORGAN TRANSPORT OF GSH IN TUMOR-BEARING MAMMALS

In rapidly growing tumors, free Cys may become limiting for GSH synthesis and cell growth. Cys concentration in blood is very low, it is extremely unstable extracellularly and rapidly autooxidizes to cystine [17, 139]. Thus, malignant cells might utilize alternative pathways to ensure Cys availability.

GSH is synthesized intracellularly and is exported from cells. Blood GSH can be used by solid tumors as a reservoir of Cys [140]. Its breakdown is initiated by the GGT located at the external surface of the plasma membrane in different cell types. GGT is the only known enzyme that cleaves the γ-glutamylcysteine peptide bond in GSH and other γ-glutamyl compounds [141]. Export of GSH functions in interorgan and intraorgan transfer of Cys moieties, and in the protection of cell membranes [142–144]. Hence GGT overexpression may provide tumor cells with a growth advantage at physiological concentrations of Cys [139]. In fact, in some tumors (i.e., for hepatocellular carcinoma or ovarian cancers), GGT is considered a tumor-related biomarker [145, 146].

Regulation of GSH levels in vivo must be looked at in terms of the entire organism, with some organs being net synthesizers of GSH, whereas others are net exporters. GSH levels in human tissues normally range from 0.1 to 10 mM, being most concentrated in liver (up to 10 mM) and in the spleen, kidney, lens, erythrocytes, and leukocytes [10]. GSH is readily oxidized nonenzymatically to GSSG, and GSSG efflux from cells contributes to a net loss of intracellular GSH. Oxidative stress may cause changes in the glutathione redox state of different tissues and, thereby, may increase the rate of GSSG release from cells [147]. As a consequence, GSH and GSSG levels in blood and the GSH/GSSG ratio in particular, may reflect changes in glutathione status in other less accessible tissues [148, 149] and provide a measure of oxidative stress in vivo.

Although the molecular mechanisms of GSH efflux have not been well identified yet, the liver is the central organ in interorgan GSH homeostasis, with sinusoidal GSH efflux as the major determinant of plasma GSH and thiol-disulfide status [150, 151]. Efflux of GSH and GSH S-conjugates from different mammalian cells is mediated by multidrug resistance proteins (MRPs) [152], among which MRP1 and MRP2 have been characterized as ATP-dependent pumps with broad specificity for GSH and glucuronic or sulfate conjugates [14, 153–155]. MRP1 and MRP2 also mediate the cotransport of unconjugated amphiphilic compounds together with free GSH, and contribute to the control of the intracellular GSSG level. Although these proteins are low-affinity GSSG transporters, they can play an essential role in the response to oxidative stress when the activity of GR becomes rate limiting [27].

GGT cleaves GSH releasing γ-glutamyl-amino acids and cysteinylglycine, which is further cleaved by membrane-bound dipeptidases into Cys and glycine (Gly) [25]. Free γ-glutamyl-amino acids, Cys and Gly entering the cell serve as GSH precursors [8]. In general, an organ with high levels of GGT activity, such as the kidney, lung, or the intestinal epithelium, can utilize plasma GSH [156]. Interorgan circulation of GSH is supported by the finding of low plasma GSH levels in the renal vein and of relatively high levels in the hepatic vein [157].

High levels of GGT in some tumors can be beneficial for surviving, since it provides abundant cyst(e)ine for uptake and synthesis of intracellular GSH [139, 158]. Most cell types have no direct system for transport of intact GSH into cells [159, 160]. In addition, if extracellular levels of glutamate are high, as may occur in patients with advanced cancer, cystine uptake is competitively inhibited, decreasing intracellular cystine availability. Under these circumstances, Cys released from extracellular GSH by GGT may play a crucial role, with tumors expressing high GGT able to degrade plasma GSH, thus providing an extra source of Cys for uptake [143, 161]. Indeed, tumor GGT activity and an intertissue flow of GSH can regulate GSH content of melanoma cells and their metastatic growth in the liver [38, 41, 162, 163]. So, GGT is a potential target in the therapy of melanoma and other tumors where an increased expression of this enzyme has been found (including human tumors of the liver, lung, breast, and ovary) [140].

19.4   GSH AND THE INTERACTION OF METASTATIC CELLS WITH THE VASCULAR ENDOTHELIUM

Formation of metastases in a secondary organ is the result of dissemination of primary cancer cells, survival in the circulation, passing through the vascular wall in a distant organ, and metastatic cell proliferation [164]. Metastases that are resistant to conventional therapies are the main cause of all cancer-related deaths in humans [165]. Cancers are biologically heterogeneous and contain subpopulations of cells with different angiogenic, invasive, and metastatic properties [164]. Tumor cell heterogeneity, which associates with genomic and phenotypic instability [166], represents a major problem for cancer therapy. Besides, additional factors such as, for example, the attack of our immune system or the organ-specific microenvironment, influence metastatic cell behavior and the response to therapy [167, 168]. Therefore, as recently proposed, therapy of metastasis should therefore be targeted against both the metastatic tumor cells and the homeostatic factors that promote metastasis [164].

Interaction of cancer and cells in capillary beds is a critical step in the initiation of metastasis [169]. Murine B16M variant tumor cell lines with low (B16M-F1) or high (B16M-F10) survival and growth potential in vivo [156] have been widely used as experimental models to study the metastatic process. It is a rapidly growing anaplasic tumor that produces melanin and can grow indefinitely in vitro under appropriate conditions. After inoculation (subcutaneous, intracardiac, intramuscular, intravenous, or intrasplenic) of the tumor into syngenic mice, it can easily colonize different organs. Early studies on the organ distribution of B16M cells showed that $<0.1\%$ of circulating cancer cells survive and may promote secondary metastatic growth [170]. Indeed, different studies have reported that the majority of cancer cells entering the microvascular bed of the liver [171] and other organs [172] are killed within the first hours due to mechanical trauma produced by blood flow [173], their inability to withstand deformation [172], locally released ROS [174], and their susceptibility to the lytic action of immunocompetent intrasinusoidal lymphocytes and macrophages [175]. Therefore the metastatic process has a very low effectivity, biologically expressed as "metastatic inefficiency" [176, 177], which implies that only specific or highly resistant cell subsets are responsible for the metastatic invasion and growth in distant organs. Experimental genetic studies using microarrays and metastatic human tumors suggest that cancer progression correlates with functional loss of proapoptotic genes (such as *BAX*, *P53*, or the death-related protein kinase *DAPK*), or with overexpression of antiapoptotic genes (e.g., *BCL2* or *NF-κB*) [21, 178, 179]. In fact it is assumed that apoptosis resistance is an acquired property of successful metastatic cells [180].

Clinical and autopsy observations on the distribution of cancer metastasis have demonstrated that liver is a common site for metastasis development [181]. Under experimental conditions, many circulating cancer cells are trapped in the liver microvasculature [176]. On the other hand, early interactions of metastatic cancer cells with hepatic sinusoidal endothelium (HSE) and Kupffer cells activate local release of pro-inflammatory cytokines (TNFα, IL-1β, IL-18) [182], which in turn promote cancer cell adhesion, invasion, and proliferation [183, 184]. Indeed, IL-1β and TNFα induce binding of very late antigen-4 (VLA-4)-expressing mouse B16M cells by upregulating vascular adhesion molecule-1 (VCAM-1) on endothelial cells [185]. Endothelial cells release harmful ROS in response to endotoxins and cytokines or in response to cancer cell contact [186–188]. Moreover, despite lethal effects on metastatic cells, oxidative stress may also create a prometastatic microenvironment at target organs by increasing cell adhesion molecule expression in both endothelial [189] and cancer cells [190]. Indeed, we know that ROS at low micromolar levels appear to act as intra- and intercellular messengers capable of promoting growth responses [19]. In fact, VCAM-1 gene transcription and expression in vascular endothelial cells is coupled to an oxidative stress-dependent mechanism [191]. Therefore, although the antioxidant capacity of cancer cells may determine their intravascular survival, surviving cells may benefit from oxidative stress-promoting metastatic mechanisms. Thus, a balance between pro-metastatic and anti-metastatic mechanisms may occur during the capillary phase of the hepatic metastatic process which may serve as one major rate regulator for its progression.

Furthermore, recent studies have identified a natural defense mechanism against metastatic cells whereby their arrest in the HSE induces endothelial NO release, leading to sinusoidal cancer cell killing and reduced hepatic metastasis formation [192]. NO, by regulating vasodilatation, platelet aggregation, angiogenesis, prostaglandin production, leukocyte proliferation, or by direct tumor cytotoxicity [193], can affect tumor cell arrest in capillaries and metastasis. NO reversibly binds to cytochrome *c* oxidase and inhibits the respiration of tumor cells, an effect that can be suppressed by GSH [194]. By interacting with metal ions or forming RNS, NO can affect the activity of different proteins, including the N-methyl-D-aspartate receptor,

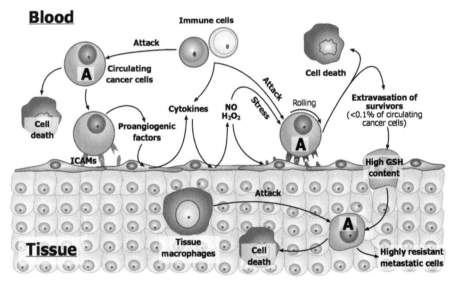

Figure 19.2   Interaction between metastatic cells and the vascular endothelium induce molecular mechanisms that lead to tumor cell death or invasion. In a first step, circulating cancer cells establish weak links with the endothelium. Metastatic growth factors induce endothelial cytokine release and, consequently, generation of cytotoxic NO and H_2O_2. Both reactive species, in cooperation with the immune system, contribute to cancer cell death. Nevertheless, some tumor cells adapted to the metastatic microenvironment survive and can colonize the extravascular tissue. Metastatic cell invaders, which will be further attacked by tissue macrophages, may follow more gene expression adaptations to enhance their resistance against stress/therapy. (A = key "adaptation" steps that may lead to a highly resistant phenotype). (See color insert.)

hemoglobin, or transcription factors (e.g., NF-κB and SoxR); and, also, by inducing S-nitrosylation of caspases, NO may switch the balance between apoptosis and necrosis [195]. Previous reports have also shown cooperative cytotoxic actions of NO and H_2O_2 in Fu5 rat hepatoma cells [196]. Hence it is possible that endothelial NO and H_2O_2 or their derived reactive species may have synergistic cytotoxic effects on cancer cells. Nevertheless, since some metastatic cells survive after interacting with the vascular endothelium, it appeared plausible that either ROS or RNS have a limited toxicity against them, or that some of these cells able to invade the liver are ROS/RNS resistant due to, for example, overexpression of their intracellular antioxidant machinery. In this respect, it has been shown that high levels of intracellular GSH protect cancer cells against ROS/RNS-induced cytotoxicity [197, 198]. By comparing B16M-F10 cells cultured to low (LD) and high density (HD), showing different GSH contents and different metastatic activities [36], we found that H_2O_2 released by the HSE was not cytotoxic; however, NO was particularly tumoricidal in the presence of the peroxide. NO-induced tumor cytotoxicity was increased by H_2O_2 due to the formation of potent oxidants, likely $OH^•$ and $ONOO^-$, via a trace metal-dependent process [37]. A high percentage of tumor cells with high GSH content survived the combined nitrosative and oxidative attack, thus representing the main task force in the metastatic invasion [37]. In agreement with this idea previous in vivo video microscopic studies on the viability of intraportally injected untreated and BSO-treated B16M-F10 cells, arrested in mouse liver microvasculature, showed that the rate of tumor cell death increased dramatically in GSH-depleted cells [199]. Therefore, indeed, GSH regulates tumor cell protection against oxidative/nitrosative stress during their intrasinusoidal arrest in vivo, contributing to the mechanism of metastatic cell survival within the microvessels [199] (Fig. 19.2).

19.5 ADAPTIVE RESPONSE IN INVASIVE CELLS

GSH, besides regulating cell death and growth (see above), may also regulate invasive potential. Transcription factors (such as NF-κB, AP-1, OxyR, or p53) are sensitive to redox changes affecting their domains [200–202], thus suggesting that GSH may play a role as DNA-binding transcriptional regulator. Moreover, a recent report, in which the role of GSH in the growth of HepG2 cells was studied, showed that changes in cell growth and DNA synthesis paralleled changes in GSH levels, suggesting a causal relationship between the two [203]. GSH may also regulate DNA synthesis, by providing reducing equivalents to glutaredoxin, necessary for ribonucleotide reductase; and mechanisms of genomic surveillance, for example, cell cycle checkpoint systems [204]. Nevertheless, GSH levels in invasive cells could be affected by microenvironment conditions, for example, Cys availability [38], heavy metals, heat shock, high glucose, NO or oxidants [204], and intercellular signals such as stress-related hormones [205]. Besides, surviving invasive cells may benefit from metastatic mechanisms already induced by oxidative stress, including activation of early growth response-1 transcription factor gene and metalloproteases and increased expression of cell adhesion molecules, manganese-containing SOD and catalase activities, and other key invasive growth-related molecules such as VEGF-A, HIF-1, and protein 8 [42]. Furthermore, it appears evident that many cellular responses to oxidative and nitrosative stress are regulated at the transcriptional level [206]. Indeed nitrosylation or oxidation of critical Cys residues in the DNA-binding domains or at allosteric sites may regulate transcription of target genes [206, 207], although the molecular mechanisms underlying redox control of mammalian gene expression still need to be elucidated. Hence, the net result of pro- and anti-metastatic ROS and RNS effects may determine the progression of invasive cells within an organ or tissue.

19.6   GSH DEPLETION AND THE SENSITIZATION OF CANCER CELLS TO THERAPY

The relationship between GSH, chemotherapy, and the radiation response has been examined in many tumor cells after treatment with different drugs, including BSO, diethylmaleate, 2-oxothiazolidine-4-carboxylate, and various radiosensitizing agents [9, 17, 27, 208]. GSH depletion only appears to be therapeutically effective when very low levels of this tripeptide can be achieved within the cancer cells [27]. But because BSO as well as other thiol-depleting agents are nonspecific, such a profound GSH depletion in vivo within a tumor will cause irreversible damage in different normal organs and tissues. Moreover, BSO-induced nonselective GSH depletion can result in DNA deletions that may further promote carcinogenesis [209]. Thus, a feasible approach, capable of decreasing GSH sufficiently in a tumor without placing normal tissues at an irreversible disadvantage, could represent a significant advantage for the treatment of different drug- and/or radiation-resistant cancers.

Efflux of GSH and GSH S-conjugates from different mammalian cells is mediated by MRPs (see above). Multidrug resistance is frequently associated with the overexpression of P-glycoprotein and/or MRP1 [210], both of which function as pumps that extrude drugs from tumor cells. MRP1 may even act in cooperation with GSTP1 to protect cancer cells from cytotoxic drugs [211]. GSH depletion by BSO resulted in a complete reversal of resistance to anticancer drugs of different cell lines overexpressing MRP1, but had no effect on P-glycoprotein-mediated multidrug resistance [212]. Moreover, cancer cells can release GSH through MRP1 even in the absence of cytotoxic drugs [41, 154]. Two mechanisms of transport of GSH by MRP1 have been suggested: passive permeability and a verapamil (VRP)-dependent active transport [213]. VRP inhibits P-glycoprotein-mediated drug efflux, is not transported by MRP1 [214], and also inhibits MRP1-mediated drug extrusion [215].

Recently we have presented evidence showing that GSH is released from highly metastatic B16M-F10 cells through MRP1 and the cystic fibrosis transmembrane conductance regulator (CFTR, a MRP1-like member of the ABC family of transport proteins) [41]. CFTR forms a phosphorylation- and ATP-dependent channel permeable to Cl^- and to other larger organic anions, including GSH [216]. Phosphorylation is mediated principally by cAMP-dependent protein kinase A (PKA) and by protein kinase C (although to a lesser degree than the activation by PKA) [217]. CFTR, which is expressed in different cell types, is sensitive to

Bcl-2-induced inhibition [41]. Different reports have shown that increased Bcl-2 levels were associated with a concomitant increase in the intracellular GSH content [27]. In fact, addition of anti-CFTR antibodies to MRP1 $-/-$ (*MRP1* knockout) B16M-F10 cells pretreated with Bcl-2 antisense oligodeoxynucleotides (Bcl-2-AS) abolished GSH efflux [41]. Nevertheless it cannot be ruled out that other GSH-channelling mechanism(s) could also be working in other cell types, or that different CFTR gene mutations could be found when comparing different cancer cells.

We assayed VRP in combination with Bcl-2-AS treatment to facilitate GSH efflux from B16M-F10 cells. A perfusion chamber, containing a suspension of B16M-F10 cells, was used as an experimental set up that mimics in vivo conditions by providing a constant supply of glucose, amino acids, and GSH at physiological plasma concentrations [41]. This set up also allows the use of drug concentrations at clinically accepted and nontoxic levels in plasma. By these means we showed that Bcl-2-AS and VRP independently increased rates of GSH efflux from perfused B16M-F10 cells. Nevertheless, loss of GSH was followed by an increase in the rate of intracellular GSH synthesis associated with GCS overexpression [41].

As mentioned above, in rapidly growing tumors cyst(e)ine, whose concentration in blood is low and is preferentially used for protein synthesis, may easily become limiting for GSH synthesis [38, 121]. Cystine is predominant outside the cell since Cys rapidly autoxidizes to cystine in the extracellular fluids, whereas once it enters the cell through the Xc- system, cystine is reduced to Cys [158]. We found that tumor GGT activity and an intertissue flow of GSH (where the liver plays a central role) increase GSH content in B16M-F10 cells and work as a tumor growth-promoting mechanism [38]. GGT cleaves extracellular GSH releasing γ-glutamyl-amino acids and cysteinylglycine, which is further cleaved by membrane-bound dipeptidases into Cys and Gly [25]. Free γ-glutamyl-amino acids, Cys, and Gly entering the cell serve as GSH precursors [25]. Thus GGT overexpression may provide cancer cells with a growth advantage at physiological concentrations of cyst(e)ine [38, 139].

Indeed when we added acivicin (ACV; an irreversible GGT inhibitor [218]), to the B16M perfusion system [41] (see above), ACV decreased GGT activity to undetectable levels, decreased GSH synthesis, but did not affect the rate of GSH efflux or the rate of cystine uptake [41]. Hence Cys availability within malignant B16M cells appears to be modulated by its GGT-dependent generation from extracellular GSH. Therefore, the Bcl-2-AS- and VRP-induced acceleration of GSH efflux, if combined with inhibition of GGT, may promote GSH depletion in B16M-F10 cells [41]. This strategy was tested and proved to be efficient under in vitro and in vivo conditions [42, 219]. Triple-combination therapy with Bcl-2-AS + VRP + ACV decreased B16M-F10 cell GSH content to $\sim$43% of control values without affecting GSH in normal tissues (including brain, heart, lung, liver, glandular stomach, kidney, pancreas, skeletal muscle, bone marrow, ovary, and erythrocytes) [42]. This indicates that the proposed treatment does not affect per se GSH levels in normal tissues. Besides, Bcl-2-AS treatment (and not treatment with a control reversed sequence) decreased Bcl-2 levels in the metastatic (liver) B16M-F10 cells in vivo to $\sim$52% of control values; whereas no significant change in Bcl-2 protein level was detected in parenchymal hepatocytes [42]. A full combination of paclitaxel, x-rays, cytokines (TNF-α and IFN-γ), and a L-Gln-enriched diet (which potentiates TNF-α-induced tumor cell toxicity and protects against different radiation-derived side effects) eliminated B16M-F10 cells from liver and all other systemic disease, leading to long-term survival (>120 days) without recurrence in 90% of mice receiving the full therapy. Toxicity was manageable; the mice recovered quickly, and hematology and clinical chemistry data was representative of accepted clinical toxicities [42]. Therefore, combined Bcl-2 and GSH depletion is a powerful approach to sensitize metastatic melanoma cells to biotherapy, chemotherapy, and/or radiation. All components in this experimental therapy can be administered at clinically tolerated doses. Thus, the application of this approach to humans appears feasible. This may help to improve the poor prognosis of melanoma patients, and likely of patients bearing other malignant tumors showing similar molecular characteristics.

Despite the potential benefits for cancer therapy of a selective GSH-depleting strategy, such a methodology had remained elusive up to now. Our results prove that acceleration of GSH efflux is a feasible way to reach selective GSH depletion in cancer cells in vivo. Nevertheless, this strategy needs to be studied further in different cancer cell types and adapted to their molecular characteristics. Figure 19.3 shows a schematic pathway that hypothetically may be useful to select the treatment of patients bearing cancers with high GSH content.

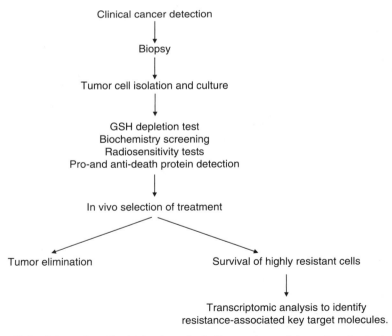

Figure 19.3 Schematic pathway that hypothetically may be useful to select the treatment of patients bearing cancers with high GSH content.

REFERENCES

1. Dickinson, D.A., Forman, H.J. (2002). Cellular glutathione and thiols metabolism. *Biochemical Pharmacology*, *64*, 1019–1026.

2. Conway, J.G., Neptun, D.A., Garvey, L.K., Popp, J.A. (1987). Carcinogen treatment increases glutathione hydrolysis by γ-glutamyl transpeptidase. *Carcinogenesis*, *8*, 999–1004.

3. Ketterer, B. (1988). Protective role of glutathione and glutathione transferases in mutagenesis and carcinogenesis. *Mutation Research*, *202*, 343–361.

4. Ames, B.N., Gold, L.S., Willett, W.C. (1995). The causes and prevention of cancer. *Proceedings of the National Academy of Sciences USA*, *92*, 5258–5265.

5. Stavrovskaya, A.A. (2000). Cellular mechanisms of multidrug resistance of tumor cells. *Biochemistry (Moscow)*, *65*, 95–106.

6. Crook, T.R., Souhami, R.L., Whyman, G.D., McLean, A.E. (1986). Glutathione depletion as a determinant of sensitivity of human leukemia cells to cyclophosphamide. *Cancer Research*, *46*, 5035–5038.

7. DeGraff, W.G., Russo, A., Mitchell, J.B. (1985). Glutathione depletion greatly reduces neocarzinostatin cytotoxicity in Chinese hamster V79 cells. *Journal of Biological Chemistry*, *260*, 8312–8315.

8. Mitchell, J.B., Russo, A. (1987), The role of glutathione in radiation and drug induced cytotoxicity. *British Journal of Cancer Supplement*, *8*, 96–104.

9. Bump, E.A., Brown, J.M. (1990). Role of glutathione in the radiation response of mammalian cells in vitro and in vivo. *Pharmacology and Therapeutics*, *47*, 117–136.

10. Estrela, J.M., Obrador, E., Navarro, J., Lasso De la Vega, M.C., Pellicer, J.A. (1995). Elimination of Ehrlich tumours by ATP-induced growth inhibition, glutathione depletion and X-rays. *Nature Medicine*, *1*, 84–88.

11. Calvert, P., Yao, K.S., Hamilton, T.C., O'Dwyer, P.J. (1998). Clinical studies of reversal of drug resistance based on glutathione. *Chemico-Biological Interactions*, *111–112*, 213–224.

12. Voehringer, D.W., Hirschberg, D.L., Xiao, J., Lu, Q., Roederer, M., Lock, C.B., Herzenberg, L.A., Steinman, L., Herzenberg, L.A. (2000). Gene microarray identification of redox and mitochondrial elements that control resistance or sensitivity to apoptosis. *Proceedings of the National Academy of Sciences USA*, *97*, 2680–2685.

13. Townsend, D.M., Tew, K.D., Tapiero, H. (2003). The importance of glutathione in human disease. *Biomedicine and Pharmacotherapy*, *57*, 145–155.

14. Gottesman, M.M., Fojo, T., Bates, S.E. (2002). Multidrug resistance in cancer: Role of ATP-dependent transporters. *Nature Reviews. Cancer*, *2*, 48–58.

15. Obrador, E., Carretero, J., Pellicer, J.A., Estrela, J.M. (2001). Possible mechanisms for tumour cell sensitivity to TNF-alpha and potential therapeutic applications. *Current Pharmaceutical Biotechnology*, *2*, 119–130.

16. Suthanthiran, M., Anderson, M.E., Sharma, V.K., Meister, A. (1990). Glutathione regulates activation-dependent DNA synthesis in highly purified normal human T lymphocytes stimulated via the CD2 and CD3 antigens. *Proceedings of the National Academy of Sciences USA*, *87*, 3343–3347.

17. Meister, A. (1991). Glutathione deficiency produced by inhibition of its synthesis, and its reversal; applications in research and therapy. *Pharmacology and Therapy*, *51*, 155–194.

18. Terradez, P., Asensi, M., Lasso de la Vega, M.C., Puertes, I.R., Viña, J., Estrela, J.M. (1993). Depletion of tumour glutathione in vivo by buthionine sulphoximine: modulation by the rate of cellular proliferation and inhibition of cancer growth. *Biochemical Journal*, *292*(Pt 2), 477–483.

19. Burdon, R.H. (1995). Superoxide and hydrogen peroxide in relation to mammalian cell proliferation. *Free Radical Biology and Medicine*, *18*, 775–794.

20. Paolicchi, A., Dominici, S., Pieri, L., Maellaro, E., Pompella, A. (2002). Glutathione catabolism as a signaling mechanism. *Biochemical Pharmacology*, *64*, 1027–1035.

21. Um, J.H., Kwon, J.K., Kang, C.D., Kim, M.J., Ju, D.S., Bae, J.H., Kim, D.W., Chung, B.S., Kim, S.H. (2004). Relationship between antiapoptotic molecules and metastatic potency and the involvement of DNA-dependent protein kinase in the chemosensitization of metastatic human cancer cells by epidermal growth factor receptor blockade. *Journal of Pharmacology and Experimental Therapy*, *311*, 1062–1070.

22. Barron, E.S. (1953). The importance of sulfhydryl groups in biology and medicine. *Texas Reports on Biology and Medicine*, *11*, 653–670.

23. Hirono, I. (1961). Mechanism of natural and acquired resistance to methyl-bis-(beta-chlorethyl)-amine N-oxide in ascites tumors. *Gann*, *52*, 39–48.

24. Chance, B., Sies, H., Boveris, A. (1979). Hydroperoxide metabolism in mammalian organs. *Physiology Review*, *59*, 527–605.

25. Meister, A. (1983). Selective modification of glutathione metabolism. *Science*, *220*, 472–477.

26. Arrick, B.A., Nathan, C.F. (1984). Glutathione metabolism as a determinant of therapeutic efficacy: A review. *Cancer Research*, *44*, 4224–4232.

27. Estrela, J.M., Ortega, A., Obrador, E. (2006). Glutathione in cancer biology and therapy. *Critical Reviews in Clinical Laboratory Sciences*, *43*, 143–181.

28. Moreadith, R.W., Lehninger, A.L. (1984). The pathways of glutamate and glutamine oxidation by tumor cell mitochondria. Role of mitochondrial NAD(P) + -dependent malic enzyme. *Journal of Biological Chemistry*, *259*, 6215–6221.

29. Mates, J.M., Perez-Gomez, C., Nunez de Castro, I., Asenjo, M., Marquez, J. (2002). Glutamine and its relationship with intracellular redox status, oxidative stress and cell proliferation/death. *International Journal of Biochemistry and Cell Biology*, *34*, 439–458.

30. Hoffman, R.M. (1985). Altered methionine metabolism and transmethylation in cancer. *Anticancer Research*, *5*, 1–30.

31. Cellarier, E., Durando, X., Vasson, M.P., Farges, M.C., Demiden, A., Maurizis, J.C., Madelmont, J.C., Chollet, P. (2003). Methionine dependency and cancer treatment. *Cancer Treatment Reviews*, *29*, 489–499.

32. Wu, G., Fang, Y.Z., Yang, S., Lupton, J.R., Turner, N.D. (2004). Glutathione metabolism and its implications for health. *Journal of Nutrition*, *134*, 489–492.

33. Rosado, J.O., Salvador, M., Bonatto, D. (2007). Importance of the trans-sulfuration pathway in cancer prevention and promotion. *Molecular and Cellular Biochemistry*, *301*, 1–12.

34. Glode, L.M., Kriegler, M.P., Livingston, D.M. (1981). Cysteine auxotrophy of human leukemic lymphoblasts is associated with decreased amounts of intracellular cystathionase protein. *Biochemistry, 20,* 1306–1311.

35. Orr, F.W., Wang, H.H., Lafrenie, R.M., Scherbarth, S., Nance, D.M. (2000). Interactions between cancer cells and the endothelium in metastasis. *Journal of Pathology, 190,* 310–329.

36. Carretero, J., Obrador, E., Anasagasti, M.J., Martin, J.J., Vidal-Vanaclocha, F., Estrela, J.M. (1999). Growth-associated changes in glutathione content correlate with liver metastatic activity of B16 melanoma cells. *Clinical and Experimental Metastasis, 17,* 567–574.

37. Carretero, J., Obrador, E., Esteve, J.M., Ortega, A., Pellicer, J.A., Sempere, F.V., Estrela, J.M. (2001). Tumoricidal activity of endothelial cells. Inhibition of endothelial nitric oxide production abrogates tumor cytotoxicity induced by hepatic sinusoidal endothelium in response to B16 melanoma adhesion in vitro. *Journal of Biological Chemistry, 276,* 25775–25782.

38. Obrador, E., Carretero, J., Ortega, A., Medina, I., Rodilla, V., Pellicer, J.A., Estrela, J.M. (2002). γ-Glutamyl transpeptidase overexpression increases metastatic growth of B16 melanoma cells in the mouse liver. *Hepatology, 35,* 74–81.

39. Gatti, L., Zunino, F. (2005). Overview of tumor cell chemoresistance mechanisms. *Methods in Molecular Medicine, 111,* 127–148.

40. Mitchell, J.B., Cook, J.A., DeGraff, W., Glatstein, E., Russo, A. (1989). Glutathione modulation in cancer treatment: Will it work? *International Journal of Radiation Oncology, Biology, Physics, 16,* 1289–1295.

41. Benlloch, M., Ortega, A., Ferrer, P., Segarra, R., Obrador, E., Asensi, M., Carretero, J., Estrela, J.M. (2005). Acceleration of glutathione efflux and inhibition of γ-glutamyltranspeptidase sensitize metastatic B16 melanoma cells to endothelium-induced cytotoxicity. *Journal of Biological Chemistry, 280,* 6950–6959.

42. Mena, S., Benlloch, M., Ortega, A., Carretero, J., Obrador, E., Asensi, M., Petschen, I., Brown, B.D., Estrela, J.M. (2007). Bcl-2 and glutathione depletion sensitizes B16 melanoma to combination therapy and eliminates metastatic disease. *Clinical Cancer Research, 13,* 2658–2666.

43. Hanahan, D., Weinberg, R.A. (2000). The hallmarks of cancer. *Cell, 100,* 57–70.

44. Vogelstein, B., Kinzler, K.W. (2004). Cancer genes and the pathways they control. *Nature Medicine, 10,* 789–799.

45. Bishop, J.M. (1991). Molecular themes in oncogenesis. *Cell, 64,* 235–248.

46. Jakobisiak, M., Lasek, W., Golab, J. (2003). Natural mechanisms protecting against cancer. *Immunology Letters, 90,* 103–122.

47. Vogelstein, B., Fearon, E.R., Kern, S.E., Hamilton, S.R., Preisinger, A.C., Nakamura, Y., White, R. (1989). Allelotype of colorectal carcinomas. *Science, 244,* 207–211.

48. Stoler, D.L., Chen, N., Basik, M., Kahlenberg, M.S., Rodriguez-Bigas, M.A., Petrelli, N.J., Anderson, G.R. (1999). The onset and extent of genomic instability in sporadic colorectal tumor progression. *Proceedings of the National Academy of Sciences USA, 96,* 15121–15126.

49. Lander, E.S., Linton, L.M., Birren, B., et al., International Human Genome Sequencing Consortium. (2001). Initial sequencing and analysis of the human genome. *Nature, 409,* 860–921.

50. Sjoblom, T., Jones, S., Wood, L.D., Parsons, D.W., Lin, J., Barber, T.D., Mandelker, D., Leary, R.J., Ptak, J., Silliman, N., Szabo, S., Buckhaults, P., Farrell, C., Meeh, P., Markowitz, S.D., Willis, J., Dawson, D., Willson, J.K., Gazdar, A.F., Hartigan, J., Wu, L., Liu, C., Parmigiani, G., Park, B.H., Bachman, K.E., Papadopoulos, N., Vogelstein, B., Kinzler, K.W., Velculescu, V.E. (2006). The consensus coding sequences of human breast and colorectal cancers. *Science, 314,* 268–274.

51. Espey, M.G., Miranda, K.M., Thomas, D.D., Xavier, S., Citrin, D., Vitek, M.P., Wink, D.A. (2002). A chemical perspective on the interplay between NO, reactive oxygen species, and reactive nitrogen oxide species. *Annals of the New York Academy of Sciences, 962,* 195–206.

52. Gutteridge, J.M., Halliwell, B. (2000). Free radicals and antioxidants in the year 2000. A historical look to the future. *Annals of the New York Academy of Sciences, 899,* 136–147.

53. Allen, R.G., Tresini, M. (2000). Oxidative stress and gene regulation. *Free Radical Biology and Medicine, 28,* 463–499.

54. Kamata, H., Hirata, H. (1999). Redox regulation of cellular signaling. *Cell Signaling, 11,* 1–14.

55. Fialkow, L., Wang, Y., Downey, G.P. (2007). Reactive oxygen and nitrogen species as signaling molecules regulating neutrophil function. *Free Radical Biology and Medicine, 42,* 153–164.

56. Valko, M., Leibfritz, D., Moncol, J., Cronin, M.T., Mazur, M., Telser, J. (2007). Free radicals and antioxidants in normal physiological functions and human disease. *International Journal of Biochemistry and Cell Biology, 39,* 44–84.

57. Dalle-Donne, I., Rossi, R., Colombo, R., Giustarini, D., Milzani, A. (2006). Biomarkers of oxidative damage in human disease. *Clinical Chemistry, 52,* 601–623.

58. Dhalla, N.S., Temsah, R.M., Netticadan, T. (2000). Role of oxidative stress in cardiovascular diseases. *Journal of Hypertension, 18,* 655–673.

59. Jenner, P. (2003). Oxidative stress in Parkinson's disease. *Annals of Neurology, 53*(Suppl 3), S26–S36; discussion S36–S38.

60. Sayre, L.M., Smith, M.A., Perry, G. (2001). Chemistry and biochemistry of oxidative stress in neurodegenerative disease. *Current Medicinal Chemistry, 8,* 721–738.

61. Cerutti, P., Shah, G., Peskin, A., Amstad, P. (1992). Oxidant carcinogenesis and antioxidant defense. *Annals of the New York Academy of Sciences, 663,* 158–166.

62. Ananthaswamy, H.N., Price, J.E., Goldberg, L.H., Bales, E.S. (1988). Detection and identification of activated oncogenes in human skin cancers occurring on sun-exposed body sites. *Cancer Research, 48,* 3341–3346.

63. Sander, C.S., Chang, H., Hamm, F., Elsner, P., Thiele, J.J. (2004). Role of oxidative stress and the antioxidant network in cutaneous carcinogenesis. *International Journal of Dermatology, 43,* 326–335.

64. Ohshima, H. (2003). Genetic and epigenetic damage induced by reactive nitrogen species: Implications in carcinogenesis. *Toxicology Letters, 140–141,* 99–104.

65. Aw, T.Y. (2005). Intestinal glutathione: Determinant of mucosal peroxide transport, metabolism, and oxidative susceptibility. *Toxicology and Applied Pharmacology, 204,* 320–328.

66. Toyokuni, S. (2006). Novel aspects of oxidative stress-associated carcinogenesis. *Antioxidants and Redox Signaling, 8,* 1373–1377.

67. Irani, K., Xia, Y., Zweier, J.L., Sollott, S.J., Der, C.J., Fearon, E.R., Sundaresan, M., Finkel, T., Goldschmidt-Clermont, P.J. (1997). Mitogenic signaling mediated by oxidants in Ras-transformed fibroblasts. *Science*, *275*, 1649–1652.

68. Polytarchou, C., Hatziapostolou, M., Papadimitriou, E. (2005). Hydrogen peroxide stimulates proliferation and migration of human prostate cancer cells through activation of activator protein-1 and up-regulation of the heparin affin regulatory peptide gene. *Journal of Biological Chemistry*, *280*, 40428–40435.

69. Okada, H., Mak, T.W. (2004). Pathways of apoptotic and non-apoptotic death in tumour cells. *Nature Reviews. Cancer*, *4*, 592–603.

70. Payne, S.L., Fogelgren, B., Hess, A.R., Seftor, E.A., Wiley, E.L., Fong, S.F., Csiszar, K., Hendrix, M.J., Kirschmann, D.A. (2005). Lysyl oxidase regulates breast cancer cell migration and adhesion through a hydrogen peroxide-mediated mechanism. *Cancer Research*, *65*, 11429–11436.

71. Pelicano, H., Carney, D., Huang, P. (2004). ROS stress in cancer cells and therapeutic implications. *Drug Resistance Update*, *7*, 97–110.

72. Trachootham, D., Zhou, Y., Zhang, H., Demizu, Y., Chen, Z., Pelicano, H., Chiao, P.J., Achanta, G., Arlinghaus, R.B., Liu, J., Huang, P. (2006). Selective killing of oncogenically transformed cells through a ROS-mediated mechanism by beta-phenylethyl isothiocyanate. *Cancer Cell*, *10*, 241–252.

73. Halliwell, B. (2007). Oxidative stress and cancer: Have we moved forward? *Biochemical Journal*, *401*, 1–11.

74. Tsuzuki, T., Egashira, A., Igarashi, H., Iwakuma, T., Nakatsuru, Y., Tominaga, Y., Kawate, H., Nakao, K., Nakamura, K., Ide, F., Kura, S., Nakabeppu, Y., Katsuki, M., Ishikawa, T., Sekiguchi, M. (2001). Spontaneous tumorigenesis in mice defective in the MTH1 gene encoding 8-oxo-dGTPase. *Proceedings of the National Academy of Sciences USA*, *98*, 11456–11461.

75. Lu, S.C. (2000). Regulation of glutathione synthesis. *Current Topics in Cellular Regulation*, *36*, 95–116.

76. Sadani, G.R., Nadkarni, G.D. (1996). Role of tissue antioxidant defence in thyroid cancers. *Cancer Letters*, *109*, 231–235.

77. Kelner, M.J., Bagnell, R.D., Uglik, S.F., Montoya, M.A., Mullenbach, G.T. (1995). Heterologous expression of selenium-dependent glutathione peroxidase affords cellular resistance to paraquat. *Archives of Biochemistry and Biophysics*, *323*, 40–46.

78. Ho, Y.S., Magnenat, J.L., Bronson, R.T., Cao, J., Gargano, M., Sugawara, M., Funk, C.D. (1997). Mice deficient in cellular glutathione peroxidase develop normally and show no increased sensitivity to hyperoxia. *Journal of Biological Chemistry*, *272*, 16644–16651.

79. Cheng, W., Fu, Y.X., Porres, J.M., Ross, D.A., Lei, X.G. (1999). Selenium-dependent cellular glutathione peroxidase protects mice against a pro-oxidant-induced oxidation of NADPH, NADH, lipids, and protein. *FASEB Journal*, *13*, 1467–1475.

80. Gresner, P., Gromadzinska, J., Wasowicz, W. (2007). Polymorphism of selected enzymes involved in detoxification and biotransformation in relation to lung cancer. *Lung Cancer*, *57*, 1–25.

81. Hines, R.N., McCarver, D.G. (2002). The ontogeny of human drug-metabolizing enzymes: Phase I oxidative enzymes. *Journal of Pharmacology and Experimental Therapy*, *300*, 355–360.

82. Jedlitschky, G., Leier, I., Buchholz, U., Center, M., Keppler, D. (1994). ATP-dependent transport of glutathione S-conjugates by the multidrug resistance-associated protein. *Cancer Research*, *54*, 4833–4836.

83. Balendiran, G.K., Dabur, R., Fraser, D. (2004). The role of glutathione in cancer. *Cell Biochemistry and Function*, *22*, 343–352.

84. Hayes, J.D., Flanagan, J.U., Jowsey, I.R. (2005). Glutathione transferases. *Annual Review of Pharmacology and Toxicology*, *45*, 51–88.

85. Yuan, J., Lipinski, M., Degterev, A. (2003). Diversity in the mechanisms of neuronal cell death. *Neuron*, *40*, 401–413.

86. Armstrong, R.N. (1997). Structure, catalytic mechanism, and evolution of the glutathione transferases. *Chemical Research in Toxicology*, *10*, 2–18.

87. Kretz-Remy, C., Arrigo, A.P. (2002). Gene expression and thiol redox state. *Methods in Enzymology*, *348*, 200–215.

88. Klatt, P., Lamas, S. (2000). Regulation of protein function by S-glutathiolation in response to oxidative and nitrosative stress. *European Journal of Biochemistry*, *267*, 4928–4944.

89. Arrigo, A.P. (1999). Gene expression and the thiol redox state. *Free Radical Biology and Medicine*, *27*, 936–944.

90. Higuchi, Y. (2004). Glutathione depletion-induced chromosomal DNA fragmentation associated with apoptosis and necrosis. *Journal of Cellular and Molecular Medicine*, *8*, 455–464.

91. Nebert, D.W., Vasiliou, V. (2004). Analysis of the glutathione S-transferase (GST) gene family. *Human Genomics*, *1*, 460–464.

92. Beeghly, A., Katsaros, D., Chen, H., Fracchioli, S., Zhang, Y., Massobrio, M., Risch, H., Jones, B., Yu, H. (2006). Glutathione S-transferase polymorphisms and ovarian cancer treatment and survival. *Gynecologic Oncology*, *100*, 330–337.

93. Dalhoff, K., Buus Jensen, K., Enghusen Poulsen, H. (2005). Cancer and molecular biomarkers of phase 2. *Methods in Enzymology*, *400*, 618–627.

94. Henderson, C.J., Wolf, C.R. (2005). Disruption of the glutathione transferase pi class genes. *Methods in Enzymology*, *401*, 116–135.

95. McIlwain, C.C., Townsend, D.M., Tew, K.D. (2006). Glutathione S-transferase polymorphisms: Cancer incidence and therapy. *Oncogene*, *25*, 1639–1648.

96. Parl, F.F. (2005). Glutathione S-transferase genotypes and cancer risk. *Cancer Letters*, *221*, 123–129.

97. Townsend, D.M., Findlay, V.L., Tew, K.D. (2005). Glutathione S-transferases as regulators of kinase pathways and anticancer drug targets. *Methods in Enzymology*, *401*, 287–307.

98. Guengerich, F.P. (2005). Activation of alkyl halides by glutathione transferases. *Methods in Enzymology*, *401*, 342–353.

99. Turella, P., Cerella, C., Filomeni, G., Bullo, A., De Maria, F., Ghibelli, L., Ciriolo, M.R., Cianfriglia, M., Mattei, M., Federici, G., Ricci, G., Caccuri, A.M. (2005). Proapoptotic activity of new glutathione S-transferase inhibitors. *Cancer Research*, *65*, 3751–3761.

100. Kim, A.L., Labasi, J.M., Zhu, Y., Tang, X., McClure, K., Gabel, C.A., Athar, M., Bickers, D.R. (2005). Role of p38 MAPK in UVB-induced inflammatory responses in the skin of SKH-1 hairless mice. *Journal of Investigative Dermatology, 124*, 1318–1325.

101. Rhee, S.G. (1999). Redox signaling: Hydrogen peroxide as intracellular messenger. *Experimental and Molecular Medicine, 31*, 53–59.

102. Egler, R.A., Fernandes, E., Rothermund, K., Sereika, S., de Souza-Pinto, N., Jaruga, P., Dizdaroglu, M., Prochownik, E.V. (2005). Regulation of reactive oxygen species, DNA damage, and c-Myc function by peroxiredoxin 1. *Oncogene, 24*, 8038–8050.

103. Park, S.H., Chung, Y.M., Lee, Y.S., Kim, H.J., Kim, J.S., Chae, H.Z., Yoo, Y.D. (2000). Antisense of human peroxiredoxin II enhances radiation-induced cell death. *Clinical Cancer Research, 6*, 4915–4920.

104. Arner, E.S., Holmgren, A. (2006). The thioredoxin system in cancer. *Seminars in Cancer Biology, 16*, 420–426.

105. Bjornstedt, M., Xue, J., Huang, W., Akesson, B., Holmgren, A. (1994). The thioredoxin and glutaredoxin systems are efficient electron donors to human plasma glutathione peroxidase. *Journal of Biological Chemistry, 269*, 29382–29384.

106. Powis, G., Montfort, W.R. (2001). Properties and biological activities of thioredoxins. *Annual Review of Pharmacology and Toxicology, 41*, 261–295.

107. Iwata, S., Hori, T., Sato, N., Hirota, K., Sasada, T., Mitsui, A., Hirakawa, T., Yodoi, J. (1997). Adult T cell leukemia (ATL)-derived factor/human thioredoxin prevents apoptosis of lymphoid cells induced by L-cystine and glutathione depletion: Possible involvement of thiol-mediated redox regulation in apoptosis caused by pro-oxidant state. *Journal of Immunology, 158*, 3108–3117.

108. Turunen, N., Karihtala, P., Mantyniemi, A., Sormunen, R., Holmgren, A., Kinnula, V.L., Soini, Y. (2004). Thioredoxin is associated with proliferation, p53 expression and negative estrogen and progesterone receptor status in breast carcinoma. *Acta Pathologica, Microbiologica, et Immunologica, Scandinavica, 112*, 123–132.

109. Iwao-Koizumi, K., Matoba, R., Ueno, N., Kim, S.J., Ando, A., Miyoshi, Y., Maeda, E., Noguchi, S., Kato, K. (2005). Prediction of docetaxel response in human breast cancer by gene expression profiling. *Journal of Clinical Oncology, 23*, 422–431.

110. Theocharis, S.E., Margeli, A.P., Koutselinis, A. (2003). Metallothionein: A multifunctional protein from toxicity to cancer. *International Journal of Biological Markers, 18*, 162–169.

111. Cherian, M.G., Jayasurya, A., Bay, B.H. (2003). Metallothioneins in human tumors and potential roles in carcinogenesis. *Mutation Research, 533*, 201–209.

112. Girnun, G.D., Naseri, E., Vafai, S.B., Qu, L., Szwaya, J.D., Bronson, R., Alberta, J.A., Spiegelman, B.M. (2007). Synergy between PPARγ ligands and platinum-based drugs in cancer. *Cancer Cell, 11*, 395–406.

113. Nakamura, Y., Colburn, N.H., Gindhart, T.D. (1985). Role of reactive oxygen in tumor promotion: Implication of superoxide anion in promotion of neoplastic transformation in JB-6 cells by TPA. *Carcinogenesis, 6*, 229–235.

114. Valko, M., Rhodes, C.J., Moncol, J., Izakovic, M., Mazur, M. (2006). Free radicals, metals, and antioxidants in oxidative stress-induced cancer. *Chemico-Biological Interactions, 160*, 1–40.

115. Dhar, A., Young, M.R., Colburn, N.H. (2002). The role of AP-1, NF-kappaB and ROS/ NOS in skin carcinogenesis: The JB6 model is predictive. *Molecular and Cellular Biochemistry, 234–235*, 185–193.

116. Kosower, N.S., Kosower, E.M. (1978). The glutathione status of cells. *International Review of Cytology, 54*, 109–160.

117. Ochoa, S. (1983). Regulation of protein synthesis initiation in eucaryotes. *Archives of Biochemistry and Biophysics, 223*, 325–349.

118. Aw, T.Y. (2003). Cellular redox: A modulator of intestinal epithelial cell proliferation. *News in Physiological Sciences, 18*, 201–204.

119. Sies, H. (1999). Glutathione and its cellular functions. *Free Radical Biology and Medicine, 27*, 916–921.

120. Lee, J.M. (1998). Inhibition of p53-dependent apoptosis by the KIT tyrosine kinase: Regulation of mitochondrial permeability transition and reactive oxygen species generation. *Oncogene, 17*, 1653–1662.

121. Estrela, J.M., Hernandez, R., Terradez, P., Asensi, M., Puertes, I.R., Viña, J. (1992). Regulation of glutathione metabolism in Ehrlich ascites tumour cells. *Biochemical Journal, 286*(Pt 1), 257–262.

122. Kang, Y.J., Enger, M.D. (1990). Glutathione content and growth in A549 human lung carcinoma cells. *Experimental Cell Research, 187*, 177–179.

123. Kerr, J.F., Wyllie, A.H., Currie, A.R. (1972). Apoptosis: A basic biological phenomenon with wide-ranging implications in tissue kinetics. *British Journal of Cancer, 26*, 239–257.

124. Baliga, B.C., Kumar, S. (2002). Role of Bcl-2 family of proteins in malignancy. *Hematological Oncology, l 20*, 63–74.

125. Takaoka, A., Adachi, M., Okuda, H., Sato, S., Yawata, A., Hinoda, Y., Takayama, S., Reed, J.C., Imai, K. (1997). Anti-cell death activity promotes pulmonary metastasis of melanoma cells. *Oncogene, 14*, 2971–2977.

126. Owen-Schaub, L.B., van Golen, K.L., Hill, L.L., Price, J.E. (1998). Fas and Fas ligand interactions suppress melanoma lung metastasis. *Journal of Experimental Medicine, 188*, 1717–1723.

127. Lowe, S.W., Lin, A.W. (2000). Apoptosis in cancer. *Carcinogenesis, 21*, 485–495.

128. Wong, C.W., Lee, A., Shientag, L., Yu, J., Dong, Y., Kao, G., Al-Mehdi, A.B., Bernhard, E.J., Muschel, R.J. (2001). Apoptosis: An early event in metastatic inefficiency. *Cancer Research, 61*, 333–338.

129. Hickman, J.A. (2002). Apoptosis and tumourigenesis. *Current Opinion in Genetics Development, 12*, 67–72.

130. Majno, G., Joris, I. (1995). Apoptosis, oncosis, and necrosis: An overview of cell death. *American Journal of Pathology, 146*, 3–15.

131. Proskuryakov, S.Y., Gabai, V.L., Konoplyannikov, A.G. (2002). Necrosis is an active and controlled form of programmed cell death. *Biochemistry (Moscow), 67*, 387–408.

132. Marzo, I., Brenner, C., Zamzami, N., Jürgensmeier, J.M., Susin, S.A., Vieira, H.L., Prévost, M.C., Xie, Z., Matsuyama, S., Reed, J.C., Kroemer, G. (1998). Bax and adenine nucleotide translocator cooperate in the mitochondrial control of apoptosis. *Science, 281*, 2027–2031.

133. Narita, M., Shimizu, S., Ito, T., Chittenden, T., Lutz, R.J., Matsuda, H., Tsujimoto, Y. (1998). Bax interacts with the permeability transition pore to induce permeability transition and cytochrome c release in isolated mitochondria. *Proceedings of the National Academy of Sciences USA, 95*, 14681–14686.

134. Pastorino, J.G., Chen, S.T., Tafani, M., Snyder, J.W., Farber, J.L. (1998). The overexpression of Bax produces cell death upon induction of the mitochondrial permeability transition. *Journal of Biological Chemistry, 273*, 7770–7775.

135. Ricci, M.S., Zong, W.X. (2006). Chemotherapeutic approaches for targeting cell death pathways. *Oncologist, 11*, 342–357.

136. Kroemer, G., Reed, J.C. (2000). Mitochondrial control of cell death. *Nature Medicine, 6*, 513–519.

137. Obrador, E., Carretero, J., Esteve, J.M., Pellicer, J.A., Pascual, A., Petschen, I., Estrela, J.M. (2001). Glutamine potentiates TNF-alpha-induced tumor cytotoxicity. *Free Radical Biology and Medicine, 31*, 642–650.

138. Arai, M., Imai, H., Koumura, T., Yoshida, M., Emoto, K., Umeda, M., Chiba, N., Nakagawa, Y. (1999). Mitochondrial phospholipid hydroperoxide glutathione peroxidase plays a major role in preventing oxidative injury to cells. *Journal of Biological Chemistry, 274*, 4924–4933.

139. Hanigan, M.H. (1995). Expression of γ-glutamyl transpeptidase provides tumor cells with a selective growth advantage at physiologic concentrations of cyst(e)ine. *Carcinogenesis, 16*, 181–185.

140. Hochwald, S.N., Harrison, L.E., Rose, D.M., Anderson, M., Burt, M.E. (1996). γ-Glutamyl transpeptidase mediation of tumor glutathione utilization in vivo. *Journal of the National Cancer Institute, 88*, 193–197.

141. Curthoys, N.P., Hughey, R.P. (1979). Characterization and physiological function of rat renal γ-glutamyltranspeptidase. *Enzyme, 24*, 383–403.

142. Meister, A. (1985). Methods for the selective modification of glutathione metabolism and study of glutathione transport. *Methods in Enzymology, 113*, 571–585.

143. Orlowski, M., Meister, A. (1970). The γ-glutamyl cycle: A possible transport system for amino acids. *Proceedings of the National Academy of Sciences USA, 67*, 1248–1255.

144. Meister, A. (1988). Glutathione metabolism and its selective modification. *Journal of Biological Chemistry, 263*, 17205–17208.

145. Yao, D.F., Dong, Z.Z., Yao, M. (2007). Specific molecular markers in hepatocellular carcinoma. *Hepatobiliary and Pancreatic Disease International, 6*, 241–247.

146. Mahata, P. (2006). Biomarkers for epithelial ovarian cancers. *Genome Informatics. International Conference on Genome Informatics, 17*, 184–193.

147. Deneke, S.M., Fanburg, B.L. (1989). Regulation of cellular glutathione. *American Journal of Physiology, 257*, L163–L173.

148. Navarro, J., Obrador, E., Pellicer, J.A., Aseni, M., Viña, J., Estrela, J.M. (1997). Blood glutathione as an index of radiation-induced oxidative stress in mice and humans. *Free Radical Biology and Medicine, 22*, 1203–1209.

149. Navarro, J., Obrador, E., Carretero, J., Petschen, I., Aviñó, J., Perez, P., Estrela, J.M. (1999). Changes in glutathione status and the antioxidant system in blood and in cancer cells associate with tumour growth in vivo. *Free Radical Biology and Medicine, 26*, 410–418.

150. Ookhtens, M., Kaplowitz, N. (1998). Role of the liver in interorgan homeostasis of glutathione and cyst(e)ine. *Seminars in Liver Disease, 18*, 313–329.

151. Ookhtens, M., Mittur, A.V., Erhart, N.A. (1994). Changes in plasma glutathione concentrations, turnover, and disposal in developing rats. *American Journal of Physiology, 266*, R979–R988.

152. Homolya, L., Varadi, A., Sarkadi, B. (2003). Multidrug resistance-associated proteins: Export pumps for conjugates with glutathione, glucuronate or sulfate. *Biofactors, 17*, 103–114.

153. Ballatori, N., Rebbeor, J.F. (1998). Roles of MRP2 and oatp1 in hepatocellular export of reduced glutathione. *Seminars in Liver Disease, 18*, 377–387.

154. Zaman, G.J., Lankelma, J., van Tellingen, O., Beijnen, J., Dekker, H., Paulusma, C., Oude Elferink, R.P., Baas, F., Borst, P. (1995). Role of glutathione in the export of compounds from cells by the multidrug-resistance-associated protein. *Proceedings of the National Academy of Sciences USA, 92*, 7690–7694.

155. Borst, P., Evers, R., Kool, M., Wijnholds, J. (2000). A family of drug transporters: The multidrug resistance-associated proteins. *Journal of the National Cancer Institute, 92*, 1295–1302.

156. Fidler, I.J., Nicolson, G.L. (1976). Organ selectivity for implantation survival and growth of B16 melanoma variant tumor lines. *Journal of the National Cancer Institute, 57*, 1199–1202.

157. Anderson, M.E., Meister, A. (1980). Dynamic state of glutathione in blood plasma. *Journal of Biological Chemistry, 255*, 9530–9533.

158. Lu, S.C. (1999). Regulation of hepatic glutathione synthesis: Current concepts and controversies. *FASEB Journal, 13*, 1169–1183.

159. O'Brien, M.L., Tew, K.D. (1996). Glutathione and related enzymes in multidrug resistance. *European Journal of Cancer, 32A*, 967–978.

160. van der Kolk, D.M., Vellenga, E., Muller, M., de Vries, E.G. (1999). Multidrug resistance protein MRP1, glutathione, and related enzymes. Their importance in acute myeloid leukemia. *Advances in Experimental Medicine and Biology, 457*, 187–198.

161. Griffith, O.W. (1999). Biologic and pharmacologic regulation of mammalian glutathione synthesis. *Free Radical Biology and Medicine, 27*, 922–935.

162. Carretero, J., Obrador, E., Pellicer, J.A., Pascual, A., Estrela, J.M. (2000). Mitochondrial glutathione depletion by glutamine in growing tumor cells. *Free Radical Biology and Medicine, 29*, 913–923.

163. Ortega, A., Ferrer, P., Carretero, J., Obrador, E., Asensi, M., Pellicer, J.A., Estrela, J.M. (2003). Down-regulation of glutathione and Bcl-2 synthesis in mouse B16 melanoma cells avoids their survival during interaction with the vascular endothelium. *Journal of Biological Chemistry, 278*, 39591–39599.

164. Fidler, I.J. (2002). Critical determinants of metastasis. *Seminars in Cancer Biology, 12*, 89–96.

165. Weigelt, B., Peterse, J.L., van't Veer, L.J. (2005). Breast cancer metastasis: Markers and models. *Nature Reviews. Cancer, 5*, 591–602.

166. Fidler, I.J., Hart, I.R. (1982). Biological diversity in metastatic neoplasms: Origins and implications. *Science, 217*, 998–1003.

167. Tassone, P., Tagliaferri, P., Fulciniti, M.T., Di Martino, M.T., Venuta, S. (2007). Novel therapeutic approaches based on the targeting of microenvironment-derived survival pathways in human cancer: Experimental models and translational issues. *Current Pharmaceutical Design*, *13*, 487–496.

168. Langley, R.R., Fidler, I.J. (2007). Tumor cell-organ microenvironment interactions in the pathogenesis of cancer metastasis. *Endocrine Reviews*, *28*, 297–321.

169. Fidler, I.J. (1990). Critical factors in the biology of human cancer metastasis: Twenty-eighth G.H.A. Clowes memorial award lecture. *Cancer Research*, *50*, 6130–6138.

170. Fidler, I.J. (1970). Metastasis: Quantitative analysis of distribution and fate of tumor emboli labeled with 125 I-5-iodo-2′-deoxyuridine. *Journal of the National Cancer Institute*, *45*, 773–782.

171. Barbera-Guillem, E., Smith, I., Weiss, L. (1993). Cancer-cell traffic in the liver. II. Arrest, transit and death of B16F10 and M5076 cells in the sinusoids. *International Journal of Cancer*, *53*, 298–301.

172. Weiss, L., Nannmark, U., Johansson, B.R., Bagge, U. (1992). Lethal deformation of cancer cells in the microcirculation: A potential rate regulator of hematogenous metastasis. *International Journal of Cancer*, *50*, 103–107.

173. Weiss, L. (1992). *Biomechanical Interactions of Cancer Cells with the Microvasculature during Hematogenous Metastasis*, Amsterdam: Springer.

174. Glaves, D. (1986). Intravascular death of disseminated cancer cells mediated by superoxide anion. *Invasion & Metastasis*, *6*, 101–111.

175. Bouwens, L., Jacobs, R., Remels, L., Wisse, E. (1988). Natural cytotoxicity of rat hepatic natural killer cells and macrophages against a syngeneic colon adenocarcinoma. *Cancer Immunology and Immunotherapy*, *27*, 137–141.

176. Weiss, L. (1990). Metastatic inefficiency. *Advances in Cancer Research*, *54*, 159–211.

177. Bockhorn, M., Jain, R.K., Munn, L.L. (2007). Active versus passive mechanisms in metastasis: Do cancer cells crawl into vessels, or are they pushed? *Lancet Oncology*, *8*, 444–448.

178. Inbal, B., Cohen, O., Polak-Charcon, S., Kopolovic, J., Vadai, E., Eisenbach, L., Kimchi, A. (1997). DAP kinase links the control of apoptosis to metastasis. *Nature*, *390*, 180–184.

179. Cairns, R.A., Khokha, R., Hill, R.P. (2003). Molecular mechanisms of tumor invasion and metastasis: An integrated view. *Current Molecular Medicine*, *3*, 659–671.

180. Mehlen, P., Puisieux, A. (2006). Metastasis: A question of life or death. *Nature Reviews. Cancer*, *6*, 449–458.

181. Sugarbaker, E.V., Weingrand, D.N., Roseman, J.M. (1982). Observations on cancer metastasis in man. In Liotta, L.A., Hart, I.R., Eds., *Tumor Invasion and Metastasis*. The Hague: Nijhoff.

182. Mendoza, L., Olaso, E., Anasagasti, M.J., Fuentes, A.M., Vidal-Vanaclocha, F. (1998). Mannose receptor-mediated endothelial cell activation contributes to B16 melanoma cell adhesion and metastasis in liver. *Journal of Cell Physiology*, *174*, 322–330.

183. Vidal-Vanaclocha, F., Amezaga, C., Asumendi, A., Kaplanski, G., Dinarello, C.A. (1994). Interleukin-1 receptor blockade reduces the number and size of murine B16 melanoma hepatic metastases. *Cancer Research*, *54*, 2667–2672.

184. Vidal-Vanaclocha, F., Alvarez, A., Asumendi, A., Urcelay, B., Tonino, P., Dinarello, C.A. (1996). Interleukin 1 (IL-1)-dependent melanoma hepatic metastasis in vivo; increased

endothelial adherence by IL-1-induced mannose receptors and growth factor production in vitro. *Journal of the National Cancer Institute, 88,* 198–205.

185. Rice, G.E., Gimbrone, M.A., Jr., Bevilacqua, M.P. (1988). Tumor cell-endothelial interactions: Increased adhesion of human melanoma cells to activated vascular endothelium. *American Journal of Pathology, 133,* 204–210.

186. Matsubara, T., Ziff, M. (1986). Increased superoxide anion release from human endothelial cells in response to cytokines. *Journal of Immunology, 137,* 3295–3298.

187. McCloskey, T.W., Todaro, J.A., Laskin, D.L. (1992). Lipopolysaccharide treatment of rats alters antigen expression and oxidative metabolism in hepatic macrophages and endothelial cells. *Hepatology, 16,* 191–203.

188. Anasagasti, M.J., Alvarez, A., Avivi, C., Vidal-Vanaclocha, F. (1996). Interleukin-1-mediated H_2O_2 production by hepatic sinusoidal endothelium in response to B16 melanoma cell adhesion. *Journal of Cell Physiology, 167,* 314–323.

189. Sellak, H., Franzini, E., Hakim, J., Pasquier, C. (1994). Reactive oxygen species rapidly increase endothelial ICAM-1 ability to bind neutrophils without detectable upregulation. *Blood, 83,* 2669–2677.

190. Anasagasti, M.J., Alvarez, A., Martin, J.J., Mendoza, L., Vidal-Vanaclocha, F. (1997). Sinusoidal endothelium release of hydrogen peroxide enhances very late antigen-4-mediated melanoma cell adherence and tumor cytotoxicity during interleukin-1 promotion of hepatic melanoma metastasis in mice. *Hepatology, 25,* 840–846.

191. Marui, N., Offermann, M.K., Swerlick, R., Kunsch, C., Rosen, C.A., Ahmad, M., Alexander, R.W., Medford, R.M. (1993). Vascular cell adhesion molecule-1 (VCAM-1) gene transcription and expression are regulated through an antioxidant-sensitive mechanism in human vascular endothelial cells. *Journal of Clinical Investigation, 92,* 1866–1874.

192. Wang, H.H., McIntosh, A.R., Hasinoff, B.B., Rector, E.S., Ahmed, N., Nance, D.M., Orr, F.W. (2000). B16 melanoma cell arrest in the mouse liver induces nitric oxide release and sinusoidal cytotoxicity: A natural hepatic defense against metastasis. *Cancer Research, 60,* 5862–5869.

193. Wink, D.A., Vodovotz, Y., Laval, J., Laval, F., Dewhirst, M.W., Mitchell, J.B. (1998). The multifaceted roles of nitric oxide in cancer. *Carcinogenesis, 19,* 711–721.

194. Nishikawa, M., Sato, E.F., Kuroki, T., Utsumi, K., Inoue, M. (1998). Macrophage-derived nitric oxide induces apoptosis of rat hepatoma cells in vivo. *Hepatology, 28,* 1474–1480.

195. Melino, G., Bernassola, F., Knight, R.A., Corasaniti, M.T., Nistico, G., Finazzi-Agro, A. (1997). S-nitrosylation regulates apoptosis. *Nature, 388,* 432–433.

196. Ioannidis, I., de Groot, H. (1993). Cytotoxicity of nitric oxide in Fu5 rat hepatoma cells: Evidence for co-operative action with hydrogen peroxide. *Biochemical Journal, 296*(Pt 2), 341–345.

197. Weisman, G.A., Lustig, K.D., Lane, E., Huang, N.N., Belzer, I., Friedberg, I. (1988). Growth inhibition of transformed mouse fibroblasts by adenine nucleotides occurs via generation of extracellular adenosine. *Journal of Biological Chemistry, 263,* 12367–12372.

198. Obrador, E., Navarro, J., Mompo, J., Asensi, M., Pellicer, J.A., Estrela, J.M. (1997). Glutathione and the rate of cellular proliferation determine tumour cell sensitivity to tumour necrosis factor in vivo. *Biochemical Journal, 325*(Pt 1), 183–189.

199. Anasagasti, M.J., Martin, J.J., Mendoza, L., Obrador, E., Estrela, J.M., McCuskey, R.S., Vidal-Vanaclocha, F. (1998). Glutathione protects metastatic melanoma cells against oxidative stress in the murine hepatic microvasculature. *Hepatology*, *27*, 1249–1256.

200. Sun, Y., Oberley, L.W. (1996). Redox regulation of transcriptional activators. *Free Radical Biology and Medicine*, *21*, 335–348.

201. Cross, J.V., Templeton, D.J. (2006). Regulation of signal transduction through protein cysteine oxidation. *Antioxidants and Redox Signaling*, *8*, 1819–1827.

202. Giles, G.I. (2006). The redox regulation of thiol dependent signaling pathways in cancer. *Current Pharmaceutical Design*, *12*, 4427–4443.

203. Huang, Z.Z., Chen, C., Zeng, Z., Yang, H., Oh, J., Chen, L., Lu, S.C. (2001). Mechanism and significance of increased glutathione level in human hepatocellular carcinoma and liver regeneration. *FASEB Journal*, *15*, 19–21.

204. Shackelford, R.E., Kaufmann, W.K., Paules, R.S. (2000). Oxidative stress and cell cycle checkpoint function. *Free Radical Biology and Medicine*, *28*, 1387–1404.

205. Lu, S.C., Kuhlenkamp, J., Garcia-Ruiz, C., Kaplowitz, N. (1991). Hormone-mediated down-regulation of hepatic glutathione synthesis in the rat. *Journal of Clinical Investigation*, *88*, 260–269.

206. Marshall, H.E., Merchant, K., Stamler, J.S. (2000). Nitrosation and oxidation in the regulation of gene expression. *FASEB Journal*, *14*, 1889–1900.

207. Oktyabrsky, O.N., Smirnova, G.V. (2007). Redox regulation of cellular functions. *Biochemistry (Moscow)*, *72*, 132–145.

208. Mistry, P., Harrap, K.R. (1991). Historical aspects of glutathione and cancer chemotherapy. *Pharmacology and Therapeutics*, *49*, 125–132.

209. Reliene, R., Schiestl, R.H. (2006). Glutathione depletion by buthionine sulfoximine induces DNA deletions in mice. *Carcinogenesis*, *27*, 240–244.

210. Zhou, D.C., Zittoun, R., Marie, J.P. (1995). Expression of multidrug resistance-associated protein (MRP) and multidrug resistance (MDR1) genes in acute myeloid leukemia. *Leukemia*, *9*, 1661–1666.

211. Depeille, P., Cuq, P., Passagne, I., Evrard, A., Vian, L. (2005). Combined effects of GSTP1 and MRP1 in melanoma drug resistance. *British Journal of Cancer*, *93*, 216–223.

212. Versantvoort, C.H., Broxterman, H.J., Bagrij, T., Scheper, R.J., Twentyman, P.R. (1995). Regulation by glutathione of drug transport in multidrug-resistant human lung tumour cell lines overexpressing multidrug resistance-associated protein. *British Journal of Cancer*, *72*, 82–89.

213. Cullen, K.V., Davey, R.A., Davey, M.W. (2001). Verapamil-stimulated glutathione transport by the multidrug resistance-associated protein (MRP1) in leukaemia cells. *Biochemical Pharmacology*, *62*, 417–424.

214. Loe, D.W., Deeley, R.G., Cole, S.P. (2000). Verapamil stimulates glutathione transport by the 190-kDa multidrug resistance protein 1 (MRP1). *Journal of Pharmacology and Experimental Therapeutics*, *293*, 530–538.

215. Tsuruo, T., Iida, H., Tsukagoshi, S., Sakurai, Y. (1981). Overcoming of vincristine resistance in P388 leukemia in vivo and in vitro through enhanced cytotoxicity of vincristine and vinblastine by verapamil. *Cancer Research*, *41*, 1967–1972.

216. Linsdell, P., Hanrahan, J.W. (1998). Glutathione permeability of CFTR. *American Journal of Physiology*, *275*, C323–C326.

217. Gadsby, D.C., Nairn, A.C. (1999). Control of CFTR channel gating by phosphorylation and nucleotide hydrolysis. *Physiological Reviews*, *79*, S77–S107.

218. Stole, E., Smith, T.K., Manning, J.M., Meister, A. (1994). Interaction of γ-glutamyl transpeptidase with acivicin. *Journal of Biological Chemistry*, *269*, 21435–21439.

219. Benlloch, M., Mena, S., Ferrer, P., Obrador, E., Asensi, M., Pellicer, J.A., Carretero, J., Ortega, A., Estrela, J.M. (2006). Bcl-2 and Mn-SOD antisense oligodeoxynucleotides and a glutamine-enriched diet facilitate elimination of highly resistant B16 melanoma cells by tumor necrosis factor-alpha and chemotherapy. *Journal of Biological Chemistry*, *281*, 69–79.

PART VI

GSH AND SULFUR AMINO ACIDS AS DRUGS AND NUTRACEUTICALS

CHAPTER 20

GSH, GSH DERIVATIVES, AND ANTIVIRAL ACTIVITY

ANNA TERESA PALAMARA, LUCIA NENCIONI, ROSSELLA SGARBANTI, and ENRICO GARACI

20.1 INTRODUCTION

The intracellular redox state is physiologically maintained in a reduced condition by several molecules, among which is glutathione (GSH), the most prevalent intracellular thiol. GSH is found in eukaryotic cells at millimolar concentrations, and it takes part directly or indirectly in many important biological phenomena, including protein synthesis, enzyme activity, metabolism, and cell protection. GSH is the most powerful intracellular antioxidant, and the reduced:oxidized glutathione ratio (GSH:GSSG) serves as a representative marker of the antioxidative capacity of the cell. In the past decade new roles for GSH have been discovered in signal transduction, gene expression, apoptosis, protein glutathionylation, and nitric oxide metabolism. An imbalance of GSH has been observed in a wide range of diseases, including cancer, neurodegenerative disorders, cystic fibrosis, hepatitis, diabetes, Parkinson's disease, and as a natural part of the aging process (reviewed in Reference 1).

Numerous studies have reported that viral infection is often associated with redox changes characteristic of oxidative stress [2–4]. A shift towards a prooxidant state has been observed in the cells and body fluids of patients infected with human immunodeficiency virus (HIV) [5–10] and the hepatitis C virus [11–13]. An alteration of the endogenous levels of GSH has been found in different experimental virus infections in vitro and in vivo [14–20]. A decrease in GSH levels and a general oxidative stress have been demonstrated also during influenza virus infection in both in vivo and in vitro studies [21–24].

Beck et al. [25] demonstrated that a nutritional deficiency of the antioxidant selenium (Se) led to greater lung pathology and altered immune function in mice infected

Glutathione and Sulfur Amino Acids in Human Health and Disease. Edited by R. Masella and G. Mazza
Copyright © 2009 John Wiley & Sons, Inc.

with influenza virus. Moreover, the same authors and others reported that one driving force for the emergence of new viral variants is the nutritional status of the host. In particular, by using two different viruses (coxsackie virus and influenza virus) it has been demonstrated that a host deficiency in either Se or vitamin E resulted in a change of viral genome, and consequently increased virulence of both viruses (reviewed in Beck et al. [26]).

Exogenous administration of molecules (i.e., GSH, GSH derivatives, GSH precursors such as glutamine or cysteine, α-lipoic acid) able to increase cellular GSH concentration inhibits the replication of different viruses, through different mechanisms (reviewed in Fraternale et al. [27]). Cai et al. [24] demonstrated that, when added extracellularly, GSH had a dose-dependent anti-influenza effect in cultured cells. The authors suggested that such an effect was probably due to an inhibition of apoptosis and subsequent release of the active virus from dead cells. Moreover, the addition of GSH to the drinking water of influenza infected mice inhibited viral titer in the trachea and lungs.

In this chapter we summarize the main results obtained in the last years about the role of intracellular GSH in the regulation of virus life cycle.

20.2 INTRACELLULAR GSH STATUS DURING VIRAL INFECTION

Modifications of endogenous GSH levels have been demonstrated in different virus/host cell systems: parainfluenza-1-Sendai virus (SV) in Madin Darby canine kidney cells (MDCK) [14], and herpes simplex virus type 1 (HSV-1) in monkey kidney cells (Vero) [15], as a model of acute infection; HIV in human monocyte-derived macrophages (M/M) [17, 18], as a model of chronic infection.

In these studies, at different time points during virus challenge (viral adsorption period) or after it, infected cells were assayed for intracellular GSH and GSSG, by HPLC. Mock-infected cells were used as control. As shown in Fig. 20.1, in all the infections, a significant decrease of intracellular GSH content was found, which shows different intensity and kinetics depending on the species of virus and the infected cell type. During acute infection (SV and HSV-1) the fall in GSH content started very early during the period of virus adsorption to the cells and reached the maximum reduction (32% of the control level) 20 to 25 min after virus challenge. After this period, but within the first hour, a slight increase in GSH concentration was consistently observed in all experiments: this was probably due to the stimulation of the GSH synthesis consequent to virus-induced depletion. This temporary increase was followed by a further and progressive reduction as compared to those measured in mock-infected cells 24 h post infection (p.i.) ($P < 0.001$). During chronic infection (HIV-1) a significant decrease in GSH intracellular levels was detected 14 days after virus infection. On the contrary, no significant difference was detected 3 and 7 days p.i. with respect to controls. In this model, no virus was detected in supernatants or in cell homogenates 3 days p.i. Indeed, the protein p-24 was determined only 7 days p.i. both intracellularly and extracellularly, and its expression reached

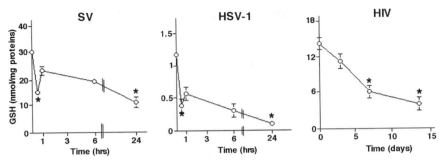

Figure 20.1 Intracellular GSH status during viral infection. Each point represents the average ± SE of duplicate samples. Results are shown for one representative experiment out of six (SV and HSV-1) or three (HIV) performed. *$P < 0.001$ vs. mock-infected cells. SV, sendai virus; HSV-1, herpes simplex virus type 1; HIV, human immunodeficiency virus.

the maximum value 14 days p.i. This is the time in which maximum GSH decrease was detected.

Moreover, our recent data indicated that, during influenza virus infection, the intracellular GSH depletion was greater in the cytoplasm than in the nucleus of infected cells (L. Nencioni et al., manuscript in preparation). It is possible that this nuclear/cytoplasmic distribution of GSH may favor the progression of viral infection. Indeed, physiologically the nucleus represents a very reducing compartment, in which GSH and thioredoxin as well as redox-sensitive factors such as redox factor 1 (Ref-1) are present at high concentrations. Some transcription factors, such as nuclear factor kappa B (NF-κB), are activated in the cytoplasm during oxidative stress, then translocate into the nucleus where, however, they bind DNA only after reduction of cysteine residues on their subunit (reviewed in Reference 28). On this basis, it could be speculated that during infection, the prooxidant conditions of the cytoplasm might contribute to the activation of some transcription factors that are essential for viral replication. At the same time, the reducing conditions of the nucleus make possible their binding to cellular DNA and the consequent activation of redox-sensitive signaling cascades. Moreover, influenza virus activates several kinases, including the four members of the mitogen activated protein kinases (MAPKs) family and the PKC cascade, that play a key role in different steps of the influenza virus life cycle [29, 30, Nencioni et al., manuscript in preparation]. It is known that these kinases are redox-sensitive. In particular, the addition of exogenous H_2O_2, and exposure to radiation or to drugs known to induce production of H_2O_2, activate the MAPKs. Moreover, the modulation of GSH levels plays a role in activating two members (JNK and p38 MAPK) of the MAPK cascade (reviewed in Reference 31). The fact that several kinases that are responsible for efficient influenza virus replication are activated by a redox unbalance suggests that the prooxidant state induced by viral infection could play a key role in their modulation during infection.

20.3   MECHANISM OF VIRUS-INDUCED GSH DEPLETION

GSH depletion may be generally caused by different mechanisms, such as oxidative stress, loss and/or extrusion from plasma membrane, or reduced synthesis. We excluded the last possibility, at least for acute infections, because the fall in GSH was too rapid to be accounted for by an inhibition of precursor uptake or biosynthesis. Then, we infected MDCK cells with SV and, since GSH depletion was a two-step process (Fig. 20.1), we performed the experiments at 20 min, in the early phase of viral infection and at 24 h, at the late stage of virus replication [32]. We demonstrated that, despite a massive and rapid GSH decrease, no significant change in the concentrations of GSSG was detected neither at 20 min or at 24 h p.i.. Thus, the glutathione loss from the GSH pool of the infected cells was not recovered in its partner redox form inside the cells. On the other hand, while 20 min p.i., large amounts of glutathione were detected in the media of infected cells predominantly as GSH, 24 h p.i. the antioxidant was detected in the medium of either infected or mock-infected cells. These results demonstrated that GSH was efficiently extruded from cells during the 24 h considered, and that infected cells did not differ from mock-infected cells. Moreover, 24 h p.i., a significant amount of GSH was found to be bound to proteins, even if the GSH equivalent present in this form represented only 10% of the total glutathione in infected cells and did not account for GSH depletion observed.

20.4   ROLE OF CONSTITUTIVE GSH LEVELS IN CONTROLLING CELL SUSCEPTIBILITY TO VIRAL INFECTION

Several data demonstrate that intracellular levels of GSH depend on the expression of the antiapoptotic protein Bcl-2. Indeed, overexpression of Bcl-2 leads to increased GSH levels [23, 33, 34], and to changes in the cell compartment distribution of the tripeptide [35].

We demonstrated that different cell populations display differential permissiveness to influenza virus infection, depending on their intracellular GSH content and Bcl-2 expression [23]. In particular, we found that cells efficiently expressing Bcl-2 had consistently higher intracellular GSH contents than Bcl-2 negative cells, and that the higher reducing conditions within Bcl-2$^+$ cells could interfere with expression and maturation of late viral proteins. For this study, we measured the GSH content in various cell populations that are characterized by different expression of Bcl-2 protein, during influenza A PR8/H1N1 virus (PR8) infection. The intracellular GSH content was measured 24 h after mock- or PR8-infection in cells that do not express detectable levels of Bcl-2 protein, that is, MDCK cells and the human pulmonary cell line, NCI-H292; and in cells that express both Bcl-2 mRNA and protein, that is, MDCK cells transfected with a vector expressing the human *bcl-2* gene (referred to hereafter as MDCKBcl-2), the neuroblastoma cell line, SH-SY5Y, and a promonocytic cell line, U937. As shown in Fig. 20.2a, GSH concentrations were significantly higher in the Bcl-2-expressing cells compared to those that do not express this protein: in

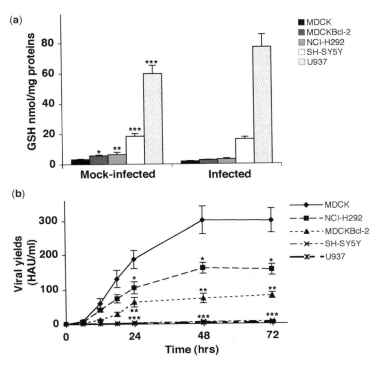

Figure 20.2 Role of constitutive GSH levels in the control of viral replication. (a) Intracellular GSH content in different cell lines was measured by HPLC, 24 h p.i. Each point represents the average $\pm$ SD of samples from five (MDCK), or three (MDCKBcl-2, NCI-H292, and U937), or six (SH-SY5Y), separate experiments, each run in duplicate. $^*P <$ 0.005; $^{**}P < 0.001$; $^{***}P < 0.0001$ vs. MDCK cells. (b) Virus released from the cells at various times p.i. was measured in the supernatant as HAU/ml. Data represent the average $\pm$ SD ($n = 10$) of results from five separate experiments, each performed in duplicate. $^*P < 0.05$; $^{**}P < 0.01$; $^{***}P < 0.0001$ vs. MDCK cells. MDCK, Madin Darby canine kidney cells; NCI-H292, human pulmonary cell line; SH-SY5Y, neuroblastoma cell line; U937, promonocytic cell line.

mock-infected MDCKBcl-2 cells GSH content was significantly higher than those of the parental line ($P < 0.005$); in SH-SY5Y and U937 the levels of the antioxidant were, respectively, 6- and 18-fold higher than those of MDCK cells ($P < 0.0001$); and in NCI-H292 cells GSH content was also approximately twice as high as that of MDCK cells, even though these cells do not express Bcl-2 ($P < 0.001$). Consistently with our previous observations, a decrease in the GSH content was documented 24 h after PR8 infection in MDCK, MDCKBcl-2, and NCI-H292 cells. Nevertheless, in infected SH-SY5Y and U937 cells the relative concentrations of GSH mirrored those of the mock-infected cells. To correlate these results with PR8 replication, hemagglutinating activity (HAU/ml) was measured in culture supernatants at different time points after virus challenge. As shown in Fig. 20.2b, viral replication in each of these cell lines was related to both Bcl-2 expression and GSH levels. In particular, in cells with high GSH contents and not expressing Bcl-2 (NCI-H292) viral replication occurred, but the virus titer in the supernatant was significantly ($P < 0.05$) lower than that of MDCK cells. The Bcl-2-expressing cells were still susceptible to PR8 infection but much less permissive to viral replication compared to that observed for MDCK cells. Indeed, PR8 replication in MDCKBcl-2 cells was significantly reduced by 66.7% to 78.8% at various time points p.i., and in SH-SY5Y and U937 cells, even if detectable virus titer was found 18 and 24 h p.i., respectively, at the end of the experiment (72 h p.i.), it was virtually unchanged, reflecting reductions in replication with respect to MDCK cells ranging from 98.5% to 99.3%.

20.5 EFFECT OF INTRACELLULAR GSH DEPLETION ON VIRAL REPLICATION

Depletion of intracellular GSH was induced by treatment of SV-infected MDCK cells and HIV-infected human M/M with buthionine sulfoximine (BSO) a specific inhibitor of GSH neosynthesis. In both cases, the treatment with BSO caused a decrease of GSH ranging between 60% and 70%. The oxidative condition induced by GSH depletion increased virus replication both in SV (Fig. 20.3a) and in HIV infection (Fig. 20.3b). Similar results were obtained during influenza virus infection [14, 18, 23].

The treatment with BSO of influenza virus-infected cells increased the expression of the viral glycoprotein hemagglutinin (HA) (Fig. 20.3c) [23]. This protein is organized as a homotrimer, and each monomer consists of two disulfide-linked subunits, HA1 and HA2 [36], and its assembly into oligomers depends on the formation of disulfide bonds, which are strongly affected by reducing agents such as GSH [37, 38]. Then, high reducing conditions within the host cell could interfere with disulfide bond formation, thus preventing the correct folding and maturation of HA and consequently its transport and insertion into the cell membrane [39]. We are currently characterizing the mechanisms that underlie the GSH inhibition of HA maturation by using a GSH derivative GSH-C4, that is able to inhibit replication of SV, HSV-1 (Fig. 20.4a and b) [40], and influenza virus (Sgarbanti et al., manuscript in preparation) with more efficacy than GSH.

For HIV, the oxidative environment could participate in the activation of NF-κB, a known enhancer of HIV transcription and replication [41].

Since typical oxidative stress is induced by several drugs of abuse in humans, mice, and primary rat culture [42, 43], we investigated whether cocaine and morphine affected SV replication through modulation of intracellular GSH levels. In MDCK cells, addition of cocaine (1 mM) or morphine (1.5 mM) induced a significant decrease of intracellular GSH in a period ranging between 3 and 6 h after treatment. GSH depletion was not the result of oxidation, since GSSG was depleted in the same way. Interestingly, when cells were pretreated with the drugs and then infected

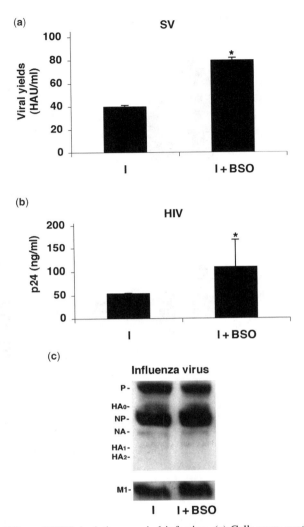

Figure 20.3 Effect of GSH depletion on viral infection. (a) Cells were continuously treated with 1 mM buthionine sulfoximine (BSO) from the 18th hour before SV infection and for 24 hours thereafter. Viral titer was measured in the supernatant as HAU/ml, 24 h p.i. Data represents the average $\pm$ SD of results from two separate experiments, each performed in duplicate. $^{*}P < 0.05$ vs. untreated cells. (b) 5 mM BSO was added every day to HIV-infected M/M from the 10th to 14th day p.i. Viral titer was measured in the supernatant as p24 antigen production, 14 days p.i. Data represents the average $\pm$ SD of results from two separate experiments, each performed in duplicate. $^{*}P < 0.05$ vs. untreated cells. (c) Cells were continuously treated with 1 mM BSO from the 18th hour before influenza virus infection and for 24 hours thereafter. Cell lysates were separated by SDS-PAGE, the gel was blotted onto a nitrocellulose membrane and stained with goat polyclonal anti-influenza A virus Abs. Results are shown for one representative experiment out of three performed. Virus proteins are indicated on the left of the figure.

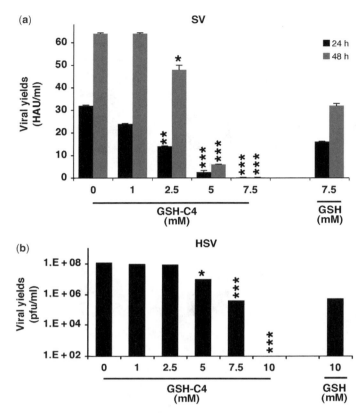

Figure 20.4 Effect of exogenous GSH-C4 on viral replication. (a) Cells were treated with different concentrations of GSH-C4 (0 to 7.5 mM range) or with 7.5 mM GSH. Data represents the viral yields detected in the supernatant as HAU/ml, at 24 and 48 h p.i. Results are shown for one representative experiment out of three performed, each performed in triplicate. *$P < 0.05$; **$P < 0.001$; ***$P < 0.0001$ vs. untreated cells. (b) Cells were treated with different concentrations of GSH-C4 (0 to 10 mM range) or 10 mM GSH. Data represents the viral yields detected in the supernatant as pfu/ml, 48 h p.i. Each point represents the average ± SD of quadruplicate samples. Results are shown for one representative experiment out of four performed. *$P < 0.05$; ***$P < 0.0001$ vs. untreated cells. SV, sendai virus; HSV, herpes simplex virus.

with SV we found a significant increase in virus released from infected cells. Such an increase was stable as long as 72 h p.i., suggesting that it was not related to an accelerated virus release (Fig. 20.5a and b). Moreover, electrophoretic analysis of viral proteins showed that cocaine significantly increased expression of all viral proteins [44, 45].

This data constitutes a further demonstration that a prooxidant state represents a favorable condition for viral replication.

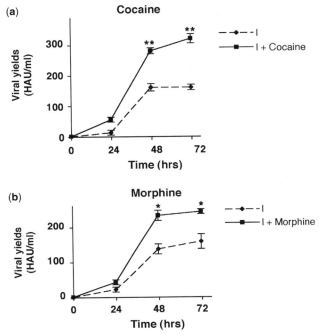

Figure 20.5 Effect of drugs of abuse on SV replication. (a) Cells were treated for 6 h with 1 mM cocaine. Virus released from the cells at various times p.i. was measured in the supernatant as HAU/ml. Each point represents the average $\pm$ SD of duplicate samples. Results are shown for one representative experiment out of six performed. $^{**}P < 0.001$ vs. untreated cells. (b) Cells were treated for 6 h with 1.5 mM morphine. Virus released from the cells at various times p.i. was measured in the supernatant as HAU/ml. Each point represents the average $\pm$ SD of duplicate samples. Results are shown for one representative experiment out of four performed. $^{*}P < 0.05$ vs. untreated cells. SV, sendai virus.

20.6 EFFECT OF EXOGENOUS GSH AND GSH DERIVATIVES ON VIRAL REPLICATION

We have demonstrated that exogenous GSH inhibits replication of SV, HSV-1, and HIV-1 viruses [14, 15, 17]. For acute infections, GSH was administered at different concentrations 1 h after virus challenge, and the supernatants were collected at 24, 48 and 72 h p.i. and tested for HAU (SV) or for plaque-forming units (p.f.u.)/ml (HSV-1). GSH caused a dose-dependent inhibition of both viruses (Fig. 20.6). Comparison of the kinetics of virus growth in untreated infected and GSH-treated infected cells proved that the inhibition was stable as long as 72 h p.i. (end of experiment), and it was not just a delay in virus burst.

For chronic infection, human M/M were challenged with 300 minimum infectious doses of a monocytotropic strain of HIV, named HIV-BaL. After removal of virus excess (2 days after virus challenge), M/M were maintained for additional 14 days,

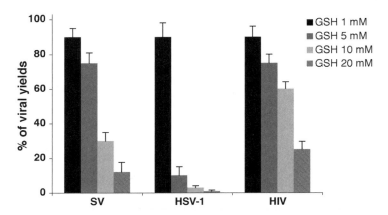

Figure 20.6   Effect of exogenous GSH on viral replication. Cells were treated with different concentrations of GSH. Data represent the viral yields detected in the supernatant as HAU/ml (SV), plaque forming units (pfu/ml) (HSV-1), p24 antigen production (HIV). Results are expressed as percentage of virus production compared to control, from four different experiments. SV, sendai virus; HSV, herpes simplex virus; HIV, human immunodeficiency virus.

when chronic infection was established. Chronically infected macrophages were treated with GSH every other day (i.e., 14, 16, 18, and 20 p.i.) for a total of four doses. As reported in Fig. 20.6, GSH suppressed HIV replication in a dose-dependent manner. In particular, 20 mM GSH decreased the release of HIV p24-gag protein (range between 60% and 73%) at all the time points tested (i.e., 15, 18, 21 days p.i., that is 1, 4, and 7 days after GSH treatment, respectively).

The antiviral activity was associated with recovery of intracellular GSH levels and consequently inhibition of the correct folding and maturation of viral envelope glycoproteins, as described above.

However, GSH is not freely transported into most cells or tissues. For this reason, we synthesized a series of GSH derivatives (with aliphatic chains of different length coupled by peptide bound to the α-NH$_2$ group of Glu) that can more easily cross the membrane of many types of cells, and we evaluated the antiviral activity of these compounds on the replication of SV and HSV-1 in MDCK and Vero cells respectively [40]. The results showed that the n-butanoyl derivative of GSH (GSH-C4) exerted remarkable antiviral activity against both viruses. Indeed, GSH-C4 inhibited replication of SV in MDCK cells in a dose-dependent manner (Fig. 20.4a). An inhibition ranging between 88% (24 h p.i.) and 93% (48 h p.i.) was found in the presence of 5 mM GSH-C4. No virus was detected in the supernatant of cells treated with 7.5 mM of the drug. The 50% inhibition of viral production (EC$_{50}$) at 48 h p.i. was obtained at the concentration of 3.6 mM compared to 7.5 mM of GSH necessary to obtain the same results. The effect of different doses of GSH-C4 on HSV-1 production in Vero cells is shown in Fig. 20.4b. Results indicate that GSH-C4 inhibited virus replication in a dose-dependent manner. A marked decrease (about 3 log) in viral replication was achieved through the addition of 7.5 mM GSH-C4. No virus particles were detected at 10 mM. The addition of GSH at the concentration of 10 mM did not induce a complete inhibition of the virus, and produced only a 2.5 log reduction of virus replication. Furthermore, differently from GSH, GSH-C4 (7.5 mM) markedly reduced the typical cytopathic effect induced by HSV-1.

The antiviral activity of GSH-C4 was evaluated also on the replication of influenza virus. Results indicate that this molecule was able to inhibit replication in a dose-dependent manner, resulting in an inhibition of 90% at the concentration of 10 mM, 24 h p.i. (Sgarbanti et al., manuscript in preparation).

At the concentrations utilized for the studies, GSH-C4 did not induce toxic effects on uninfected cells as confirmed by microscopic examination of the monolayers and by trypan blue exclusion.

20.7 IN VIVO EFFECTS OF SYSTEMIC AND TOPIC GSH ADMINISTRATION

20.7.1 Murine AIDS (MAIDS)

To determine whether GSH is able to exert any antiviral activity in vivo, we investigated the efficacy and toxicity of the administration of reduced GSH on an animal model of immunodeficiency (C57BL/6 mice infected with the retroviral complex LP-BM5). GSH (50 or 100 mg/day) was administered intramuscularly 5 days a week.

As shown in Table 20.1, after 10 weeks from infection GSH significantly reduced splenomegaly and lymphoadenopathy in a dose-dependent manner. Thus, since enlargement of lymph nodes and spleen correlate with viral replication, we suggested that GSH reduces the formation of new viral particles in MAIDS. Moreover, the antiviral activity of GSH was confirmed by several in vitro data [46].

20.7.2 HSV-1-Induced Keratitis

The therapeutic effect of topical administration of GSH was studied in HSV-1-induced keratitis in rabbits by evaluating the clinical signs of the disease and the corneal redox state [19]. Animals were infected and treated with GSH (200 mM administered as eyedrops, 100 μL per eye, four times daily, for 2 weeks) or with placebo. On day 7 p.i.,

TABLE 20.1 GSH Significantly Reduced Splenomegaly and Lymphoadenopathy in a Dose-Dependent Manner

	Spleen Weight (g)	Lymph Node Weight (g)
Control	0.08 ± 0.01	0.02 ± 0.01
I	0.66 ± 0.06	1.39 ± 0.31
I + GSH 50 mg	0.34 ± 0.05*	0.52 ± 0.15*
I + GSH 100 mg	0.2 ± 0.11*	0.25 ± 0.25*

I, infected animals; I + GSH, infected animals treated with GSH.

TABLE 20.2 GSH Content Significantly Decreased in Infected Corneas Compared to Those of Mock-Infected Animals; on the Contrary, Levels of GSSG Were Not Affected by Infection

Control		HSV-1		HSV-1 + GSH	
GSH	GSSG	GSH	GSSG	GSH	GSSG
11.32 ± 1.24	0.85 ± 0.24	$4.44 \overset{**}{\pm} 1.05$	1.03 ± 0.42	$7.8 \overset{*}{\pm} 1.81$	1.44 ± 0.3

when corneal involvement was at its maximum, levels of GSH and GSSG were measured in the corneas. As shown in Table 20.2, GSH content significantly decreased in infected corneas compared to those of mock-infected animals. On the contrary, levels of GSSG were not affected by infection, suggesting that the decrease in GSH was not primarily due to its oxidation. In the GSH-treated animals, corneal GSH content was significantly higher with respect to the placebo treated group even though it was not completely restored to its physiological levels. Then, to evaluate whether the restoration of corneal redox state was also associated with an improvement of the clinical signs of the disease, the corneal involvement of 24 animals after ocular HSV-1 infection and treatment with GSH or placebo was examined. As shown in Fig. 20.7, on days 4, 7, and 9 p.i., the mean keratitis score of the GSH-treated animals was

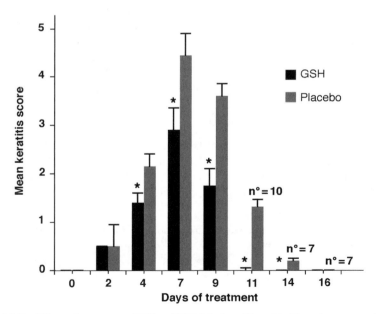

Figure 20.7 Effect of exogenous GSH on HSV-1-induced keratitis. Data shows mean keratitis scores $\pm$ SD ($n = 12$/group until day 9). Starting from day 11, some animals died in the placebo-treated group. The number of surviving animals is indicated in the figure for each day. $^*P < 0.01$ vs. placebo.

significantly reduced with respect to the placebo-treated group. On day 11 p.i., none of the animals in the GSH-treated group showed signs of keratitis. On the contrary, in the placebo-treated group countable lesions persisted until day 14. Moreover, in this group five animals died showing signs of neurological involvement, while, in a follow-up lasting one month, none of the GSH-treated animals died. The clinical efficacy paralleled the significant reduction of virus titer in the corneal tissue of infected-GSH treated animals with respect to the control group.

REFERENCES

1. Townsend, D.M., Kenneth, D.T., Tapiero, H. (2003). The importance of glutathione in human disease. *Biomedicine and Pharmacotherapy, 57*, 145–155.
2. Peterhans, E. (1997). Oxidants and antioxidants in viral diseases: Disease mechanisms and metabolic regulation. *Journal of Nutrition, 127*, S962–S965.
3. Beck, M.A., Handy, J., Levander, O.A. (2000). The role of oxidative stress in viral infections. *Annals of the New York Academy of Science, 917*, 906–912.
4. Kaul, P., Biagioli, M.C., Singh, I., Turner, R.B. (2000). Rhinovirus-induced oxidative stress and interleukin-8 elaboration involves p47-*phox* but is independent of attachment to intercellular adhesion molecule-1 and viral replication. *Journal of Infectious Diseases, 181*, 1885–1890.
5. Eck, H.P., Gmunder, H., Hartmann, M., Petzoldt, D., Daniel, V., Droge, W. (1989). Low concentrations of acid-soluble thiol (cysteine) in the blood plasma of HIV-1-infected patients. *Biological Chemistry Hoppe-Seyler, 370*, 101–108.
6. Buhl, R., Jaffe, H.A., Holroyd, K.J., Wells, F.B., Mastrangeli, A., Saltini, C., Cantin, A.M., Crystal, R.G. (1989). Systemic glutathione deficiency in symptom-free HIV-seropositive individuals. *Lancet, 2*, 1294–1298.
7. Staal, F.J.T., Roederer, M., Herzenberg, L.A., Herzenberg, L.A. (1990). Intracellular thiols regulate activation of nuclear factor kB and transcription of human immunodeficiency virus. *Proceedings of the National Academy of Science USA, 87*, 9943–9947.
8. Herzenberg, L.A., De Rosa, S.C., Dubs, J.G., Roederer, M., Anderson, M.T., Ela, S.W., Deresinski, S.C., Herzenberg, L.A. (1997). Glutathione deficiency is associated with impaired survival in HIV disease. *Proceedings of the National Academy of Sciences USA, 94*, 1967–1972.
9. Banki, K., Hutter, E., Gonchoroff, N.J., Perl, A. (1998). Molecular ordering in HIV-induced apoptosis oxidative stress, activation of caspases, and cell survival are regulated by transaldolase. *Journal of Biological Chemistry, 273*, 11944–11953.
10. Elbim, C., Pillet, S., Prevost, M.H., Preira, A., Girard, P.M., Rogine, N., Matusani, H., Hakim, J., Israel, N., Gougerot-Pocidalo, M.A. (1999). Redox and activation status of monocytes from human immunodeficiency virus-infected patients: Relationship with viral load. *Journal of Virology, 73*, 4561–4566.
11. Barbaro, G., Di Lorenzo, G., Soldini, M., Parrotto, S., Bellomo, G., Belloni, G., Grisorio, B., Barbarini, G. (1996). Hepatic glutathione deficiency in chronic hepatitis C: Quantitative evaluation in patients who are HIV positive and HIV negative and correlations with plasmatic and lymphocytic concentrations and with the activity of the liver disease. *American Journal of Gastroenterology, 91*, 2569–2573.

12. Boya, P., de la Pena, A., Beloqui, O., Larrea, E., Conchillo, M., Castelruiz, Y., Civeira, M.P., Prieto, J. (1999). Antioxidant status and glutathione metabolism in peripheral blood mononuclear cells from patients with chronic hepatitis C. *Journal of Hepatology*, *31*, 808–814.

13. Gong, G., Waris, G., Tanveer, R., Siddiqui, A. (2001). Human hepatitis C virus NS5A protein alters intracellular calcium levels, induces oxidative stress, and activates STAT-3 and NF-kappa B. *Proceedings of the National Academy of Sciences USA*, *98*, 9599–9604.

14. Garaci, E., Palamara, A.T., Di Francesco, P., Favalli, C., Ciriolo, M.R., Rotilio, G. (1992). Glutathione inhibits replication and expression of viral proteins in cultured cells infected with Sendai virus. *Biochemical and Biophysical Research Communications*, *188*, 1090–1096.

15. Palamara, A.T., Perno, C.F., Ciriolo, M.R., Dini, L., Balestra, E., D'Agostini, C., Di Francesco, P., Favalli, C., Rotilio, G., Garaci, E. (1995). Evidence for antiviral activity of glutathione: *In vitro* inhibition of herpes simplex virus type 1 replication. *Antiviral Research*, *27*, 237–253.

16. Mihm, S., Galter, D., Dröge, W. (1995). Modulation of transcription factor NF kappa B activity by intracellular glutathione levels and by variations of the extracellular cysteine supply. *FASEB Journal*, *9*, 246–252.

17. Palamara, A.T., Perno, C.F., Aquaro, S., Buè, M.C., Dini, L., Garaci, E. (1996). Glutathione inhibits HIV replication by acting at late stages of the virus life cycle. *AIDS Research and Human Retroviruses*, *12*, 1537–1541.

18. Garaci, E., Palamara, A.T., Ciriolo, M.R., D'Agostini, C., Abdel-Latif, M.S., Aquaro, S., Lafavia, E., Rotilio, G. (1997). Intracellular GSH content and HIV replication in human macrophages. *Journal of Leukocyte Biology*, *62*, 54–59.

19. Nucci, C., Palamara, A.T., Ciriolo, M.R., Nencioni, L., Savini, P., D'Agostini, C., Rotilio, G., Cerulli, L., Garaci, E. (2000). Imbalance in corneal redox state during herpes simplex virus 1-induced keratitis in rabbits. Effectiveness of exogenous glutathione supply. *Experimental Eye Research*, *70*, 215–220.

20. Choi, J., Liu, R.M., Kundu, R.K., Sangiorgi, F., Wu, W., Maxson, R., Forman, H.J. (2000). Molecular mechanism of decreased glutathione content in human immunodeficiency virus type 1 TAT-transgenic mice. *Journal of Biological Chemistry*, *275*, 3693–3698.

21. Hennet, T., Peterhans, E., Stocker, R. (1992). Alterations in antioxidant defences in lung and liver of mice infected with influenza A virus. *Journal of General Virology*, *73*, 39–46.

22. Mileva, M., Tancheva, L., Bakalova, R., Galabov, A., Savov, V., Ribarov, S. (2000). Effect of vitamin E on lipid peroxidation and liver monooxigenase activity in experimental influenza virus infection. *Toxicology Letters*, *114*, 39–45.

23. Nencioni, L., Iuvara, A., Aquilano, K., Ciriolo, M.R., Cozzolino, F., Rotilio, G., Garaci, E., Palamara, A.T. (2003). Influenza A virus replication is dependent on an antioxidant pathway that involves GSH and Bcl-2. *FASEB Journal*, *17*, 758–760.

24. Cai, J., Chen, Y., Seth, S., Furukawa, S., Compans, R.W., Jones, D.P. (2003). Inhibition of influenza infection by glutathione. *Free Radical Biology and Medicine*, *34*, 928–936.

25. Beck, M.A., Nelson, H.K., Shi, Q., Van Dael, P., Schiffrin, E.J., Blum, S., Barclay, D., Levander, O.A. (2001). Selenium deficiency increases the pathology of an influenza virus infection. *FASEB Journal*, *15*, 1481–1483.

26. Beck, M.A., Handy, J., Levander, O.A. (2004). Host nutritional status: The neglected virulence factor. *Trends in Microbiology, 12*, 417–423.

27. Fraternale, A., Paoletti, M.F., Casabianca, A., Oiry, J., Clayette, P., Vogel, J.U., Cynatl, J., Jr., Palamara, A.T., Sgarbanti, R., Garaci, E., Millo, E., Benfatti, U., Magnani, M. (2006). Antiviral and immunomodulatory properties of new pro-glutathione (GSH) molecules. *Current Medicinal Chemistry, 13*, 1749–1755.

28. Filomeni, G., Rotilio, G., Ciriolo, M.R. (2005). Disulfide relays and phosphorylative cascades: Partners in redox-mediated signaling pathways. *Cell Death and Differentiation, 12*, 1555–1563.

29. Palamara, A.T., Nencioni, L., Aquilano, K., De Chiara, G., Hernandez, L., Cozzolino, F., Ciriolo, M.R., Garaci, E. (2005). Resveratrol inhibits influenza A virus replication in vitro and in vivo. *Journal of Infectious Diseases, 191*, 1719–1729.

30. Ludwig, S., Pleschka, S., Planz, O., Wolff, T. (2006). Ringing the alarm bells: Signaling and apoptosis in influenza virus infected cells. *Cellular Microbiology, 8*, 375–386.

31. Nencioni, L., Sgarbanti, R., De Chiara, G., Garaci, E., Palamara, A.T. (2007). Influenza virus and redox mediated cell signaling: A complex network of virus/host interaction. *New Microbiology, 30*, 367–375.

32. Ciriolo, M.R., Palamara, A.T., Incerpi, S., Lafavia, E., Bué, M.C., De Vito, P., Garaci, E., Rotilio, G. (1997). Loss of GSH, oxidative stress, and decrease of intracellular pH as sequential steps in viral infection. *Journal of Biological Chemistry, 272*, 2700–2708.

33. Mirkovic, N., Voehringer, D.W., Story, M.D., McConkey, D.J., McDonnell, T.J., Meyn, R.E. (1997). Resistance to radiation-induced apoptosis in Bcl-2-expressing cells is reversed by depleting cellular thiols. *Oncogene, 15*, 1461–1470.

34. Meredith, M.J., Cusick, C.L., Soltaninassab, S., Sekhar, K.S., Lu, S., Freeman, M.L. (1998). Expression of Bcl-2 increases intracellular glutathione by inhibiting methionine-dependent GSH efflux. *Biochemical and Biophysical Research Communications, 248*, 458–463.

35. Voehringer, D.W., Meyn, R.E. (2000). Redox aspects of Bcl-2 function. *Antioxidants and Redox Signaling, 2*, 537–550.

36. Lamb, R.A., Krug, R.M. (2001). Orthomyxoviridae: The viruses and their replication. In Fields, B.N., Knipe, D.M., and Howley, P.M., eds., *Virology*, 3rd ed., Vol. 1, pp. 1487–1531. Philadelphia: Lippincott-Raven Publishers.,,

37. Lukacs, N., Thiel, H.J., Mettenleiter, T.C., Rziha, H.J. (1985). Demonstration of three major species of pseudorabies virus glycoproteins and identification of a disulfide-linked glycoprotein complex. *Journal of Virology, 53*, 166–173.

38. Vidal, S., Mottet, G., Kolakofsky, D., Roux, L. (1989). Addition of high-mannose sugars must precede disulfide bond formation for proper folding of Sendai virus glycoproteins. *Journal of Virology, 63*, 892–900.

39. Braakman, I., Helenius, J., Helenius, A. (1992). Role of ATP and disulphide bonds during protein folding in the endoplasmic reticulum. *Nature, 356*, 260–262.

40. Palamara, A.T., Brandi, G., Rossi, L., Millo, E., Benatti, U., Nencioni, L., Iuvara, A., Garaci, E., Magnani, M. (2004). New synthetic glutathione derivatives with increased antiviral activities. *Antiviral Chemistry and Chemotherapy, 15*, 83–91.

41. Schreck, R., Rieber, P., Baeuerle P.A. (1991). Reactive oxygen intermediates as apparently widely used messengers in the activation of the NF-kappa B transcription factor and HIV-1. *EMBO Journal, 10*, 2247–2258.

42. Kanel, G.C., Cassidy, W. (1990). Cocaine-induced liver cell injury: Comparison of morphological features in man and in experimental models. *Hepatology*, *11*, 646–651.

43. Wiener, H.L., Reith, M.E.A. (1990). Differential effects of daily administration of cocaine on hepatic and cerebral glutathione in mice. *Biochemical Pharmacology*, *40*, 1763–1768.

44. Palamara, A.T., Di Francesco, P., Ciriolo, M.R., Buè, C., Lafavia, E., Rotilio, G., Garaci, E. (1996b). Cocaine increases Sendai virus replication in cultured epithelial cells: Critical role of the intracellular redox status. *Biochemical and Biophysical Research Communications*, *228*, 579–585.

45. Macchia, I., Palamara, A.T., Buè, C., Savini, P., Ciriolo, M.R., Gaziano, R., Di Francesco, P. (1999). Increased replication of Sendai virus in morphine-treated epithelial cells: Evidence for the involvement of the intracellular levels of glutathione. *International Journal of Immunopharmacology*, *21*, 185–193.

46. Palamara, A.T., Garaci, E., Rotilio, G., Ciriolo, M.R., Casabianca, A., Fraternale, A., Rossi, L., Schiavano, G.F., Chiarantini, L., Magnani, M. (1996). Inhibition of murine AIDS by reduced glutathione. *AIDS Research and Human Retroviruses*, *12*, 1373–1381.

CHAPTER 21

N-ACETYL CYSTEINE AND CYTOPROTECTIVE EFFECTS AGAINST BRONCHOPULMONARY DAMAGE: FROM IN VITRO STUDIES TO CLINICAL APPLICATION

RICHARD DEKHUIJZEN

21.1 INTRODUCTION

N-acetyl-L-cysteine (NAC) is the *N*-acetyl derivative of the naturally occurring amino acid L-cysteine. The solubility of NAC is higher than that of cysteine both in water and in buffered solutions at different pH values. The acetyl substituted amino group makes the molecule less easily oxidized and more stable in solution than cysteine. NAC has been widely used in clinical practise, administered orally, by nebulisation, and intramuscular (i.m.) and intravenous (i.v.) routes. Its safety is well documented (Table 21.1).

NAC is widely used as a mucolytic agent in the treatment of respiratory tract disorders. Its free sulfydryl group (-SH) interacts with the disulfide bonds of mucoproteins of bronchial mucus, breaking them and thus making mucus more fluid and consequently more easily eliminated by the mucociliary mechanism.

More importantly, NAC can also act as a direct antioxidant agent due to the -SH group. The drug can easily penetrate into the cells where it is deacetylated to L-cysteine, thus supporting the biosynthesis of glutathione (GSH). GSH is a tripeptide composed of L-glutamic acid, L-cysteine, and L-glycine, and is crucial to protect cellular components from damage induced by reactive oxygen species (ROS) and xenobiotics. GSH maintains a reducing environment inside cells and the overall result of enzymatic reactions is the oxidation of glutathione (GSSG). The enzyme GSH reductase then uses NADPH, as a donor of H^+, to reduce GSSG to two

TABLE 21.1   Physical, Chemical and Pharmaceutical Properties of *N*-Acetylcysteine

Int. Non-Proprietary Name (INN):	*N*-acetyl-L-cysteine (NAC)
Other names:	*N*-acetylcysteine, *N*-acetyl-3-mercapto-L-alanine
IUPAC denomination:	*R*-2-acetamido-3-mercapto-propionic acid
Laboratory code:	NAC
Brand name:	Fluimucil®, Lysomucil®, Hidonac®
Molecular formula:	$C_5H_9NO_3S$
Chemical structure:	$HS\text{-}CH_2\text{-}CH\text{-}COOH$ $\mid$ $NH\text{-}COCH_3$
Molecular weight:	163.2
Color:	White
Physical state:	Crystalline powder
Melting point:	106–110°C
Odor:	Slightly sulfurous
Storage:	In well-closed containers kept far from humidity, heat, and light
Solubility:	Highly soluble in water, soluble in alcohol, insoluble in methylene chloride and diethylether

molecules of GSH. GSH is also the substrate for GSH peroxidase, an enzyme that scavenges ROS produced inside cells. However, GSH can also nonenzymatically scavenge free radicals by hydrogen atom transfer. Finally, xenobiotic chemicals (e.g., organic halides, epoxides, and alkenes) are conjugated with GSH through the mediation of the GSH *S*-transferases and excreted as mercapturates from the body.

This chapter focuses on the protective effects of NAC against cytotoxicity. The main focus is on its applicability in respiratory disorders, since the use of NAC as an antioxidant has been studied most widely and applied in chronic obstructive pulmonary disease (COPD) [1] and idiopathic pulmonary fibrosis (IPF) [2]. In addition, information relevant to its activity as an antioxidant agent in other pathological conditions (e.g., IPF, paracetamol intoxication, and nephrotoxicity induced by radiocontrast medium) is presented. In view of its focus on pulmonary disorders, a brief overview of the presence of oxidative stress and it consequences in COPD is presented.

21.2   OXIDATIVE STRESS IN COPD

Several reviews have summarized the available data on the presence (Table 21.2) and consequences (Table 21.3) of oxidative stress in the lungs of healthy smokers and smokers with COPD [3–6]. Cigarette smoke is a major source of oxidants, for example, free radicals, including semiquinone and hydroxyl radicals, nitric oxide, and hydrogen peroxide, in the lungs. Furthermore, cigarette smoke promotes the influx and activation of neutrophils and macrophages. Leukocytes from smokers release more oxidants, such as the superoxide anion and H_2O_2, than leukocytes from nonsmokers [7]. The alveolar macrophages of smokers contain increased amounts

TABLE 21.2   Indices of Increased Oxidative Stress in Chronic Obstructive Pulmonary Disease

Biochemical Marker
Elevated breath hydrogen peroxide and 8-isoprostane levels
Decreased plasma antioxidant capacity
Elevated plasma lipid peroxides (TBARS) levels
Plasma protein sulhydryl oxidation
Increased exhaled carbon monoxide
Release of ROS from peripheral blood neutrophils and alveolar macrophages
Increased urinary isoprostane F2-alpha-IH levels

of iron and release more free iron than those of nonsmokers [8]. The presence of free iron facilitates the generation of very reactive hydroxyl radicals. An important part of the pulmonary antioxidant defense is located in the epithelial lining fluid (ELF). Vitamin C and E levels in ELF are depleted in smokers, but GSH levels are increased [7, 9]. These effects are dependent on the time course of exposure to tobacco smoke. Acute exposure causes marked depletion of antioxidants in plasma, intracellular GSH in erythrocytes, and GSH in ELF [1].

Oxidative stress may cause alterations in essential components of the lung, contributing to pathological abnormalities and functional changes (Table 21.2). Increased amounts of ROS have been shown to reduce the synthesis of elastin and collagen [10]. Fragmentation of these major constituents of the lung skeleton may also occur. In addition, ROS may affect the structure of components of the extracellular matrix, such as hyaluronate [11]. Depolymerization of the proteoglycans in the lung

TABLE 21.3   Alterations in Components of the Lung Caused by Oxidative Stress

Airway wall	Contraction of airway smooth muscle
	Impairment of β-adrenoceptor function
	Stimulation of airway secretion
	Pulmonary vascular smooth muscle relaxation or contraction
	Activation of mast cells
Alveolar epithelial cell layer	>Permeability by detachment
	<Adherence
	>Cell lysis
Lung matrix	<Elastin synthesis and fragmentation
	<Collagen synthesis and fragmentation
	Depolymerization of proteoglycans
Antiproteases	Inactivation of α-1-proteinase inhibitor
	Inactivation of secretory leukoprotease inhibitor
Pulmonary microcirculation	>Permeability
	(polymorphonuclear neutrophil) PMN sequestration
	>PMN adhesion to endothelium of arterioles and venules
Transcription factors	Switch-on of genes for TNF-α, interleukin-8, other inflammatory proteins

reduces the viscosity of the extracellular matrix. Oxidative stress may also initiate or amplify alterations in the airway wall. Lipid peroxidation may initiate the release of arachidonic acid from membrane phospholipids, leading to release of prostaglandins and leukotrienes. Increased levels of ROS may also increase interleukine (IL)-1 and -8 production in several cell systems [12, 13]. Other changes include changes in protein structure, leading to altered antigenicity and thus immune responses, contraction of smooth muscle, impairment of beta-adrenoceptor function, stimulation of airway secretion, pulmonary vascular smooth muscle relaxation or contraction, and activation of mast cells [11]. Antiproteases such as alpha-1-proteinase inhibitor (a1-PI) and secretory leukoprotease inhibitor may be inactivated by ROS [14]. In particular, oxidation of the active site of a1-PI, the so-called methionine residue, reduces the ability of a1-PI to inactivate neutrophil elastase [15].

Changes in the alveolar epithelial cell layer occur both as a direct result of inhaled ROS and through the abovementioned alterations [16]. The permeability of this part of the lung is increased by detachment of the cellular layer, reduced adherence of cells, and increased cell lysis. Sequestration of neutrophils, initiated by inhaled tobacco smoke, may occur in the lung microcirculation [17]. Both a reduction in the deformability of neutrophils and an increase in neutrophil adhesion to the vascular endothelium, due to increased levels of adhesion molecules, are involved in this pulmonary sequestration. The increased numbers and prolonged presence of these inflammatory cells contributes to the cycle of locally increased ROS production, attraction of new inflammatory cells, etc.

Finally, oxidative stress activates the transcription factor nuclear factor kappa B (NF-κB), which switches on the genes for tumor necrosis factor (TNF)-α, IL-8, and other inflammatory proteins, enhancing inflammation [6, 18]. Taken together, these data strongly suggest that oxidative stress is an important pathogenetic factor in the alterations in the lungs of patients with COPD.

21.3   PHARMACOLOGY OF *N*-ACETYLCYSTEINE

NAC exhibits direct and indirect antioxidant properties. Its free thiol group is capable of interacting with the electrophilic groups of ROS [19, 20]. This interaction with ROS leads to intermediate formation of NAC thiol, with NAC disulfide as a major end product [21]. In addition, NAC exerts an indirect antioxidant effect related to its role as a GSH precursor. GSH is a tripeptide made up of glutamic acid, cysteine, and glycine. It serves as a central factor in protecting against internal toxic agents (such as cellular aerobic respiration and metabolism of phagocytes) and external agents (such as NO, sulfur oxide, and other components of cigarette smoke, and pollution). The sulfydryl group of cysteine neutralizes these agents. Maintaining adequate intracellular levels of GSH is essential to overcoming the harmful effects of toxic agents. GSH synthesis takes place mainly in the liver (which acts as a reservoir) and the lungs. Synthesis takes place in the cellular cytoplasm in two separate enzymatic stages. In the first, the amino acids glutamic acid and cysteine are combined by c-glutamylcysteine synthetase, and, in the second, GSH synthetase adds glycine to the dipeptide c-glutamylcysteine to form GSH. In vitro, NAC acts as a precursor of GSH as it can penetrate cells easily and is subsequently deacylated to form cysteine [19]. The availability of amino acids for GSH synthesis is a fundamental factor in its regulation. Cellular levels of glutamic acid and glycine, but not cysteine, are plentiful. Consequently, GSH synthesis depends on the availability of cysteine. In the case of (relative) depletion of GSH levels or increased demand, GSH levels may be increased by delivering additional cysteine via NAC. However, it is impossible to administer the active form of cysteine, L-cysteine, because of low intestinal absorption, poor water solubility, and rapid hepatic metabolism. NAC, with the acetyl radical linked to amine function, eliminates these disadvantages. The required quantity of cysteine may thus be administered to maintain adequate levels of GSH in the lungs. Other cysteine derivatives, in which the sulfydryl group is blocked (carboxymethylcysteine), do not have this precursor action.

NAC is rapidly absorbed after oral administration in both animals and humans [22–24]. Following a single oral dose of 200 to 600 mg NAC, peak plasma concentrations of 2 to 17 µM can be achieved approximately one hour after drug intake. Subsequently, the plasma concentrations decrease with an apparent half-life of approximately one to six hours. After i.v. administration of 600 to 18,000 mg NAC, the elimination half-life from plasma is two to six hours. The pharmacokinetics of free and total NAC appeared to be dose independent up to a dose of 4 g. Protein binding of NAC is approximately 50% at 4 hours, and approximately 20% at 12 hours after drug administration. The absolute bioavailability of oral NAC is 4% and 9% for the free and total forms, respectively. Approximately 70% of total body clearance is nonrenal. After oral administration of ^{35}S-NAC, radioactivity was rapidly absorbed. At least 13% to 38% of the radioactive dose was absorbed and recovered in urine. Radioactivity was found in the lung in the free form for at least five hours at concentrations that were comparable to those found in plasma. The presence of radioactivity in the bronchial secretion indicates that the drug and/or its metabolites pass into the mucus.

NAC is effectively metabolized in vitro to cysteine by the cytosolic fraction obtained from human liver homogenates but also in human plasma and buffer (containing cystine), indicating that the enzymatic deacetylation is not the only mechanism by which cysteine is released from NAC; the other mechanism acts by reduction of cystine by NAC with formation of mixed disulfides of NAC and cysteine and release of a molecule of cysteine. The pharmacokinetics of intravenous NAC is not different in subjects treated for paracetamol overdosing with or without liver damage, indicating that the elimination of NAC is not impaired by severe liver damage [25].

NAC cannot be detected in plasma or bronchoalveolar lavage fluid (BALF) following oral administration for 5 to 14 days [26, 27]. In contrast, cysteine and GSH levels were increased transiently in plasma and lung after oral administration of 600 mg NAC once daily [26, 27]. In patients with COPD, however, plasma concentrations of GSH were unchanged after this dose of NAC, whereas 600 mg three times daily increased plasma GSH levels [28]. With this higher dose, administered for five days to patients who underwent lung resection surgery ($n = 11$), cysteine and GSH levels were increased by $\sim$50% compared to untreated patients ($n = 11$). This difference was, however, not significant, which was probably due to the high variation in concentrations of cysteine and GSH. Nevertheless, the data suggests that there is a transient dose-dependent effect of NAC on lung cysteine and GSH levels.

21.4   PULMONARY ANTIOXIDANT AND ANTI-INFLAMMATORY EFFECTS

The efficacy of NAC as a precursor in GSH synthesis has been studied in isolated mouse lungs [19]. Cigarette smoke administered directly to the lung through the trachea caused a dose-dependent reduction in total pulmonary GSH. Administering NAC together with cigarette smoke prevented the loss of pulmonary GSH and abolished the effects of cigarette smoke. NAC reduced H_2O_2-induced damage to epithelial cells in vitro and NF-κB activation in some cells [29]. In addition, NAC treatment reduced cigarette smoke-induced abnormalities in polymorphonuclear neutrophils (PMNs), alveolar macrophages, fibroblasts, and epithelial cells in vitro [30–34]. Treatment with NAC also attenuated rat secretory cell hyperplasia induced by tobacco smoke [35] and prevented hypochlorous acid-mediated inactivation of a1-PI in vitro [36]. In a rat model of cigarette smoke-induced alterations in small airways, NAC prevented thickening of the airway wall and improved distribution of ventilation [37].

In addition to its effects on PMNs, NAC also influences the morphology and markers of oxidative stress in red blood cells (RBCs). An increased percentage of RBCs in COPD patients is morphologically damaged, with high concentrations of H_2O_2 and lowered levels of thiols [38]. These alterations were correlated with reduced oxygen exchange [39]. Treatment of COPD patients with 1.2 or 1.8 g/day NAC for two months improved RBC shape, reduced H_2O_2 concentrations by 38% to 54% and increased thiol levels by 50% to 68% [40].

Treatment with NAC may alter lung oxidant-antioxidant imbalance. NAC (600 mg/day) given orally increased lung lavage GSH levels, reduced O_2^- production by alveolar macrophages and decreased BALF PMN chemiluminescence in vitro [27, 32, 41]. In addition, 600 mg/day NAC in COPD patients reduced sputum eosinophil cationic protein concentrations and the adhesion of PMNs [42]. In vitro, NAC reduced adhesion of *Haemophilus influenzae* and *Streptococcus pneumoniae* to oropharyngeal epithelial cells [43].

21.4.1   Effects on Cigarette Smoke-Induced Changes

Three studies have investigated the effects of 600 mg/day NAC given orally on parameters of inflammation in the BALF of "healthy" smokers [32, 44, 45]. NAC resulted in a tendency towards normalization of the cell composition, with an increase in lymphocyte concentration ($p < 0.05$) [32]. In addition, improvements were observed in the phagocytic activity of alveolar macrophages, and an increase in secretion of leukotriene B4 ($p < 0.05$), which shows a chemotactic activity that represents an important defense mechanism against aggressive agents. In addition, NAC reduced the stimulated production of O_2^- (from $p < 0.01$ to $p < 0.05$, depending on the type of stimulus) [44]. Finally, a reduction in the levels of various markers of inflammatory activity, such as eosinophil cationic protein, lactoferrin, and antichymotrypsin ($p < 0.05$), was observed after administration of NAC [45].

21.4.2 Effects on Elastase Activity

Treatment with NAC resulted in a considerable reduction in elastase activity, in both the bronchoalveolar cavity and plasma, related to its property of scavenging HOCl [20].

21.4.3 Modulatory Effect on Genes

Redox signaling forms part of the fundamental mechanisms of inflammation, such as cytokine induction, proliferation, apoptosis, and gene regulation for cell protection. Oxidants act as mediators of signal transduction, for example, activation of NF-κB and activation protein-1. NAC has been shown to inhibit activation of NF-κB, which controls the cellular genes for intracellular adhesion molecules in intact cells [29]. In addition, NAC has been shown to inhibit the expression of vascular cell adhesion molecule-1 in human endothelial cells [46].

21.4.4 Effects on Oxidative Stress Induced by Viruses

Oxidant production in respiratory cells rises when they become infected with pathogenic viruses, and the oxidative stress is accompanied by increased production of a variety of inflammatory mediators. NAC has been shown to play a protective role in increasing the resistance of mice to influenza virus [47]. Influenza virus increased the production of ROS in epithelial cells and activated NF-κB transcription factor [48]. Pretreatment with NAC attenuated virus-induced NF-κB and IL-8 release. Mice infected intranasally with influenza virus APR/8 showed high BALF levels of xanthine oxidase, TNF-α, and IL-6 as early as 3 days after infection [49]. Xanthine oxidase levels were also elevated in serum and lung tissue. Administration orally of 1 g/kg body weight/day NAC significantly reduced the mortality rate of the infected mice ($p < 0.005$). Rhinoviruses also stimulated increased production of H_2O_2 and oxidative stress of human respiratory epithelial cells [50]. Oxidative stress, in turn, caused activation of NF-κB and release of IL-8, and this effect was blocked by NAC in a dose-dependent manner.

21.4.5 Effect on Exhaled Biomarkers of Oxidative Stress

Increased levels of H_2O_2 in exhaled breath condensate (EBC) have been shown in stable COPD patients, with a further increase during exacerbations [51]. Treatment with 600 mg NAC once daily for 12 months reduced the concentration of H_2O_2 in EBC compared to placebo in stable COPD patients [52]. This effect was observed in the second six months of the treatment period. A higher dose of NAC (1.2 g once daily) reduced the concentration of H_2O_2 in EBC within a period of 30 days, suggesting that there is a dose-dependent effect on this marker of oxidative stress [53].

21.4.6   Mucolytic Effects

In addition to these antioxidant actions, NAC exhibits mucolytic properties by destroying the disulfide bridges of mucoprotein macromolecules after inhalation. This pharmacological action is due to the presence of a free sulfydryl group in the NAC molecule [54, 55]. Mucus viscosity is reduced in vitro in human tracheobronchial secretions [56]. NAC also decreased the viscosity of canine tracheal mucus, leading to improved mucociliary transport [57]. In an animal model of chronic bronchitis, oral NAC inhibited smoke-induced goblet cell hyperplasia [58] and associated mucus hypersecretion [59]. In addition, NAC reduced the time to recovery of goblet cell numbers after smoking cessation [60].

21.5   NONPULMONARY EFFECTS

21.5.1   Prevention of Kidney Damage

The protection of renal tissue against oxidative and hypoxic damage, as well as radio contrast medium-induced damage, was tested in vitro using isolated mouse renal tubule segments and a human tubular cell line. In this test a protection against radio contrast medium-induced and oxidative damage was seen. In vivo the protection against radio contrast medium-induced renal tubule vacuolization by NAC was tested in rats, but no protection was found. In contrast in another study in rats the hystologically visible renal tubular lesions caused by the administration of radio contrast medium were significantly improved by NAC.

21.5.2   Antidotic/Cytoprotective Activities

When administered at high doses, NAC is a potent antidote to prevent hepatotoxicity induced by paracetamol, since it replenishes the GSH supplies exhausted by the formation of intermediate reactive products. This effect was demonstrated both in animals and in humans.

NAC improved post-transplant survival in pigs, in spite of the warm liver ischemia [61].

A cytoprotective effect of NAC was observed in an experimental model of myocardial ischemia [62]. Pretreatment with NAC limited in a dose-dependent way the reduction of GSH and protein sulfydryl groups and eliminated the accumulation of GSSG in the heart of rabbits after 60 min of ischemia. The integrity of the intracellular thiol pool is essential for cell protection against exogenous and endogenous damaging agents. In dogs with experimental myocardial infarct, NAC reduces the extent of necrosis and the incidence of arrhythmias [63].

NAC has both growth-promoting and antiapoptotic activities. As recently reviewed by Sadowska et al. [64], NAC blocks lipopolysaccharides (LPS)-induced apoptosis of endothelial cells [65] and TNF-α- and thrombin-induced neuronal cell death at 0.5 mM [66]. In addition, NAC prevented the cytotoxic effects of agents like paraquat [67], cadmium [68], and cisplatin [69]. At high concentrations, NAC has cytotoxic effects that are cell-type specific. At concentrations of 30 mM, NAC was not cytotoxic to Kupffer cells [70]. The same concentration prevented WISH cells from cadmium-induced cytotoxicity [68]. Similarly, NAC at concentrations of 5 to 40 mM did not affect cell viability in 3T3 fibroblast cultures where NAC was used to inhibit paraquat-induced ROS production [67]. Moreover, concentration of 15 mM did not affect the viability of human fetal membranes [71].

In endothelial cells the effects of NAC are divergent. In porcine aortic endothelial cells viability was decreased by 5 mM NAC [72], while no adverse effects were reported for 20 mM NAC in human dermal microvascular cells [73] or at concentrations of 7.5 to 30 mM on the ECV-304 cell line [74]. Moreover, the viability of aortic endothelial cells was not affected at concentrations as high as 50 mM NAC [75]. Epithelial cells remained unaffected by concentrations of NAC up to 10 mM [76]. In contrast, NAC exerted toxic effects at concentrations ≥ 30 mM in vascular smooth muscle cells, monocytes, and neutrophils [77–80]. These reports are in line with recent observations that the viability of human neutrophils was decreased by concentration ≥ 30 mM NAC [81]. In in vivo studies high concentrations of NAC (950 mg/kg for 48 h) administered to rats before endotoxin challenge resulted in a higher mortality rate than after endotoxin alone, while low concentrations (275 mg/kg) had a beneficial influence on survival. On the other hand, NAC did not have any direct effect on survival when administered in those high dosages in the absence of endotoxin [82].

21.5.3 Effects on Immunological Parameters

GSH is required for immune function and particularly in T cell proliferation and activation [83]. Reduced levels of serum cysteine and intracellular GSH in peripheral blood mononuclear cells (PBMC) have been found in subjects with HIV infection [83]. In vitro studies using blood from HIV-infected patients showed that NAC at a concentration of 10^{-5} M significantly enhanced formation of T cell colony-forming cells (T-CFC), partly through its action on GSH levels [84].

21.5.4 Effects on Tumor Necrosis Factor-Alpha (TNF-α)

NAC (0.5 to 1 g/kg p.o.) significantly inhibited the increase of TNF-α plasma levels assayed 1 hour after LPS administration in mice. Decreased plasma TNF-α levels in NAC-pretreated mice were associated with protective effect of NAC on LPS toxicity (lethality and hepatotoxicity) [85].

21.5.5 Antiviral Activity

In vitro studies demonstrated that 30 mM NAC reduces HIV replication in infected MOLT (acute lymphoblastic leukaemia cell line, derived from human peripheral blood) and PBMC. HIV replication was measured by p24 antigen levels in response to phorbol 12-myristate 13-acetate (PMA) and TNF-α. Pretreatment of chronically infected monocytic U1 cells with NAC also suppressed HIV expression mediated by TNF, PMA, and IL-6, with a dose-dependent response [86].

The stimulation of HIV-1 replication by TNF-α or PMA resulted in a decrease of intracellular GSH and blocked the PMA- or GSH TNF-α-induced stimulation of HIV (measured either as transcription of the reporter gene lacZ directed by the HIV promoter or as replication of HIV in acutely infected human PBMC). These findings implicate GSH in the regulation of HIV expression and in the control of NF-κB activity. At high concentrations, NAC antagonized the PMA- and TNF-α-induced stimulation of the HIV long terminal repeat (LTR)-directed gene expression in a 293.27.2 cell line clone [87].

The effect of NAC has been investigated in a model of influenza infection in mice [88]. In animals treated with the drug at a dose of 1000 mg/kg given from one day before infection to day 8 post-infection, a reduction of mortality was observed, for example, 8% survival in the control group versus 45% in the NAC group. In a second study NAC at a dose of 1000 mg/kg was given with a different therapeutic schedule, that is, starting four hours after infection until day 4 after infection, to mice intranasally infected with influenza virus APR/8. The endpoint was 14 days survival. In this study NAC was given also associated to ribavirin (100 mg/kg i.p.). With this schedule survival in infected animals (17%) was not significantly changed by NAC (25%). Survival increased to 58% with ribavirin and to 92% with the combined treatment ribavirin + NAC. Mean survival time (days) was: control 10, NAC 9, ribavirin 21, ribavirin + NAC 108. The data suggests that the antioxidant therapy with NAC can improve survival and the combination therapy can also improve the therapeutic efficacy of ribavirin.

21.5.6 Chemoprevention

NAC has been shown to have chemopreventive effects in experimental systems; this effect is thought to be related to its action as a precursor of GSH, an intracellular scavenger of free radicals and electrophil metabolites of carcinogens. In addition, NAC proved to be effective in preventing hemorrhagic cystitis caused by cyclophosphamide and isofosfamide administration [89, 90].

21.6 CLINICAL EFFICACY OF *N*-ACETYLCYSTEINE IN COPD

The clinical efficacy of NAC has been investigated in a number of both open and double-blind studies of patients with chronic bronchitis, with and without COPD. The effects on symptoms, viral and bacterial infections, number and severity of exacerbations, and lung function decline are discussed separately.

21.6.1 Clinical Symptoms

An open clinical trial including 1392 patients demonstrated the efficacy of NAC at a dose of 600 mg/day in reducing the viscosity of expectorations, promoting expectoration, and reducing the severity of cough [91]. After two months of treatment with NAC, the viscosity of expectorations improved in 80% of cases, the nature of the expectorations improved in 59%, difficulty in expectorating improved in 74%, and the severity of cough improved in 71%. Improvement in clinical symptoms as a result of treatment with NAC has been shown in a placebo-controlled trial with 744 patients [92]. The results confirmed the efficacy of NAC regarding the parameters related to bronchial hypersecretion.

21.6.2 Bronchial Bacterial Colonization

In an open cross-sectional study performed in 22 smokers with no chronic bronchitis, 19 smokers with chronic bronchitis, with or without airway obstruction, and 14 healthy nonsmokers, the bacterial flora and effect of NAC on bacterial numbers were investigated [93]. The number of bacterial colonies was highest in smokers with chronic bronchitis. In addition, the number of intrabronchial bacteria was significantly lower in patients treated with NAC compared to other patients. This effect was more obvious in patients with chronic obstructive bronchitis.

21.6.3 *N*-Acetylcysteine and Viruses

The effects of NAC on influenza and influenza-like episodes have been studied in 262 patients suffering from nonrespiratory chronic degenerative diseases [94]. Compared to placebo, NAC, 600 mg twice daily for six months, resulted in a significant decrease in both the frequency and severity of influenza-like episodes. Local and systemic symptoms were also significantly reduced in the group receiving NAC. Although seroconversion towards influenza virus was similar in the two groups, only 25% of virus-infected subjects treated with NAC developed the symptomatic form of the condition compared with 79% of the placebo group.

21.6.4 Lung Function Decline

In an open observational survey in Sweden, the decline in forced expiratory volume (FEV1) in COPD patients who took NAC for two years was less than that in a reference group receiving usual care [95]. This favorable effect was particularly apparent in COPD patients older than 50 years (annual decline in FEV1 of 30 mL) compared to the reference group (annual decline in FEV1 of 54 mL). After five years, the reduction in FEV1 in the NAC group was less than that in the reference group (B. Lundback, Unit for Lung and Allergy Research, National Institute of Environmental Medicine, Karolinska Institutet, Stockholm, Sweden, personal communication).

Recently, the Bronchitis Randomized on NAC Cost-Utility Study (BRONCUS) trial was conducted, testing the hypothesis that treatment with NAC would reduce the rate of lung function decline, reduce yearly exacerbation rate, and improve outcome variables [96]. Patients were recruited from 50 different centers in 10 European countries. Patients were 62 ± 8 years old and consisted of 239 (48%) current smokers. Patients allocated to NAC treatment ($n = 256$) had on the average 2.4 ± 0.7 exacerbations per year during the last two years; patients allocated to placebo ($n = 267$) had on the average 2.5 ± 0.9 exacerbations per year in the last two years. Predicted FEV1 was on average 57% ± 9% in both groups, and the reversibility after 400 μg of Salbutamol averaged 4% ± 4% of predicted values in both groups. Patients were treated for three years and the following endpoints were considered: decline in FEV1 and exacerbation rate as primary outcome variables, quality of life and cost utility as secondary outcome variables. In the NAC group 186 patients completed the treatment and 168 in the placebo group. Compliance with treatment was a mean of 94% of prescribed tablets in the NAC group and 92% for placebo. Analysis was by intention to treat.

The rate of decline in FEV1 or vital capacity (VC) was not different in the 256 patients in the NAC group and the 267 patients in the placebo group. Secondary analysis in patients completing the trial showed that after three years, functional residual capacity (FRC) was decreased (-0.374 L) in the NAC group, while it was slightly increased ($+0.008$ L) in the placebo group ($p = 0.008$).

21.6.5 Exacerbations

In a recent systematic review by Stey et al. [97], data on prevention of exacerbation, improvement of symptoms, and adverse effects were extracted from original reports. The relative benefit and number needed to treat were calculated for both individual trials and the combined data. Of the 39 trials retrieved, 11 (2011 patients analyzed), published between 1976 and 1994, were regarded as relevant and valid according to preset criteria. Except for one study, these were placebo-controlled, randomized trials. In nine of the studies, 351 of 723 (48.5%) patients receiving NAC showed no exacerbation compared with 229 of 733 (31.2%) patients receiving placebo (relative benefit 1.56 [95% confidence interval (CI) 1.37–1.77], number needed to treat 5.8 [95% CI 4.5–8.1]). There was no evidence of any effect of study period (12 to 24 weeks) or cumulative dose of NAC on efficacy. In five of the trials, 286 of 466 (61.4%) patients receiving NAC reported improvement of their symptoms compared with 160 of 462 (34.6%) patients receiving placebo (relative benefit 1.78 [95% CI 1.54–2.05], number needed to treat 3.7 [95% CI 3.0–4.9]). These findings are in line with the outcomes of two previous meta-analyses using less precise selection of these studies [98, 99], and confirm that NAC has a clinically significant effect on the number and impact of exacerbations. Again, it should be stressed that the patients included in these studies were not characterized in as detailed a fashion as would currently be demanded according to international guidelines.

In the abovementioned BRONCUS trial, the yearly exacerbation rate was not influenced by NAC, but the hazard ratio for an exacerbation decreased significantly by 22% in patients not taking inhaled corticosteroids treated with NAC ($p = 0.040$) [96].

It may be questioned if NAC 600 mg once daily is the right dose for an optimal effect in patients with COPD. The abovementioned studies on exhaled biomarkers indicate that NAC in a dose of 1200 mg daily is superior in reducing oxidative stress, measured by the concentration of exhaled H_2O_2. A recent study compared

NAC 1200 mg daily, 600 mg daily, and placebo on markers of systemic inflammation and symptoms in patients with COPD GOLD II-III [100]. NAC 1200 mg daily significantly reduced C-reactive protein (CRP) and IL-8 levels compared to NAC 600 mg daily and placebo. Besides, both dosages were well tolerated.

21.6.6   Side Effects

With NAC, 68 of 666 (10.2%) patients reported gastrointestinal adverse effects compared to 73 of 671 (10.9%) taking placebo [97]. With NAC, 79 of 1207 (6.5%) patients withdrew from the study due to adverse effects, compared to 87 of 1234 (7.1%) receiving placebo.

21.7   IDIOPATHIC PULMONARY FIBROSIS

Idiopathic pulmonary fibrosis (IPF) is a chronic progressive interstitial pneumonia and an oxidant-antioxidant imbalance is believed to be of key importance in the disease process. A multinational, double-blind, randomized parallel group trial (IFIGENIA-Idiopathic Pulmonary Fibrosis International Group Exploring N-Acetylcysteine I Annual) was conducted to test the hypothesis that a high dose of NAC administered over a period of one year, in addition to prednisone and azathioprine, would slow the functional deterioration in patients with IPF [2]. A total of 182 patients were randomly assigned to treatment (92 to NAC and 90 to placebo); 155 out of 182 (80 assigned to NAC and 75 to placebo) had usual interstitial pneumonia as confirmed by high resolution computed tomography and histological findings.

The 80 patients of the NAC group were aged 62 ± 9 years and the 75 of the placebo group 64 ± 9 years. The treatment consisted of 600 mg NAC three times a day or placebo, for one year. The patients also received prednisone and azathioprine. In the NAC group 57 patients (71%) and 51 of the placebo group (68%) completed one year of treatment. The primary endpoints were changes between baseline and months 12 in vital capacity and in single breath carbon monoxide diffusing capacity (DLCO). NAC slowed the deterioration of vital capacity and DLCO. At 12 months the absolute difference in the change from baseline between NAC and placebo were 0.18 L (95% CI, 0.03–0.32), or a relative difference of 9%, for vital capacity ($p = 0.02$), and 0.75 mmol per minute per kilopascal (95% CI, 0.27–1.23), or 24 %, for DCLO ($p = 0.003$). Mortality during the study was 9% among patients taking NAC and 11% among those taking placebo ($p = 0.69$). There were no significant differences in the type or severity of adverse events between patients of the NAC group and those taking placebo, except for a significantly lower rate of myelotoxic effects in the group taking NAC ($p = 0.03$).

This study showed that NAC at a dose of 600 mg three times daily added to prednisone and azathioprine in patients with IPF preserved vital capacity and DCLO better than standard therapy alone.

21.8   OTHER DISORDERS

21.8.1   Paracetamol Overdosing

Paracetamol (acetaminophen) is an analgesic-antipyretic drug that is metabolized in the liver through the cytochrome P-450 system. Its highly reactive metabolite, N-acetyl-p-benzoquinonimine, is normally neutralized by GSH. However, the increased production of this intermediate following paracetamol overdosing can deplete GSH stores, allowing the metabolite to react with and destroy hepatocytes and other cells. NAC acts as an antidote to paracetamol toxicity by enhancing GSH stores and inducing nontoxic sulfate conjugation. In addition NAC, acting as antioxidant, maintains the hepatic microcirculation by inhibiting neutrophil accumulation and plugging [101] and is effective also against the complications of severe intoxications, such as renal failure, hepatic failure [102], metabolic acidosis, and encephalopathy.

The favorable effects of NAC on organ function and survival have also been explained by the improvement in the cardiac function, tissue oxygen delivery, and oxygen consumption in patients with fulminant hepatic failure induced by paracetamol overdosing [103]. Standard treatment of paracetamol overdosing intoxication consists of 300 mg/kg administered intravenously over a 20-hour period in Europe and Canada and of 1330 mg/kg given orally over a 72-hour period in the United States. As documented in a wide retrospective analysis on 2540 subjects, NAC (140 mg/kg orally followed by 70 mg/kg every four hours for an additional 17 doses) has been found to be as effective as the 20 hour intravenous regimen on hepatotoxicity induced by paracetamol metabolism and hepatic failure [104].

21.8.2   Renal Failure and End Stage Renal Disease

Convincing evidence indicates that in uremic patients an overproduction of free oxygen radicals and a profound disturbance in antioxidant defense occur [105], with abnormalities in plasma and intracellular amino acid concentration caused by kidney defective synthesis, degradation, or clearance. In addition hyperhomocysteinemia, present in uremic patients and in hemodialysis patients [106], mainly due to a reduction of plasma homocysteine clearance, is considered a risk factor for atherosclerosis; hyperhomocysteinemia may also predispose to cardiovascular diseases by altering the vascular endothelium through a mechanism that involves generation of reactive oxygen species [107].

These data underline the importance of the antioxidant therapy in uremic and hemodialysis patients. The oxidative stress in chronic renal failure and hemodialysis patients increases RBC membrane lipid peroxidation, an important mechanism causing hemolysis and shortened RBC survival. Reduced glutathione has been shown to be of importance in the treatment of anemic status in patients suffering from chronic renal failure and undergoing hemodialysis [108]. Furthermore, NAC was effective in reducing the formation of (carboxymethyl)lysine in peritoneal dialysate. A study confirmed NAC and glutathione (among other various chemicals) as new additive to dialysate in order to inhibit the formation of glucose degradation products and advance glycation end products [109].

21.8.3 Kidney Protection from Radio Contrast Medium-Induced Nephrotoxicity

Radio contrast medium-induced nephrotoxicity is an important cause of acute renal failure. This topic is of paramount importance considering that in the presence of risk factors (such as diabetes, preexisting renal dysfunction, dehydration) a radio contrast-induced renal toxicity may be present in a significant percentage of patients; in the absence, however, of such risk factors, nephrotoxicity occurs in less than 10% of patients exposed to this risk. NAC may prevent radio contrast-induced nephropathy by preventing oxidative damage through GSH synthesis and its direct antioxidant activity. In patients with baseline renal insufficiency the prophylactic use of oral NAC significantly reduced the risk of a reduction in renal function induced by radiographic contrast agent [110].

21.8.4 HIV Infection

Based on in vitro studies [111, 112], it has been shown that normal lymphocyte function and viability may depend on the ability of the host to sustain normal levels of intracellular GSH. Intracellular GSH is directly dependent on the level of thiol compounds (cysteine) in the surrounding environment and is inversely affected by the level of extracellular glutamate. Patients with AIDS have been found to have markedly reduced serum thiol concentrations in association with elevated serum glutamate levels. Thus, it has been proposed that restoration towards normal levels of depleted serum thiol levels in patients with AIDS or ARC (AIDS-related complex), could increase lymphocyte intracellular GSH levels and thus lead to improved lymphocyte function. Additionally, NAC has been found to inhibit the stimulation of HIV-1 replication by TNF-α or PMA (phorbol 12-myristate 13-acetate) in acutely infected human PBMC, as determined by the p24 antigen assay [113].

NAC has been evaluated in the treatment of HIV-infected patients [114]. Oral NAC 9.6 g/day was both safe and well tolerated when administered daily for periods up to 12 months. In this study the effect of intravenously administered NAC was associated with substantial toxicity at the two highest doses studied, 100 mg/kg and 250 mg/kg, each given over one hour. These toxicities included features of both anaphylactic and anaphylactoid reactions and were frequently dose limiting. The increase of infusion time from one hour to three to four hours permitted the safe infusion of the same total dose of NAC, suggesting that the reactions are related to peak systemic drug concentrations rather than to total body drug exposure.

21.9 CONCLUSIONS

Oxidative stress is considered to be an important part of the inflammatory response to both environmental and internal signals. Transcription factors such as NF-κB and activation protein 1 are activated by oxidative stress, and, in turn, amplify the inflammatory response to noxious stimuli. In this way, both oxidative stress and inflammation are involved in the complex pathophysiology of COPD, in terms of both pathogenesis and progression of the disease. The benefits of ICS in severe COPD are limited, and no effects have been found in mild and moderate COPD. In vitro and in vivo data show that *N*-acetylcysteine protects the lungs against toxic agents by increasing pulmonary defense mechanisms through its direct antioxidant properties and indirect role as a precursor in glutathioine synthesis. In patients with COPD, treatment with *N*-acetylcysteine at a dose of at least 600 mg once daily reduces the risk of exacerbations and improves symptoms compared to placebo.

REFERENCES

1. Dekhuijzen, P.N.R. (2004). Antioxidant properties of N-acetylcysteine: Their relevance in relation to chronic obstructive pulmonary disease. *European Respiratory Journal, 23,* 629–636.

2. Demedts, M., Behr, J., Buhl, R., Costabel, U., Dekhuijzen, P.N.R., Jansen, H.M., MacNee, W., Thomeer, M., Wallaert, B., Laurent, F., Nicholson, A.G., Verbeken, E.K., Verschakelen, J., Flower, C.D., Capron, F., Petruzzelli, S., De Vuyst, P., van den Bosch, J.M., Rodriguez-Becerra, E., Corvasce, G., Lankhorst, I., Sardina, M., Montanari, M. IFIGENIA Study Group. (2005). IFIGENIA Study Group. High-dose acetylcysteine in idiopathic pulmonary fibrosis. *New England Journal of Medicine, 353,* 2229–2242.

3. Repine, J.E., Lankhorst, I.L.M., Debacker, W.A., Oxidative Stress Study Group (1997). Oxidative stress in chronic obstructive pulmonary disease. *American Journal of Respiratory and Critical Care Medicine, 156,* 341–357.

4. Rahman, I., MacNee, W. (1999). Lung glutathione and oxidative stress: Implications in cigarette smoke-induced airway disease. *American Journal of Physiology, 27(7),* L1067–L1088.

5. MacNee, W., Rahman, I. (1999). Oxidants and antioxidants as therapeutic targets in chronic obstructive pulmonary disease. *American Journal of Respiratory and Critical Care Medicine, 160,* S58–S65.

6. Barnes, P.J. (2000). Chronic obstructive pulmonary disease. *New England Journal of Medicine, 343,* 269–280.

7. Morrison, D., Rahman, I., Lannan, S., MacNee, W. (1999). Epithelial permeability, inflammation, and oxidant stress in the air spaces of smokers. *American Journal of Respiratory and Critical Care Medicine, 159,* 473–479.

8. Mateos, F., Brock, J.H., Perez-Arellano, J.L. (1998). Iron metabolism in the lower respiratory tract. *Thorax, 53,* 594–600.

9. Cantin, A.M., North, S.L., Hubbard, R., Crystal, R.G. (1987). Normal alveolar epithelial lining fluid contains high levels of glutathione. *Journal of Applied Physiology, 63,* 152–157.

10. Laurent, P., Janoff, A., Kagan, H.M. (1983). Cigarette smoke blocks cross-linking of elastin *in vitro. American Review of Respiratory Disease, 127,* 189–192.

11. Warren, J.S., Johnson, K.J., Ward, P.A. (1997). Consequences of oxidant injury. In Crystal, R.G., West, J.B., Weibel, E.R., Barnes, P.J., Eds., *The Lung,* pp. 2279–2288. New York: Scientific Foundations, Raven Press.

12. Ghezzi, P., Dinarello, C.A., Bianchi, M., Rosandich, M.E., Repine, J.E., White, C.W. (1991). Hypoxia increases production of interleukin-1 and tumor necrosis factor by human mononuclear cells. *Cytokine*, *3*, 189–194.

13. Metinko, A.P., Kunkel, S.L., Standiford, T.J., Strieter, R.M. (1992). Anoxia-hyperoxia induces monocyte-derived interleukin-8. *Journal of Clinical Investigation*, *90*, 791–798.

14. Abboud, R.T., Fera, T., Richter, A., Tabona, M.Z., Johal, S. (1985). Acute effect of smoking on the functional activity of a1 protease inhibitor in bronchoalveolar lavage fluid. *American Review of Respiratory Disease*, *131*, 79–85.

15. Maier, K.L., Leuschel, L., Costabel, U. (1992). Increased oxidized methionine residues in BAL fluid proteins in acute or chronic bronchitis. *European Respiratory Journal*, *5*, 651–658.

16. Cotgreave, I.A., Moldeus, P. (1987). Lung protection by thiol containing antioxidants. *Bulletin of European Physiopathological Respiratory*, *23*, 275–277.

17. MacNee, W., Wiggs, B., Belzberg, A.S., Hogg, J.C. (1989). The effect of cigarette smoking on neutrophil kinetics in human lungs. *New England Journal of Medicine*, *321*, 924–928.

18. Rahman, I., MacNee, W. (2000). Oxidative stress and regulation of glutathione in lung inflammation. *European Respiratory Journal*, *16*, 534–554.

19. Moldeus, P., Cotgreave, I.A., Berggren, M. (1986). Lung protection by a thiol-containing antioxidant: *N*-acetylcysteine. *Respiration*, *50*, 31–42.

20. Aruoma, O.I., Halliwell, B., Hoey, B.M., Butler, J. (1989). The antioxidant action of *N*-acetylcysteine: Its reaction with hydrogen peroxide, hydroxyl radical, superoxide, and hypochlorous acid. *Free Radical Biology and Medicine*, *6*, 593–597.

21. Cotgreave, I.A. (1997). *N*-acetylcysteine: Pharmacological considerations and experimental and clinical applications. *Advances in Pharmacology*, *38*, 205–227.

22. Sheffner, A.L., Medler, E.M., Bailey, K.R., Gallo, D.G., Mueller, A.J., Sarett, H.P. (1966). Metabolic studies with acetylcysteine. *Biochemical Pharmacology*, *15*, 1523–1535.

23. Rodenstein, D., DeCoster, A., Gazzaniga, A. (1978). Pharmacokinetics of oral acetylcysteine: Absorption, binding and metabolism in patients with respiratory disorders. *Clinical Pharmacokinetic*, *3*, 247–254.

24. Borgstrom, L., Kagedal, B., Paulsen, O. (1986). Pharmacokinetics of *N*-acetylcysteine in man. *European Journal of Clinical Pharmacology*, *31*, 217–222.

25. Prescott, L.F., Donovan, J.W., Jarvie, D.R., Proudfoot, A.T. (1989). The disposition and kinetics of intravenous *N*-acetylcysteine in patients with paracetamol overdosage. *European Journal of Clinical Pharmacology*, *37*, 501–506.

26. Cotgreave, I.A., Eklund, A., Larsson, K., Moldeus, P. (1987). No penetration of orally administered *N*-acetylcysteine into bronchoalveolar lavage fluid. *European Journal of Respiratory Diseases*, *70*, 73–77.

27. Bridgeman, M.M., Marsden, M., MacNee, W., Flenley, D.C., Ryle, A.P. (1991). Cysteine and glutathione concentrations in plasma and bronchoalveolar lavage fluid after treatment with *N*-acetylcysteine. *Thorax*, *46*, 39–42.

28. Bridgeman, M.M., Marsden, M., Selby, C., Morrison, D., MacNee, W. (1994). Effect of *N*-acetyl cysteine on the concentrations of thiols in plasma, bronchoalveolar lavage fluid, and lung tissue. *Thorax*, *49*, 670–675.

29. Schreck, R., Albermann, K., Baeuerle, P.A. (1992). Nuclear factor κB: An oxidative stress-responsive transcription factor of eukaryotic cells. *Free Radical Research Communications, 17*, 221–237.

30. Bridges, R.B. (1985). Protective action of thiols on neutrophil function. *European Journal of Respiratory Diseases, 66*(Suppl 139), 40–48.

31. Voisin, C., Aerts, C., Wallaert, B. (1987). Prevention of *in vitro* oxidant-mediated alveolar macrophage injury by cellular glutathione and precursors. *Bulletin Européen de Physiopathologie Respiratoire, 23*, 309–313.

32. Linden, M., Wieslander, E., Eklund, A., Larsson, K., Brattsand, R. (1988). Effects of oral N-acetylcysteine on cell content and macrophage function in bronchoalveolar lavage from healthy smokers. *European Respiratory Journal, 1*, 645–650.

33. Moldeus, P., Berggren, M., Graffstrom, R. (1985). N-Acetylcysteine protection against the toxicity of cigarette smoke and cigarette smoke condensates in various tissues and cells *in vitro*. *European Journal of Respiratory Diseases, 66*(Suppl 139), 123–129.

34. Drost, E., Lannan, S., Bridgeman, M.M., Brown, D., Selby, C., Donaldson, K., MacNee, W. (1991). Lack of effect of N-acetylcysteine on the release of oxygen radicals from neutrophils and alveolar macrophages. *European Respiratory Journal, 4*, 723–729.

35. Jeffery, P.K., Rogers, D.F., Ayers, M.M. (1985). Effect of oral acetylcysteine on tobacco smoke-induced secretory cell hyperplasia. *European Journal of Respiratory Disease, 66*(Suppl 139), 117–122.

36. Borregaard, N., Jensen, H.S., Bjerrum, O.W. (1987). Prevention of tissue damage: Inhibition of myeloperoxidase mediated inactivation of a1-proteinase inhibitor by N-acetyl cysteine, glutathione, and methionine. *Agents and Actions, 22*, 255–260.

37. Rubio, M.L., Sanchez-Cifuentes, M.V., Ortega, M., Peces-Barba, G., Escolar, J.D., Verbanck, S., Paiva, M., González Mangado, N. (2000). N-Acetylcysteine prevents cigarette smoke induced small airways alterations in rats. *European Respiratory Journal, 15*, 505–511.

38. Santini, M.T., Straface, E., Cipri, A., Peverini, M., Santulli, M., Malorni, W. (1997). Structural alterations in erythrocytes from patients with chronic obstructive pulmonary disease. *Haemostasis, 27*, 201–210.

39. Cuzzocrea, S., Mazzon, E., Dugo, L., Serraino, I., Ciccolo, A., Centorrino, T., De Sarro, A., Caputi, A.P. (2001). Protective effects of N-acetylcysteine on lung injury and red blood cell modification induced by carrageenan in the rat. *FASEB Journal, 15*, 1187–1200.

40. Straface, E., Matarrese, P., Gambardella, L., Forte, S., Carlone, S., Libianchi, E., Schmid, G., Malorni, W. (2000). N-Acetylcysteine counteracts erythrocyte alterations occurring in chronic obstructive pulmonary disease. *Biochemical and Biophysical Research Communications, 279*, 552–556.

41. Jankowska, R., Passowicz-Muszynska, E., Medrala, W., Banas, T., Marcinkowska, A. (1993). The influence of N-acetylcysteine on chemiluminescence of granulocytes in peripheral blood of patients with chronic bronchitis. *Pneumonologia i Alergologia Polska, 61*, 586–591.

42. De Backer, W., van Overveld, F., Vandekerckhove, K. (1997). Sputum ECP levels in COPD patients decrease after treatment with N-acetylcysteine (NAC). *European Respiratory Journal, 12*, 225s.

43. Riise, G.C., Qvarfordt, I., Larsson, S., Eliasson, V., Andersson, B.A. (2000). Inhibitory effect of *N*-acetylcysteine on adherence of *Streptococcus pneumoniae* and *Haemophilus influenzae* to human oropharyngeal epithelial cells *in vitro*. *Respiration*, *67*, 552–558.

44. Bergstrand, H., Björnson, A., Eklund, A., Hernbrand, R., Larsson, K., Linden, M., Nilsson, A. (1986). Stimuli-induced superoxide radical generation *in vitro* by human alveolar macrophages from smokers: Modulation by *N*-acetylcysteine treatment *in vivo*. *Free Radical Biology and Medicine*, *2*, 119–127.

45. Eklund, A., Eriksson, O., Hakansson, L., Larsson, K., Ohlsson, K., Venge, P., Bergstrand, H., Björnson, A., Brattsand, R., Glennow, C. (1988). Oral *N*-acetylcysteine reduces selected humoral markers of inflammatory cell activity in BAL fluid from healthy smokers: Correlation to effects on cellular variables. *European Respiratory Journal*, *1*, 832–838.

46. Marui, N., Offermann, M.K., Swerlick, R., Kunsch, C., Rosen, C.A., Ahmad, M., Alexander, R.W., Medford, R.M. (1993). Vascular cell adhesion molecule-1 (VCAM-1) gene transcription and expression are regulated through an antioxidant-sensitive mechanism in human vascular endothelial cells. *Journal of Clinical Investigation*, *92*, 1866–1874.

47. Streightoff, F., Redman, C.E., DeLong, D.C. (1966). *In vivo* antiviral chemotherapy. II. Anti-influenza action of compounds affecting mucous secretions. *Antimicrobial Agents and Chemotherapy*, *6*, 503–508.

48. Knobil, K., Choi, A.M., Weigand, G.W., Jacoby, D.B. (1998). Role of oxidants in influenza virus-induced gene expression. *American Journal of Physiology*, *274*, L134–L142.

49. Akaike, T., Ando, M., Oda, T., Doi, T., Ijiri, S., Araki, S., Maeda, H. (1990). Dependence on O^{2-} generation by xanthine oxidase of pathogenesis of influenza virus infection in mice. *Journal of Clinical Investigation*, *85*, 739–745.

50. Biagioli, M.C., Kaul, P., Singh, I., Turner, R.B. (1999). The role of oxidative stress in rhinovirus induced elaboration of IL-8 by respiratory epithelial cells. *Free Radical Biology and Medicine*, *26*, 454–462.

51. Dekhuijzen, P.N.R., Aben, K.K., Dekker, I., Aarts, L.P., Wielders, P.L., van Herwaarden, C.L., Bast, A. (1996). Increased exhalation of hydrogen peroxide in patients with stable and unstable COPD. *American Journal of Respiratory and Critical Care Medicine*, *154*, 813–816.

52. Kasielski, M., Nowak, D. (2001). Long-term administration of *N*-acetylcysteine decreases hydrogen peroxide exhalation in subjects with chronic obstructive pulmonary disease. *Respiratory Medicine*, *95*, 448–456.

53. De Benedetto, F., Aceto, A., Dragani, B., Spacone, A., Formisano, S., Pela, R., Donner, C.F., Sanguinetti, C.M. (2005). Long-term oral N-acetylcysteine reduces exhaled hydrogen peroxide in stable COPD. *Pulmonary Pharmacology Therapeutics*, *18*, 41–47.

54. Braga, P.C., Allegra, L. (1989). *Drugs in Bronchial Mucology*. New York: Raven Press.

55. Nightingale, J.A., Rogers, D.F. (2002). Should drugs affecting mucus properties be used in COPD? Clinical evidence. In Similowski, T., Whitelaw, W.A., Derenne, J.P., Eds., *Clinical Management of Chronic Obstructive Pulmonary Disease*, pp. 405–425. New York: Marcel Dekker.

56. Sheffner, A.L., Medler, E.M., Jacobs, L.W., Sarett, H.P. (1964). The *in vitro* reduction in viscosity of human tracheobronchial secretions by acetylcysteine. *American Review of Respiratory Disease*, *90*, 721–729.

57. Martin, R., Litt, M., Marriott, C. (1980). The effect of mucolytic agents on the rheologic and transport properties of canine tracheal mucus. *American Review of Respiratory Disease, 121*, 495–500.

58. Rogers, D.F., Jeffery, P.K. (1986). Inhibition by oral *N*-acetylcysteine of cigarette smoke-induced "bronchitis" in the rat. *Experimental Lung Research, 10*, 267–283.

59. Rogers, D.F., Turner, N.C., Marriott, C., Jeffery, P.K. (1989). Oral *N*-acetylcysteine or *S*-carboxymethylcysteine inhibit cigarette smoke-induced hypersecretion of mucus in rat larynx and trachea *in situ*. *European Respiratory Journal, 2*, 955–960.

60. Rogers, D.F., Godfrey, R.W., Majumdar, S., Jeffery, P.K. (1988). Oral *N*-acetylcysteine speeds reversal of cigarette smoke-induced mucous cell hyperplasia in the rat. *Experimental Lung Research, 14*, 19–35.

61. Regueira, F.M., Hernández, J.L., Sola, I., Cienfuegos, J.A., Pardo, F., Díez-Caballero, A., Sierra, A., Nwose, E., Espí, A., Baixaúli, J., Rotellar, F. (1997). Ischemic damage prevention by acetylcysteine treatment of the donor before orthotopic liver transplant. *Transplantation Proceedings, 29*, 3347–3349.

62. Ceconi, C., Curello, S., Cargnoni, A., Ferrari, R., Albertini, A., Visioli, O. (1988). The role of glutathione status in the protection against ischemia and reperfusion damage: Effect of N-acetylcysteine. *Journal of Molecular and Cellular Cardiology, 20*, 5–13.

63. Sochman, J., Kolc, J., Vrána, M., Fabián, J. (1990). Cardioprotective effects of N-acetylcysteine: The reduction of the extent of infarction and occurrence of reperfusion arrhythmias in the dog. *International Journal of Cardiology, 28*, 191–196.

64. Sadowska, A.M., Manuel, Y., Keenoy, B., De Backer, W.A. (2007). Antioxidant and anti-inflammatory efficacy of NAC in the treatment of COPD: Discordant in vitro and in vivo dose-effects: A review. *Pulmonary Pharmacology Therapeutics, 20*, 9–22.

65. Abello, P.A., Fidler, S.A., Buchman, T.G. (1994). Thiol reducing agents modulate induced apoptosis in porcine endothelial cells. *Shock, 2*, 79–83.

66. Talley, A.K., Dewhurst, S., Perry, S.W., Dollard, S.C., Gummuluru, S., Fine, S.M., New, D., Epstein, L.G., Gendelman, H.E., Gelbard, H.A. (1995). Tumor necrosis factor alpha-induced apoptosis in human neuronal cells: Protection by the antioxidant N-acetylcysteine and the genes bcl-2 and crmA. *Molecular and Cellular Biology, 15*, 2359–2366.

67. Hong, S.Y., Yang, J.O., Lee, E.Y., Lee, Z.W. (2003). Effects of N-acetyl-L-cysteine and glutathione on antioxidant status of human serum and 3T3 fibroblasts. *Journal of Korean Medical Science, 18*, 649–654.

68. Abe, T., Yamamura, K., Gotoh, S., Kashimura, M., Higashi, K. (1998). Concentration-dependent differential effects of N-acetyl-cysteine on the expression of HSP70 and metallothionein genes induced by cadmium in human amniotic cells. *Biochimica et Biophysica Acta—General Subjects, 1380*, 123–132.

69. Wu, Y.J., Muldoon, L.L., Neuwelt, E.A. (2005). The chemoprotective agent N-acetylcysteine blocks cisplatin-induced apoptosis through caspase signaling pathway. *Journal of Pharmacology and Experimental Therapeutics, 312*, 424–431.

70. Fox, E.S., Brower, J.S., Bellezzo, J.M., Leingang, K.A. (1997). N-Acetylcysteine and alpha-tocopherol reverse the inflammatory response in activated rat Kupffer cells. *Journal of Immunology, 158*, 5418–5423.

71. Lappas, M., Permezel, M., Rice, G.E. (2003). N-Acetylcysteine inhibits phospholipid metabolism, proinflammatory cytokine release, protease activity and nuclear factor-κB deoxyribonucleic acid-binding activity in human fetal membranes in vitro. *Journal of Clinical Endocrinology, 88*, 1723–1729.

72. Tsou, T.C., Yeh, S.C., Tsai, F.Y., Chang, L.W. (2004). The protective role of intracellular GSH status in the arsenite-induced vascular endothelial dysfunction. *Chemical Research in Toxicology, 17,* 208–217.

73. Chan, E.L., Murphy, J.T. (2003). Reactive oxygen species mediate endotoxin-induced human dermal endothelial NF-[κ]B activation. *Journal of Surgery Research, 111,* 120–126.

74. Pajonk, F., Riess, K., Sommer, A., McBride, W.H. (2002). N-acetyl-L-cysteine inhibits 26S proteasome function: Implications for effects on NF-[κ]B activation. *Free Radical Biology and Medicine, 32,* 536–543.

75. Atkins, K.B., Lodhi, I.J., Hurley, L.L., Hinshaw, D.B. (2000). N-Acetylcysteine and endothelial cell injury by sulfur mustard. *Journal of Applied Toxicology, 20*(Suppl 1), S125–S128.

76. Hashimoto, S., Gon, Y., Takeshita, I., Matsumoto, K., Jibiki, I., Takizawa, H., Kudoh, S., Horie, T. (2000). Diesel exhaust particles activate p38 MAP kinase to produce interleukin 8 and RANTES by human bronchial epithelial cells and N-acetylcysteine attenuates p38 MAP kinase activation. *American Journal of Respiratory and Critical Care Medicine, 161,* 280–285.

77. Jiang, B., Haverty, M., Brecher, P. (1999). N-Acetyl-L-cysteine enhances interleukin-1beta-induced nitric oxide synthase expression. *Hypertension, 34,* 574–579.

78. Vulcano, M., Rosa, M.F.A., Breyer, I., Isturiz, M.A. (1998). Hydroxyl radical scavengers inhibit TNF-α production in mononuclear cells but not in polymorphonuclear leukocytes. *International Journal of Immunopharmacology, 20,* 709–722.

79. Peters, M.J., Dixon, G., Kotowicz, K.T., Hatch, D.J., Heyderman, R.S., Klein, N.J. (1999). Circulating platelet–neutrophil complexes represent a subpopulation of activated neutrophils primed for adhesion, phagocytosis and intracellular killing. *British Journal of Haematology, 106,* 391–399.

80. Kharazmi, A., Nielsen, H., Schiotz, P.O. (1988). N-Acetylcysteine inhibits human neutrophil and monocyte chemotaxis and oxidative metabolism. *International Journal of Immunopharmacology, 10,* 39–46.

81. Sadowska, A.M., Manuel-y-Keenoy, B., Vertongen, T., Schippers, G., Radomska-Lesniewska, D., Heytens, E., De Backer, W.A. (2006). Effect of N-acetylcysteine on neutrophil activation markers in healthy volunteers: In vivo and in vitro study. *Pharmacology Research, 53*(3), 216–225.

82. Sprong, R.C., Winkelhuyzen-Janssen, A.M., Aarsman, C.J., van Oirschot, J.F., van der Bruggen, T., van Asbeck, B.S. (1998). Low-dose N-acetylcysteine protects rats against endotoxin-mediated oxidative stress, but high-dose increases mortality. *American Journal of Respiratory and Critical Care Medicine, 157,* 1283–1293.

83. Fidelus, R.K., Tsan, M. (1986). Enhancement of intracellular glutathione promotes lymphocyte activation by mitogen. *Cellular Immunology, 97,* 155–163.

84. Wu, J., Levy, E.M., Black, P.H. (1989). 2-Mercaptoethanol and N-acetylcysteine enhance T-cell colony formation in AIDS and ARC. *Clinical and Experimental Immunology, 77,* 7–10.

85. Peristeris, P., Clark, B., Gatti, S., Faggioni, R., Mantovani, A., Mengotti, M., Orencole, S.F., Sironi, M., Ghezzi, P. (1992). N-Acetylcysteine and glutatione as inhibitors of tumor necrosis factor production. *Cellular Immunology, 140,* 390–399.

86. Staal, F.J.T., Ela, S., Roederer, M. (1992). Glutathione deficiency and human immunodeficiency virus infection. *Lancet, 399,* 909–912.

87. Roederer, M., Syaal, F.J.K., Raju, P.A., Ela, S.W., Herzenberg, L.A. (1990). Cytokine-stimulated human immunodeficiency virus replication is inhibited by N-acetylcysteine. *Proceedings of the National Academy of Sciences USA*, *87*, 4884–4888.

88. NEW: Fluimucil (N-acetyl-L-cysteine). Expert report on the clinical documentation. May 1998. *Zambon, data on file*.

89. Morgan, L., Holdiness, M., Gillen, L. (1983). N-Acetylcysteine: Its availability and interaction with ifosfamide metabolites. *Seminars in Oncology*, *10*, 56–61.

90. Holoye, P.Y., Duelge, J., Hansen, R.M., Ritch, P.S., Anderson, T. (1983). Prophylaxis of ifosfamide toxicity with oral acetylcysteine. *Seminars in Oncology*, *10*, 66–71.

91. Tattersall, A.B., Bridgman, K.M., Huitson, A. (1983). Acetylcysteine (Fabrol) in chronic bronchitis. A study in general practice. *Journal of Internal Medicine Research*, *11*, 279–284.

92. Multicenter Study Group. (1980). Long-term oral acetylcysteine in chronic bronchitis. A double-blind controlled study. *European Journal of Respiratory Diseases*, *61*(Suppl 111), 93–108.

93. Riise, G.C., Larsson, S., Larsson, P., Jeansson, S., Andersson, B.A. (1994). The intrabronchial microbial flora in chronic bronchitis patients: A target for *N*-acetylcysteine therapy? *European Respiratory Journal*, *7*, 94–101.

94. De Flora, S., Grassi, C., Carati, L. (1997). Attenuation of influenza symptomatology and improvement of immunological parameters due to long-term treatment with *N*-acetylcysteine. *European Respiratory Journal*, *10*, 1535–1541.

95. Lundbäck, B., Lindström, M., Andersson, S., Nyström, L., Rosenhall, L., Stjernberg, N. (1992). Possible effect of acetylcysteine on lung function. *European Respiratory Journal*, *5*(Suppl 15), 289s.

96. Decramer, M., Dekhuijzen, P.N., Troosters, T., van Herwaarden, C., Rutten-van Molken, M., van Schayck, C.P., Olivieri, D., Lankhorst, I., Ardia, A. (2001). The Bronchitis Randomized On NAC Cost-Utility Study (BRONCUS): Hypothesis and design. BRONCUS-trial Committee. *European Respiratory Journal*, *17*, 329–336.

97. Stey, C., Steurer, J., Bachmann, S., Medici, T.C., Tramer, M.R. (2000). The effect of oral *N*-acetylcysteine in chronic bronchitis: A quantitative systematic review. *European Respiratory Journal*, *16*, 253–262.

98. Grandjean, E.M., Berthet, P., Ruffmann, R., Leuenberger, P. (2000). Efficacy of oral long-term *N*-acetylcysteine in chronic bronchopulmonary disease: A meta-analysis of published double-blind, placebo-controlled clinical trials. *Clinical Therapy*, *22*, 209–221.

99. Poole, P.J., Black, P.N. (2001). Oral mucolytic drugs for exacerbations of chronic obstructive pulmonary disease: Systematic review. *British Medical Journal*, *322*, 1271–1274.

100. Zuin, R., Palamidese, A., Negrin, R., Catozzo, L., Scarda, A., Balbinot, M. (2005). High-dose N-acetylcysteine in patients with exacerbations of chronic obstructive pulmonary disease. *Clinical Drug Investigation*, *25*(6), 401–408.

101. Jensen, T., Kharazmi, A., Schiøtz, P.O., Nielsen, H., Stenvang Pedersen, S., Stafanger, G., Koch, C., Høiby, N. (1988). Effect of oral N-acetylcysteine administration on human blood neutrophil and monocyte function. *Acta Pathologica, Microbiologica, et Immunologica Scandinavica*, *96*(1), 62–67.

102. Kirsch, B.M., Lam, N., Layadent, T.J., Wiley, T.E. (1995). Diagnosis and management of fulminant hepatic failure. *Comprehensive Therapy*, *21*, 166–171.

103. Harrison, P.M., Wendom, J.A., Gimson, A.E.S., Alexander, G.J.M., Williams, R. (1991). Improvement by acetylcysteine of haemodynamics and oxygen transport in fulminant hepatic failure. *New England Journal of Medicine*, *324*, 1852–1857.

104. Smilkstein, M.J., Knapp, G.L., Kulig, K.W., Rumack, B.H. (1988). Efficacy of oral N-acetylcysteine in the treatment of acetaminophen overdose. *New England Journal of Medicine*, *319*, 1557–1562.

105. Massy, Z.A., Ceballos, I., Chadefaux-Vekemens, B., Nguyen-Khoa, T., Descamps-Latscha, B., Drüeke, T.B., Jungers, P. (2001). Homocyst(e)ine, oxidative stress and endothelium function in uremic patients. *Kidney International*, *59*, S78, 243–245.

106. Bostom, A.G., Culleton, B.F. (1999). Hyperhomocysteinemia in chronic renal diseases. *Journal of the American Society of Nephrology*, *10*, 891–900.

107. LoScalzo, J. (1996). The oxidant stress of hyperhomocyst(e)inemia. *Clinical Investigation*, *98*, 5–7.

108. Costagliola, C., Romano, L., Scibelli, G., de Vincentiis, A., Sorice, P., Di Benedetto, A. (1992). Anemia and chronic renal failure: A therapeutical approach by reduced glutathione parenteral administration. *Nephron*, *61*, 404–408.

109. Asahi, S., Masaaki, N. (2001). Sodium sulphite and N-acetylcysteine: New additives to dialysates for inhibition of formation of glucose degradation products and glication end products. *Advances in Peritoneal Dialysis*, *17*, 66–67.

110. Tepel, M., Van Dergiet, M., Schwartzfeld, C., Laufer, U., Liermann, D., Zidek, W. (2000). Prevention of radiographic contrast-agent-induced reduction in renal function by acetylcysteine. *New England Journal of Medicine*, *343*(3), 180–184.

111. Eck, H., Gmunder, H., Hartmann, M., Petzoldt, D., Daniel, V., Droge, W. (1989). Low concentration of acid-soluble thiol (cysteine) in the blood plasma of HIV-1-infected patients. *Biological Chemistry Hoppe-Seyler*, *370*, 101–108.

112. Eck, H., Droge, W. (1989). Influence of the extracellular glutamate concentration on the intracellular cyst(e)ine concentration in macrophages and on the capacity to release cysteine. *Biological Chemistry Hoppe-Seyler*, *370*, 109–113.

113. Schreck, R., Rieber, P., Baeuerle, P.A. (1991). Reactive oxygen intermediates as apparently widely used messengers in the activation of the NFkB transcription factor and HIV-1. *EMBO Journal*, *10*, 2247–2258.

114. Walker, R.E., Lane, H.C., Boenning, C.M., Polis, M.A., Kovacs, J.A., Fallon, J., Davey, R.T., Gavel, L., Correa-Coronas, R., Masur, H., Fauci, A.S. (1992). The safety, pharmacokinetics and antiviral activity of NAC in HIV infected individuals. Presented at VIII International Conference on AIDS, Amsterdam, Netherlands, July.

CHAPTER 22

TAURINE AS DRUG AND FUNCTIONAL FOOD COMPONENT

RAMESH C. GUPTA, MASSIMO D'ARCHIVIO, and ROBERTA MASELLA

22.1 INTRODUCTION

The concept of food changes all the time but for the majority of the people it is still a source to feed the hungry, while for some others, it is also a medium for socialization. Recently, food has acquired an additional value: to be able to reduce the risk of diseases. The new term "functional food" has been coined to indicate food that shows health-promoting and/or disease-preventing properties beyond its basic function of supplying nutrients [1, 2]. To be defined as "functional," food has to demonstrate its beneficial effects on one or more target functions in the body, thus improving health, strengthening well-being, or contributing to a reduction of the risk of diseases [3]. Functional food can still be regarded as natural food, even when the nature and/or the bioavailability of one or more of its active components have been modified in order to acquire new properties. This may be beneficial for an entire population or for groups of people selected on the basis of their health status and need. Functional food ingredients include many phytochemicals, vitamins, minerals, amino acids, and several plant and animal extracts [3].

Sulfur amino acids (SAA) play an important metabolic and functional role in human health and disease prevention. Also, SAA provide elemental sulfur required for growth and development [4, 5]. Pathological conditions are often determined by increased oxidative activities, a reduction in the host defense system, and a presence of other risk-promoting substances. Taurine is a well-known SAA and has been recognized as a protective agent against such events. Perhaps it is one biomolecule involved in many of the prevention and protection activities of various organ dysfunctions [6] and because of this it is known as a polyfunctional molecule [7].

With regards to amino acids, taurine does not participate in protein formation but it has a major role in human development [8]. Taurine also participates in a variety of biological processes, such as bile salt formation, osmoregulation, oxidative stress inhibition, immunomodulation, maintenance of cellular functions, and a variety of actions on the central nervous system (CNS) and cardiovascular system (CVS), diabetes, atherosclerosis, and many other biological actions [7–14]. For these reasons taurine is now part of many energy drinks, antiaging and antidiabetic formulas, baby food, pet food, and more.

22.2   THE UNIQUE CHARACTER OF TAURINE: BASIS FOR DISTINGUISHED BEHAVIOR

22.2.1   Taurine Chemistry and Physical Properties

Taurine (2-aminoethanesulfonic acid) is a naturally occurring β-amino acid containing sulfur (Fig. 22.1). It is one of the most abundant free amino acids in animal tissues, and in humans represents about 1% of the body weight.

Generally, the bioactivity of a substance is the cumulative index of its chemical and physical properties. Furthermore, chemicals can change their behavior according to the environment. Taurine is a monobasic acid that has unique physical constants compared to other neuroactive amino acids. The uniqueness of taurine is mainly due to the functional group containing sulfur, the sulfonic group, unlike the carboxylic group typical of all the other natural amino acids. This difference may provide the rationale behind the unique biological nature of taurine which is not shared with other neuroactive amino acids [15]. With its sulfonate group, it is a stronger acid (pKa 1.5) than glycine, aspartic acid, β-alanine, and γ-aminobutyric acid (GABA). Similarly, having a pKb value of 8.82, it is less basic than GABA, β-alanine, and glycine. Its solubility in water is 10.48 g/100 mL at 25°C, which is lower than that of β-alanine, GABA, or glycine.

The high acidity of taurine almost gives it a zwitterionic character, which makes it highly hydrophilic with very low lipophilicity. Consequently, the diffusion of taurine through lipophilic membrane is slower than for other carboxylic neuroactive amino acids, thus explaining its extremely high concentration gradient across cell membranes. Its isoelectric point is similar to carboxylic ω-amino acids like GABA, β-alanine, and glycine, and acidic amino acids like aspartate and glutamate. The membrane modulating activity of taurine and its interaction with Ca^{2+} and other cations is probably due to its unique ionic character [16].

Conformational analyses indicate three different conformational forms of taurine, among which the cyclic form is the most stable [16]. There is evidence of

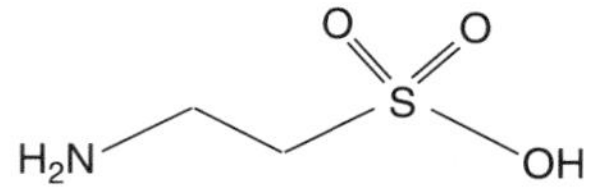

Figure 22.1   Chemical structure for taurine.

intramolecular hydrogen binding of taurine, which has a lower proton affinity of the amino groups, enabling taurine to penetrate the blood–brain barrier (BBB) but at a lower rate. Its precursor hypotaurine has a folded conformation and its proton affinity is similar to that of GABA, which enables it to cross the BBB more easily [16].

22.2.2 Taurine Biosynthesis

Taurine synthesis, which mainly occurs in the liver, can be produced from several pathways and be derived from different compounds [17–19]. Two biosynthesis pathways start with methionine being converted to cysteine which is then oxidized to cysteine sulfinic acid (CSA) by a cysteine dioxygenase. CSA can be decarboxylated to hypotaurine by a rate-limiting enzyme, cysteine sulfinic acid decarboxylase (CSAD) which requires pyridoxyl phosphate, and finally, hypotaurine is oxidized to taurine. Alternatively, CSA is converted to cysteic acid and then to taurine. Two other pathways start from cysteamine and cystine, respectively, and through the production of a number of intermediates, produce hypotaurine and taurine. In another pathway, sulfate is reduced to a sulfite intermediate and this is converted to cysteic acid which is then converted to taurine (Fig. 22.2).

However, the capability of synthesizing taurine is species specific, being very high in rodent and very low in humans and cats, and as a consequence taurine must be obtained through dietary sources. Taurine concentration in food varies widely, from 40 to 400 mg/100 g and it is present at higher concentrations in animal products than in plants, with the exception of some algae.

Fish is a good source of taurine and tests for taurine content for a variety of fish have been constructed. The content in some common species is as follows: albacore tuna, 155 mg/100 g wet weight; ray wing, 128; plaice, 126; cod, 93; mackerel, 69; farmed salmon, 53; wild salmon, 53; siki shark, 44; whiting, 35; Greenland halibut, 28; round-nose grenadier, 6; and bairds smooth-head, 5. This data indicates that the fish species have different levels of inherent functionality (in term of taurine status), with albacore tuna having the highest level.

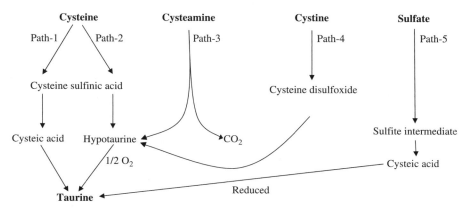

Figure 22.2 Biosynthetic pathways of taurine biosynthesis. See the text for details.

22.2.3 Taurine Bioavailability, Transport across the Membranes, and Metabolism

Taurine is found in most organs in mammals, with the highest concentration in the heart and brain, and the lowest level in the plasma and cerebrospinal fluid. Taurine accumulation in tissues is due to two efficient transport systems, which differ only in their affinity for taurine [20, 21]. The uptake of taurine by cells is Na^+ dependent, while other ions, such as Cl^-, Ca^{2+}, or Mg^{2+}, also have an effect in its transport in specific cases [22]. A third nonsaturable transport system, attributable to simple diffusion across the membrane, has also been reported [23]. This uptake is temperature sensitive and is influenced by the membrane lipid composition. It is the major determinant of the "leaking of taurine," which is the most common mechanism of taurine release by the cells. Finally, taurine is excreted as such or in the form of a bile salt conjugate.

22.3 FUNCTIONAL PROPERTIES OF TAURINE

The physicochemical properties of taurine make it fit to exert some of the observed functional activities such as antioxidation and enhancement of host defenses. The pathogenetic mechanisms of several diseases are not fully understood, but involve a variety of events that are responsible for tissue damage. Particularly, the production of reactive oxygen species (ROS) and inflammatory mediators, such as cytokines, among which tumor necrosis factor-α (TNF-α), interleukin (IL)-1β and IL-6, by activated cells, has been shown to be responsible for cellular damage [24, 25]. Consequently, any agent able to deactivate cells and/or inactivate oxidative/inflammatory mediators can exert beneficial effects, such as physiological antioxidant/anti-inflammatory responses, and taurine may participate in counteracting tissue damages [26, 27].

22.3.1 Oxidative Process and Myeloperoxidase Activity

Neutrophilic polymorphonuclear leukocytes (neutrophils) are circulating cells that exert defensive antimicrobial, cytotoxic, and cytolytic activities, releasing a complete armamentarium of reactive oxygen intermediates.

The oxidation of organic substances occurs in parallel with the stepwise reduction of oxygen into water. In general, the complete reduction of oxygen to water requires four electrons (e^-) and the overall reaction proceeds by four single-electron steps, generating sequentially superoxide, hydrogen peroxide di-anion and hydroxyl radical as intermediates (Fig. 22.3). They are more reactive than oxygen itself and are primarily responsible for the toxicity of oxygen. Hydrogen peroxide (H_2O_2) is a strong oxidant but it reacts slowly; on the contrary the hydroxyl radical is indiscriminately reactive in biological systems. In most tissues protection from oxygen toxicity is provided by a combination of three enzymes: superoxide dismutase, catalase, and glutathione peroxidase. Superoxide dismutase increases many-fold to convert superoxide to H_2O_2 and the other two enzymes rapidly convert H_2O_2 to water. Taurine has been recognized as an antioxidant capable of scavenging both ROS and nitrogenous radicals. These radicals also combine with halogen ions such as chloride, in a reaction

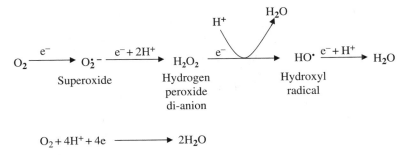

Figure 22.3 Reduction of oxygen by four single-electron steps.

catalyzed by the enzyme myeloperoxidase (MPO) producing hypohalo acids (Fig. 22.4a) [28]. The strongly nucleophilic amino group of taurine is able to react with these compounds, converting them to taurine haloamines, which are long-lived, less reactive, and much less toxic (Fig. 22.4b) [29].

Activated neutrophils and monocytes mainly generate H_2O_2, and secrete MPO, an enzyme characterized by powerful prooxidative and pro-inflammatory properties [30]. MPO catalyzes the conversion of chloride and H_2O_2 to a highly reactive hypochlorite

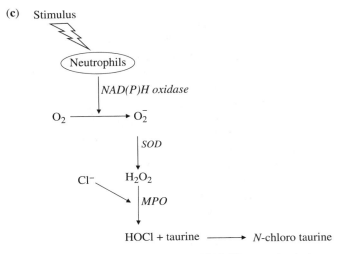

Figure 22.4 The respiratory burst and formation of *N*-chloro taurine in human neutrophils. MPO, myeloperoxidase; SOD, superoxide dismutase.

(HOCl) which is paradoxically both beneficial and detrimental to the host. The production of HOCl is necessary for bacterial killing, but it is a major player in host tissue damage following inflammatory cell activation. In fact, it is able to induce structural modifications in lipids, DNA, and proteins. It also catalyzes amino acid halogenation, deamination, and decarboxylation. MPO acts in both intracellular and extracellular environments. Intracellularly MPO induces IgG and C3b production, while extracellular MPO upregulates TNF-α secretion by macrophages which, in turn, also generate ROS [30].

22.3.2 *N*-Chloro Taurine Formation and Its Protective Role

Experimental data have indicated that taurine plays a role in host defense by interacting with MPO-derived HOCl [31–33]. Specifically, it has been shown that an exogenous supply of taurine is able to reduce luminal-dependent chemiluminescence due to increased MPO activity in human neutrophils. This reduced activity of taurine is likely related to its ability to react with HOCl forming less toxic derivatives, among which is the *N*-chloro taurine sodium salt (NCT-Na). It is a weak oxidant produced in high amounts (20 to 50 μM) by stimulated human granulocytes and monocytes [34] and plays an important role in the destruction of pathogens during inflammation [35]. The synthesis of taurine chloromine, or *N*-chloro taurine (NCT), by neutrophils, depends on several factors, such as taurine concentration, time, number of cells, and availability of chlorine. Furthermore, NCT synthesis can be inhibited by catalase and MPO blockers. Human neutrophils utilize the H_2O_2-MPO-Cl system to produce NCT, as shown in Fig. 22.4c.

The removal of HOCl, through the formation of NCT, inevitably reduces its potential for host tissue damage and also helps in minimizing the oxidizing equivalents available to render pathogens effective in perpetuating host inflammatory consequences. Although NCT is quite stable, it spontaneously undergoes transformation to sulfoacetaldehyde, which increases its stability when stored at very low temperature (−20°C).

NCT as a weak oxidant reacts only with thiols with activated CH functions and amines but not with amides and alcohols. Furthermore it has been suggested that NCT, more than taurine itself, is able to reduce nitric oxide (NO). The synthesis of TNF-α, as well as of IL-1β, IL-6, and IL-8, in activated phagocytes occurs in a dose-dependent manner by a mechanism involving transcriptional and translational events [36–39] modulated by different signaling pathways, such as NF-κB [39], which is still poorly understood. A schematic representation of the role of taurine in disease prevention through *N*-chloro taurine formation is shown in Fig. 22.5.

Whatever the mechanism involved, NCT could act as a neutrophil-derived signaling molecule responsible for the downregulation of inflammatory mediators produced by macrophages and neutrophils [40].

Finally, it is worth noting that taurine represents 76% of the amino acid content of human granulocytes and neutrophils. Taurine is generally not redistributed even after long-term parental nutrition without supplementation.

Taurine represents a competitive inhibitor of the MPO-H_2O_2-Cl complex. It can directly or indirectly, through NCT, participate in attenuating oxidative stress and

Primary insult: free radicals, toxic chemicals, microbial activities

Secondary insult: neutrophil activation and accumulation

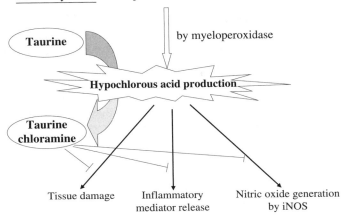

Figure 22.5   Role of taurine in disease prevention.

the production of inflammatory mediators, and hence have a pivotal role in host defense resulting in the alleviation of cellular damage [41].

22.4 TAURINE DEFICIENCY

Taurine availability can be affected by the reduction of plasma taurine transport to the cells, restricting dietary supply or using transport inhibitors and antagonists [20, 22, 42, 43]. Studies of taurine knockout mice have been particularly useful to unravel its role in the development and maintenance of normal organ functions [44]. Such studies have demonstrated significant effects on retinal degeneration [45], cardiac dysfunction, cardiomyopathy [46], and platelet hyperaggregation [47]. The decline of tissue taurine content during aging has been demonstrated and could exacerbate age-related increase of oxidative stress and related morbidity [48–50].

Studies on taurine deprivation have also provided surprising results on growth and development [51]. Taurine is essential for growth and survival of mammalian cells, as well as fetus development and development of the newborn and during childhood [52, 53]. Lymphoblastoid cells do not grow and myocytes have poor viability in the absence of taurine [54, 55].

22.5 TAURINE CONCENTRATION IN FETAL DEVELOPMENT AND NEONATAL GROWTH

Deprivation of taurine to embryos in vitro proves to be toxic to cellular development [56]. The human fetus has no ability to synthesize taurine, but considerably high levels of taurine have been recorded, and this may be due to a very efficient placental transport system for taurine. Reduction in the placental transport of taurine, typically seen in intrauterine growth restriction or in mothers affected by diabetes, results in low plasma taurine concentrations, which subsequently compromise the availability of amino acids for cellular processes [56–58].

Taurine has a dose-dependent trophic effect on the human fetal brain cell. In low birth-weight infants, taurine supplementation up to the time of discharge from the hospital increased plasma taurine concentrations yielding better auditory evoked responses as well as a healthier latency of the response interval compared to infants who were not supplemented [59]. Taurine is indispensable to proper neurological development and neuromuscular function [60]. Very low birth-weight delivery complicates the taurine availability in infancy. In fact, with these infants, the kidney is not yet fully developed and is unable to conserve taurine through renal reabsorption. As a result, these infants are more at risk of taurine depletion than their larger preterm or full-term counterparts. Taurine has the ability to promote fat emulsification via conjugation of bile acids and hence taurine level is directly related to the ability to properly absorb lipids. In children with cholestasis decrease in taurine has been observed [61]. However, the homeostasis of taurine in the fetus and neonate is not fully known yet, as well as its importance to fetal and neonatal growth.

During pregnancy, taurine accumulates in the maternal tissues, from where it is periodically released to the fetus via the placenta. In infants, taurine is acquired through the mother's milk. This is the stage when taurine accumulates more in fetal and neonatal brain. A low maternal taurine concentration will lead to low fetal taurine concentration. Such taurine deficiency may result in retarded growth in the child and also impair the prenatal CNS and endocrine pancreas development. When such a child becomes an adult, it can show signs of impaired neurological function, glucose tolerance, and vascular dysfunction [62]. Furthermore, there is a high possibility that these offspring, in turn, may develop gestational diabetes, transmitting the adverse effects to the next generation. Thus, this trans-generation effect of taurine deficiency in prenatal periods must be checked and also requires in-depth study.

The amount of taurine was found to be very high in human breast milk compared to cow's milk, on which a large portion of infants are fed, and this may be due to the high concentration of taurine in placenta. Thus, taurine is now added to many infant formulas to provide improved nourishment [63, 64]. Several types of organ dysfunction develop from abnormalities of taurine levels in growing children. In neonatal cardiomyocytes (as in adult ones), taurine functions as an organic osmolyte. When taurine is lost, the cardiac cells are found to be smaller in size and changed in form, as well as configuration [65].

Neurological disorders correspond to a certain characteristic of amino acid levels measured in the cerebrospinal fluid (CSF) [36]. While excitatory and inhibitory amino acids can be widely distributed across brain tissue, CSF amino acids reveal a different makeup. In bacterial meningitis and encephalitis, taurine levels are increased [66, 67]. Abnormal levels of neurotransmitter amino acids are also found in autistic children with increase in taurine level [68]. This may be due to the deliberate responsive efforts by the cells of the CNS to modulate osmotic changes in these diseases by promoting increased taurine levels. While this finding provides insight into the pathology of meningitis and encephalitis, it remains to be seen whether the administration of taurine has any therapeutic value.

22.6 BENEFICIAL ACTIONS OF TAURINE

Taurine has been used as a therapeutic supplement for the past 30 years. It has proven to be beneficial in relieving a number of diseases, such as epilepsy [69, 70], cardiovascular diseases [71, 72], myocardial infarction [73], hypertension [74], diabetes [75], ischemia [76, 77], alleviation of the noxious effects of smoking [78], reduction of alcoholic craving after detoxification [79], and also the prevention of neurodegeneration in the elderly [80]. More often, it is used as a nutritional supplement, as an anti-aging agent, and a mood modifier. It is also a part of health drinks, booster, eyes and ear drops, and much more.

However, with taurine being an amino acid, it is poorly absorbed in the gastrointestinal tract and is highly lost through renal excretion. In addition taurine has very strong hydrophilic nature, lipophobic character and a fast rate of extraction by urine. Consequently, the ratio between doses administered orally and those available at tissue level are very unfavorable. This prompted researchers to find ways to improve taurine availability by synthesizing suitable pro-drugs of taurine. In the last 25 years, a large number of analogs have been synthesized and evaluated for their biological activity, sometimes with great success [81].

22.6.1 Taurine and the CNS

22.6.1.1 Neurological Activities   Taurine is the most abundant amino acid in the brain after glutamate, and it is found in all cell types in the CNS. A high concentration of taurine occurs in the developing brain, but with maturity, its levels fall to 30%. Various reports have suggested that taurine is a neurotransmitter, but the evidence is not yet conclusive [14, 82, 83]. Taurine is extensively involved in neurological activities, including protection, modulation of neural excitability, maintenance of cerebellar functions, and modulation of motor behavior through interaction with dopaminergic, adrenergic, serotonergic, and cholinergic receptors [84–86] and through glutamate [87–89].

The activity of taurine is probably mediated by binding to GABA or glycine receptors [90], but this still lacks convincing evidence. Taurine modulates the release of GABA but their biochemical actions are different. Taurine and glycine have several similar activities but they work on different receptors. A putative taurine receptor has been studied and described [91, 92].

Free radicals are particularly detrimental to brain tissue where there is a high concentration of lipids, suitable target for oxidation. Taurine is now being explored for its capacity to protect tissues against oxidative stress. In cerebellar neurons, stimulation by excitatory agents was effectively countered by taurine. While taurine may not directly decrease the levels of free radicals, it does increase cell viability. This may become an important alternate protective mechanism against free radical damage to brain cells.

In addition, the oxidation of catecholamine catalyzed by metals, such as iron, is thought to play a role in neurodegenerative diseases. Taurine directly inhibits levodopa (L-DOPA) oxidation catalyzed by ferric chloride, and as such decreases the oxidative damage of proteins [93]. On the other hand, taurine can exert neuroprotection by reducing membrane depolarization responsible for increased intracellular calcium content, which is the principal sign of abnormal stimulation of neurons [94]. Finally, it is worth noting that decreased taurine concentration has been found in the brain and cerebrospinal fluid of patients affected by Alzheimer's disease (AD) [95, 96]. Recently, it has been proposed that taurine could prevent the neurotoxicity of β-amyloid peptide, which is the main component of senile plaque found in the brain of AD patients [97, 98]. In addition, a taurine derivative, tauroursodeoxycholic acid (TUDCA), has been found to potently inhibit apoptosis. This could be a possible therapeutic agent in pathological conditions, such as AD, in which apoptosis could play a relevant role [99].

In short, taurine is involved in many brain functions, for example, as an anticonvulsant [70, 100], modulator of neuronal excitability [12, 84], cerebellar function [101], central regulation of cardiorespiratory responses [102, 103], and thermoregulation [104–106]. It exerts antinociceptive responses [36, 83, 107], antiaggressive actions [108], antianxiety effects [109, 110], and improves resistance to anoxia/hypoxia [111–114]. Finally, taurine counteracts the alteration in sleeping duration [115, 116], learning [117, 118], and may suppress appetite [119–123].

22.6.1.2 Seizure/Epilepsy
Seizures are the result of electrical miscommunication between brain neurons. The onset of the seizure event is now correlated to significant changes in the levels of amino acids in the hippocampal region of the brain. The levels of the excitatory amino acids, glutamate and aspartate, as well as the inhibitory amino acids, GABA and taurine, were found to be increased during seizure [70]. The antiepileptic action is the most prominent activity of taurine. A number of taurine analogs have been synthesized and evaluated for their anticonvulsant action [70, 81, 100, 124] which occurs through the interaction with the GABA binding site in the brain.

22.6.1.3 Hypoxia and Ischemia
Hypoxia is a condition in which tissues fail to receive sufficient oxygen. The CNS is the least tolerant to hypoxic conditions. Symptoms include changes in the mental state, confusion or encephalopathy, and coma or death. Brain death usually occurs in 3 to 5 min in an anoxic state. Taurine has been shown to act as a preventive agent against the disturbance associated with hypoxia [111]. Taurine modulates the enzymes involved in energy metabolism in the brain, restoring adenine and ATP while reducing ADP and AMP levels [117]. In addition, through its ability to preserve the glutathione peroxide system and for its potent antioxidant capabilities, taurine protects cells from lipid peroxidation and deleterious membrane structure changes [125].

22.6.2 Taurine and the Liver

22.6.2.1 Promoter of Bile Salts Formation
Besides processing blood, the liver is also involved in the absorption of nutrients from food by secreting bile.

Liver synthesizes bile, which is a mixture of bile acids, salts, bilirubin, cholesterol, and fatty acids, stored in the gallbladder. It is also responsible for the detoxification of harmful substances, but only if available in sufficient quantities. The bile acids act as detergents to solubilize or emulsify food into digestible components. This detergent action is due to the presence of both lipophilic and hydrophilic ends in the bile acids. The hydrophilic regions include sulfonates or carboxylate backbones. Mammals mainly use taurine and, to a lesser extent glycine, as the major amino acids that conjugate with bile acids to form biliary salts. Among the tauro-conjugates, tauro-cholic acid (TC), taurodeoxycholic acid (TDC), taurolithocholic acid (TLC), and taur-ocheno-deoxycholic acid (TCDC), can act as cholagogues (agents that promote the flow of bile into the intestine) or choleretics (agents that stimulate the liver to increase production of bile) [126].

The ratio between tauro-conjugates and glycocholate in humans is about 3 : 1 and this ratio is adversely affected in cases of low taurine supply. In the absence of TC, bile salts can precipitate and form gallstones [127].

The removal of cholesterol from the body is generally done by the formation of TC. Reduced taurine supply will result in lower quantities of TC and will severely affect the removal rate of cholesterol, leading to its accumulation in the body. Any agent that will increase the availability of taurine will make cholesterol more extractable [128]. Therefore, the role of taurine as a potent lipid metabolizer cannot be overlooked or underestimated.

22.6.2.2 *Taurine, Cholesterolemia and Liver Diseases*

In blood, choles-terol is carried in low density lipoproteins (LDL) and high density lipoproteins (HDL). Elevated LDL levels are implicated in a range of heart and vascular diseases, including myocardial infarction (heart attack) and atherosclerosis (clogging of the arteries). Taurine can attenuate the increased levels in total and LDL cholesterol in animals con-suming a high fat, high cholesterol diet [129]. High fat diets produce hypercholester-olemia, atherosclerosis, and accumulation of lipids on the aortic valve of the heart. Dietary taurine supplements are known to be beneficial in situations when the body cholesterol status is high, as well as normal. In particular, it has been demonstrated that taurine is capable of reducing plasma lipid concentration and visceral fat in dia-betic rats [130] as well as in obese humans [131, 132]. In children with simple obesity, taurine supplements trigger improvements in liver enzyme levels, independent of weight loss control measures [133, 134].

Taurine conjugates of all bile acids suppress very low density lipoprotein (VLDL) secretion. Taurine exhibits a high reactivity with aldehydes, thus it acts to inhibit protein modification of LDL from undergoing oxidative modification. With regard to HDL, taurine treatments enhance serum HDL concentration in a dose-dependent manner and lower serum LDL and VLDL considerably [135–138]. Taurine also decreases the presence of cholesterol in the liver [139].

The cholesterol-lowering action of taurine may lie in its ability to promote the con-version of potentially detrimental cholesterol to relatively harmless bile acids. This represents a way to protect the liver from cholesterol-induced cytotoxicity, which results in hepatocyte destruction and apoptosis, characteristic signs of liver pathology [140, 141].

A new drug, sodium tauroursodeoxycholate (TUDC), has been synthesized to treat cholestasis, with beneficial results [142]. In severe cholesterol diseases, hydrophobic bile-induced injury is due to cytolysis, in which the cell dissolves. In moderate cholesterolemia, apoptosis is the main mechanism in which bile acid toxicity is expressed. The taurine conjugate TUDC is able to reduce both cytolysis and apoptosis by exerting a direct protective effect against hydrophobic bile acids cytotoxicity [143]. Taurine itself also has a role in the prevention of hepatocyte apoptosis and necrosis [144]. This effect can be partially linked to the taurine antioxidant activity not only by directly reacting with the free radical intermediates but also by inhibiting the inducible nitric oxide synthase (iNOS) mRNA expression [145].

Taken all together, these findings can offer a scientific base to explain the protective effects of taurine on liver disorders and diseases, including hepatitis and cirrhosis [140, 146].

22.6.2.3 Taurine and Occupational/Environmental Liver Damage

Exposure to toxic chemicals, which is a common hazard for industrial workers, has been linked to birth defects, sterility, headache, chronic fatigue, arthritic-like inflammation, and many other symptoms. These chemicals have a deleterious effect on the liver and taurine is able to moderate the extent and severity of their side. Furthermore, it reduces the number of cancer antigen-positive hepatocytes, and in several cases of chemical exposure, taurine also protected against DNA damage [141].

22.7 TAURINE AND DIABETES

Type 2 diabetes mellitus is one of the most common human diseases and its prevalence is constantly growing. This pathology is characterized by the reduced sensitivity of the cellular targets, mainly adipose and muscle cells, to insulin stimulation. Such alteration can lead to insulin resistance, hyperinsulinemia, hyperglycemia, and several other metabolic dysfunctions. Lifestyle, dietary habits, and environment can influence the appearance of diabetes [147]. Taurine supplements administered to patients with type 2 diabetes were proven to be beneficial [148, 149]. Also, taurine alleviates clinical complications of diabetes, having beneficial effects on nephropathy and retinopathy [150]. In animal models of experimental insulin resistance, it has been demonstrated that the metabolic alterations associated with diabetes are ameliorated by taurine administration [151, 152].

Several papers have reported different activities of taurine on insulin comprising insulin-like and insulinogenic actions, as well as stimulation of insulin release from the pancreas and improvement of insulin producing apparatus [149, 153]. Increased insulin secretion has been recorded with addition of taurine to a low protein diet, suggesting a direct relationship between taurine supplementation and insulin secretion from the pancreatic islets [154–156]. Taurine also amplifies the effects of insulin binding to its receptor [157].

In patients with type 2 diabetes, taurine level was found to be significantly lower both in the plasma and platelets [75]. This is mostly believed to be due to the altered transport of taurine which further leads to reduced uptake of taurine in diabetic patients. This hypothesis was proposed by several studies demonstrating that the system responsible for taurine transport is selectively impaired in diabetics [158].

Finally, reduced taurine level was recorded in urine of children with diabetic ketoacidosis (DKA), and it has been postulated that the altered taurine level may be due to the DKA-induced alteration in the metabolic state and renal functions [159].

22.7.1 Taurine Concentration in Diabetes and Diseases of Fetal Origin

Many studies have been done to evaluate the relationship between taurine concentration, diabetic mothers, and their offspring. Taurine seems to be essential for the fetuses and neonates because deprivation during growth may result in the development of type 2 diabetes, obesity, and other metabolic diseases [160, 161].

The importance of taurine can be judged by the first report published in 1975, the earliest clinical study performed on diabetic mothers who were pregnant [57]. In the clinical examination, five cases of diabetic pregnant mothers were shown to have a lower taurine concentration compared to the nine cases of healthy pregnant mothers. However, taurine concentration in newborn infants of diabetic mothers did not show significant differences from infants of healthy mothers. A higher level of taurine has been recorded in amniotic fluid of diabetic mothers subsequent to the spontaneous rupture of membranes in the 40th week of pregnancy [162].

It has been observed that alterations in placental transport, which have been demonstrated to be decreased in human intrauterine growth restriction [58], are further complicated by diabetes [163].

22.8 TAURINE AND THE CARDIOVASCULAR SYSTEM

Taurine concentration is high in the mammalian heart. In the human heart, taurine levels range from 5 to 20 μmol/g (wet wt), with no noticeable differences with respect to age or sex [164]. The maintenance of cardiac taurine content is governed by a series of processes, which include transport, accumulation, binding, release, as well as metabolism. The availability of taurine in cardiac tissue is generally dependent on the transport process, because of its limited ability to be effectively synthesized in the cardiac tissue. However, limited taurine synthesis in the heart has been reported, through the classical pathway involving CSAD.

The transportation process is a vital source of taurine accumulation in cardiac tissue, which is generally taken from the blood. This is mediated by taurine transporters that are Na^+ and Cl^- dependent, which use the sodium gradient across the plasma membrane to allow intracellular taurine accumulation [165]. The taurine content in the cardiac tissue generally remain constant, even with a low taurine diet, and any increase in the amount of taurine ultimately results in a faster degradation. Normally, taurine degradation is a slow and uniform process. Heart taurine concentration shows noticeable variations with the use of transport inhibitors, like β-alanine, without reaching a level of taurine deficiency that could promote severe pathology [166].

The maintenance of cardiac taurine contents appears thus to be governed by a complex network of processes which include, besides the transport, also the accumulation, binding, and release, as well the metabolism.

Taurine deficiency may possibly be linked to cardiomyopathy, as it has been well reported in cats. A cat having plasma taurine concentration below 40 nmol^{-1} can be considered taurine deficient and it is desirable to add taurine to the diet [167]. Furthermore, conclusive evidence of the relationship between taurine and heart health was provided by studies with transgenic mice knocked out of its taurine transporter [168]. This study suggests that taurine has multiple roles such as osmoregulation, regulation of mitochondrial protein expression, and inhibition of apoptosis, which collectively, were able to protect the cardiac structure and function. In fact, the knockout mice exhibited a deficiency in myocardial taurine content and were associated with cardiomyocyte atrophy, ultrastructural cellular damage, and severe cardiac dysfunction.

22.8.1 Cardiovascular Protective Mechanisms

Taurine functions as a cardiotonic and protective agent against heart stress and it has been classified as an inotropic agent. The cardio-protective properties of taurine have been well studied, and in particular, after stress produced by chemical agents. The cardio-protective nature of taurine is the result of its in situ involvement in the mediation of cardiac actions, for example, as an inotropic, antiarrhythmic, osmoregulator, hypotensive and other related actions. These actions are believed to be mediated via a specific taurine-type or glycine-like receptor. Apart from the above, taurine also produces antagonistic effects on angiotensin II through intraventricular administration [169].

It is believed that taurine interacts mostly with cations, specifically with Ca^{2+}, rather than anions, and takes part in the stabilization of membrane. A fascinating hypothesis of taurine interaction in membrane stabilization was formulated by Huxtable and Sebring [170], who have provided a link to membrane phospholipids. In particular, acidic phospholipids are important Ca^{2+} binding sites on the membrane bilayer and regulate Ca^{2+} entry in the cells. Taurine, which is more similar to neutral phospholipids, intercalates with the head group of membrane phospholipids and modifies its environment and the cation binding capacity of acidic phospholipids. Other hypotheses proposed by Schaffer et al. [171] suggest that taurine actions are mediated through the interaction with sarcolemmal proteins and by the inhibition of calmodulin, an important calcium modulator.

Apart from its major involvement with Ca^{2+}, taurine interactions with other cations, like Na^+, K^+, and Mg^{2+}, have been formulated. Calcium homeostasis is critical for myocardial contractile function as it transmits several biofunctional expressions through its mobilization. Any noticeable alteration in Ca^{2+} content also produces stress in the cell. For example, an overload of calcium may cause the cell to be dysfunctional. Calcium entry into the myocardial cells is regulated by the sarcolemma, which provides a barrier between intra- and extracellular Ca^{2+} concentrations. The sarcolemma is the site where several pharmacological agents, such as Ca^{2+} antagonists, blockers, exert their actions. The role of taurine in Ca^{2+} management is established and exhibits dual inotropic actions [171]. At high Ca^{2+} concentrations, taurine produces negative inotropic effects, but at low Ca^{2+}, it exhibit positive inotropic properties. The calcium modulation and the contractility action of taurine are dose dependent and are not affected by agents like propranolol and indomethacin. The protective role of taurine is even observed under calcium paradox condition. In an age-dependent response of chick heart to calcium paradox, taurine restores the cardiac abnormalities to a considerable extent [172]. In hamsters with genetic cardiomyopathia, taurine decreased the heart calcium reversing the symptoms associated with calcium overload and necrosis [173].

Use of taurine as therapeutic agents for congestive heart failure (CHF) is well recorded [71, 72]. The first study reported the case of a 60-year-old woman clinically in class III, IV of the New York Heart Association (NYHA) classification. After a four-week taurine treatment (2 g, twice a day) the patient was lowered to NYHA class I, II. Similarly, in a related study, 58 patients of both sexes in different NYHA classes underwent taurine treatments and overall have improved considerably with increased urinary output and reduced body weight. Also, a higher taurine dosage, 6 g per day, was found to improve the patient's condition while reducing the NYHA class [174].

Recently, taurine has been found to be an effective nutrient with therapeutic relevance to heart failure [175]. Also, several taurine analogs have been synthesized and tested for their effects on the cardiovascular system. Some results have shown only partial effect, while others have become therapeutic agents [81]. In particular, the taurineamide derivatives, propionylcarnitine-taurineamide (PCTA) and butirylcarnitine-taurineamide (BCTA) exhibited cardioprotective activity at a lower concentration than taurine. A phenylalkyl taurine derivative, TAU-5, infused intravenously during electrostimulation normalizes the abnormal hemodynamic characters such as increased peripheral resistance, decreased cardiac output, and aortic pressure. It is also capable of increasing the stability of the heart with respect to hypoxia and anoxia, thus exerting a protective role against ischemic damage.

Although the benefits of taurine therapy can be obtained from an exogenous source, there are several groups studying ways to increase the endogenous taurine level by enhancing its biosynthesis, especially through the leg exchange of amino acid via physical exercise. In humans, exercise stimulates the production of taurine due to increases of cysteine and cystein levels, which may increase taurine biosynthesis [176].

22.9   TAURINE AND ENDOTHELIAL DYSFUNCTION

Endothelial dysfunction is common among cardiovascular diseases and diabetes and it is known as one of the primary events in the development of atherosclerosis and diabetic angiopathies. Monocyte-endothelial interactions have been implicated in the initiation of endothelial dysfunction. This dysfunction is partially attributed to the impaired activity of endothelial-derived NO and overproduction of a cytokine, endothelin-1 (ET-1). NO activity is critical in modulating many potentially protherogenic processes, namely monocyte adhesion, platelet aggregation, vascular smooth muscle proliferation, and oxidative modification of LDL [177].

Taurine has been shown to be a protector of endothelial structure and function after exposure to inflammatory cells, their mediators, or other chemicals. Treatment of activated macrophages with taurine inhibits the generation of NO and other inflammatory mediators [41]. Taurine, which is present in high amounts in inflammatory cells, seems to be uniquely capable of modifying homeostasis in both target and receptor cells through antioxidant calcium flux and the osmoregulatory pathway. Finally, taurine was proven to protect endothelial cells from damage induced by hyperglycemia and oxidized LDL [178].

Taurine analogs, which could probably suppress the inflammation process much better, offer new tools in the treatment of inflammatory diseases. Both hypotaurine and homotaurine have demonstrated their superior ability in protecting the cells against oxidative damage of DNA by free radicals [179].

22.10 TAURINE AND LUNG DYSFUNCTION

The depletion of taurine is particularly harmful to pulmonary tissue. Alveolar macrophages, which reside on the surface of lung alveoli, ingest inhaled particulates to clear the alveolar spaces. However, alveolar macrophages, much like the general macrophages, become more susceptible to ROS and more pro-inflammatory when deprived of the antioxidant protective capacity that taurine provides.

In particular, taurine possesses beneficial activities in people afflicted with cystic fibrosis (CF). CF is an inherited condition that affects the respiratory and digestive systems. Patients with CF produce thick mucus that clogs their pulmonary system and also are afflicted by liver disease, a complication that often leads to death. In CF patients with poor liver function, treatment with taurine provides a notable increase in serum pre-albumin and a reduction in fat malabsorption, without having severe side effects. Also, with the taurine treatments, these patients have an increased stimulation of bile synthesis [180, 181].

However, most patients affected by CF suffer from nutrient malabsorption, due to the damage in the ileum. Since the terminal ileum serves as the main absorption site for the enterohepatic recycling of approximately 80% of bile acids, they are malabsorbed as well. Taurine supplementation has been shown to decrease the severity of steatorrhea associated with many CF cases. Children with CF showed decreased fecal excretion of fatty acids and sterols while taking taurine. This ability to correct absorption makes taurine a novel valuable aid for CF treatment [182].

Fibrosis may also result from toxic chemical exposure. There are numerous factors responsible for toxin-induced damage to lung cells and tissue in animal models of induced interstitial pulmonary fibrosis [183]. In several cases, the administration of taurine, niacin, or a combination of both, yielded promising results, and can reverse increased lung lipid peroxidation. Furthermore, the ability to scavenge ROS and to stabilize cell membranes contributed to the suppression of lung collagen accumulation and oxidative stress damage.

Asthma is a chronic disease characterized by bronchial obstruction and airway hyperreactivity with neutrophil accumulation. There is increasing evidence that excessive production of ROS along with defective endogenous antioxidant defense mechanisms may be responsible for asthma [184]. In an animal model of allergic asthma, taurine content was found to be reduced and oral treatment with taurine produced anti-inflammatory responses. Similar effects have also been demonstrated in humans [185].

Finally, radiation exposure may also cause lung fibrosis, characterized by endothelial cell damage. Taurine significantly attenuates endothelial cell necrosis and apoptosis due to oxidative stress, with similar efficacy. This may also be due to taurine's ability to regulate intracellular calcium flux. In this regard, taurine has great potential for its therapeutic value for any type of inflammatory lung condition.

22.11   TAURINE AND THE KIDNEY

In the kidneys, taurine is found at a high concentration, which is regulated by the reabsorption at the modulating proximal tubule according to its dietary intake. Taurine's role in the development of renal diseases can be recognized by the lower level of taurine contents in kidney. This may be due to the impairment in the transport mechanism of taurine resulting in altered levels and decreased accumulation. Taurine's immunohistochemical localization in rat renal tissues further proves its involvement in kidney pathologies. Normally, taurine is found in medullary tubules, concentrated at the proximal tubules and glomerulus regions, but in a diseased condition, taurine is distributed in a much larger area, covering almost the entire medullary tubules. This extended distribution area might have some recuperative effect to maintain normal renal functions, even under chronic pathological conditions [186].

As taurine seems to act through volume regulation and, to some extent, antioxidation, the study of taurine content in endothelium and epithelium kidney cells is essential to formulate its concentration in diseased states of the kidneys and to further exploit taurine as a preventive agent [187].

Finally, kidney dysfunction is common in chronic diabetic patients. As stated above (see Section 22.7), taurine supplements provide beneficial effects [148, 149], in alleviating clinical complications due to diabetes, including nephropathy [150]. Taurine treatments ameliorate diabetic nephropathy by reducing oxidant injury with decreased lipid peroxidation and lower the accumulation of advanced glycation end products (AGEs) in the kidney. In alleviating the diabetic nephropathy, taurine serves as an osmolyte, an endogenous antioxidant and an inhibitor of phosphokinase C (PKC) in mesangial cells [188]. The beneficial effects of taurine may be due to its well-known antioxidative, anti-inflammatory, and antiapoptotic activities.

22.12   RETINAL PROTECTION

Among all amino acids, taurine concentration is the highest (10 to 50 mM) in the retina and taurine is involved in the protection of retinal structure and functions [150]. Taurine is required for normal vision because any deficiencies lead to retinal degeneration and blindness. Such phenomena were observed in cats, rats, and monkeys, but in humans it is still a subject of debate. However, abnormal electroretinograms were seen in children who received long-term parental nutrition poor in taurine [189, 190].

The activity of taurine may be due to the regulation of the excitation threshold of the modulating calcium fluxes. In particular, taurine was seen to influence the binding and transport of calcium ions in retinal membrane preparation. This finding suggests that taurine may contribute to membrane stabilization by altering calcium mobilization during depolarization [191]. Furthermore, the modulation of calcium uptake can promote the transmission of visual signals from the retina to the brain.

Lens transparency is a function of the amino acids available in the lens itself. Lenses in oxidative stress exhibited lower taurine level and subsequently, it causes temporary and permanent changes in lens transparency. The common eye disease cataract demonstrates the importance of lens condition. It is speculated that cataract formation may be largely due to the oxidation of protein in the lens. Consequently, a lack of antioxidants could be a major factor in the development of cataracts. Since taurine acts as an antioxidant directly, it prevents changes in the levels of glutathione, ATP, and insoluble proteins, molecular factors that predispose to cataract formation [192].

Furthermore, taurine plays a critical role in the structure and function of the photoreceptors, specifically rods, which are responsible for seeing in both low illumination and night conditions [193].

Taurine is important for the regeneration of damaged cells in the retina and could have some effects in treating retinal dystrophy, an age-related degenerative disease that alters the pigmented epithelium and photoreceptors of the retina. The promotional effect of taurine in cellular regeneration is compromised with drugs that induce the activation of PKC or phosphate inhibitors [194].

Retinitis pigmentosa (RP) is characterized by visual field loss and night blindness. Nutritional factors are now recognized as important factors in the reversal of RP. Experimental finding suggests that RP patients recover their visual capacities with the addition of nutrients, including taurine, which has been found to be beneficial. Taurine and zinc interact with each other to influence the development of the retinal structure and function in the eye. Both molecules promote the healthy oscillatory potentials necessary for vision. Deficiency of taurine has been identified as the cause of all these diseases and clearly demonstrates its vital role in vision [195, 196].

22.13 ANTICANCER ACTIVITY OF TAURINE

Modifying nucleic acid structures through the interactions of sulfur substances with guanosine is now a century-old story. It has been observed that sulfates and sulfonic acids interact with RNA and DNA and exert their protective effects against alkylating agents, radiation, and other carcinogens. Such sulfur substances may participate in the regulation of the conformational states of nucleic acids, thus alleviating the toxic effects of chemical mutagens. Taurine, being a sulfonic acid, can behave in a similar way. Indeed, it has been found that taurine has radioprotective properties and antimutagenic effect, reducing nucleic acid damage [197, 198].

The chemopreventive activity of taurine and, in particular, 1-(2-chloroethyl)-3(2-dimethyl sulfony) ethyl-11-nitrosourea derivative (e.g., tauromustine), have been used against colon and hepatic cancers [199, 200]. In hepatocarcinogenesis, the degree of membrane damage and the fall in glutathione function were reduced when oral taurine was given prior to exposure to carcinogens. These findings suggest that taurine, by inhibiting lipoperoxidation and preserving the glutathione antioxidant system, offers protection against membrane breakdown.

Recombinant interleukin-2 immunotherapy is utilized as a therapeutic approach in certain types of cancers. However, it may produce a cytotoxic effect on both tumor cells and healthy vascular endothelial cells. In such cancer therapy programs, taurine reduces interleukin endothelial cell cytotoxicity without compromising the antitumor activity of the immunotherapy. In addition, when taurine is used in conjunction with interleukin, it actually increases the tumor cytotoxicity [201].

For the treatment of intraperitoneal (abdominal) tumors, researchers have studied a taurine derivative, taurolidine, as both an alternative and an adjunct to heparin, a standard substance used to prolong the clotting time of blood [202]. It appears that taurolidine can produce a significant decrease in the growths of both tumor cells and intraperitoneal tumors.

In certain cancers, the amino acid profile yields data about the disease that is useful to better assess the therapeutic approach. Colorectal cancer patients exhibit a characteristic amino acid profile with significantly lower intracellular levels of taurine, glutamic acid, methionine, and ornithine, and elevated levels of valine. Likewise, squamous cell carcinoma of the head and neck exhibit a profile that is marked by decreased taurine [203].

22.14 TAURINE IN BONE TISSUE FORMATION AND INHIBITION OF BONE LOSS

Bone provides both mechanical support to vital organs and protection to bone marrow. It also serves as a reservoir of calcium and phosphate ions which play a major role in maintaining serum homeostasis. Bone tissue contains cells and the extracellular matrix, which is composed of collagen fibers and noncollagenous proteins.

Bone tissue contains three types of cells: (1) osteoblasts, bone forming cells; (2) osteoblast-derived osteocytes, constituents of calcified bone that reduce metabolic activity; and (3) osteoclasts, bone resorption cells [204, 205]. The osteoblasts, rich in alkaline phosphatase, are involved mainly in the formation of matrix constituents, specifically collagen and noncollagen proteins. In addition, the osteoblasts regulate the bone structure and provide regulatory factors for mineralization. The entire process of bone formation is under hormonal control. With the parathyroid hormone, it mediates ion and amino acid transport and stimulates enzymatic activities such as alkaline phosphatase. The formation of the matrix also depends on amino acids availability, as demonstrated by Ishikawa et al [206]. In particular, the maximum enhancing effect was obtained with five amino acids, including taurine.

In bone tissue, taurine is found in high concentration, similar to that found in the liver and kidneys. This taurine-bone interaction is one of the latest added to its long list of actions [207]. In bones, taurine acts as a double agent. It is involved in both bone formation and inhibition of bone loss. In addition to these two major actions, taurine has beneficial effects in wound healing and bone repair.

Taurine enhances bone tissue formation which is evidenced by increased matrix formation and collagen synthesis. Evidence was obtained by Park et al. [208], who reported increased alkaline phosphatase activity and collagen synthesis in osteoblast-like cells treated with taurine (10 mM), which probably activated the mitogen activated protein kinase ERK2. Actually, the key action of taurine seems to be to modulate the sequential intracellular protein kinase cascade, which promotes mineralization and the anabolism of the bone.

Besides stimulating bone tissue formation, taurine also prevents bone loss by inhibiting bone resorption and osteoclast formation. It is known that bone resorption is mediated by osteoclasts and is positively influenced by lipopolysaccharide (LPS) and inflammatory mediators, such as IL-1 and prostaglandin E2 (PGE2), which have been demonstrated to be potent stimulators of osteoclast differentiation [204]. Taurine was shown to inhibit the stimulation of bone resorption and osteoclast differentiation induced by LPS of periodontopathic microorganisms. In particular, in experimental periodontitis, hamsters treated with taurine demonstrated inhibited alveolar bone resorption, suggesting it is an effective agent in preventing inflammatory bone resorption [205].

One of the most widespread diseases connected to bone loss is osteoporosis. It is a disease in which bones become fragile and prone to breakage. If not prevented or treated, osteoporosis can progress until bone breaks. Taurine can be used as a preventive and therapeutic agent for osteoporosis since it is capable of suppressing the amount of calcium liberated from bones, through the stimulation of human parathyroid hormones and prostaglandins, and it is excellent in suppressing bone resorption and also safe even if used for a long period. Since it is a naturally available molecule, it can be used as a preventive and therapeutic agent and may be a choice for sound bone health [207].

22.15 TAURINE AND SMOKING

Cigarette smoking interacts adversely with the cardiovascular system at many different sites. Recently, taurine has been patented in alleviating some of the noxious effects of cigarette smoking and, thus, taurine (6 ppm) is incorporated in the cigarette filter. Apart from this, daily supplements of taurine have also lessened the harmful effects on blood vessels caused by smoking. In fact, many vasculopathies are linked to chronic cigarette smoking. Taurine doses, comparable to those achievable with the daily intake of 100 g of fish, would restore flow-mediated dilatation (FMD) response to normal in otherwise-healthy, young, chronic cigarette smokers. This effect is mediated by the restoration of the normal expression of iNOS, an enzyme responsible for the production of NO from L-arginine within the endothelial cell [209].

It should be noted that young smokers treated with a daily dose of 1.5 g of taurine, orally, for 5 days, showed FMD responses in the brachial artery comparable with those seen in healthy normal controls and in the same group of smokers who were given 2 g of vitamin C daily for 5 days [210]. The beneficial effect of taurine was also recorded on the in vitro expression of iNOS and the release of NO and ET-1 from human umbilical vein endothelial cells (HUVECs), when co-cultured from 24 to 48 hours with conditioned medium from monocytes derived from smokers. Studies suggest that taurine supplements have a beneficial impact on macrovascular endothelial function of the iNOS protein expression.

22.16 TAURINE AS AN ANTIALCOHOL MOLECULE

Study of the effect of taurine on a variety of behavioral and pharmacological properties of ethanol showed numerous responses depending on the mode of administration, combination of doses, the route and length of treatment employed, and certain other conditions. The literature reveals conflicting reports on whether or not sleeping time was altered, or any changes that occurred in the blood or brain ethanol levels. Taurine and ethanol are known to share certain central depressant actions, like hypoactivity and hypothermia. Taurine is considered to antagonize some effects of ethanol in a person's behavior [79], likely by potentiating GABA and glycine receptors functions, and inhibiting excitatory amino acid receptors. This can also be the mechanism by which taurine plays a role during ethanol withdrawal from chronic alcohol intoxication when the CNS neurons become hyperexcitable and can cause convulsions. Also, taurine modulates the Ca^{2+} channel function in the same way as ethanol does [211]. It is interesting to note that the morphological and neurological abnormalities associated with taurine deficiency in alcohol-exposed offspring include hydrocephalus, cell failure in the cerebella external granule cell layer, retinal degeneration, and abnormal visual codex development [212].

Supplements of taurine in the diet of alcoholic mothers were found to have beneficial effects in preventing some alcohol-induced fetal alterations and alcohol-induced oxidative damage [213].

However, without understanding the diversity of the mechanisms underlying ethanol toxicity, it is difficult to provide any definite mechanism of protection. Ethanol directly induces its adverse effects through redox alterations, membrane and cellular defects, hormonal and neuron-hormonal disturbances [213, 214]. On the other hand, its first oxidative metabolite, acetaldehyde, induces more damaging effect on multiple targets. For example, it increases synthesis and release of catecholamine, binds to proteins and enzymes, particularly in blood and other tissues, alters membrane and mitochondrial functions, and causes the formation of free radicals, which further interferes with the physiology of neurotransmitters [215]. Taurine can increase alcohol metabolism, specifically, it can enhance the oxidation of acetaldehyde by activating its degradation enzyme, aldehyde dehydrogenase. It is also able to modify the adverse actions of glutamate, possibly through the osmolarity changes, and by modifying the activity of the enzyme involved in ethanol metabolism. Taurine prevents calcium loss from the brain during acute ethanol administration. The calcium stabilizing effect in brain could also evoke a partial explanation for the sleeping time reduction.

Taurine can reverse the liver damage caused by alcoholism [216]. Due to excess drinking, fat builds up in the liver, causing steatosis, which can eventually evolve into alcoholic cirrhosis. In experiments with rats fed with alcohol, taurine administration for a month before alcohol consumption protected the rat liver from the lipid accumulation. More surprisingly, when administered to rats after drinking alcohol, taurine continued to reverse the liver damage. Similar results have been seen in rats administered with alcohol intragastrically [217]. Because of these findings, it is possible that adding taurine to alcohol drinks could help minimize liver damage and ward off hangover.

Taurine seems to exert the following actions in counteracting alcohol effects:

- Increases the capacity of metabolizing alcohol
- Enhances the oxidation of the first alcohol metabolite, acetaldehyde, by activating its degradative enzyme
- Reduces ethanol-induced sleeping time
- Prevents calcium loss during generalized electrolyte depletion, such as that induced in the brain after acute ethanol administration
- Protects against the fatty liver and lipid peroxidation
- Acts as an osmolarity regulator during ethanol intoxication

22.17   TAURINE AS FUNCTIONAL FOOD AND SUPPLEMENT

22.17.1   Energy Drink

In many countries taurine is a component of energy drinks sold under various brands. These energy drinks generally include taurine and caffeine among the ingredients and significantly improve aerobic endurance. Significant improvements in mental performance include choice reaction time, concentration, and memory, and increased subjective alertness [218, 219].

Besides providing extra energy, taurine has been evaluated as an antimanic agent and mood modifier [220]. Caffeinated and taurine-containing beverage produced improved attention and verbal reasoning than with sugar-free and sugar-containing drinks. Another important finding was the reduction in the variability of intentional performance between participants.

Today the entire global market is flooded with products containing taurine only or in combination with oriental medicine to modern medicine and herbal products. These taurine-containing products are generally in the form of capsules, tablets, or drinks.

However, some papers have indicated that consumption of these products, in excess, is associated with undesirable effects such as increase in the mean arterial blood pressure and lower heart rate [221]. Very recently, a study involving four subjects reported individuals had discrete seizure on several occasions following high consumption of energy drink. The symptoms disappeared when the subjects stopped consuming those beverages [222].

22.17.2 Meat and Fish Enrichment with Taurine

In several cases, tumbling food has been used to introduce additional value in food. For example in the meat industry, meat pieces are treated in a solution (e.g., brine or pickle) to enrich it with some component of the solution. Meat or other foods are positioned in a slow, rotating stainless steel cylinder under vacuum for a certain time. In the case of taurine-enriched fish, tumbling in a solution of taurine (7.5% w/v), with polyphosphate, is used to introduce additional taurine into different fish. Tuna was the first fish to be treated in this manner. After the tumbling treatment, the fish were then subjected to four post-tumbling process treatments: frozen at 90°C (5 days); chilled at 4°C (6 days); freeze-chilled at -20°C (5 days) and 4°C (6 days); and cooked at 90°C (10 min). The level of taurine retention was measured in cooked (microwaved) and uncooked samples. A taurine content of about 800 to 1000 mg/100 g (w/w) was achieved in the tumbled tuna portions that underwent the post-tumbling process treatment. With these processes, taurine content can increase considerably, and have been found in the following order: plaice, 100 to 160 mg/100 g (w/w); cod, 60 to 100; mackerel, 60 to 80; farmed salmon, 40 to 60.

22.17.3 γ-Glutamyl Taurine

Another example of enrichment is represented by a natural peptide of taurine, γ-glutamyl-taurine (γGT) which takes part in magnesium homeostasis [223]. Along with taurine, it is also a candidate of inherent functionality. A technique for manufacturing γGT-enriched fish sauce has been developed. A salt-free sauce was produced by mixing alkalase, fermented fish meat, soy sauce koji, glucose, and dried yeast. An enzyme solution was prepared by hydrolyzing wheat gluten and defatted soybeans, in the presence of alkalase and peptidase. By incubating the salt-free sauce and the enzyme solution with glutaminase, extracted from bread flour and skimmed milk, the γGT-enriched fish sauce was produced. The salt-free fish sauce was found to contain 10 to 20 times more γGT than regular fish sauce.

22.18 CONCLUSIONS

Food and its functional nature are now well defined, and many agents have been identified as functional food components. Sulfur amino acids are one such group of biochemicals that have been shown to offer health benefits and disease prevention. Of the several sulfur amino acids, taurine belongs to a special class. Taurine was proven to have beneficial actions and is involved in regulation mechanisms of a wide spectrum of physiological events from vision to neurological actions and from liver metabolism to osmoregulation. However, it is best known for its antioxidant and anti-inflammatory properties, and is thus able to counteract the principal mechanisms involved in the pathogenesis of several diseases.

The functional nature of taurine has been well addressed in a variety of organs and tissues, such as the brain and central nervous system, heart and cardiovascular system, liver, lungs, and kidneys. In particular, it has preventive and therapeutic roles in diabetes and metabolic bone diseases. Finally, the devastating effects of taurine deficiency during fetal life show its prominent role in normal embryo and newborn development.

Considering the beneficial activity of taurine, a large number of taurine derivatives/ analogs and functional food products have been produced and analyzed for their functional properties. However, this growing field of research needs expansion and enlargement, especially more extended clinical trials, in order to highlight the real potential of this fascinating amino acid.

REFERENCES

1. Arai, S., Morinaga, Y., Yoshikawa, T., Ichiishi, E., Kiso, Y., Yamazaki, M., Morotomi, M., Shimizu, M., Kuwata, T., Kaminogawa, S. (2002). Recent trends in functional food science and the industry in Japan. *Bioscience, Biotechnology, and Biochemistry*, 66(10), 2017–2029.

2. Bellisle, F., Diplock, A.T., Hornstra, G., Koletzoko, M. (1998). Functional food science in Europe. *British Journal of Nutrition*, 80, S1–SI93.

3. Carlos, K.B.F. (2004). Functional foods, herbs, and nutraceuticals towards biochemical mechanisms of healthy aging. *Biogerontology*, 5, 275–289.

4. Van de Poll, M.C., Dejong, C.H., Soeters, P.B. (2006). Adequate range for sulfur-containing amino acids and biomarkers for their excess: Lessons from enteral and parenteral nutrition. *Journal of Nutrition*, 136(Suppl), 1694S–1700S.

5. Fukagawa, N.K. (2006). Sparing of methionine requirements: Evaluation of human data takes sulfur amino acids beyond protein. *Journal of Nutrition*, 136(Suppl), 1676S–1681S.

6. Heird, W.C. (2004). Taurine in neonatal nutrition-revisited. *Archives of Disease in Childhood. Fetal and Neonatal Edition*, 89, F473–F474.

7. Gupta, R.C., Kim, S.J. (2003). Role of taurine in organs' dysfunction and in their alleviation. *Critical Care and Shock*, 6, 171–175.

8. Sturman, J.A. (1993). Taurine in development. *Physiological Reviews*, 73, 119–147.

9. Spaeth, D.G., Schneider, D.L., Sarett, H.P. (1974). Taurine synthesis, concentration, and bile salt conjugation in rat, guinea pig, and rabbit. *Proceedings of the Society for Experimental Biology and Medicine*, 147, 855–858.

10. Chorazy-Massalska, M., Kontny, E., Kornatka, A., Rell-Bakalarska, M., Marcinkiewicz, J., Maśliński, W. (2004). The effect of taurine chloromine on pro-inflammatory cytokine production by peripheral blood mononuclear cell isolated from rheumatoid arthritis and osteoarthritis patients. *Clinical and Experimental Rheumatology*, 22(6), 692–698.

11. Kontny, E., Szczepanska, K., Kowalczewski, J., Kurowska, M., Janicka, I., Marcinkiewicz, J., Maslinski, W. (2000). The mechanism of taurine chloramine inhibition of cytokine (interleukin-6, interleukin-8) production by rheumatoid fibroblast-like synoviocytes. *Arthritis and Rheumatism*, 43, 2169–2177.

12. Schaffer, S., Takahashi, K., Azuma, J. (2000). Role of osmoregulation in the actions of taurine. *Amino Acids*, 19(3–4), 527–546.

13. Redmond, H.P., Stapleton, P.P., Neary, P., Bouchier-Hayes, D. (1998). Immunonutrition: The role of taurine. *Nutrition*, 14, 599–604.

14. Huxtable, R.J. (1989). Taurine in the central nervous system and the mammalian actions of taurine. *Progress in Neurobiology, 32*, 471–533.

15. Huxtable, R.J. (1992). Physiological action of taurine. *Physiochemical Reviews, 72*, 101–163.

16. Huxtable, R.J. (1981). Physio-chemical properties of taurine. *Advanced Experimental Medicine and Biology, 139*, 1–4.

17. Huxtable, R.J. (1986). Taurine and the oxidative metabolism of cysteine. In Huxtable, R.J., ed., *Biochemistry of Sulfur*, pp. 121–198. New York: Plenum Press.

18. Tang, X.W., Hsu, C.C., Schloss, J.V., Morris, D.F., Faiman, M.D., Wu, E., Yang, C.Y., Wu, J.Y. (1997). Protein phosphorylation and taurine biosynthesis in vivo and in vitro. *Journal of Neuroscience, 17*, 6947–6951.

19. Wu, J., Chen, W.C., Tang, X.W., Jin, H., Foos, T., Schloss, J.V., Davis, K., Faiman, M.D., Hsu, C.C. (2000). Mode of action of taurine and regulation dynamics of its synthesis in the CNS. In Della Corte, L., Huxtable, R.J., Sgaragli, G., Tipton, K.F., eds., *Taurine*, 4th edition, pp. 35–44. New York: Kluwer Academic.

20. Huxtable, R.J., Laird, H., Lippincott, S.E. (1979). The transport of taurine in the heart and the rapid depletion of tissue taurine content by guanidinoethyl sulfonate. *Journal of Pharmacological Experiments and Therapy, 211*(3), 465–471.

21. Leibach, J.W., Cool, D.R., Dal Monte, M.A., Granapathy, V., Leibach, F.H., Miyamoto, Y. (1993). Properties of taurine transport in a human retinal pigment epithelial cell line. *Current Eye Research, 12*, 29–36.

22. Holopainen, I., Kontro, P., Frey, H.J., Oja, S.S. (1983). Taurine, hypotaurine, and GABA uptake by cultured neuroblastoma cells. *Journal of Neuroscience Research, 10*(1), 83–92.

23. Yan, C.C., Masella, R., Sun, Y., Cantafora, A. (1991). Transport and function of taurine in mammalian cells and tissue. *Acta Toxicologica et Therapeutica, 12*, 277–298.

24. Libby, P. (2007). Inflammatory mechanisms: The molecular basis of inflammation and disease. *Nutrition Reviews, 65*, S140–S146.

25. Ho, H.Y., Cheng, M.L., Chiu, D.T. (2007). Glucose-6-phosphate dehydrogenase: From oxidative stress to cellular functions and degenerative diseases. *Redox Report: Communications in Free Radical Research, 12*, 109–118.

26. Fang, Y.Z., Yang, S., Wu, G. (2002). Free radicals, antioxidants, and nutrition. *Nutrition, 18*, 872–879.

27. Evans, P., Halliwell, B. (2001). Micronutrients: Oxidant/antioxidant status. *British Journal of Nutrition, 85*(2), S67–S74.

28. Andrews, P.C., Krinky, N.I. (1982). A kinetic analysis of the interaction of human myeloperoxidase with hydrogen peroxide, chloride ions, and protons. *Journal of Biological Chemistry, 257*, 13240–13245.

29. Schaffer, S., Azuma, J., Takahashi, K., Mozzafari, M. (2003). Why is taurine cytoprotective? *Advances in Experimental Medicine and Biology, 526*, 307–321.

30. Malle, E., Furtmuller, P.G., Sattler, W., Obinger, C. (2007). Myeloperoxidase: A target for a new drug development? *British Journal of Pharmacology, 152*, 838–854.

31. Cantin, A.M. (1994). Taurine modulation of hypochlorous acid-induced lung epithelial cell injury in vitro. Role of anion transport. *Journal of Clinical Investigation, 93*, 606–614.

32. Marcinkiewicz, J., Grabowska, A., Bereta, J., Stelmaszynska, T. (1995). Taurinechloramine, a product of activated neutrophils inhibits in vitro generation of

nitric oxide and other macrophage inflammatory mediators. *Journal of Leukocyte Biology*, *58*, 667–674.

33. Lima, L. (1999). Taurine and its tropic effects in the retina. *Neurochemical Research*, *25*, 1333–1338.

34. Stapleton, P.P., O'Flaherty, L., Redmond, A.P., Boucher-Hays, D.J. (1998). Host defense. A role for the amino acid taurine? *Journal of Parenteral and Enteral Nutrition*, *22*, 42–48.

35. Weiss, S.J., Lampert, M.B., Test, S.T. (1983). Long-lived oxidants generated by human neutrophils: Characterization and bioactivity. *Science*, *222*, 625–628.

36. Gupta, R.C., Seki, Y., Yosida, J. (2006). Role of taurine in spinal cord injury. *Current Neurovascular Research*, *3*, 225–235.

37. Schuller-Levis, G.B., Park, E. (2004). Taurine and its chloramine: Modulators of immunity. *Neurochemistry Research*, *29*, 117–126.

38. Kim, J.W., Kim, C. (2005). Inhibition of LPS-induced NO production by taurine chloramine in macrophages is mediated through Ras-ERK-NF-κB. *Biochemical Pharmacology*, *70*, 1352–1360.

39. Quinn, M.R., Park, E., Schuller-Levis, G. (1996). Taurine chloramine inhibits prostaglandin E_2 production in activated macrophages RAW 2647 cells by posttranscriptional effects on inducible cycloxigenase expression. *Immunology Letters*, *50*, 185–188.

40. Park, E., Alberti, J., Quinn, M.R., Schuller-Levis, G. (1998). Taurine chloramine inhibits the production of superoxide anion, IL-6 and IL-8 in activated human polymorphonuclear leukocytes. *Advances in Experimental Medicine and Biology*, *442*, 177–182.

41. Kontny, E., Wojtecka-Lukasik, E., Rell-Bakalarska, K., Dziewczopolski, W., Maśliński, W., Maślinski, S. (2002). Impaired generation of taurine chloramine by synovial fluid neutrophils of rheumatoid arthritis patients. *Amino Acids*, *23*, 415–418.

42. Yarbrough, G.G., Singh, D.K., Taylor, D.A. (1979). Neuropharmacological characterization of taurine antagonist. *Journal of Pharmacological Experiments and Therapy*, *219*(3), 604–613.

43. Braghiroli, D., Di Bella, M., Zanoli, P., Truzzi, C., Baraldi, M. (1990). Rigid analogs of taurine as potential taurine antagonists. *Farmaco*, *45*(6), 631–635.

44. Warskulat, U., Heller-Stilb, B., Oermann, E., Zilles, K., Haas, H., Lang, F., Haussinger, D. (2007). Phenotype of the taurine transporter knockout mouse. *Methods in Enzymology*, *428*, 439–458.

45. Militante, J., Lombardini, J.B. (2004). Age-related retinal degeneration in animal models of aging: Possible involvement of taurine deficiency and oxidative stress. *Neurochemistry Research*, *29*, 151–160.

46. Schaffer, S., Solodushko, V., Azuma, J. (2000). Taurine-deficient cardiomyopathy: Role of phospholipids, calcium and osmotic stress. *Advances in Experimental Medicine and Biology*, *483*, 57–69.

47. McCarty, M.F. (2004). Sub-optimal taurine status may promote platelet hyperaggregability in vegetarians. *Medical Hypotheses*, *63*, 426–433.

48. Dawson, J.K. (2003). Taurine in aging and models of neurodegeneration. *Advances in Experimental Medicine and Biology*, *526*, 537–544.

49. Dawson, R., Jr., Liu, S., Eppler, B., Patterson, T. (1999). Effects of dietary taurine supplementation or deprivation in aged male Fischer 344 rats. *Mechanisms of Ageing and Development*, *107*, 73–91.

50. Pierno, S., De Luca, A., Camerino, C., Huxtable, R.J., Camerino, C.D. (1998). Chronic administration of taurine to aged rats improves the electrical and contractile properties of skeletal muscles fibres. *Journal of Pharmacology and Experimental Therapeutics*, *286*, 1183–1190.

51. Warskulat, U., Borsch, E., Reinehr, R., Heller-Stilb, B., Roth, C., Witt, M., Haussinger, D. (2007). Taurine deficiency and apoptosis: Findings from the taurine transporter knockout mouse. *Archives of Biochemistry and Biophysics*, *462*(2), 202–209.

52. Sturman, J.A., Moretz, R.C., French, J.H., Wisniewski, H.M. (1985). Taurine deficiency in the developing cat: Persistence of the cerebellar external granule cell layer. *Journal of Neuroscience Research*, *13*(3), 405–416.

53. Aerts, L., Van Assche, F.A. (2002). Taurine and taurine-deficiency in the perinatal period. *Journal of Perinatal Medicine*, *30*(4), 281–286.

54. Gaull, G.E., Wright, C.E., Tallan, H.H. (1983). Taurine in human lymphoblastoid cells: Uptake and role in proliferation. *Progress in Clinical Biology Research*, *125*, 297–303.

55. Hunter, E.G. (1986). Adult ventricular myocytes isolated from CHF 146 and CHF 147 cardiomyopathic hamsters. *Canadian Journal of Physiology and Pharmacology*, *64*(12), 1503–1506.

56. Guerin, P., El Mouatassim, S., Menezo, Y. (2001). Oxidative stress and protection against reactive oxygen species in the pre-implantation embryo and its surroundings. *Human Reproduction Update*, *7*, 175–189.

57. Mansani, F.E., Cavatorta, E., Ceruti, M., Condemi, V.C. (1975). Maternal and foetal amino acidaemia and amino acids contents of amniotic fluid in normal, gestosic and diabetic pregnancy. *L'Ateneo Parmense. Acta Bio-Medica*, *46*(6), 545–569.

58. Roos, S., Powell, T.L., Jansson, T. (2004). Human placental taurine transporter in uncomplicated and IUGR pregnancies: Cellular localization, protein expression, and regulation. *American Journal of Physiology. Regulatory, Integrative, and Comparative Physiology*. *287*(4), R886–R893.

59. Dhillon, S.K., Davies, W.E., Hopkins, P.C., Rose, S.J. (1998). Effects of dietary taurine on auditory function in full term infants. *Advances in Experimental Medicine and Biology*, *442*, 507–514.

60. Wharton, B.A., Morley, R., Isaacs, E.B., Cole, T.J., Lucan, A. (2004). Low plasma taurine and later neurodevelopment. *Archives of Disease in Childhood. Fetal and Neonatal Edition*, *89*, F497–F498.

61. Howard, D., Thompson, D.F. (1992). Taurine: An essential amino acid to prevent cholestasis in neonates? *Annals of Pharmacotherapy*, *26*, 1390–1392.

62. Aerts, L., Van Assche, F.A. (2001). Low taurine, γ-aminobutyric acid and carnosine levels in plasma of diabetic pregnant rats: Consequences for the offspring. *Journal of Perinatal Medicine*, *29*(1), 81–84.

63. Rivero Urgell, M., Santamaría Orleans, A., Rodríguez-Palmero Seuma, M. (2005). The importance of functional ingredients in pediatric milk formulas and cereals. *Nutrición Hospitalaria*, *20*, 135–146.

64. Eshach Adiv, O., Berant, M., Shamir, R. (2004). New supplements to infant formulas. *Pediatric Endocrinology Reviews*, *2*(2), 216–224.

65. Schaffer, S.W., Solodushko, V., Kakhniashvili, D. (2002). Beneficial effect of taurine depletion on osmotic sodium and calcium loading during chemical hypoxia. *American Journal of Physiology. Cell Physiology*, *282*(5), C1113–C1120.

66. Shen, E.Y., Lai, Y.J., Ho, C.S., Lee, Y.L. (1999). Excitatory and inhibitory amino acid levels in the cerebrospinal fluids of children with neurological disorders. *Acta Paediatrica Taiwanica*, *40*(2), 65–69.

67. Qureshi, G.A., Baig, S.M., Bednar, I., Halawa, A., Parvez, S.H. (1998). The neurochemical markers in cerebrospinal fluid to differentiate between aseptic and tuberculous meningitis. *Neurochemistry International*, *32*(2), 197–203.

68. Moreno-Fuenmayor, H., Borjas, L., Arrieta, A., Valera, V., Socorro-Candanoza, L. (1996). Plasma excitatory amino acids in autism. *Investigación Clínica*, *37*(2), 113–128.

69. Barbeau, A., Donaldson, J. (1974). Zinc, taurine, and epilepsy. *Archives of Neurology*, *30*(1), 52–58.

70. Airaksinen, E.M., Oja, S.S., Marnela, K.M., Leino, E., Paakkonen, L. (1980). Effect of taurine treatment on epileptic patients. *Progress in Clinical and Biological Research*, *39*, 157–166.

71. Azuma, J., Hasegawa, H., Sawamura, A., Awata, N., Ogura, K., Harada, H., Yamamura, Y., Kishimoto, S. (1983). Therapy of congestive heart failure with orally administered taurine. *Clinical Therapeutics*, *5*, 398–408.

72. Azuma, J., Takihara, K., Awata, N., Ohta, H., Sawamura, A., Harada, H., Kishimoto, S. (1984). Beneficial effect of taurine on congestive heart failure induced by chronic aortic regurgitation in rabbits. *Research Communications in Chemical Pathology and Pharmacology*, *45*, 261–270.

73. Singh, R.B., Kartikey, K., Charu, A.S., Niaz, M.A., Schaffer, S. (2003). Effect of taurine and coenzyme Q10 in patients with acute myocardial infarction. *Advances in Experimental Medicine and Biology*, *526*, 41–48.

74. Militante, J.D., Bombardini, J.B. (2002). Treatment of hypertension with oral taurine: Experimental and clinical studies. *Amino Acids*, *23*, 381–393.

75. Franconi, F., Bennardini, F., Mattana, A., Miceli, M., Ciuti, M., Mian, M., Gironi, A., Anichimi, R., Seghieri, G. (1995). Plasma and platelet taurine are reduced in subjects with insulin-dependent diabetes mellitus: Effects of taurine supplementation. *American Journal of Clinical Nutrition*, *61*, 1115–1119.

76. McCarty, M.F. (1999). The reported clinical utility of taurine in ischemic disorders may reflect a down-regulation of neutrophil activation and adhesion. *Medical Hypothesis*, *53*(4), 290–299.

77. McCarty, M.F. (2004). A taurine-supplemented vegan diet may blunt the contribution of neutrophil activation to acute coronary events. *Medical Hypothesis*, *63*, 419–425.

78. Fennessy, F.M., Moneley, D.S., Wang, J.S., Kelly, C.J., Bouchier-Hayes, D.J. (2002). Taurine and vitamin C modify monocyte and endothelial dysfunction in young smokers. *Circulation*, *107*, 410–415.

79. Olive, M.F. (2002). Interactions between taurine and ethanol in the central nervous system. *Amino Acids*, *23*, 345–357.

80. Barbeau, A., Inoue, N., Tsukada, Y., Butterworth, R.F. (1975). The neuropharmacology of taurine. *Life Science*, *17*, 669–677.

81. Gupta, R.C., Win, T., Bittner, S. (2005). Taurine analogues a new class of therapeutics: Retrospect and prospects. *Current Medicinal Chemistry*, *12*, 2021–2039.

82. Huxtable, R.J. (1981). Insights on function: Metabolism and pharmacology of taurine in the brain. *Progress in Clinical and Biological Research*, *68*, 53–97.

83. Wu, J., Kohno, T., Georgiev, S.K., Ikoma, M., Ishii, H., Petrenko, A.B., Baba, H. (2008). Taurine activates glycine and γ-aminobutyric acid A receptors in rat substantia gelatinosa neurons. *Neuroreport, 19*(3), 333–337.

84. Jia, F., Yue, M., Chandra, D., Keramidas, A., Goldstein, P.A., Homanics, G.E., Harrison, N.L. (2008). Taurine is a potent activator of extrasynaptic GABA(A) receptors in the thalamus. *Journal of Neuroscience, 28*(1), 106–115.

85. Lima, L., Obregon, F., Cubillos, S., Fazzino, F., Jaimes, I. (2001). Taurine as a micronutrient in development and regeneration of the central nervous system. *Nutritional Neuroscience, 4*(6), 439–443.

86. Hussy, N., Deleuze, C., Bres, V., Moos, F.C. (2000). New role of taurine as an osmomediator between glial cells and neurons in the rat supraoptic nucleus. *Advances in Experimental Medicine and Biology, 483*, 227–237.

87. Howland, R.H. (2007). Glutamate-modulating drugs and the treatment of mental disorders. *Journal of Psychosocial Nursing and Mental Health Services, 45*(1), 11–14.

88. Coyle, J.T. (2006). Substance use disorders and schizophrenia: A question of shared glutamatergic mechanisms. *Neurotoxicity Research, 10*(3–4), 221–233.

89. Garcia Dopico, J., Perdomo Diaz, J., Alonso, T.J., Gonzales Hernandez, T., Castro Fuentes, R., Rodriguez Diaz, M. (2004). Extracellular taurine in the substantia nigra: Taurine-glutamate interaction. *Journal of Neuroscience Research, 76*(4), 528–538.

90. Albrecht, J., Schousboe, A. (2005). Taurine interaction with neurotransmitter receptors in the CNS. An update. *Neurochemistry Research, 30*, 1615–1621.

91. Van Gelder, M.N. (1983). A central mechanism of action for taurine, osmoregulation, bivalent cations, and excitation threshold. *Neurochemical Research, 8*, 687–699.

92. Konto, P., Oja, S.S. (1981). Properties of hypotaurine uptake in mouse brain slices. *Advances in Experimental Medicine and Biology, 139*, 115–126.

93. Biasetti, M., Dawson, R., Jr. (2002). Effects of sulfur containing amino acids on iron and nitric oxide stimulated catecholamine oxidation. *Amino Acids, 22*(4), 351–368.

94. Wu, H., Jin, Y., Wei, J., Jin, H., Sha, D., Wu, J.Y. (2005). Mode of action of taurine as a neuroprotector. *Brain Research, 1038*(2), 123–131.

95. Arai, H., Kobayashi, K., Ichimiya, Y., Kosaka, K., Iizuka, R. (1984). A preliminary study of free amino acids in the postmortem temporal cortex from Alzheimer-type dementia patients. *Neurobiology of Aging, 5*, 319–321.

96. Alom, J., Mahy, J.N., Brandi, N., Tolosa, E. (1991). Cerebrospinal fluid taurine in Alzheimer's disease. *Annals of Neurology, 30*, 735.

97. Louzada, P.R., Lima, A.C., Mendonca-Silva, D.L., Noel, F., De Mello, F.G., Ferreira, S.T. (2004). Taurine prevents the neurotoxicity of beta-amyloid and glutamate receptor agonists: Activation of GABA receptors and possible implications for Alzheimer's disease and other neurological disorders. *FASEB Journal, 18*, 511–518.

98. Santa-Maria, I., Hernandez, F., Moreno, F.J., Avila, J. (2007). Taurine, an inducer for tau polymerization and a weak inhibitor for amyloid-beta-peptide aggregation. *Neuroscience Letters, 429*(2–3), 91–94.

99. Ramalho, R.M., Viana, R.J., Low, W.C., Steer, C.J., Rodrigues, C.M. (2008). Bile acids and apoptosis modulation: An emerging role in experimental Alzheimer's disease. *Trends in Molecular Medicine, 14*, 54–62.

100. Gaby, A.R. (2007). Natural approaches to epilepsy. *Alternative Medicine Review. 12*(1), 19–24.

101. Trenkner, E., El Idrissi, A., Harris, C. (1996). Balanced interaction of growth factors and taurine regulate energy metabolism, neuronal survival, and function of cultured mouse cerebellar cells under depolarizing conditions. *Advances in Experimental Medicine and Biology*, *403*, 507–517.

102. Hehre, D.A., Devia, C.J., Bancalari, E., Suguihara, C. (2008). Brainstem amino acid neurotransmitters and ventilatory response to hypoxia in piglets. *Pediatric Research*, *63*, 46–50.

103. Petty, M.A., Di Francesco, G.F. (1989). The cardiovascular effects of centrally administered taurine in anaesthetised and conscious rats. *European Journal of Pharmacology*, *162*, 359–364.

104. Frosini, M., Ricci, L., Saponara, S., Palmi, M., Valoti, M., Sgaragli, G. (2006). GABA-mediated effects of some taurine derivatives injected i.c.v. on rabbit rectal temperature and gross motor behavior. *Amino Acids*, *30*(3), 233–242.

105. Sgaragli, G.P., Palmi, M. (1985). The role and mechanism of action of taurine in mammalian thermoregulation. *Progress in Clinical and Biological Research*, *179*, 343–357.

106. Frosini, M. (2007). Changes in CSF composition during heat stress and fever in conscious rabbits. *Progress in Brain Research*, *162*, 449–457.

107. Pellicer, F., Lopez-Avila, A., Coffeen, U., Manuel-Ortega-Legaspi, J., Angel, R.D. (2007). Taurine in the anterior cingulate cortex diminishes neuropathic nociception: A possible interaction with the glycine(A) receptor. *European Journal of Pain*, *11(4)*, 444–451.

108. Mandel, P., Gupta, R.C., Bourguignon, J.J., Wermuth, C.G., Molina, V., Gobaille, S., Ciesielski, L., Similer, S. (1985). Effect of taurine and taurine analogs on aggressive behavior. *Progress in Clinical and Biological Research*, *179*, 449–458.

109. McCool, B.A., Chappell, A. (2007). Strychnine and taurine modulation of amygdala-associated anxiety-like behavior is "state" dependent. *Behavioural Brain Research*, *178*(1), 70–81.

110. Zhang, C.G., Kim, S.J. (2007). Taurine induces anti-anxiety by activating strychnine-sensitive glycine receptor in vivo. *Annals of Nutrition and Metabolism*, *51*(4), 379–386.

111. Canas, P.E. (1992). The role of taurine and its derivatives on cellular hypoxia: A physiological view. *Acta Physiologica, Pharmacologica et Therapeutica Latinoamericana*, *42*, 133–137.

112. Nakada, T., Hida, K., Kwee, I.L. (1992). Brain pH and lactic acidosis: Quantitative analysis of taurine effect. *Neuroscience Research*, *15*(1–2), 115–123.

113. Saransaari, P., Oja, S.S. (2007). Taurine release in mouse brain stem slices under cell-damaging conditions. *Amino Acids*, *32*(3), 439–446.

114. Zhao, P., Qian, H., Xia, Y. (2005). GABA and glycine are protective to mature but toxic to immature rat cortical neurons under hypoxia. *European Journal of Neuroscience*, *22*(2), 289–300.

115. Ferko, A.P. (1987). Ethanol-induced sleep time: Interaction with taurine and a taurine antagonist. *Pharmacology, Biochemistry, and Behavior*, *27*(2), 235–238.

116. Kukorelli, T., Feuer, L., Juhasz, G., Detari, L. (1986). Effect of glutaurine on sleep-wakefulness cycle and aggressive behaviour in the cat. *Acta Physiologica Hungarica*, *67*(1), 31–35.

117. El Idrissi, A. (2008). Taurine improves learning and retention in aged mice. *Neuroscience Letters*, *436*(1), 19–22.

118. Suge, R., Hosoe, N., Furube, M., Yamamoto, T., Hirayama, A., Hirano, S., Nomura, M. (2007). Specific timing of taurine supplementation affects learning ability in mice. *Life Science*, *81*(15), 1228–1234.

119. Kranzler, H.R., Gage, A. (2008). Acamprosate efficacy in alcohol-dependent patients: Summary of results from three pivotal trials. *American Journal on Addictions*, *17*(1), 70–76.

120. Rosner, S., Leucht, S., Lehert, P., Soyka, M. (2008). Acamprosate supports abstinence, naltrexone prevents excessive drinking: Evidence from a meta-analysis with unreported outcomes. *Journal of Psychopharmacology*, *22*(1), 11–23.

121. Han, D.H., Lyool, I.K., Sung, Y.H., Lee, S.H., Renshaw, P.F. (2008). The effect of acamprosate on alcohol and food craving in patients with alcohol dependence. *Drug Alcohol Depend*, *93*(3), 279–283.

122. Laaksonen, E., Koski-Jannes, A., Salaspuro, M., Ahtinen, H., Alho, H. (2008). A randomized, multicentre, open-label, comparative trial of disulfiram, naltrexone and acamprosate in the treatment of alcohol dependence. *Alcohol*, *43*(1), 53–61.

123. Boothby, L.A., Doering, P.L. (2005). Acamprosate for the treatment of alcohol dependence. *Clinical Therapeutics*, *27*(6), 695–714.

124. Sgaragli, G., Frosini, M., Palmi, M., Bianchi, L., Della-Corte, L. (1994). Calcium and taurine interaction in mammalian brain metabolism. *Advances in Experimental Medicine and Biology*, *359*, 299–308.

125. Vohra, B.P., Hui, X. (2001). Taurine protects against carbon tetrachloride toxicity in the cultured neurons and in vivo. *Archives of Physiology and Biochemistry*, *109*(1), 90–94.

126. Nakai, T., Katagiri, K., Hoshino, M., Hayakawa, T., Ohiwa, T. (1992). Microtubule-independent choleresis and anti-cholestatic action of tauroursodeoxycholate in colchicines rat liver. *Biochemical Journal*, *288*, 613–617.

127. Haslewood, G.A.D. (1978). The biological importance of bile salts. *Quarterly Review of Biology*, *54*(4), 445–446.

128. Leuschner, U. (1992). Oral bile acid treatment of biliary cholesterol stones. *Recenti Progressi in Medicina*, *83*, 392–399.

129. Murakami, S., Kondo, Y., Nagate, T. (2000). Effects of long-term treatment with taurine in mice fed a high-fat diet: Improvement in cholesterol metabolism and vascular lipid accumulation by taurine. *Advances in Experimental Medicine and Biology*, *483*, 177–186.

130. Tsuboyama-Kasaoka, N., Shozawa, C., Sano, K., Kamei, Y., Kasaoka, S., Hosokawa, Y., Ezaki, O. (2006). Taurine (2-aminoethanesulfonic acid) deficiency creates a vicious circle promoting obesity. *Endocrinology*, *147*(7), 3276–3284.

131. Zhang, M., Bi, L.F., Fang, J.H., Su, X.L., Da, G.L., Kuwamori, T., Kagamimori, S., (2004). Beneficial effects of taurine on serum lipids in overweight or obese non-diabetic subjects. *Amino Acids*, *26*(3), 267–271.

132. Brons, C., Spohr, C., Storgaard, H., Dyerberg, J., Vaag, A. (2004). Effect of taurine treatment on insulin secretion and action, and on serum lipid levels in overweight men with a genetic predisposition for type II diabetes mellitus. *European Journal of Clinical Nutrition*, *58*(9), 1239–1247.

133. Lee, M.Y., Cheong, S.H., Chang, K.J., Choi, M.J., Kim, S.K. (2003). Effect of the obesity index on plasma taurine levels in Korean female adolescents. *Advances in Experimental Medicine and Biology*, *526*, 285–290.

134. Obinata, K., Maruyama, T., Hayashi, M., Watanabe, T., Nittono, H. (1996). Effect of taurine on the fatty liver of children with simple obesity. *Advances in Experimental Medicine and Biology*, *403*, 607–613.

135. Yokogoshi, H., Mochizuki, H., Nanami, K., Hida, Y., Miyachi, F., Oda, H. (1999). Dietary taurine enhances cholesterol degradation and reduces serum and liver cholesterol concentrations in rats fed a high-cholesterol diet. *Journal of Nutrition*, *129*(9), 1705–1712.

136. Choi, M.J., Kim, J.H., Chang, K.J. (2006). The effect of dietary taurine supplementation on plasma and liver lipid concentrations and free amino acid concentrations in rats fed a high-cholesterol diet. *Advances in Experimental Medicine and Biology*, *583*, 235–242.

137. Mochizuki, H., Oda, H., Yokogoshi, H. (1998). Increasing effect of dietary taurine on the serum HDL-cholesterol concentration in rats. *Bioscience, Biotechnology, and Biochemistry*, *62*(3), 578–579.

138. Kishida, T., Ishikawa, H., Tsukaoka, M., Ohga, H., Ogawa, H., Ebihara, K. (2003). Increase of bile acids synthesis and excretion caused by taurine administration prevents the ovariectomy-induced increase in cholesterol concentrations in the serum low-density lipoprotein fraction of Wistar rats. *Journal of Nutritional Biochemistry*, *14*(1), 7–16.

139. Yokogoshi, H., Oda, H. (2002). Dietary taurine enhances cholesterol degradation and reduces serum and liver cholesterol concentrations in rats fed a high-cholesterol diet. *Amino Acid*, *23*, 433–439.

140. Hu, Y.H., Lin, C.L., Huang, Y.W., Liu, P.E., Hwang, D.F. (2008). Dietary amino acid taurine ameliorates liver injury in chronic hepatitis patients. *Amino Acids*, *35*, 469–473.

141. Wu, C., Miyagawa, C., Kennedy, D.O. (1997). Involvement of polyamines in the protection of taurine against the cytotoxicity of hydrazine or carbon tetrachloride in isolated rat hepatocytes. *Chemico-Biological Interactions*, *103*, 213–224.

142. Baiocchi, L., Tisone, G., Russo, M.A., Longhi, C., Palmieri, G., Volpe, A., Almerighi, C., Telesca, C., Carbone, M., Toti, L., Leonardis, F.D., Angelico, M. (2008). TUDCA prevents cholestasis and canalicular damage induced by ischemia-reperfusion injury in the rat, modulating PKCalpha-ezrin pathway. *Transplant International*, *21*, 792–800.

143. Puls, T., Vennegeerts, T., Wimmer, R., Denk, G.U., Beuers, U., Rust, C. (2008). Tauroursodeoxycholic acid reduces bile acid-induced apoptosis by modulation of AP-1. *Biochemical and Biophysical Research Communications*, *367*(1), 208–212.

144. Waters, E., Wang, J.H., Redmond, H.P., Wu, Q.D., Kay, E., Bouchier-Hayes, D. (2001). Role of taurine in preventing acetaminophen-induced hepatic injury in the rat. *American Journal of Physiology. Gastrointestinal and Liver Physiology*, *280*(6), G1274–G1279.

145. Gurijeyalakshmi, G., Wang, Y., Giri, S.N. (2000). Suppression of bleomicin-induced nitric oxide production in mice by taurine and niacin. *Nitric Oxides*, *4*(4), 399–411.

146. Miyazaki, T., Karube, M., Matsuzaki, Y., Ikegami, T., Doy, M., Tanaka, N., Bouscarel, B. (2005). Taurine inhibits oxidative damage and prevents fibrosis in carbon tetrachloride-induced hepatic fibrosis. *Journal of Hepatology*, *43*(1), 117–125.

147. Kelly, G.S. (2000). Insulin resistance: Lifestyle and nutritional interventions. *Alternative Medicine Review*, *5*, 109–132.

148. Franconi, F., Loizzo, A., Ghirlanda, G., Seghieri, G. (2006). Taurine supplementation and diabetes mellitus. *Current Opinion in Clinical Nutrition and Metabolic Care*, *9*, 32–36.

149. Kim, S.J., Gupta, R.C., Lee, H.W. (2007). Taurine-diabetes interaction: From involvement to protection. *Journal of Biological Regulators and Homeostatic Agents*, *21*(3–4), 63–77.

150. Hansen, S.H. (2001). The role of taurine in diabetes and the development of diabetic complications. *Diabetes and Metabolism Research Reviews, 17*, 330–346.

151. Nandhini, A.T., Thirunavukkarasu, V., Ravichandran, M.K., Anuradha, C.V. (2005). Effects of taurine on biomarkers of oxidative stress in tissues of fructose-fed insulin-resistant rats. *Singapore Medical Journal, 46*, 82–87.

152. Tenner, T.E., Jr., Zhang, X.L., Lombardini, J.B. (2003). Hypoglycemic effects of taurine in the alloxan-treated rabbit: A model for type 1 diabetes. *Advances in Experimental Medicine and Biology, 526*, 97–106.

153. Lampson, W.G., Kramer, J.H., Schaffer, S.W. (1983). Potentiation of the actions of insulin by taurine. *Canadian Journal of Physiology and Pharmacology, 61*, 457–463.

154. Dokshina, G.A., Silaeva, T.I. (1976). Effect of taurine on insulin secretion by the isolated pancreatic tissue of intact and irradiated rats. *Radiobiologiia, 16*, 446–449.

155. Hardikar, A.A., Risbud, M.V., Remacle, C., Reusens, B., Hoct, J.J., Bhonde, R.R. (2001). Islet cryopreservation: Improved recovery following taurine pretreatment. *Cell Transplantion, 10*, 247–253.

156. Cherif, H., Reusens, B., Dahri, S., Remacle, C., Hoet, J.J. (1998). Effects of taurine on the insulin secretion by fetal islets cultured in vitro. *Journal of Endocrinology, 151*, 501–506.

157. Kulakowski, E.C., Maturo, J. (1990). Does taurine bind to the insulin binding site of the insulin receptor? *Progress in Clinical and Biological Research, 351*, 95–102.

158. Nakashima, E., Pop-Busui, R., Towns, R., Thomas, T.P., Hosaka, Y., Nakamura, J., Greene, D.A., Killen, P.D., Schroeder, J., Larkin, D.D., Ho, Y.L., Stevens, M.J. (2005). Regulation of the human taurine transporter by oxidative stress in retinal pigment epithelial cells stably transformed to overexpress aldose reductase. *Antioxidants & Redox Signaling, 7*(11–12), 1530–1542.

159. Szabo, A., Kenesei, E., Korner, A., Miltenyi, M., Szucs, L., Nagy, I. (1991). Changes in plasma and urinary amino acid levels during diabetic ketoacidosis in children. *Diabetes Research and Clinical Practice, 12*, 91–97.

160. Hultman, K., Alexanderson, C., Manneras, L., Sandberg, M., Holmang, A., Jansson, T. (2007). Maternal taurine supplementation in the late pregnant rat stimulates postnatal growth and induces obesity and insulin resistance in adult offspring. *Journal of Physiology, 15*, 823–833.

161. Aerts, L., Van Assche, F.A. (2006). Animal evidence for the transgenerational development of diabetes mellitus. *International Journal of Biochemistry and Cell Biology, 38*, 894–903.

162. Horská, S., Rázová, M., Vondrácek, J. (1980). Amino acids in the amniotic fluid of diabetic mothers. *Biology of the Neonate, 37*, 204–208.

163. Jansson, T., Erkstrand, Y., Bjom, C., Wennergren, M., Powell, T.L. (2002). Alterations in the activity of placental amino acid transporters in pregnancies complicated by diabetes. *Diabetes, 51*, 2214–2219.

164. Chapman, R.A., Suleiman, M.S., Earm, Y.E. (1993). Taurine and the heart. *Cardiovascular Research, 27*, 358–363.

165. Takahashi, K., Azuma, M., Yamada, T., Ohyabu, Y., Takahashi, K., Schaffer, S.W., Azuma, J. (2003). Taurine transporter in primary cultured neonatal rat heart cells: A comparison between cardiac myocytes and nonmyocytes. *Biochemical Pharmacology, 65*, 1181–1187.

166. Takihara, K., Azuma, J., Awata, N., Ohta, H., Hamagichi, T., Sawamura, A., Tanaka, Y., Kishimoto, S., Sperelakis, N. (1986). Beneficial effect of taurine in rabbits with chronic congestive heart failure. *American Heart Journal, 112*, 1278–1284.

167. Hayes, K.C., Trautwein, E.A. (1989). Taurine deficiency syndrome in cats. *Veterinary Clinics of North America. Small Animal Practice, 19*(3), 403–413.

168. Ito, T., Kimura, Y., Uozumi, Y., Takai, M., Muraoka, S., Matsuda, T., Ueki, K., Yoshiyama, M., Ikawa, M., Okabe, M., Schaffer, S.W., Fujio, Y., Azuma, J. (2008). Taurine depletion caused by knocking out the taurine transporter gene leads to cardiomyopathy with cardiac atrophy. *Journal of Molecular and Cellular Cardiology, 44*, 927–937.

169. Takahahsi, K., Azuma, M., Baba, A., Schaffer, S., Azuma, J. (1998). Taurine improves angiotensin II-induced hypertrophy of cultured neonatal rat heart cells. *Advances in Experimental Medicine and Biology, 442*, 129–135.

170. Huxtable, R.J., Sebring, L.A. (1986). Towards a unifying theory for the action of taurine. *Trends in Pharmacological Science, 7*, 481–485.

171. Schaffer, S.W., Punna, S., Duan, J, Harada, H., Hamaguchi, T., Azuma, J. (1992). Mechanism underlying physiological modulation of myocardial contraction by taurine. *Advances in Experimental Medicine and Biology, 315*, 193–198.

172. Huxtable, R.J., Sebring, L.A. (1989). Taurine and the heart: the phospholipid connection. In: Iwata, H., Lombardini, J.B., Segawa, T., eds., *Taurine and the Heart*, pp. 31–42. New York: Kluwer Academic Publishers.

173. Welty, M.C., Welty, J.D., McBroom, M.J. (1982). Effect of isoproterenol and taurine on heart calcium in normal and cardiomyopathic hamsters. *Journal of Molecular and Cellular Cardiology, 14*, 353–357.

174. Azuma, J., Sawamura, A., Awata, N. (1992). Usefulness of taurine in chronic congestive heart failure and its prospective application. *Japanese Circulation Journal, 56*(1), 95–99.

175. Allard, M.L., Jeejeebhoy, K.N., Sole, M.J. (2006). The management of conditioned nutritional requirements in heart failure. *Heart Failure Reviews, 11*(1), 75–82.

176. Ahn, C.S., Kim, E.S. (2003). Effect of alpha-tocopherol and taurine supplementation on oxidized LDL levels of middle aged Korean women during aerobic exercise. *Advances in Experimental Medicine and Biology, 526*, 269–276.

177. Pechanova, O., Simko, F. (2007). The role of nitric oxide in the maintenance of vasoactive balance. *Physiological Research, 56*(2), S7–S16.

178. Ulrich-Merzenich, G., Zeitler, H., Vetter, H., Bhonde, R.R. (2007). Protective effects of taurine on endothelial cells impaired by high glucose and oxidized low density lipoproteins. *European Journal of Nutrition, 46*, 431–438.

179. Mehta, T.R., Dawson, R., Jr. (2001). Taurine is a weak scavenger of peroxynitrite and does not attenuate sodium nitroprusside toxicity to cells in culture. *Amino Acids, 20*(4), 419–433.

180. Smith, L.J., Lacaille, F., Lepage, G., Ronco, N., Lamarre, A., Roy, C.C. (1991). Taurine decreases fecal fatty acid and sterol excretion in cystic fibrosis. A randomized double-blind trial. *American Journal of Diseases of Children, 145*(12), 1401–1404.

181. Colombo, C., Battezzati, P.M., Podda, M., Bettinardi, N., Giunta, A. (1996). Ursodeoxycholic acid for liver disease associated with cystic fibrosis: A double-blind multicenter trial. The Italian Group for the Study of Ursodeoxycholic Acid in Cystic Fibrosis. *Hepatology, 23*(6), 1484–1490.

182. Carrasco, S., Codoceo, R., Prieto, G., Lama, R., Polanco, I. (1990). Effect of taurine supplements on growth, fat absorption and bile acid on cystic fibrosis. *Acta Universitatis Carolinae Medica, 36,* 152–156.

183. Schuller-Levis, G.B., Gordon, R.E., Wang, C., Park, E. (2003). Taurine reduces lung inflammation and fibrosis caused by bleomycin. *Advances in Experimental Medicine and Biology, 526,* 395–402.

184. Santangelo, F., Cortijo, J., Morcillo, E. (2003). Taurine and the lung: Which role in asthma? *Advances in Experimental Medicine and Biology, 526,* 403–410.

185. Kim, C. (2006). Accumulation of taurine in tumor and inflammatory lesions. *Advances in Experimental Medicine and Biology, 583,* 213–217.

186. Trachtman, H., Lu, P., Sturman, J.A. (1993). Immunohistochemical localization of taurine in rat renal tissue: Studies in experimental disease states. *Journal of Histochemistry and Cytochemistry, 41,* 1209–1216.

187. Suliman, M.E., Barany, P., Divino Filho, J.C., Qureshi, A.R., Stenvinkel, P., Heimbürger, O., Anderstam, B., Lindholm, B., Bergström, J. (2002). Influence of nutritional status on plasma and erythrocytes sulphur amino acids, sulphhydryls and inorganic sulphate in end-stage renal diseases. *Nephrology, Dialysis, Transplantation, 17,* 1050–1056.

188. Studer, R.K., Craven, P.A., De Rubertis, F.R. (1997). Antioxidant inhibition of protein kinase C-signaled increases in transforming growth factor-beta in mesangial cells. *Metabolism, 46*(8), 918–925.

189. Kozumbo, W.J., Agarwal, S., Koren, H.S. (1992). Breakage and binding of DNA by reaction products of hypochlorous acid with aniline, I-naphthylamine or I-naphthol. *Toxicology and Applied Pharmacology, 115,* 107–115.

190. Reccia, R., Pignalosa, B., Grasso, A., Campanella, G. (1980). Taurine treatment in retinitis pigmentosa. *Acta Neurologica, 18,* 132–136.

191. Head, K.A. (1999). Natural therapies for ocular disorders, part one: Diseases of the retina. *Alternative Medicine Review, 5,* 342–359.

192. Kilic, F., Bhardwaj, R., Caulfeild, J., Trevithick, J.R. (1999). Modelling cortical cataractogenesis 22: Is in vitro reduction of damage in model diabetic rat cataract by taurine due to its antioxidant activity? *Experimental Eye Research, 69*(3), 291–300.

193. Di Leo, M.A., Ghirlanda, G., Gentiloni Silveri, N., Giardina, B., Franconi, F., Santini, S.A. (2003). Potential therapeutic effect of antioxidants in experimental diabetic retina: A comparison between chronic taurine and vitamin E plus selenium supplementations. *Free Radical Research, 37,* 323–330.

194. Di Leo, M.A., Santini, S.A., Cercone, S., Lepore, D., Gentiloni Silveri, N., Caputo, S., Greco, A.V., Giardina, B., Franconi, F., Ghirlanda, G. (2002). Chronic taurine supplementation ameliorates oxidative stress and $Na^+ K^+$ ATPase impairment in the retina of diabetic rats. *Amino Acids, 23*(4), 401–406.

195. Lindholm, B., Alvestrand, A., Furst, P., Bergstrom, J. (1989). Plasma and muscle free amino acids during continuous ambulatory peritoneal dialysis. *Kidney International, 35,* 1219–1226.

196. Alvestrand, A., Furst, P., Bergstrom, J. (1982). Plasma and muscle free amino acids in uremia: Influence of nutrition with amino acids. *Clinical Nephrology, 18,* 297–305.

197. Desai, T.K., Maliakkal, J., Kinzie, J.L., Ehrinpreis, M.N., Luk, G.D., Ceika, J. (1992). Taurine deficiency after intensive chemotherapy and/or radiation. *American Journal of Clinical Nutrition, 55,* 708–711.

198. Laidlaw, S.A., Dietrich, M.F., Lamtenzan, M.P., Vargas, H.I., Block, J.B., Kopple, J.D. (1989). Antimutagenic effects of taurine in a bacterial assay system. *Cancer Research*, *49*, 6600–6604.

199. Molineus, G., Schofield, R., Testa, N.G. (1978). Hematopoietic effects of TCNU in mice. *Cancer Treatment Reports*, *71*, 837–841.

200. Hartley-Asp, B. (1992). Genotoxicity of tauromustine, a new water soluble taurine-based nitrosourea I. Mutagenic and clastogenic activity of tauromustine in vitro. *Mutagenesis*, *7*(6), 427–431.

201. Maher, S.G., Condron, C.E., Bouchier-Hayes, D.J., Toomey, D.M. (2005). Taurine attenuates CD3/interleukin-2-induced T cell apoptosis in an in vitro model of activation-induced cell death (AICD). *Clinical and Experimental Immunology*, *139*(2), 279–286.

202. Opitz, I., Van der Veen, H., Witte, N., Braumann, C., Mueller, J.M., Jacobi, C.A. (2007). Instillation of taurolidine/heparin after laparotomy reduces intraperitoneal tumour growth in a colon cancer rat model. *European Surgical Research*, *39*(3), 129–135.

203. Daigeler, A., Chromic, A.M., Geisler, A., Bulut, D., Hilgert, C., Krieg, A., Klein-Hitpass, L., Lehnhardt, M., Uhl, W., Mittelkotter, U. (2008). Synergistic apoptotic effects of taurolidine and TRAIL on squamous carcinoma cells of the esophagus. *International Journal of Oncology*, *32*(6), 1205–1220.

204. Mundy, G.R. (1996). Regulatory mechanisms of osteoclast differentiation and function. *Journal of Bone and Mineral Metabolism*, *14*, 59–64.

205. Koide, M., Okahashi, N., Tanaka, R., Kazuno, K., Shibasaki, K., Yamazaki, Y., Kaneko, K., Ueda, N., Ohguchi, M., Ishihara, Y., Noguchi, T., Nishihara, T. (1999). Inhibition of experimental bone resorption and osteoclast formation and survival by 2-aminoethanesulphonic acid. *Archives of Oral Biology*, *44*(9), 711–719.

206. Ishikawa, Y.I., Chin, J.E., Schalk, E.M., Wuthier, R.E. (1986). Effect of amino acid levels on matrix vesicle formation by epiphyseal growth plate chondrocytes in primary culture. *Journal of Cellular Physiology*, *126*, 399–406.

207. Kim, S.J., Lee, H.W., Gupta, R.C. (2008). Taurine, bone growth and bone development. *Current Nutrition and Food Science*, *4*(2), 135–144.

208. Park, S., Kim, H., Kim, S.J. (2001). Stimulation of ERK2 by taurine with enhanced alkaline phosphatase activity and collagen synthesis in osteoblast like UMR-106 cells. *Biochemical Pharmacology*, *62*, 1107–1111.

209. Narahashi, T., Soderpalm, B., Ericson, M., Olausson, P., Engel, J.A., Zhang, X., Nordberq, A., Marszalec, W., Aistrup, G.L., Schmidt, L.G., Kalouti, U., Smolka, M., Hedlund, L. (2001). Mechanisms of alcohol-nicotine interactions: Alcoholics versus smokers. *Alcoholism Clinical and Environmental Research*, *25*(5), 152S–156S.

210. Fennessy, F.M., Moneley, D.S., Wang, J.H., Kelly, C.J., Bouchier-Hayes, D.J. (2002). Taurine and vitamin C modify monocyte and endothelial dysfunction in young smokers. *Circulation*, *107*, 410–415.

211. Olive, M.F., Mehmert, K.K., Hodge, C.W. (2000). Modulation of extracellular neurotransmitter levels in the nucleus accumbens by a taurine uptake inhibitor. *European Journal of Pharmacology*, *409*(3), 291–294.

212. Murillo-Fuentes, M.L., Murillo, M.L., Carreras, O. (2003). Effects of maternal ethanol consumption during pregnancy or lactation on intestinal absorption of folic acid in suckling rats. *Life Science*, *12*, 2199–2209.

213. Olive, M.F. (2002). Interactions between taurine and ethanol in the central nervous system. *Amino Acids*, *23*(4), 345–357.

214. Kerai, M.D., Waterfield, C.J., Kenyon, S.H., Asker, D.S., Timbrell, J.A. (1998). Taurine: Protective properties against ethanol-induced hepatic steatosis and lipid peroxidation during chronic ethanol consumption in rats. *Amino Acids*, *5*(1–2), 53–76.

215. Hipolito, L., Sanchez, M.J., Polache, A., Granero, L. (2007). Brain metabolism of ethanol and alcoholism: An update. *Current Drug Metabolism*, *8*(7), 716–727.

216. Spanagel, R., Zieglgänsberger, W. (1997). Anti-craving compounds for ethanol: New pharmacological tools to study addictive processes. *Trends in Pharmacological Sciences*, *18*(2), 54–59.

217. Wu, G., Yang, J., Sun, C., Luan, X., Shi, J., Hu, J. (2009). Effect of taurine on alcoholic liver disease in rats. *Advanced Experimental Medicine and Biology*, *643*, 313–322.

218. Seidl, R., Peyrl, A., Nicham, R., Hauser, E. (2000). A taurine and caffeine-containing drink stimulates cognitive performance and well-beings. *Amino Acids*, *19*, 635–642.

219. Warburton, D.M., Bersellini, E., Sweeney, E. (2001). An evaluation of a caffeinated taurine drink on mood memory and information processing in healthy volunteers without caffeine abstinence. *Psychopharmacology*, *158*, 322–328.

220. Alford, C., Cox, H., Wescott, R. (2001). The effect of Red Bull energy drink on human performance and mood. *Amino Acids*, *21*, 139–150.

221. Bichler, A., Swenson, A., Harris, M.A. (2006). A combination of caffeine and taurine has no effect on short term memory but induces changes in heart rate and mean arterial blood pressure. *Amino Acids*, *31*(4), 471–476.

222. Iyadurai, S.J., Chung, S.S. (2007). New-onset seizures in adults: Possible association with consumption of popular energy drinks. *Epilepsy and Behavior*, *10*, 504–508.

223. Bittner, S., Win, T., Gupta, R.C. (2005). γ-L-glutamyltaurine. *Amino Acids*, *28*, 343–356.

SUBJECT INDEX